RC 901.8 .U755   Urinary tract infections : molecular pathogenesis

# URINARY TRACT INFECTIONS

*Molecular
Pathogenesis and
Clinical Management*

# URINARY TRACT INFECTIONS

*Molecular Pathogenesis and Clinical Management*

*Editors*

Harry L. T. Mobley, Ph.D., and
John W. Warren, M.D.

Division of Infectious Diseases
Department of Medicine
University of Maryland School of Medicine
Baltimore, Maryland

**ASM PRESS**
Washington, D.C.

Copyright © 1996 American Society for Microbiology
1325 Massachusetts Ave, N.W.
Washington, DC 20005

**Library of Congress Cataloging-in-Publication Data**

Urinary tract infections : molecular pathogenesis and clinical
 management / edited by Harry L. T. Mobley and John W. Warren.
  p.   cm.
  Includes index.
  ISBN 1-55581-093-4
  1. Urinary tract infections—Molecular aspects.  2. Urinary tract
infections—Pathogenesis.  3. Urinary tract infections—
Microbiology.  I. Mobley, Harry L. T.  II. Warren, John W. (John
Windiate)
  [DNLM: 1. Urinary Tract Infections—microbiology. 2. Urinary
Tract Infections—physiopathology.  3. Urinary Tract Infections—
therapy.   WJ 151 U763 1996]
RC901.8.U755  1996
616.6—dc20
DNLM/DLC
for Library of Congress                                              95-24719
                                                                        CIP

All Rights Reserved
Printed in the United States of America

*Cover photo:* A uropathogenic *Escherichia coli* strain, CFT073, adheres to a cultured human renal proximal tubular epithelial cell, as revealed by transmission electron microscopy. The original photo was taken and kindly provided by our colleague Anna L. Trifillis, Department of Pathology, University of Maryland School of Medicine.

*To
Natalie, Anne, and Blake
and
Nanny, Gus, and Abby*

# CONTENTS

*Contributors* ix
*Preface* xiii

## I  CLINICAL ASPECTS OF URINARY TRACT INFECTIONS

### 1. Clinical Presentations and Epidemiology of Urinary Tract Infections
*John W. Warren, M.D.*
3

### 2. Diagnostic Microbiology for Bacteria and Yeasts Causing Urinary Tract Infections
*Janice Eisenstadt, D.O., and John A. Washington, M.D.*
29

### 3. The Vaginal Flora and Urinary Tract Infections
*Thomas M. Hooton, M.D., and Walter E. Stamm, M.D.*
67

### 4. Treatment and Prevention of Urinary Tract Infections
*James R. Johnson, M.D.*
95

### 5. Urinary Tract Infections Due to *Candida* Species
*Jack D. Sobel, M.D., and Jose A. Vazquez, M.D.*
119

## II  MOLECULAR MECHANISMS OF BACTERIAL PATHOGENESIS IN URINARY TRACT INFECTIONS

### 6. Virulence Determinants of Uropathogenic *Escherichia coli*
*Michael S. Donnenberg, M.D., and Rodney A. Welch*
135

7. **Structure, Function, and Assembly of Adhesive P Pili**
*C. Hal Jones, Ph.D., Karen Dodson, Ph.D., and Scott J. Hultgren, Ph.D.*
175

8. **Host Resistance to Urinary Tract Infection**
*William Agace, B.Sc. (Hons), Hugh Connell, Ph.D., and Catharina Svanborg, M.D., Ph.D.*
221

9. **Virulence of *Proteus mirabilis***
*Harry L. T. Mobley, Ph.D.*
245

10. ***Proteus mirabilis* Swarmer Cell Differentiation and Urinary Tract Infection**
*Robert Belas, Ph.D.*
271

11. **Virulence Determinants of Uropathogenic *Klebsiella pneumoniae***
*Carleen M. Collins, Ph.D., and Sarah E. F. D'Orazio, Ph.D.*
299

12. **Virulence Factors of *Staphylococcus saprophyticus*, *Staphylococcus epidermidis*, and Enterococci**
*Sören G. Gatermann, M.D., Ph.D.*
313

13. **In Vitro Models for the Study of Uropathogens**
*Bogdan J. Nowicki, M.D., Ph.D.*
341

14. **Animal Models of Urinary Tract Infection**
*David E. Johnson, Ph.D., and Robert G. Russell, D.V.M., Ph.D.*
377

15. **Prospects for Urinary Tract Infection Vaccines**
*Peter O'Hanley, M.D., Ph.D.*
405

**Index**
427

# CONTRIBUTORS

**William Agace**
Division of Clinical Immunology, Department of Medical Microbiology, Lund University, Lund, Sweden

**Robert Belas**
Center of Marine Biotechnology, University of Maryland Biotechnology Institute, Baltimore, Maryland 21202

**Carleen M. Collins**
Department of Microbiology and Immunology, University of Miami School of Medicine, Miami, Florida 33101

**Hugh Connell**
Division of Clinical Immunology, Department of Medical Microbiology, Lund University, Lund, Sweden

**Karen Dodson**
Department of Molecular Microbiology, Washington University Medical School, St. Louis, Missouri 63110-1093

**Michael S. Donnenberg**
Division of Infectious Diseases, University of Maryland School of Medicine, Baltimore, Maryland 21201

**Sarah E. F. D'Orazio**
Department of Microbiology and Immunology, University of Miami School of Medicine, Miami, Florida 33101

**Janice Eisenstadt**
Department of Internal Medicine, Division of Infectious Diseases, Sinai Hospital of Detroit, Detroit, Michigan 48235

**Sören G. Gatermann**
Institut für Medizinische Mikrobiologie, Hochhaus am Augustusplatz, 55101 Mainz, Germany

**Thomas M. Hooton**
Department of Medicine, University of Washington School of Medicine, Harborview Medical Center, Seattle, Washington 98104

**Scott J. Hultgren**
Department of Molecular Microbiology, Washington University Medical School, St. Louis, Missouri 63110-1093

**David E. Johnson**
Research Service, Veteran's Administration Medical Center, Baltimore, Maryland 21201

**James R. Johnson**
Division of Infectious Diseases, University of Minnesota School of Medicine, Minneapolis, Minnesota 55455

**C. Hal Jones**
Department of Molecular Microbiology, Washington University Medical School, St. Louis, Missouri 63110-1093

**Harry L. T. Mobley**
Division of Infectious Diseases, University of Maryland School of Medicine, Baltimore, Maryland 21201

**Bogdan J. Nowicki**
Department of Obstetrics and Gynecology and Department of Microbiology and Immunology, University of Texas Medical Branch, Galveston, Texas 77555-1062

**Peter O'Hanley**
Homeless Veterans Rehabilitation Program, Medicine Service, Palo Alto Veterans Affairs Medical Center, Palo Alto, California 94306, and Department of Medicine, Division of Infectious Diseases and Geographic Medicine, and Department of Microbiology and Immunology, Stanford University School of Medicine, Stanford, California 94305

**Robert G. Russell**
Department of Comparative Medicine, University of Maryland School of Medicine, Baltimore, Maryland 21201

**Jack D. Sobel**
Division of Infectious Diseases, Department of Internal Medicine, Wayne State University School of Medicine, Detroit Medical Center, Detroit, Michigan 48201

**Walter E. Stamm**
Department of Medicine, University of Washington School of Medicine, Harborview Medical Center, Seattle, Washington 98104

**Catharina Svanborg**
Division of Clinical Immunology, Department of Medical Microbiology, Lund University, Lund, Sweden

**Jose A. Vazquez**
Division of Infectious Diseases, Department of Internal Medicine, Wayne State University School of Medicine, Detroit Medical Center, Detroit, Michigan 48201

**John W. Warren**
Division of Infectious Diseases, Department of Medicine, University of Maryland School of Medicine, Baltimore, Maryland 21201

**John A. Washington**
Division of Pathology and Laboratory Medicine, The Cleveland Clinic Foundation, Cleveland, Ohio 44195

**Rodney A. Welch**
Department of Microbiology and Immunology, University of Wisconsin School of Medicine, Madison, Wisconsin 53706

# PREFACE

The urinary tract is a complicated epithelium-lined tube with an opening to the body surface, making it susceptible to infection by exogenous organisms. Most urinary tract infections (UTIs) occur in otherwise healthy people with normal urinary tracts and no systemic diseases predisposing them to bacterial infections. *Escherichia coli* is the most common pathogen, causing 80% or more of these uncomplicated UTIs, and isolates generally express a number of well-studied virulence factors for UTI. The balance of infections is caused by very few species, including *Proteus mirabilis, Klebsiella pneumoniae,* and, especially in young women, *Staphylococcus saprophyticus.*

In a landmark study published in the *Lancet* in 1976, Svanborg and her colleagues demonstrated that *E. coli* causing acute pyelonephritis adhered in greater numbers in vitro to uroepithelial cells obtained from the urine of volunteers than did strains causing asymptomatic bacteriuria. This work rapidly led a number of investigators to the identification of a new fimbria that binds to the P blood group antigen. The development of molecular genetic techniques then allowed isolation of the *pap* gene sequences that encoded this "pyelonephritis-associated pilus." Work that ensued on fimbrial biogenesis, using P fimbria as a model, established many of the general principles that govern the assembly and function of these adherence organelles. One startling finding was that the adhesin itself is present in only a few copies at the tip of the fimbria, where it can most easily gain access to the uroepithelial digalactoside receptor. Other adhesins have been identified since, but none have supplanted P fimbria in its predominance in acute pyelonephritis.

However, while adherence may define tropism to and within the urinary tract, subsequent events mediated by the bacterium and the host are necessary for symptomatic infection to become manifest. Bacterial factors such as hemolysin and cytotoxic necrotizing factor may perturb the epithelium, an important step among a series of events which results in symptomatic disease. Virulence factors probably work in combination and in sequence; indeed, some may be genetically linked on "pathogenicity islands." However, because some pyelonephritogenic strains do not produce P fimbriae and many do not secrete hemolysin and most do not produce cytotoxic necrotizing factor, these strains must employ other virulence factors, some known and some as yet undiscovered. Indeed, uropathogenic *E. coli* may have several profiles of virulence determinants and therefore may be more similar to diarrheagenic *E. coli* strains, which have several distinct and well-defined pathogeneses, than to *Vibrio cholerae*, for which one mechanism predominates.

Infection requires not only a microorganism but also a susceptible host. The effects of exposure to microbes may depend on the host's hereditary properties, such as secretor status or expression of specific blood group antigens, or the presence of congenital or acquired anatomical defects of the urinary tract. An inflammatory response may be triggered by adherence-mediated cytokine induction resulting in polymorphonuclear leukocyte infiltration and the development of cell-mediated and humoral immunity. The outcome of infection depends on the balance of bacterial virulence and host response.

The battle between microorganism and host is complex, and to be understood it must be broken down into discrete subjects. In this book, we have asked leaders in the field to review topics pertinent to clinical management of UTI, including epidemiology, microbiology, diagnostic procedures, therapy, and the emerging relevance of the vaginal flora in development of UTI. With this practical information as a background, we then turn our attention to the molecular mechanisms by which uropathogens infect the urinary tract and cause the diseases that require physician intervention. This section includes an updated and provocative description of what constitutes a uropathogenic *E. coli* strain. The molecular biology of other uropathogenic bacterial species, including *P. mirabilis, K. pneumoniae,* staphylococci, and enterococci, is also discussed in detail. Finally, we review methods for in vitro and in vivo investigations of experimental UTI. It is our hope that the details that follow will not only be informative but also serve as stimuli for future research.

HARRY L. T. MOBLEY
JOHN W. WARREN

# CLINICAL ASPECTS OF URINARY TRACT INFECTIONS

# CLINICAL PRESENTATIONS AND EPIDEMIOLOGY OF URINARY TRACT INFECTIONS

*John W. Warren, M.D.*

# 1

## OVERVIEW

Urinary tract infection (UTI) is the most common kidney and urologic disease in the United States and one of the most common bacterial infections of any organ system. Its magnitude can be judged either by visits to physicians, estimated as high as 8 million/year in the United States, or by hospital discharge diagnoses, 1.5 million/year (138). Admission to hospitals, presumably mostly for acute pyelonephritis, are estimated at more than 100,000/year (64, 100), and the urinary tract is usually identified as the most common source of bacteremia in the community, hospital, and nursing home (43, 70, 92, 108, 153).

## Bacteriuria

Bacteriuria is the presence of bacteria in the urine. Since the function of the urinary tract is to produce urine, this complex epithelium-lined tube is continually flushed, and infecting organisms are usually delivered in a urine specimen to the waiting clinician or investigator. There are some exceptions. Hematogenous infections can present without bacteriuria. Some patients with symptomatic UTI may not have recognizable bacteriuria even when bacteria can be seen or cultured from their bladder mucosa (28). However, for epidemiologic and most clinical purposes, bacteriuria is an excellent representation of the presence of bacteria in the urinary tract.

## Ascending UTI

By far the greatest majority of organisms infect the urinary tract by the ascending route. Ascending UTI refers to one of two processes. The first is the ascent of organisms from the periurethral area through the urethra into the bladder. The second is their ascent from the bladder through the ureter(s) to the kidney(s). In both circumstances, bacterial movement appears to be through the lumen of the urinary tract. There is little evidence for ascent from the bladder to the kidneys via periurinary lymphatics.

Hematogenous UTI refers to the small percentage of infections in which the organism is delivered to the urinary tract, usually to one or both kidneys, by the bloodstream. Such infections are generally caused by a handful of species, including *Staphylococcus aureus, Salmonella* spp., and

---

*John W. Warren,* Division of Infectious Diseases, Department of Medicine, University of Maryland Medical Center, 10 South Pine Street, Baltimore, Maryland 21201-1192.

*Candida* spp. (each of which, however, can also cause ascending infections).

## Uncomplicated UTI

Most UTIs occur in otherwise healthy people. These hosts have normal urinary tracts and do not have systemic diseases predisposing them to bacterial infections. *Escherichia coli* is the most common pathogen, causing 80% or more of uncomplicated UTIs, and isolates generally express a number of well-studied virulence factors for UTI. Most of the balance is caused by a very few species, including *Proteus mirabilis, Klebsiella pneumoniae,* and, especially in young women, *Staphylococcus saprophyticus*. These infections are quite responsive to antibiotic therapy, and recurrences are usually reinfections with organisms that enter the bladder through the urethra.

## Complicated UTI

Complicated UTIs generally occur in one of two groups of patients. The first group comprises those with complicated urinary tracts, i.e., one containing a foreign body or not functioning normally because of anatomic or functional defects. The second group includes hosts generally susceptible to infections, such as patients with immunosuppression. The characteristics of complicated UTIs are that the spectrum of organisms is broader, the *E. coli* strains that are isolated are less likely to express putative virulence factors, response to antibiotic therapy is less certain, and relapse with the same organism may occur.

## CLINICAL SYNDROMES

UTI generally manifests itself in one of three clinical presentations: cystitis, acute pyelonephritis, or asymptomatic bacteriuria. The interpretation of quantitative bacteriuria must consider these presenting syndromes.

## Cystitis

Cystitis is characterized by dysuria, frequency and urgency of urination, and sometimes suprapubic pain. This presentation accounts for 95% of all visits to physicians for UTIs (29). Although the name implies that the infection is restricted to the bladder, localization tests such as bladder washouts and ureteral catheterizations have demonstrated that of "cystitis" patients, 15 to 25% may actually have bacteria above the bladder (18). Because the same organism found in bladder urine can be isolated from the urethra and because some women with symptoms of cystitis have sterile bladder urine yet positive urethral cultures, a portion of women with cystitis symptoms may have urethritis (32).

Quantitative bacteriuria is helpful in making the diagnosis of cystitis. Stamm et al. demonstrated that in young women, concentrations as low as $10^2$ bacteria per ml of urine are significantly associated with symptoms of cystitis (125, 127, 128). Recently, Kunin and colleagues confirmed these findings and further demonstrated that stepwise increases in bacterial counts are associated with increased prevalences of symptoms and pyuria (75). If they are left untreated, some women with this low-count bacteriuria will several days later yield bacteriuria of $\geq 10^5$ CFU/ml (6). A consensus definition of quantitative bacteriuria for cystitis has been generated by the Infectious Diseases Society of America (IDSA) (110). Although proposed for antibiotic studies, bacteriuria of $\geq 10^3$ CFU/ml of urine is quite suitable to confirm the diagnosis of cystitis in a woman with compatible symptoms. This quantitation yields a specificity of 90% and a sensitivity of 80% (110).

## Acute Pyelonephritis

Acute pyelonephritis is clinically identified by flank pain and fever and is often accompanied by nausea, vomiting, sweats, and malaise. Elevated levels of C-reactive protein in serum or elevated erythrocyte sedimentation rate and diminished renal concentrating ability have been used in its diagnosis. Cystitis symptoms may or may not be present. Acute pyelonephritis can be complicated by bacteremia in about 30% of cases (56). The term pyelonephritis refers to inflammation of the renal pelvis and kidney. However, the aforementioned localization techniques revealed that 30 to 50% of patients with the acute pyelonephritis syndrome have bacteria only in the lower urinary tract (18).

For those who do have an infection of the kidney(s), the means by which bacteria have ascended through the ureter(s) is unclear. Vesicoureteral reflux in the normal adult urinary tract is uncommon and even among children with acute pyelonephritis is present in only a minority (146). Whether bacteria ascend by progressively colonizing the luminal surface, swimming against the stream of urine, moving in the slower turbulent urine along the mucosa, or exploiting a disordered ureteral peristalsis during infection is unclear.

The IDSA group suggested that the criterion for bacteriuria in acute pyelonephritis be $\geq 10^4$ CFU/ml. Of patients with acute pyelonephritis, 90 to 95% will have bacteriuria of this concentration (110).

## Asymptomatic Bacteriuria

Some population screenings for asymptomatic bacteriuria indicate that a small percentage of persons with this finding actually have symptoms (47, 98). However, in a study of aged women, the population with the highest prevalence of this entity, this syndrome is truly asymptomatic. Those with bacteriuria have no higher prevalence of urinary or general symptoms than those without bacteriuria (11). Localization studies indicate that bacteria may frequently be in the kidney as well as in the bladder (97, 134). The IDSA group endorsed the decades-old criterion for asymptomatic bacteriuria as two consecutive urine cultures with $\geq 10^5$ of the same organism per ml. This count yields a specificity of more than 95% and a sensitivity of more than 80% (110).

## EPIDEMIOLOGY

The epidemiology of UTI can be analyzed in several ways. One means of analysis is by organism. For instance, the species causing a UTI may be a clue as to whether the infection is an uncomplicated or a complicated UTI. The molecular pathogeneses of uncomplicated UTI caused by *E. coli, S. saprophyticus, K. pneumoniae,* and *P. mirabilis* make up a substantial proportion of the chapters in this book. In the complicated urinary tract, *E. coli* is less prominent and may even cause a minority of cases. Most of the infections are caused by the other organisms mentioned plus additional gram-negative rods such as *Enterobacter, Pseudomonas, Providencia,* and *Morganella* species; gram-positive organisms such as *Enterococcus, Streptococcus,* and *Staphylococcus* species; and yeasts, particularly *Candida* species.

Another way to describe the epidemiology of UTI and the one to be used here is by the nature of the host. A graph helpful in understanding the relationships between sex, age, and symptomatic infection and asymptomatic bacteriuria is a venerable one by Kunin (Fig. 1) (74).

## CHILDREN

The epidemiology and natural history of UTI in children were well investigated by Jan Winberg and his colleagues in a series of studies begun in 1960. These investigations were performed in Göteborg, Sweden, and represent well-organized population-based studies of symptomatic and asymptomatic bacteriuria in children. In this section, except as noted, the data are from their reports (62, 145).

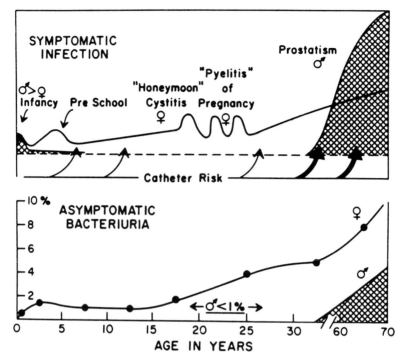

**FIGURE 1** Overview of the incidence of symptomatic UTI and the prevalence of asymptomatic bacteriuria according to age and sex (curves, females; hatched areas, males) (74).

## Symptomatic Infection

### BOYS

Winberg's studies suggest that 1% of boys have at least one symptomatic UTI during their first 10 years of life. The highest incidence is within the first month (Fig. 2 and 3). Most episodes among these infants are associated with fever and are assumed to be acute pyelonephritis (Fig. 4); 75 to 85% of the episodes are caused by *E. coli* (Table 1). The prevalence of congenital abnormalities resulting in obstruction to urine flow is 10 to 20% among boys with UTIs in the first 2 months of life (107, 145). The male/female ratio of symptomatic UTI is 2.5:1 in the first month of life and gradually changes to 1:20 by the age of 10 years. Interestingly, in older boys, *P. mirabilis* is as common as *E. coli* (Table 1). UTIs recur in about 25% of boys with first-time UTI, usually within a year of the initial infection; multiple recurrences are uncommon.

Other investigators demonstrated that uncircumcised males in their first year of life have an incidence of UTI 10 to 20 times greater than circumcised boys (50, 147, 148).

### GIRLS

About 3% of girls have symptomatic UTI within the first 10 years of life. The highest incidence of first-time UTI is within the first year but, unlike in boys, is distributed throughout the year (Fig. 2). In subsequent years, girls show a slowly decreasing incidence of first episodes of symptomatic UTI (Fig. 3). UTIs with fever make up the majority of their infections until girls reach the age of 8 to 10 years (Fig. 4). *E. coli* is isolated in more than 80% of cases in

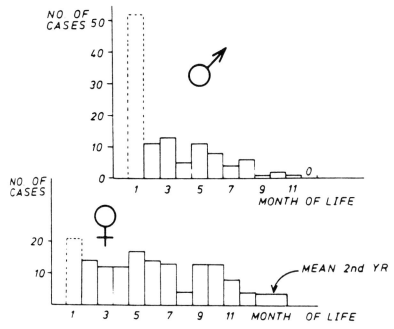

**FIGURE 2** First-time UTI in children during the first year of life. Reprinted from reference 145 with permission.

young girls but in only 60% of teenagers, in whom *S. saprophyticus* becomes more prominent (Table 1). Only about 2% of girls receiving imaging studies for symptomatic UTI have pertinent urinary obstruction. About 40% of girls experience recurrent UTI, usually within a year after the initial infection. Multiple recurrences, over years, are more common in girls than boys and are associated with increased periurethral colonization and in vitro bacterial adherence to the girls' harvested periurethral and uroepithelial cells (65, 135).

## RENAL SCARRING

Scarring of the kidney is observed at the site of infection in about one-third of children with acute pyelonephritis (60, 112). The incidence of such scarring is highest within the first years of age (146); the appearance of new scars is rare after the age of 10 (144). However, renal scarring may have an impact for many years. Children with UTI and renal scarring who were followed to adulthood (58a) and individuals first identified with renal scarring as adults (26, 58) appear to be at risk for hypertension, renal dysfunction, and renal failure. The reason for this progression may be the development of glomerular disease in the remaining functional kidney tissue (5, 26, 144).

Renal scarring in children with febrile UTIs is epidemiologically associated with vesicoureteral reflux, recurrent pyelonephritis, infection with non-*E. coli*, infection with *E. coli* lacking P fimbriae, and host nonsecretor status.

Vesicoureteral reflux, the reflux of urine from the bladder into one or both kidneys, occurs in some children because the physiologic "valve" afforded by the location of the ureter in the wall of the contracting bladder may be immature, thus allowing passage of urine into the ureter during urination. The most severe cases allow urine under pressure to reflux into the pelvis and even the collecting ducts of the kidney (57). Fortunately, reflux disappears spontaneously in 80% of ureters as the child

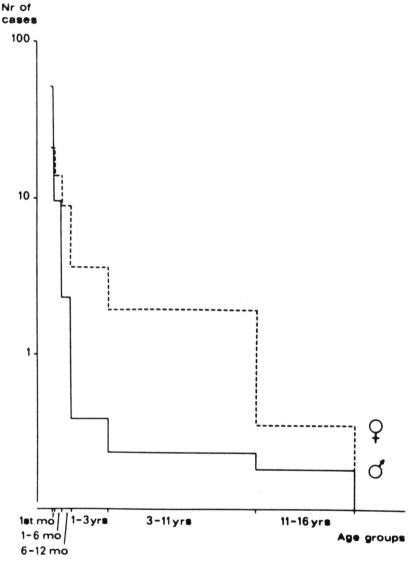

**FIGURE 3** Number of first-time UTIs by age in children up to 16 years of age. Reprinted from reference 145 with permission.

grows older (25). Such cures, however, are inversely proportional to severity: reflux disappears in 85% of ureters of normal dimension but in only about 40% of those with more severe reflux, as indicated by dilated ureters (25). About one-third of male and female infants presenting with acute pyelonephritis have vesicoureteral reflux; in 10%, the reflux is high grade, with dilatation of the ureter, pelvis, and calices. A number of studies have demonstrated that the greater the severity of reflux, the higher the prevalence of renal scarring (60, 62, 82) (Table 2). Indeed, for

1. CLINICAL PRESENTATIONS AND EPIDEMIOLOGY ■ 9

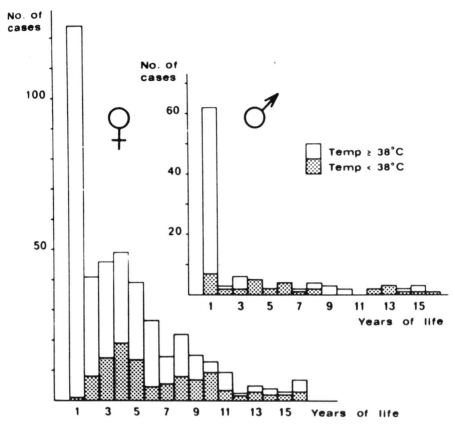

**FIGURE 4** Febrile and nonfebrile UTIs among children up to 16 years of age. Reprinted from reference 145 with permission.

**TABLE 1** Bacteria isolated from children with first UTI[a]

| Infecting organism | % of infected: | | | | |
| --- | --- | --- | --- | --- | --- |
| | Neonates of both sexes ($n = 73$) | Boys | | Girls | |
| | | 1 mo–1 yr ($n = 62$) | 1–16 yr ($n = 42$) | 1 mo–10 yr ($n = 389$) | 10–16 yr ($n = 30$) |
| E. coli | 75 | 85 | 33 | 83 | 60 |
| Klebsiella spp. | 11 | 2 | 2 | <1 | 0 |
| Proteus spp. | 0 | 5 | 33 | 3 | 0 |
| Enterococci | 3 | 0 | 2 | 2 | 0 |
| Staphylococci | 1 | 0 | 12 | <1 | 30 |

[a] Data are from Winberg et al. (145).

**TABLE 2** Renal scarring and vesicoureteral reflux among children with UTI[a]

| Reflux grade | No. (%) of kidneys with scarring |
|---|---|
| 0 | 23/119 (19) |
| 1–2 | 5/17 (29) |
| ≥3 | 9/16 (56) |

[a] Data are from Jakobsson et al. (60).

a while, this observation prompted use of the term "reflux nephropathy" for kidneys with deformed calices and associated parenchymal scarring.

However, such scarred kidneys have been identified in nonrefluxing urinary tracts (60, 62, 81, 112, 144). Jakobsson et al., while confirming an association of renal scarring with reflux severity, pointed out that the majority of children with renal scarring do not have reflux (60) (Table 2). They and others found that renal scarring is epidemiologically associated with recurrent pyelonephritis (60, 62). This finding has been interpreted by recent investigators as suggesting that the term reflux nephropathy is a misnomer and that reflux is associated with renal scarring because it is associated with the development of acute pyelonephritis (60, 112).

Relatively nonvirulent organisms are associated with renal scarring in children. Non-*E. coli* and *E. coli* lacking putative virulence factors are overrepresented in pyelonephritis associated with reflux (82, 83). Similarly, in children with acute pyelonephritis, the frequency of renal scarring is significantly higher with non-*E. coli* (60, 85, 112) and with *E. coli* strains that do not possess certain putative virulence determinants (84, 85, 103).

### Asymptomatic Bacteriuria

Jodal reported the results of screening for bacteriuria among more than 3,500 newborns in the Göteborg area (62). Asymptomatic bacteriuria was present on at least one of three screenings before the age of 10 months in 2.5% of boys and 0.9% of girls. The prevalence of reflux among these children was 11%, and the reflux was usually low grade. On follow-up, the great majority of these bacteriurias cleared spontaneously. Three years after entry into the study, most patients subjected to radiographic studies revealed no renal scarring.

After the first year of life, asymptomatic bacteriuria diminishes in boys but is still prevalent in girls. Estimates are that 5 to 10% of girls have asymptomatic bacteriuria at least one time before the age of 10. In most, the infection is dynamic, with spontaneous cure or changes of organisms. In some, however, the bacteriuria may be quite stable, with the same strain persisting for many months (46, 99). Persistent asymptomatic bacteriuria in normal urinary tracts, however, results in little risk of renal damage or acute pyelonephritis (76). Some school-age girls with asymptomatic bacteriuria reveal mild urinary symptoms upon careful questioning and may have functional bladder abnormalities with increased residual urine (47).

Data indicating that breast feeding is associated with a decreased incidence of UTI, both symptomatic and asymptomatic, are emerging (88, 101).

## ADULT WOMEN

Among adults with normal urinary tracts who are otherwise healthy, women represent 90% of patients with urinary tract infections (29).

### Cystitis

Of women going to physicians for a UTI, 95% do so for symptoms of cystitis (29). The incidence of cystitis becomes prominent at the time of puberty and may occur throughout adulthood. Estimates are that 40% of adult women will experience symptoms of cystitis sometime during their lifetime. *E. coli* makes up 75 to 80% of causative organisms (Table 3), although

**TABLE 3** Causes of community-acquired UTI among adults

| Infecting organism | % Symptomatic[a] | | % Asymptomatic | |
| --- | --- | --- | --- | --- |
| | Women (330 episodes) | Men (25 episodes) | Elderly women[b] (68 episodes) | Elderly men[c] (29 episodes) |
| E. coli | 75 | 63 | 79 | 17 |
| Klebsiella spp. | 2 | 4 | 12 | 7 |
| Proteus spp. | 1 | 0 | 1 | 7 |
| Staphylococcus spp. | 6[d] | 8[d] | 0 | 53[e] |
| Streptococcus spp. | 0 | 4 | 1 | 10 |

[a] Data are from Ferry et al. (29).
[b] Data are from Boscia et al. (12).
[c] Data are from Mims et al. (90).
[d] S. saprophyticus.
[e] S. epidermidis is prominent.

its incidence may be lower among young women as S. saprophyticus emerges in a distant second position (Table 4).

## SEXUAL ACTIVITY

A number of clinical studies indicate that sexual intercourse is associated with UTI in young women (37, 106, 133). These investigations demonstrate a strong link between UTI, recent sexual activity, and frequency of sexual activity. Strom et al. demonstrated that new sexual activity, defined as changes in duration, position, or type of activity, is associated with UTI (133). Remis et al. calculated that the incidence of UTI among the population of university-aged women whom they studied was 7/100 woman-years for those who never had intercourse versus 52/100 woman-years for those who were sexually active (106).

Diaphragm use has been associated with UTI, even after adjustment for sexual activity (33, 37, 106, 133). Fihn and colleagues found that urethral and vaginal colonization with E. coli is greater in diaphragm users than in nonusers and that diaphragm users with a history of UTI have a higher prevalence of urethral and vaginal coliforms than those without such a history (31). They demonstrated that nonoxynol-9, a spermicide used with diaphragms, may be the important component in this predisposition. Obtaining cultures within hours before and after intercourse, they noted a marked increase in E. coli vaginal colonization and bacteriuria rates among the nonoxynol-9–diaphragm users as well as a significant increase in the group using condoms and nonoxynol-9 compared to oral contraceptive users (52). They began to explore mechanisms by showing that nonoxynol-9 has a greater bactericidal effect on the common vaginal organisms (lactobacilli and Gardnerella vaginalis) than on E. coli and that the spermicide enhances the adherence of microorganisms, including E. coli, to vaginal epithelial cells (51). These data led them to postulate that nonoxynol-9 offers E. coli a selective advantage in coloni-

**TABLE 4** Distribution of community-acquited UTIs by bacterial species and patient age[a]

| Age (yr)[b] | % of infections caused by: | |
| --- | --- | --- |
| | E. coli | S. saprophyticus |
| 0–14 | 89 | 0 |
| 15–44 | 63 | 15 |
| 45–64 | 80 | 1 |
| ≦65 | 81 | 1 |

[a] Data are from Ferry et al. (29).
[b] Mostly females.

zation of the vagina, thus affording these organisms opportunity for entry into the bladder during intercourse. Additionally, their recent evidence suggests that nonoxynol-9 use is associated with vaginal colonization with other uropathogens such as other gram-negative rods, group D and B streptococci, and *Candida* species (53).

Urination after sexual activity has a protective effect against UTI (37, 133). Presumably, this procedure washes out organisms that enter the bladder during intercourse.

Although there are occasional reports of sexual partners experiencing UTIs caused by what appears to be the same organism (8, 49, 124, 150), UTIs are not generally considered to be sexually transmitted diseases. Consistent with this stance is that the number of sexual partners is not associated with UTI (37, 133). By aspiration of bladder urine before and after manipulation of the urethra at operation, Bran et al. demonstrated entry of organisms into the bladder; they suggested that such entry could occur during intercourse (13). The association with sexual activity, then, is more likely related to transmission through the urethra of organisms, uropathogens or not (17), that are already colonizing the perianal or periurethral area.

## NONSEXUAL RISK FACTORS

Risk factors for symptomatic UTI among young women that are not associated with sexual activity have been identified. These factors include previous UTIs (36, 106, 133) and family history of UTI, particularly in the mother (133). Foxman and Chi demonstrated a protective effect of vitamin C (37), a finding that Strom et al. did not confirm (133). A number of factors are not associated with UTI. These include wearing of pants instead of skirts, use of menstrual tampons instead of pads, bicycle riding, direction of wiping after defecation, number of urinations per day, volume and types of fluids consumed (coffee, tea, alcohol, cranberry juice), ingestion of a variety of food items, constipation, diarrhea, use of laxatives or douches, showers, tub baths, bubble baths, and tight or loose clothing (37, 106, 133).

## Recurrent UTI

Following a first episode, about 30% of women experience recurrent UTI over the succeeding 6 to 12 months (36, 87). The peak recurrence is within 60 days following the index episode, and incidence of recurrence diminishes thereafter (36, 87, 96, 126). Of identified recurrent episodes, about 75% are symptomatic, and of those, 95% are cystitis and 5% are acute pyelonephritis (126). Some women experience frequent recurrences: Mabeck found that 70% of recurrent UTIs were experienced by one-sixth of the patients (87). Daily urine cultures show a significant association of recurrent UTI with sexual activity (96). Among women with prior UTIs, cotton underwear was associated with protective effect in one study (36). Less than 5% of recurrent UTIs have evidence of predisposing anatomic or functional abnormalities of the urinary tract (34, 55, 87).

*E. coli* makes up 65% of the organisms causing recurrent UTIs, a somewhat lower frequency than in first-time episodes. The aforementioned uropathogens make up the balance (126). Most recurrences are caused by organisms entering the urinary tract through the urethra, and the organism may be different from or the same as those that caused earlier episodes (14, 87, 113, 124). Russo et al. demonstrated by pulsed-field gel electrophoresis that in a given woman, the same strain could cause recurrent UTI and presented evidence that these strains persist in the feces (113).

In women with recurrent UTI, periurethral colonization with the infecting organism often precedes the UTI (124). Moreover, women with recurrent UTI not only have more frequent periurethral colonization but also are colonized with higher numbers of organisms and for a longer duration (123). Indeed, periurethral, vaginal (35, 116), and even buccal (116) epithelial cells harvested from women with recurrent UTI allow significantly greater numbers of *E. coli* to adhere; findings in girls with periurethral and voided uroepithelial cells are similar (65, 135).

## NONSECRETORS

Colonization and particularly in vitro adherence studies suggest a hereditary predisposition to recurrent UTI. Consistent with this thesis is the finding that persons who are nonsecretors of blood group antigens are susceptible to recurrent UTI. The blood group antigens A, B, H, and Lewis (Le$^a$ and Le$^b$) are biochemically related and are under the regulatory control of a number of genes. The Se gene is necessary to express these antigens on epithelial surfaces and in secretions such as saliva. Persons who do not secrete blood group antigens in their saliva are known as nonsecretors. Nonsecretors demonstrate substantially lower expression of these antigens on urinary tract epithelium than secretors do (19).

Kinane et al. discovered that the nonsecretor phenotype is overrepresented among women with recurrent UTIs (67). Others not only confirmed this finding (118) but also revealed that nonsecretors (and/or the corresponding Lewis antigen phenotypes) are overrepresented among children with febrile UTIs (61, 86), among women with renal scarring (59), and among children with structural urinary abnormalities who have had UTIs (117). Stapleton et al. discovered that the frequency of rectal colonization with F-fimbriated *E. coli* is higher in nonsecretors with UTI than in nonsecretors without UTI and secretors with UTI (129). Lomberg et al. demonstrated that uropathogenic *E. coli* adheres in greater numbers to squamous epithelial cells from voided urine of nonsecretors than to those from secretors (80). The cellular and molecular bases for the association between nonsecretor status and UTI are being pursued (38, 93, 130).

## POSTMENOPAUSAL WOMEN

In some older women, recurrent symptomatic UTI is a problem and may be associated with hormonally caused changes in the vaginal flora. The rationale is the following: decreased systemic estrogen is associated with a diminished vaginal colonization of lactobacilli, which allows colonization by *E. coli,* making possible a consequent higher incidence of *E. coli* entry into the bladder and leading to bacteriuria and UTI. A powerful test of this premise was a prospective, randomized, placebo-controlled trial of topical estriol cream applied to the vagina (105). Women using the placebo cream had an average of six UTIs per patient-year compared to 0.5 UTIs in the estriol group. A longitudinal review of vaginal flora revealed that two-thirds of the women treated with placebo but only one-third of the women receiving topical estrogen continued to be colonized with members of the family *Enterobacteriaceae*.

### Asymptomatic Bacteriuria

Beginning at puberty, the prevalence of asymptomatic bacteriuria goes up by about one percentage point per decade of life through the sixth decade (Fig. 1). Some evidence suggests that in young women, diaphragm use is associated with asymptomatic bacteriuria (133). After the age of 60, the prevalence of asymptomatic bacteriuria accelerates, and women this age and older have prevalences of 15 to 25% and higher (2, 10, 12). Women in nursing homes and hospitals generally have even higher prevalences (94).

The consequences of asymptomatic bacteriuria have been investigated. Gaymans et al. studied it in two large general practices in Holland and found that women who had asymptomatic bacteriuria at the beginning of the study had a higher incidence of symptomatic UTI in the succeeding year (41). Two populations of women with asymptomatic bacteriuria have been well studied: pregnant women and elderly women.

## PREGNANT WOMEN

Asymptomatic bacteriuria occurs in 3 to 10% of pregnant women (44, 66, 109, 114). Women who as children had asymptomatic bacteriuria are more likely to have this syndrome during pregnancy (23, 114). Two clinical problems may be consequences. The first is that, if untreated, asymptomatic bacteriuria results in an incidence of acute pyelonephritis of 25 to 50% during the pregnancy (66). This incidence may be a result of the dilatation of ureters and renal pelvises caused by hormonal as well as mechanical changes of pregnancy, with presumed easier ascent of bacteria from bladder to kidneys.

Additionally, an association of maternal asymptomatic bacteriuria with premature delivery and low birth weight has frequently been reported (91). Romero et al. reviewed by meta-analysis the English language literature addressing this issue (109). Their assessment was that asymptomatic bacteriuria during pregnancy, if left untreated, is significantly associated with low birth weight and preterm delivery. Recognizing that bacteriuria may be a marker for confounding variables, they also evaluated reported randomized clinical trials of antibiotic treatment. Their conclusion was that antibiotic therapy of asymptomatic bacteriuria significantly reduces the risk of low birth weight.

## ELDERLY WOMEN

Estimates are that the majority of elderly women will at one time or another have an episode of asymptomatic bacteriuria (10). Most are caused by gram-negative rods, among which *E. coli* is the most common (Table 3). The bacteriuria spontaneously appears and disappears, and only a few individuals are continuously bacteriuric (2, 12). As demonstrated by restriction fragment length polymorphism, recurrence of asymptomatic bacteriuria in aged women is usually by reinfection with new strains (79). In elderly women, asymptomatic bacteriuria has been associated with fecal incontinence (15), vaginal descensus, uterine prolapse, and cystocele or urethrocele (121); diabetes mellitus is relatively common in this population and may result in autonomic neuropathy and urine retention (16, 27).

Prospective studies show a somewhat increased incidence of symptomatic UTI among women who at the beginning of longitudinal investigations have asymptomatic bacteriuria (7, 136). However, other consequences of asymptomatic bacteriuria in aged women appear not to be serious. This is an important assertion, because in the 1950s and 1960s, merely the identification of bacteriuria of $\geq 10^5$ CFU/ml over several examinations caused clinicians and investigators to assume that the patient had chronic renal infection and that the consequences could be dire. Nevertheless, in the absence of structural or functional urologic abnormalities, the development of renal damage or dysfunction or of hypertension has not been convincingly associated with asymptomatic bacteriuria.

However, several studies in the 1960s and 1970s suggested that asymptomatic bacteriuria in the elderly is associated with a higher mortality rate. This disturbing concept became less of a concern when a well-designed investigation of 70-year-old people in Sweden followed for 10 years revealed no difference in mortality between initially bacteriuric and nonbacteriuric individuals (98). A recently reported study, actually two investigations, confirmed this finding. This study was an observational investigation of almost 1,500 older women followed for up to 9 years and, nested within that study, a controlled trial of antimicrobial agents for bacteriuria. Both studies demonstrated no increased mortality with untreated bacteriuria (1). Taken together, these studies provide persuasive evidence that asymptomatic bacteriuria in elderly women does not have a direct effect on mortality.

**ADULT MEN**
Lipsky et al. demonstrated that first-voided urine and clean-catch midstream urine in men are quite accurate for identifying bladder bacteriuria as defined by suprapubic or urethral catheterization (78). The dry periurethral epidermis of a man is presumably less often colonized with uropathogenic organisms than the moist mucosa of the periurethral area of a woman; thus, contamination of voided specimens is less common. The IDSA group suggested $\geq 10^4$ CFU/ml as the criterion for UTI in a man (110).

**Symptomatic UTIs**

NORMAL URINARY TRACTS
After infancy, the incidence of symptomatic infection and the prevalence of asymptomatic bacteriuria markedly diminish in males and are close to but not zero (Fig. 1). The traditional wisdom has been that a UTI in a male of any age is a complicated infection that requires thorough evaluation to rule out anatomic abnormality, obstruction, etc. (74, 77).

However, two studies suggest that a low incidence of UTI occurs in otherwise healthy men. Over a 6-year period, Krieger et al. studied 38 men who presented to a university health clinic with UTI, representing a mean incidence of five symptomatic UTI per year per 10,000 men enrolled in the university (73). Almost all had lower urinary tract symptoms; additionally, 14 of the men had fever and 7 had flank pain. Six had a urethral discharge; of the five tested, none revealed chlamydiae or *Neisseria gonorrhoeae*. *E. coli* caused 37 of the 40 infections. Almost 90% of the patients were circumcised. Most were interviewed about sexual habits: about 90% had been sexually active within the previous month, each with one female sex partner; none acknowledged ever having had insertive rectal intercourse or sex with a man. Only one was diagnosed with chronic bacterial prostatitis. Eleven agreed to radiologic and functional investigations, and all of the results were normal. This study suggests that symptomatic UTIs occur at a low incidence in young, heterosexual, circumcised men with apparently normal urinary tracts.

The second report is of 88 men enrolled over a 10-year period in a series of studies of community-acquired symptomatic *E. coli* UTIs in Göteborg (137). The patients were divided into cases of acute pyelonephritis-febrile UTI ($n = 74$) and cystitis ($n = 14$). Fifty-six men underwent excretory urography, and four had ultrasonography. Factors defining complicated UTIs were recognized in only 25 patients: urologic abnormalities in 15 and diabetes mellitus in 10. The role of prostatic diseases in this retrospective study is unclear. The infecting *E. coli* strains carried putative virulence factors at frequencies higher than occur in fecal strains: P fimbriation (50%), hemolysin (75%), and O serotypes commonly found in UTIs (78%). These high prevalences of putative virulence factors are consistent with the concept that at least some of these men had uncomplicated urinary tracts.

Risk factors for UTIs in men with normal urinary tracts are being sought. A study of men presenting to a clinic for sexually transmitted diseases suggests that lack of circumcision may be associated with UTI (122). Urethritis without evidence of chlamydiae or *N. gonorrhoeae* infection was present in two-thirds. *E. coli* caused about 60% of these UTIs and tended to express putative virulence factors. The role of heterosexual sex in fostering penile colonization is unclear. Occasional cases of apparent heterosexual transmission of uropathogenic organisms have been reported (8, 49, 124, 150). Studies as to whether sexually active homosexual men are predisposed to symptomatic UTI compared to heterosexual men show conflicting results (9, 122, 143).

## PROSTATE

The male urinary tract is different from the female tract, and associated structures can become infected. Infection of the prostate gland may occur through retrograde passage of organisms and may result in focal inflammation presenting as perineal, lower back, or lower abdominal pain with intermittent symptoms of cystitis. A culture process using segmented urine specimens with prostatic massage can help in making this diagnosis. A poorly defined proportion of men with recurrent UTI have prostatitis and probably should be classified as having complicated UTIs (71, 72, 77, 78, 120). Prostatic hypertrophy in aged men can result in obstruction and is associated with complicated UTIs (see below).

## ASYMPTOMATIC BACTERIURIA

After infancy, the prevalence of asymptomatic bacteriuria in males is close to zero until the elderly age ranges are reached. Among community-living men, the prevalence in those over 85 years is about 15% (90); of aged men admitted to hospitals and nursing homes, the rate may be up to 42% (94, 149). Most of the men are indeed asymptomatic, but perhaps 10% have dysuria, a slight but significantly greater prevalence than that in abacteriuric men (90). Gram-positive organisms are a substantially larger proportion of causative bacteria in men than in women, making up 30 to 60% of asymptomatic bacteriuric strains (12, 90, 149) (Table 3). Bacteriuria tends to be intermittent with frequent spontaneous resolution (90). Wolfson et al. identified several predisposing factors, including prostatic hypertrophy, a history or presence of urinary stones and a history of urinary surgery, instrumentation, or previous urinary infection. Although these factors were associated with asymptomatic bacteriuria over all ages combined, the prevalences of these putative risk factors in men over the age of 70 with and without UTI were high but equivalent (149). The already-cited Swedish longitudinal study showed, after exclusion of those with cancer, no association between bacteriuria and mortality in men (98).

## COMPLICATED UTIs

The ability of an organism to cause symptomatic UTI is the net result of effects of the bacteria and responses of the host. If the host is unable to prevent colonization, inhibit bacterial growth, clear the organism from the body, contain the invader or its effects, or kill the organism, then the host is susceptible to UTI. Certain characteristics of the host may put the individual at a disadvantage in performing one or more of these functions. These characteristics are thus associated with an increased incidence of UTIs and, because of the complicated host, are known as complicated UTIs. These UTIs can be grouped into two large categories. The first comprises patients with functional or anatomic abnormalities of the urinary tract. The second is composed of individuals with certain medical situations that yield an increased incidence or severity of UTI; these situations include chronic renal failure (115), diabetes mellitus, immunocompromising illnesses, or use of immunosuppressive agents (63, 69).

In practical terms, a complicated UTI usually manifests itself by lack of response to antibiotic therapy, relapse with the same organism following an antibiotic course, or infection with a non-*E. coli* organism. Of non-*E. coli* organisms, *P. mirabilis* stands out because of its production of urease. Expression of this enzyme causes the elaboration of ammonia from urea, prompting a local rise in urine pH and a consequent precipitation of struvite and apatite crystals. These crystals may coalesce into stones in the bladder, ureter, or kidney. By this means, *P. mirabilis* can make a complicated urinary tract even more complicated.

## Complicated Urinary Tracts

The epidemiology of complicated UTIs includes the epidemiology of complicated urinary tracts, a topic beyond the purview of this chapter. These urinary tracts include anatomic and functional abnormalities as well as instrumentation such as catheterization. Such abnormalities result in bacterial access to the urinary tract, obstruction to urine flow, high intraluminal pressures, sequestration of organisms, and/or presence of a foreign body, each of which can predispose to UTI. Examples of pertinent urinary tract abnormalities, excluding instrumentation, can be derived from trials of antibiotic treatment of complicated UTIs (Table 5). Our understanding of complicated UTIs is limited, in part because of the heterogeneity of these urologic abnormalities. This lack of understanding is unfortunate, because the combination of infection, even with relatively avirulent organisms, and an obstructed urinary tract

**TABLE 5** Examples of complicated urinary tracts in antibiotic trials[a]

| Complicating factor | No. of patients with abnormality |
|---|---|
| Urethral stricture | 126 |
| Prostatic hypertrophy | 84 |
| Neurogenic bladder | 77 |
| Urinary stones | 69 |
| Urologic malignancy | 36 |
| Other obstruction | 30 |

[a] Data are from Allais et al. (4), Cox (20, 20a), and Mattina et al. (89).

**TABLE 6** Organisms causing complicated UTIs[a]

| Infecting organism | Distribution (%) |
|---|---|
| E. coli | 37 |
| K. pneumoniae | 13 |
| P. mirabilis | 12 |
| P. aeruginosa | 9 |
| Enterobacter spp. | 7 |
| Citrobacter spp. | 3 |
| Serratia spp. | 3 |
| Enterococcus spp. | 3 |
| S. aureus | 2 |
| Other | 9 |

[a] Data are from Allais et al. (4), Cox (20, 20a), and Mattina et al. (89).

or one at high intraluminal pressures can result in substantial renal damage. An intriguing finding is that among children who have had operations for urologic abnormalities, nonsecretor status is associated with UTI (117).

One of the clear conclusions of assessments of UTIs in complicated urinary tracts is that *E. coli* is not nearly as prominent as it is in normal urinary tracts (Table 6). Moreover, of *E. coli* causing these UTIs, the isolated strains are relatively avirulent, less commonly expressing virulence determinants such as P fimbriae and hemolysin, which are carried by strains infecting normal urinary tracts (63, 82, 83).

The urologic abnormalities listed in Table 5 have excluded instrumentation. Infections associated with one type of instrumentation, i.e., catheterization, are among the best studied of complicated UTIs.

## URETHRAL CATHETERS

The majority of organisms causing catheter-associated bacteriuria are from the patient's own colonic flora (22) and may be native inhabitants or new immigrants, i.e., exogenous organisms from the environment, often a hospital or nursing home. As in the pathogenesis of UTI in noncatheterized patients, these bacteria may colonize the periurethral area, especially in women (39). Once in or on the patient or on the surface of the catheter system, organisms may enter the bladder through one of three ways: (i) at the time of catheter insertion, (ii) through the catheter lumen, or (iii) along the catheter-urethral interface. With appropriate catheter care, the catheter-urethral interface is estimated to be the route of entry for 70 to 80% of episodes of bacteriuria in women and 20 to 30% of episodes in men (22). The majority of bacterial strains that enter are able to multiply to high concentrations within a day or so (131).

Millions of patients in general hospitals have a catheter in place sometime during their stay. The mean and median durations are between 2 and 4 days (141). With an incidence of 5 to 10% bacteriuria per day, 15 to 30% of catheterized patients will become bacteriuric, usually with a single species (40, 141). E. coli is a common isolate but causes only a minority of the bacteriurias (Table 7). Furthermore, consistent with our knowledge that complicated urinary tracts can be infected with relatively avirulent organisms, of E. coli strains causing nosocomial UTI with fever, i.e., comparable to community-acquired pyelonephritis, only 10% express P fimbriae, a frequency similar to what one would expect in feces of control persons. Other common organisms are Pseudomonas aeruginosa, K. pneumoniae, P. mirabilis, Staphylococcus epidermidis, and enterococci (Table 7). Particularly when antibiotics are in use, yeast cells may be isolated as well (141).

At any given time, more than 100,000 patients in American nursing homes have urethral catheters in place. Many of these patients have been catheterized for months and in some cases years. Even with excellent care, all patients eventually become bacteriuric if catheterized long enough. This high prevalence of bacteriuria in long-term catheterization is a function of two related phenomena (132, 139, 142). The first is an incidence of new episodes of bacteriuria similar to that seen in short-term catheterized patients. The second is the ability of some of these strains to persist for weeks or months. Two of the most persistent organisms are E. coli and Providencia stuartii. These phenomena result in polymicrobial bacteriuria, with sometimes as many as six to eight species, each at $\geq 10^5$ CFU/ml, in up to 95% of urine specimens from long-term catheterized patients (139). These species include common uropathogens such as E. coli and P. mirabilis as well

TABLE 7 Organisms causing catheter-associated bacteriuria

| Infecting organism | Distribution (%) | |
| --- | --- | --- |
| | Short term[a] (incidence) | Long term[b] (weekly prevalance) |
| Escherichia coli | 24 | 14 |
| Klebsiella spp. | 8 | 4 |
| Proteus spp. | 6 | 15 |
| Pseudomonas aeruginosa | 9 | 12 |
| Providencia stuartii | | 24 |
| Morganella morganii | | 7 |
| Other gram-negative bacilli | 7 | 6 |
| Enterococcus spp. | 7 | 11 |
| Coagulase-negative staphylococci | 8 | 3 |
| Other gram-positive bacteria | 4 | 4 |
| Yeasts | 26 | |

[a] Data are from Platt et al. (102) for hospitalized patients with mean and median durations of 2 to 4 days.
[b] Data are from Warren et al. (142) for nursing home patients with duration of >30 days.

Chronic granulomatous disease, caused by hereditary defects in the respiratory burst of granulocytes, is associated with an increased incidence and severity of UTI (3).

## AIDS

Men with AIDS may have a somewhat increased incidence of UTI, including symptomatic UTI. Severe episodes that resulted in septicemia and death have been reported (24).

## SUMMARY

Infection is the most common disease affecting the urinary tract; almost all cases occur by the ascending route and are identified in otherwise healthy persons with normal urinary tracts. These are uncomplicated UTIs and are common in females, presumably because of an anatomy that allows uropathogen colonization of the vagina and the mucosa adjacent to the relatively short urethra. In girls, the highest incidence is in the first year. The incidence of symptomatic UTI rises again in young women and is epidemiologically associated with several factors related to sexual activity. UTIs recur in about 30% of patients; nonsecretors of blood group antigens are predisposed to recurrences. Asymptomatic bacteriuria in the absence of urinary tract structural or functional abnormality does not appear to place the individual at risk for hypertension, renal failure, or mortality. In one group, however, it may be serious: pregnant women with asymptomatic bacteriuria have a substantial risk of acute pyelonephritis, premature delivery, and low infant birth weight.

Among males, UTIs occur with substantial incidence only at the extremes of life. One percent of boys may have a symptomatic UTI, most presenting within their first month. Whether the presence of a prepuce warrants a diagnosis of a complicated urinary tract is definitional; uncircumcised infants are at 10 to 20 times the risk of UTI. After infancy, the incidence of UTI among males is low, but infections do occur and some episodes may be complicated by prostatitis. In older men, symptomatic infection and asymptomatic bacteriuria are often complicated UTIs, usually attributable to benign prostatic hypertrophy. As in women, there appears to be no direct association between asymptomatic bacteriuria and mortality.

Complicated UTIs occur in two groups of patients. One group comprises those with certain medical illnesses that predispose the individual to a higher incidence or severity of UTI. The second is of patients with complicated urinary tracts. Among infants with UTI, 10 to 20% of boys and 2% of girls have anatomic obstructions of some type, and about one-third of each group have vesicoureteral reflux, a functional abnormality that in most children reverses with growth. Children with reflux have a high risk of renal scarring, although reflux is neither necessary nor sufficient for this consequence of infection. Among adults, bladder outflow obstruction, neurogenic bladder, urinary stones, urinary tract malignancies, and urologic instrumentation including catheterization are common predispositions to complicated UTIs. An understanding of the pathogeneses of complicated UTIs is at an early stage.

## REFERENCES

1. **Abrutyn, E., J. Mossey, J. A. Berlin, J. Boscia, M. Levison, P. Pitsakis, and D. Kaye.** 1994. Does asymptomatic bacteriuria predict mortality and does antimicrobial treatment reduce mortality in elderly ambulatory women? *Ann. Intern. Med.* **120:** 827–833.
2. **Abrutyn, E., J. Mossey, M. Levison, J. Boscia, P. Pitsakis, and D. Kaye.** 1991. Epidemiology of asymptomatic bacteriuria in elderly women. *J. Am. Geriatr. Soc.* **39:** 388–393.
3. **Aliabadi, H., R. Gonzalez, and P. G. Quie.** 1989. Urinary tract disorders in patients with chronic granulomatous disease. *N. Engl. J. Med.* **321:**706–708.

as less familiar species such as *Providencia stuartii* and *Morganella morganii* (Table 7).

Most patients with catheter-associated bacteriuria are asymptomatic. However, complications in two categories do occur. The first category includes symptomatic UTIs and occurs in the short- and long-term catheterized patient: fever, acute pyelonephritis, and bacteremia. Some of these episodes end in death (42, 48, 111, 140). The second group is more often witnessed in long-term catheterized patients: catheter obstruction, urinary tract stone, local periurinary infection, chronic interstitial nephritis, chronic pyelonephritis, renal failure, and, over years, bladder cancer (138a).

## EXTERNAL COLLECTION DEVICES

For men with urinary incontinence, condoms that empty through a collection tube into a drainage bag are widely used. Although these avoid the problems of a tube in the urinary tract, urine within these condom catheters may develop high concentrations of organisms, the urethra and skin may be colonized with uropathogens, and bladder bacteriuria may develop (30). To distinguish bladder bacteriuria from skin contamination, careful collection of urine in a new condom by well-trained individuals is necessary (95).

## INTERMITTENT CATHETERIZATION

Insertion of a sterile or only clean catheter every 3 to 6 h by caregivers or the patient, drainage of urine, and immediate removal of the catheter provide periodic bladder emptying (151). Intermittent catheterization is the standard of urinary care for spinal injury patients (45). The incidence of bacteriuria is about 1 to 3% per catheterization. At four catheterizations per day, a new episode of bacteriuria occurs every 1 to 3 weeks (68).

## Medical Illnesses

The second group of patients with complicated UTIs are those with certain illnesses that predispose an individual to UTI or, if UTI develops, to an infection of greater severity (69).

## DIABETES MELLITUS

There has been controversy as to whether diabetes mellitus is associated with an increased frequency of UTI. A number of studies suggest that the prevalence of asymptomatic bacteriuria is greater in diabetic than in nondiabetic women but is equivalent in diabetic and nondiabetic men (152). The relative incidence of symptomatic UTI among diabetics and nondiabetics remains unclear. However, when they do occur, UTIs may be more severe in diabetics and may result in renal and perirenal abscesses, papillary necrosis, and emphysematous pyelonephritis.

## SOLID-ORGAN TRANSPLANTS

The incidence of UTI following solid-organ transplantation and the attendant immunosuppression appears to be proportional to the duration of perioperative urinary catheterization and the absence of antibiotic use. Female recipients are at greater risk than males. The incidence of UTI rapidly decreases after the first 2 to 3 months following transplantation (21, 54, 104).

## GRANULOCYTOPENIA

Among patients who are granulocytopenic because of bone marrow transplantation, myelosuppression for treatment of malignancy, or acute leukemia or aplastic anemia, the risk of UTI is present but not high, perhaps in part because catheterization is generally minimized in these patients. It is interesting that in patients with granulocytopenia and UTI, irritative bladder symptoms such as dysuria, frequency, and urgency are uncommon manifestations yet fever and flank pain are common (119).

4. **Allais, J. M., L. C. Preheim, T. A. Cuevas, J. S. Roccaforte, M. A. Mellencamp, and M. J. Bittner.** 1988. Randomized, double-blind comparison of ciprofloxacin and trimethoprim-sulfamethoxazole for complicated urinary tract infections. *Antimicrob. Agents Chemother.* **32:**1327–1330.
5. **Anonymous.** 1991. Prevention of reflux nephropathy. *Lancet* **338:**1050.
6. **Arav-Boger, R., L. Leibovici, and Y. L. Danon.** 1994. Urinary tract infections with low and high colony counts in young women. Spontaneous remission and single-dose vs. multiple-day treatment. *Arch. Intern. Med.* **154:**300–304.
7. **Asscher, A. W., S. Chick, and N. Radford.** 1973. Natural history of asymptomatic bacteriuria (ASB) in non-pregnant women, p. 51–60. *In* W. Brumfitt and A. W. Asscher (ed.), *Urinary Tract Infection.* Oxford University Press, London.
8. **Bailey, R. R., B. A. Peddie, C. P. Swainson, and D. Kirkpatrick.** 1986. Sexual acquisition of urinary tract infection in a man. *Nephron* **44:**217–218.
9. **Barnes, R. C., R. Daifuku, R. E. Roddy, and W. E. Stamm.** 1986. Urinary-tract infection in sexually active homosexual men. *Lancet* **i:**171–173.
10. **Boscia, J. A., and D. Kaye.** 1987. Asymptomatic bacteriuria in the elderly. *Infect. Dis. Clin. North Am.* **1:**893–905.
11. **Boscia, J. A., W. D. Kobasa, E. Abrutyn, M. E. Levison, A. M. Kaplan, and D. Kaye.** 1986. Lack of association between bacteriuria and symptoms in the elderly. *Am. J. Med.* **81:**979–982.
12. **Boscia, J. A., W. D. Kobasa, R. A. Knight, E. Abrutyn, M. E. Levison, and D. Kaye.** 1986. Epidemiology of bacteriuria in an elderly ambulatory population. *Am. J. Med.* **80:**208–213.
13. **Bran, J. L., M. E. Levison, and D. Kaye.** 1972. Entrance of bacteria into the female urinary bladder. *N. Engl. J. Med.* **286:**626–629.
14. **Brauner, A., S. H. Jacobson, and I. Kühn.** 1992. Urinary *Escherichia coli* causing recurrent infections—a prospective follow-up of biochemical phenotypes. *Clin. Nephrol.* **38:**318–323.
15. **Brocklehurst, J. C., P. Bee, D. Jones, and M. K. Palmer.** 1977. Bacteriuria in geriatric hospital patients: its correlates and management. *Age Ageing* **6:**240–245.
16. **Buck, A. C., P. I. Reed, Y. K. Siddiq, G. D. Chisholm, and T. R. Fraser.** 1976. Bladder dysfunction and neuropathy in diabetes. *Diabetologia* **12:**251–258.
17. **Buckley, R. M., Jr., M. McGuckin, and R. R. MacGregor.** 1978. Urine bacterial counts after sexual intercourse. *N. Engl. J. Med.* **298:**321–324.
18. **Busch, R., and H. Huland.** 1984. Correlation of symptoms and results of direct bacterial localization in patients with urinary tract infections. *J. Urol.* **132:**282–285.
19. **Cordon-Cardo, C., K. O. Lloyd, C. L. Finstad, M. E. McGroarty, V. E. Reuter, N. H. Bander, L. J. Old, and M. R. Melamed.** 1986. Immunoanatomic distribution of blood group antigens in the human urinary tract. *Lab. Invest.* **55:**444–454.
20. **Cox, C. E.** 1989. Ofloxacin in the management of complicated urinary tract infections, including prostatitis. *Am. J. Med.* **87:**61S–68S.
20a. **Cox, C. E.** 1992. A comparison of the safety and efficacy of lomefloxacin and ciprofloxacin in the treatment of complicated or recurrent urinary tract infections. *Am. J. Med.* **92:**82S–86S.
21. **Cuvelier, R., Y. Pirson, G. P. J. Alexandre, and C. V. de Strihou.** 1985. Late urinary tract infection after transplantation: prevalence, predisposition and morbidity. *Nephron* **40:**76–78.
22. **Daifuku, R., and W. Stamm.** 1984. Association of rectal and urethral colonization with urinary tract infection in patients with indwelling catheters. *JAMA* **252:**2028–2030.
23. **Davison, J. M., M. S. Sprott, and J. B. Selkon.** 1984. The effect of covert bacteriuria in school girls on renal function at 18 years and during pregnancy. *Lancet* **ii:**651–655.
24. **De Pinho, A. M. F., G. S. Lopes, C. F. Ramos-Filho, O. D. R. Santos, M. P. B. De Oliverira, M. Halpern, C. A. B. Gouvea, and M. Schechter.** 1994. Urinary tract infection in men with AIDS. *Genitourin. Med.* **70:**30–34.
25. **Edwards, D., I. C. S. Normand, N. Prescod, and J. M. Smellie.** 1977. Disappearance of vesicoureteric reflux during long-term prophylaxis of urinary tract infection in children. *Br. Med. J.* **2:**285–288.
26. **El-Khatib, M. T., G. J. Becker, and P. S. Kincaid-Smith.** 1990. Reflux nephropathy and primary vesicoureteric relux in adults. *Q. J. Med.* **77:**1241–1253.
27. **Ellenberg, M.** 1966. Diabetic neurogenic vesical dysfunction. *Arch. Intern. Med.* **117:**348–354.

28. Elliott, T. S. J., C. B. Slack, and M. C. Bishop. 1986. Scanning electron microscopy and bacteriology of the human bladder in acute and chronic urinary tract infections, p. 31–46. *In* A. W. Asscher and W. Brumfitt (ed.), *Microbial Diseases in Nephrology*. John Wiley & Sons, Ltd., London.
29. Ferry, S., L. G. Burman, and S. E. Holm. 1988. Clinical and bacteriological effects of therapy of urinary tract infection in primary health care: relation to *in vitro* sensitivity testing. *Scand. J. Infect. Dis.* **20:** 535–544.
30. Fierer, J., and M. Ekstrom. 1981. An outbreak of *Providencia stuartii* urinary tract infections. Patients with condom catheters are a reservoir of the bacteria. *JAMA* **245:** 1553–1555.
31. Fihn, S. D., C. Johnson, C. Pinkstaff, and W. E. Stamm. 1986. Diaphragm use and urinary tract infections: analysis of urodynamic and microbiological factors. *J. Urol.* **136:**853–856.
32. Fihn, S. D., C. Johnson, and W. E. Stamm. 1988. *Escherichia coli* urethritis in women with symptoms of acute urinary tract infection. *J. Infect. Dis.* **157:**196–199.
33. Fihn, S. D., R. H. Latham, P. Roberts, K. Running, and W. E. Stamm. 1985. Association between diaphragm use and urinary tract infection. *JAMA* **254:**240–245.
34. Fowler, J. E., Jr., and E. T. Pulaski. 1981. Excretory urography, cystography, and cystoscopy in the evaluation of women with urinary-tract infection. A prospective study. *N. Engl. J. Med.* **304:**462–465.
35. Fowler, J. E., Jr., and T. A. Stamey. 1977. Studies of introital colonization in women with recurrent urinary infections. VII. The role of bacterial adherence. *J. Urol.* **117:**472–476.
36. Foxman, B. 1990. Recurring urinary tract infection: incidence and risk factors. *Am. J. Public Health.* **80:**331–333.
37. Foxman, B., and J.-W. Chi. 1990. Health behavior and urinary tract infection in college-aged women. *J. Clin. Epidemiol.* **43:** 329–337.
38. Gaffney, R. A., A. J. Schaeffer, B. E. Anderson, and J. L. Duncan. 1994. Effect of Lewis blood group antigen expression on bacterial adherence to COS-1 cells. *Infect. Immun.* **62:**3022–3026.
39. Garibaldi, R. A., J. P. Burke, M. R. Britt, W. A. Miller, and C. B. Smith. 1980. Meatal colonization and catheter-associated bacteriuria. *N. Engl. J. Med.* **303:** 316–318.
40. Garibaldi, R. A., J. P. Burke, M. L. Dickman, and C. B. Smith. 1974. Factors predisposing to bacteriuria during indwelling urethral catheterization. *N. Engl. J. Med.* **291:**215.
41. Gaymans, R., H. A. Valkenburg, M. J. Haverkorn, and W. R. O. Goslings. 1976. A prospective study of urinary-tract infections in a Dutch general practice. *Lancet* **ii:** 674–677.
42. Gordon, D., A. Bune, B. Grime, P. J. McDonald, V. R. Marshall, J. Marsh, and G. Sinclair. 1983. Diagnostic criteria and natural history of catheter-associated urinary tract infections after prostatectomy. *Lancet* **i:** 1269–1271.
43. Gransden, W. R., S. J. Eykyn, I. Phillips, and B. Rowe. 1990. Bacteremia due to *Escherichia coli*: a study of 861 episodes. *Rev. Infect. Dis.* **12:**1008–1018.
44. Gratacós, E., P.-J. Torres, J. Vila, P. L. Alonso, and V. Cararach. 1994. Screening and treatment of asymptomatic bacteriuria in pregnancy prevent pyelonephritis. *J. Infect. Dis.* **169:**1390–1392.
45. Guttmann, L., and H. Frankel. 1966. The value of intermittent catheterization in the early management of traumatic paraplegia and tetraplegia. *Paraplegia* **4:**63.
46. Hansson, S., D. Caugant, U. Jodal, and C. Svanborg-Edén. 1989. Untreated asymptomatic bacteriuria in girls. I. Stability of urinary isolates. *Br. Med. J.* **298:**853–855.
47. Hansson, S., K. Hjälmås, U. Jodal, and R. Sixt. 1990. Lower urinary tract dysfunction in girls with untreated asymptomatic or covert bacteriuria. *J. Urol.* **143:**333–335.
48. Hartstein, A. I., S. B. Garber, T. T. Ward, S. R. Jones, and V. H. Morthland. 1981. Nosocomial urinary tract infection: a prospective evaluation of 108 catheterized patients. *Infect. Control* **2:**380–386.
49. Hebelka, M., K. Lincoln, and T. Sandberg. 1993. Sexual acquisition of acute pyelonephritis in a man. *Scand. J. Infect. Dis.* **25:**141–143.
50. Herzog, L. W. 1989. Urinary tract infections and circumcision. A case-control study. *Am. J. Dis. Child.* **143:**348–350.
51. Hooton, T. M., C. L. Fennell, A. M. Clark, and W. E. Stamm. 1991. Nonoxynol-9: differential antibacterial activity and enhancement of bacterial adherence to vaginal epithelial cells. *J. Infect. Dis.* **164:** 1216–1219.
52. Hooton, T. M., S. Hillier, C. Johnson, P. L. Roberts, and W. E. Stamm. 1991.

*Escherichia coli* bacteriuria and contraceptive method. *JAMA* **265**:64–69.
53. **Hooton, T. M., P. L. Roberts, and W. E. Stamm.** 1994. Effects of recent sexual activity and use of a diaphragm on the vaginal microflora. *Clin. Infect. Dis.* **19**:274–278.
54. **Hoy, W. E., S. M. Kissel, R. B. Freeman, and W. A. Sterling, Jr.** 1985. Altered patterns of posttransplant urinary tract infections associated with perioperative antibiotics and curtailed catheterization. *Am. J. Kidney Dis.* **6**:212–216.
55. **Ikäheimo, R., A. Siitonen, U. Kärkkäinen, P. Kuosmanen, and P. H. Mäkelä.** 1993. Characteristics of *Escherichia coli* in acute community-acquired cystitis of adult women. *Scand. J. Infect. Dis.* **25**:705–712.
56. **Ikäheimo, R., A. Siitonen, U. Kärkkäinen, J. Mustonen, T. Heiskanen, and P. H. Mäkelä.** 1994. Community-acquired pyelonephritis in adults: characteristics of *E. coli* isolates in bacteremic and non-bacteremic patients. *Scand. J. Infect. Dis.* **26**:289–296.
57. **International Reflux Study Committee.** 1981. Medical versus surgical treatment of primary vesicoureteral reflux: a prospective international reflux study in children. *J. Urol.* **125**:277–283.
58. **Jacobson, S. H.** 1991. A five-year prospective follow-up of women with nonobstructive pyelonephritic renal scarring. *Scand. J. Urol. Nephrol.* **25**:51–57.
58a. **Jacobson, S. H., O. Eklöf, C. G. Eriksson, L.-E. Lins, B. Tidgren, and J. Winberg.** 1989. Development of hypertension and uraemia after pyelonephritis in childhood: 27 year follow up. *Br. Med. J.* **299**:703–706.
59. **Jacobson, S. H., and H. Lomberg.** 1990. Overrepresentation of blood group nonsecretors in adults with renal scarring. *Scand. J. Urol. Nephrol.* **24**:145–150.
60. **Jakobsson, B., U. Berg, and L. Svensson.** 1994. Renal scarring after acute pyelonephritis. *Arch. Dis. Child.* **70**:111–115.
61. **Jantausch, B. A., V. R. Criss, R. O'Donnell, B. L. Wiedermann, M. Majd, H. G. Rushton, R. S. Shirey, and N. L. C. Luban.** 1994. Association of Lewis blood group phenotypes with urinary tract infection in children. *J. Pediatr.* **124**:863–868.
62. **Jodal, U.** 1987. The natural history of bacteriuria in childhood. *Infect. Dis. Clin. North Am.* **1**:713–729.
63. **Johnson, J. R., P. L. Roberts, and W. E. Stamm.** 1987. P fimbriae and other virulence factors in *Escherichia coli* urosepsis: association with patients' characteristics. *J. Infect. Dis.* **156**:225–228.
64. **Johnson, J. R., and W. E. Stamm.** 1989. Urinary tract infections in women: diagnosis and treatment. *Ann. Intern. Med.* **111**:906–917.
65. **Källenius, G., and J. Winberg.** 1978. Bacterial adherence to periurethral epithelial cells in girls prone to urinary-tract infections. *Lancet* **ii**:540–543.
66. **Kass, E. H.** 1962. Pyelonephritis and bacteriuria: a major problem in preventive medicine. *Ann. Intern. Med.* **56**:46–53.
67. **Kinane, D. F., C. C. Blackwell, R. P. Brettle, D. M. Weir, F. P. Winstanley, and R. A. Elton.** 1982. ABO blood group, secretor state, and susceptibility to recurrent urinary tract infection in women. *Br. Med. J.* **285**:7–9.
68. **King, R. B., C. E. Carlson, J. Mervine, Y. Wu, and G. M. Yarkony.** 1992. Clean and sterile intermittent catheterization methods in hospitalized patients with spinal cord injury. *Arch. Phys. Med. Rehabil.* **73**:798–802.
69. **Korzeniowski, O. M.** 1991. Urinary tract infection in the impaired host. *Med. Clin. North Am.* **75**:391–404.
70. **Kreger, B. E., D. E. Craven, P. C. Carling, and W. R. McCabe.** 1980. Gram-negative bacteremia. III. Reassessment of etiology, epidemiology and ecology in 612 patients. *Am. J. Med.* **68**:332–355.
71. **Krieger, J. N.** 1984. Prostatitis syndromes: pathophysiology, differential diagnosis, and treatment. *Sex. Transm. Dis.* **11**:100–112.
72. **Krieger, J. N., and L. A. McGonagle.** 1989. Diagnostic considerations and interpretation of microbiological findings for evaluation of chronic prostatitis. *J. Clin. Microbiol.* **27**:2240–2244.
73. **Krieger, J. N., S. O. Ross, and J. M. Simonsen.** 1993. Urinary tract infections in healthy university men. *J. Urol.* **149**:1046–1048.
74. **Kunin, C. M.** 1987. *Detection, Prevention and Management of Urinary Tract Infections*, 4th ed. Lea & Febiger, Philadelphia.
75. **Kunin, C. M., L. V. White, and T. H. Hua.** 1993. A reassessment of the importance of "low-count" bacteriuria in young women with acute urinary symptoms. *Ann. Intern. Med.* **119**:454–460.

76. Lindberg, U., I. Claesson, L. Å. Hanson, and U. Jodal. 1978. Asymptomatic bacteriuria in schoolgirls. VIII. Clinical course during a 3-year follow-up. *J. Pediatr.* **92:**194–199.
77. Lipsky, B. A. 1989. Urinary tract infections in men: epidemiology, pathophysiology, diagnosis, and treatment. *Ann. Intern. Med.* **110:**138–150.
78. Lipsky, B. A., R. C. Ireton, S. D. Fihn, R. Hackett, and R. E. Berger. 1987. Diagnosis of bacteriuria in men: specimen collection and culture interpretation. *J. Infect. Dis.* **155:**847–854.
79. LiPuma, J. J., T. L. Stull, S. E. Dasen, K. A. Pidcock, D. Kaye, and O. M. Korzeniowski. 1989. DNA polymorphisms among *Escherichia coli* isolated from bacteriuric women. *J. Infect. Dis.* **159:**526–532.
80. Lomberg, H., B. Cedergren, H. Leffler, B. Nilsson, A.-S. Carlström, and C. Svanborg-Edén. 1986. Influence of blood group on the availability of receptors for attachment of uropathogenic *Escherichia coli*. *Infect. Immun.* **51:**919–926.
81. Lomberg, H., P. de Man, and C. Svanborg-Edén. 1989. Bacterial and host determinants of renal scarring. *APMIS* **97:**193–199.
82. Lomberg, H., L. Å. Hanson, B. Jacobsson, U. Jodal, H. Leffler, and C. Svanborg-Edén. 1983. Correlation of P blood group, vesicoureteral reflux, and bacterial attachment in patients with recurrent pyelonephritis. *N. Engl. J. Med.* **308:**1189–1192.
83. Lomberg, H., M. Hellström, U. Jodal, H. Leffler, K. Lincoln, and C. Svanborg-Edén. 1984. Virulence-associated traits in *Escherichia coli* causing first and recurrent episodes of urinary tract infection in children with or without vesicoureteral reflux. *J. Infect. Dis.* **150:**561–569.
84. Lomberg, H., M. Hellström, U. Jodal, I. Ørskov, and C. Svanborg-Edén. 1989. Properties of *Escherichia coli* in patients with renal scarring. *J. Infect. Dis.* **159:**579–582.
85. Lomberg, H., M. Hellström, U. Jodal, and C. Svanborg-Edén. 1986. Renal scarring and non-attaching *Escherichia coli*. *Lancet* **ii:**1341.
86. Lomberg, H., U. Jodal, H. Leffler, P. de Man, and C. Svanborg. 1992. Blood group non-secretors have an increased inflammatory response to urinary tract infection. *Scand. J. Infect. Dis.* **24:**77–83.
87. Mabeck, C. E. 1972. Treatment of uncomplicated urinary tract infection in nonpregnant women. *Postgrad. Med. J.* **48:**69–75.
88. Mårild, S., U. Jodal, and L. Å. Hanson. 1990. Breastfeeding and urinary-tract infection. *Lancet* **ii:**942.
89. Mattina, R., C. E. Cocuzza, M. Cesana, and the Italian Multicentre UTI Rufloxacin Group. 1993. Rufloxacin once daily versus ofloxacin twice daily for treatment of complicated cystitis and upper urinary tract infections. *Infection* **21:**106–111.
90. Mims, A. D., D. C. Norman, R. H. Yamamura, and T. T. Yoshikawa. 1990. Clinically inapparent (asymptomatic) bacteriuria in ambulatory elderly men: epidemiological, clinical, and microbiological findings. *J. Am. Geriatr. Soc.* **38:**1209–1214.
91. Mittendorf, R., M. A. Williams, and E. H. Kass. 1992. Prevention of preterm delivery and low birth weight associated with asymptomatic bacteriuria. *Clin. Infect. Dis.* **14:**927–932.
92. Muder, R. R., C. Brennen, M. M. Wagener, and A. M. Goetz. 1992. Bacteremia in a long-term-care facility: a five-year prospective study of 163 consecutive episodes. *Clin. Infect. Dis.* **14:**647–654.
93. Navas, E. L., M. F. Venegas, J. L. Duncan, B. E. Anderson, C. Kanerva, J. S. Chmiel, and A. J. Schaeffer. 1994. Blood group antigen expression on vaginal cells and mucus in women with and without a history of urinary tract infections. *J. Urol.* **152:**345–349.
94. Nicolle, L. E. 1993. Urinary tract infections in long-term care facilities. *Infect. Control Hosp. Epidemiol.* **14:**220–225.
95. Nicolle, L. E., G. K. M. Harding, J. Kennedy, M. McIntyre, F. Aoki, and D. Murray. 1988. Urine specimen collection with external devices for diagnosis of bacteriuria in elderly incontinent men. *J. Clin. Microbiol.* **26:**1115–1119.
96. Nicolle, L. E., G. K. M. Harding, J. Preiksaitis, and A. R. Ronald. 1982. The association of urinary tract infection with sexual intercourse. *J. Infect. Dis.* **146:**579–583.
97. Nicolle, L. E., P. Muir, G. K. M. Harding, and M. Norris. 1988. Localization of urinary tract infection in elderly, institutionalized women with asymptomatic bacteriuria. *J. Infect. Dis.* **157:**65–70.
98. Nordenstam, G. R., C. Å. Brandberg, A. S. Odén, C. M. Svanborg Edén, and A. Svanborg. 1986. Bacteriuria and mortality in an elderly population. *N. Engl. J. Med.* **314:**1152–1156.
99. Olling, S., K. Verrier Jones, R. Mackenzie, E. R. Verrier Jones, L. A. Hanson,

99. and A. W. Asscher. 1981. A four-year follow-up of schoolgirls with untreated covert bacteriuria: bacteriological aspects. *Clin. Nephrol.* **16:**169–171.
100. Patton, J. P., D. B. Nash, and E. Abrutyn. 1991. Urinary tract infection: economic considerations. *Med. Clin. North Am.* **75:**495–513.
101. Pisacane, A., L. Graziano, G. Mazzarella, B. Scarpellino, and G. Zona. 1992. Breast-feeding and urinary tract infection. *J. Pediatr.* **120:**87–89.
102. Platt, R., B. F. Polk, B. Murdock, and B. Rosner. 1986. Risk factors for nosocomial urinary tract infection. *Am. J. Epidemiol.* **124:**977–985.
103. Plos, K., H. Lomberg, S. Hull, I. Johansson, and C. Svanborg. 1991. *Escherichia coli* in patients with renal scarring: genotype and phenotype of Gal$\alpha$1-4Gal$\beta$-, Forssman- and mannose-specific adhesins. *Pediatr. Infect. Dis. J.* **10:**15–19.
104. Prát, V., M. Horiková, K. Matoušovic, M. Hatala, and M. Liška. 1985. Urinary tract infection in renal transplant patients. *Infection* **13:**207–210.
105. Raz, R., and W. E. Stamm. 1993. A controlled trial of intravaginal estriol in postmenopausal women with recurrent urinary tract infections. *N. Engl. J. Med.* **329:**753–756.
106. Remis, R. S., M. J. Gurwith, D. Gurwith, N. T. Hargrett-Bean, and P. M. Layde. 1987. Risk factors for urinary tract infection. *Am. J. Epidemiol.* **126:**685–694.
107. Ring, E., and G. Zobel. 1988. Urinary infection and malformations of urinary tract in infancy. *Arch. Dis. Child.* **63:**818–820.
108. Roberts, F. J., I. W. Geere, and A. Coldman. 1991. A three-year study of positive blood cultures, with emphasis on prognosis. *Rev. Infect. Dis.* **13:**34–46.
109. Romero, R., E. Oyarzun, M. Mazor, M. Sirtori, J. C. Hobbins and M. Bracken. 1989. Meta-analysis of the relationship between asymptomatic bacteriuria and preterm delivery/low birth weight. *Obstet. Gynecol.* **73:**576–582.
110. Rubin, R. H., E. D. Shapiro, V. T. Andriole, R. J. Davis, and W. E. Stamm. 1992. Evaluation of new anti-infective drugs for the treatment of urinary tract infection. *Clin. Infect. Dis.* **15:**S216–S227.
111. Rudman, D., A. Hontanosas, Z. Cohen, and D. E. Mattson. 1988. Clinical correlates of bacteremia in a Veterans Administration extended care facility. *J. Am. Geriatr. Soc.* **36:**726–732.
112. Rushton, H. G., M. Majd, B. Jantausch, B. L. Wiedermann, and A. B. Belman. 1992. Renal scarring following reflux and nonreflux pyelonephritis in children: evaluation with $^{99m}$technetium-dimercaptosuccinic acid scintigraphy. *J. Urol.* **147:**1327–1332.
113. Russo, T. A., A. Stapleton, S. Wenderoth, T. M. Hooton, and W. E. Stamm. 1995. Chromosomal restriction fragment length polymorphism analysis of *Escherichia coli* strains causing recurrent urinary tract infections in young women. *J. Infect. Dis.* **172:**440–445.
114. Sacks, S. H., K. V. Jones, R. Roberts, A. W. Asscher, and J. G. G. Ledingham. 1987. Effect of symptomless bacteriuria in childhood on subsequent pregnancy. *Lancet* **ii:**991–994.
115. Saitoh, H., K. Nakamura, M. Hida, and T. Satoh. 1985. Urinary tract infection in oliguric patients with chronic renal failure. *J. Urol.* **133:**990–993.
116. Schaeffer, A. J., J. M. Jones, and J. K. Dunn. 1981. Association of *in vitro* Escherichia coli adherence to vaginal and buccal epithelial cells with susceptibility of women to recurrent urinary-tract infections. *N. Engl. J. Med.* **304:**1062–1066.
117. Sheinfeld, J., C. Cordon-Cardo, W. R. Fair, D. D. Wartinger, and R. Rabinowitz. 1990. Association of type 1 blood group antigens with urinary tract infections in children with genitourinary structural abnormalities. *J. Urol.* **144:**469–473.
118. Sheinfeld, J., A. J. Schaeffer, C. Cordon-Cardo, A. Rogatko, and W. R. Fair. 1989. Association of the Lewis blood-group phenotype with recurrent urinary tract infections in women. *N. Engl. J. Med.* **320:**773–777.
119. Sickles, E. A., W. H. Greene, and P. H. Wiernik. 1975. Clinical presentation of infection in granulocytopenic patients. *Arch. Intern. Med.* **135:**715–719.
120. Smith, J. W., S. R. Jones, W. P. Reed, A. D. Tice, R. H. Deupree, and B. Kaijser. 1979. Recurrent urinary tract infections in men. Characteristics and response to therapy. *Ann. Intern. Med.* **91:**544–548.
121. Sourander, L. B., I. Ruikka, and M. Gronroos. 1965. Correlation between urinary tract infection, prolapse conditions and function of the bladder in aged female hospital patients. *Gerontol. Clin.* **7:**179–184.
122. Spach, D. H., A. E. Stapleton, and W. E. Stamm. 1992. Lack of circumcision increases the risk of urinary tract infection in young men. *JAMA* **267:**679–681.

123. Stamey, T. A., and C. C. Sexton. 1975. The role of vaginal colonization with enterobacteriaceae in recurrent urinary infections. *J. Urol.* **113:**214–217.
124. Stamey, T. A., M. Timothy, M. Millar, and G. Mihara. 1971. Recurrent urinary infections in adult women. The role of introital enterobacteria. *Calif. Med.* **115:**1–19.
125. Stamm, W. E., G. W. Counts, K. R. Running, S. Fihn, M. Turck, and K. K. Holmes. 1982. Diagnosis of coliform infection in acutely dysuric women. *N. Engl. J. Med.* **307:**463–468.
126. Stamm, W. E., M. McKevitt, P. L. Roberts, and N. J. White. 1991. Natural history of recurrent urinary tract infections in women. *Rev. Infect. Dis.* **13:**77–84.
127. Stamm, W. E., K. Running, M. McKevitt, G. W. Counts, M. Turck, and K. K. Holmes. 1981. Treatment of the acute urethral syndrome. *N. Engl. J. Med.* **304:**956–958.
128. Stamm, W. E., K. F. Wagner, R. Amsel, E. R. Alexander, M. Turck, G. W. Counts, and K. K. Holmes. 1980. Causes of the acute urethral syndrome in women. *N. Engl. J. Med.* **303:**409–415.
129. Stapleton, A., T. M. Hooton, C. Fennell, P. L. Roberts, and W. E. Stamm. 1995. Effect of secretor status on vaginla and rectal colonization with fimbriated *Escherichia coli* in women with and without recurrent urinary tract infection. *J. Infect. Dis.* **171:**717–720.
130. Stapleton, A., E. Nudelman, H. Clausen, S. Hakomori, and W. E. Stamm. 1992. Binding of uropathogenic *Escherichia coli* R45 to glycolipids extracted from vaginal epithelial cells is dependent on histo-blood group secretor status. *J. Clin. Invest.* **90:**965–972.
131. Stark, R. P., and D. G. Maki. 1984. Bacteriuria in the catheterized patient. What quantitative level of bacteriuria is relevant? *N. Engl. J. Med.* **311:**560–564.
132. Steward, D. K., G. L. Wood, R. L. Cohen, J. W. Smith, and P. A. Mackowiak. 1985. Failure of the urinalysis and quantitative urine culture in diagnosing symptomatic urinary tract infections in patients with long-term urinary catheters. *Am. J. Infect. Control.* **13:**154–160.
133. Strom, B. L., M. Collins, S. L. West, J. Kreisberg, and S. Weller. 1987. Sexual activity, contraceptive use, and other risk factors for symptomatic and asymptomatic bacteriuria. *Ann. Intern. Med.* **107:**816–823.
134. Suntharalingam, M., V. Seth, and B. Moore-Smith. 1983. Site of urinary tract infection in elderly women admitted to an acute geriatric assessment unit. *Age Ageing* **12:**317–322.
135. Svanborg-Edén, C., and U. Jodal. 1979. Attachment of *Escherichia coli* to urinary sediment epithelial cells from urinary tract infection-prone and healthy children. *Infect. Immun.* **26:**837–840.
136. Tencer, J. 1988. Asymptomatic bacteriuria—a long-term study. *Scand. J. Urol. Nephrol.* **22:**31–34.
137. Ulleryd, P., K. Lincoln, F. Scheutz, and T. Sandberg. 1994. Virulence characteristics of *Escherichia coli* in relation to host response in men with symptomatic urinary tract infection. *Clin. Infect. Dis.* **18:**579–584.
138. U.S. Department of Health and Human Services, Public Health Service, National Institutes of Health. 1990. *The National Kidney and Urologic Diseases Advisory Board 1990 Long-Range Plan—Window on the 21st Century.* NIH publication no. 90-583. National Institutes of Health, Bethesda, Md.
138a. Warren, J. W. 1991. The catheter and urinary tract infection. *Med. Clin. North Am.* **75:**481–493.
139. Warren, J. W., D. Damron, J. H. Tenney, J. M. Hoopes, B. Deforge, and H. L. Muncie. 1987. Fever, bacteremia, and death as complications of bacteriuria in women with long-term urethral catheters. *J. Infect. Dis.* **155:**1151–1158.
140. Warren, J. W., H. L. Muncie, Jr., and M. Hall-Craggs. 1988. Acute pyelonephritis associated with the bacteriuria of long-term catheterization: a prospective clinicopathological study. *J. Infect. Dis.* **158:**1341–1346.
141. Warren, J. W., R. Platt, R. J. Thomas, B. Rosner, and E. H. Kass. 1978. Antibiotic irrigation and catheter-associated urinary-tract infections. *N. Engl. J. Med.* **299:**570.
142. Warren, J. W., J. H. Tenney, J. M. Hoopes, and H. L. Muncie. 1982. A prospective microbiologic study of bacteriuria in patients with chronic indwelling urethral catheters. *J. Infect. Dis.* **146:**719–723.
143. Wilson, A. P. R., S. J. Tovey, M. W. Adler, and R. N. Grüneberg. 1986. Prevalence of urinary tract infection in homosexual and heterosexual men. *Genitourin. Med.* **62:**189–190.
144. Winberg, J. 1992. Commentary: progressive renal damage from infection with or without reflux. *J. Urol.* **148:**1733–1734.
145. Winberg, J., H. J. Andersen, T. Bergström, B. Jacobsson, H. Larson, and K.

Lincoln. 1974. Epidemiology of symptomatic urinary tract infection in childhood. *Acta Paediatr. Scand.* **252**(Suppl.):3–20.
146. **Winberg, J., I. Bollgren, G. Källenius, R. Möllby, and S. B. Svenson.** 1982. Clinical pyelonephritis and focal renal scarring. *Pediatr. Clin. North Am.* **29**:801–814.
147. **Wiswell, T. E., and J. D. Roscelli.** 1986. Corroborative evidence for the decreased incidence of urinary tract infections in circumcised male infants. *Pediatrics* **78**:96–99.
148. **Wiswell, T. E., F. R. Smith, and J. W. Bass.** 1985. Decreased incidence of urinary tract infections in circumcised male infants. *Pediatrics* **75**:901–903.
149. **Wolfson, S. A., G. M. Kalmanson, M. E. Rubini, and L. B. Guze.** 1965. Epidemiology of bacteriuria in a predominantly geriatric male population. *Am. J. Med. Sci.* **250**:168–173.
150. **Wong, E. S., and W. E. Stamm.** 1983. Sexual acquisition of urinary tract infection in a man. *JAMA* **250**:3087–3088.
151. **Wyndaele, J.-J., and D. Maes.** 1990. Clean intermittent self-catheterization: a 12-year followup. *J. Urol.* **143**:906–908.
152. **Zhanel, G. G., G. K. M. Harding, and L. E. Nicolle.** 1991. Asymptomatic bacteriuria in patients with diabetes mellitus. *Rev. Infect. Dis.* **13**:150–154.
153. **Ziegler, E. J., C. J. Fisher, Jr., C. L. Sprung, R. C. Straube, J. C. Sadoff, G. E. Foulke, C. H. Wortel, M. P. Fink, R. P. Dellinger, N. N. H. Teng, I. E. Allen, H. J. Berger, G. L. Knatterud, A. F. LoBuglio, C. R. Smith, and the HA-1A Sepsis Study Group.** 1991. Treatment of gram-negative bacteremia and septic shock with HA-1A human monoclonal antibody against endotoxin. *N. Engl. J. Med.* **324**:429–436.

# DIAGNOSTIC MICROBIOLOGY FOR BACTERIA AND YEASTS CAUSING URINARY TRACT INFECTIONS

*Janice Eisenstadt, D.O., and John A. Washington, M.D.*

# 2

Urine samples make up the largest category of specimens submitted for microbiological study. The large volume of specimens arriving daily at the microbiology laboratory reflects the high incidence of urinary tract infections (UTIs) occurring in the community and in the hospital. In the United States in 1991, urinary symptoms resulted in more than 6 million office visits to physicians (155). Office visits to urologists from 1989 to 1990 for UTIs numbered almost 270,000 annually (197). UTIs are the most common cause of nosocomial infection (15, 83), occurring in 2 to 3% of hospitalized patients in the United States (and accounting for 42% of all nosocomial infections [50]). UTIs "necessitate or complicate more than 1 million admissions to the hospital in the U.S. annually" (130). Despite the high incidence of UTIs, most specimens submitted to the microbiology laboratory lack evidence of infection. The enormous workload associated with processing these specimens, the need for cost containment, and the need for rapid and reliable results have motivated the continuing development of new methods for urine screening and culturing and for antimicrobial susceptibility testing.

## DEVELOPMENT OF THE CONCEPT OF "SIGNIFICANT BACTERIURIA" IN QUANTITATIVE CULTURE

The predictors of UTI are pyuria and bacteriuria. Screening methods for detecting pyuria and bacteriuria are discussed in detail below. Pyuria can be accurately detected by microscopy or other rapid detection systems. The detection of bacteriuria by these methods is not as reliable as the quantitative culture of "significant" numbers of bacteria in specimens.

Since urine is normally a sterile body fluid, the presence of bacteria (bacteriuria), fungi (funguria), mycobacteria, or viruses is defined as infection. The term "infection" does not imply the presence or absence of associated symptoms, and patients are often asymptomatic. Infection of the urinary tract may occur anywhere along its course. Infection of the lower urinary tract refers generally to superficial infections of the bladder, the urethra, or both. Infections

---

*Janice Eisenstadt,* Department of Internal Medicine, Division of Infectious Diseases, Sinai Hospital of Detroit, Detroit, Michigan 48235.   *John A. Washington,* Division of Pathology and Laboratory Medicine, The Cleveland Clinic Foundation, 9500 Euclid Avenue, Cleveland, Ohio 44195.

may also occur in the upper urinary tract, causing pyelonephritis or intrarenal abscess, or in associated glands and tissues, producing prostatitis, epididymitis, or perirenal abscess.

In voiding, urine must past through the distal urethra and (in females) over the perineum, and it is contaminated by the flora of these external surfaces. Since the work of Kass and Finland (72, 75) and Sanford et al. (70, 152), quantitative cultures of urine have become an established clinical tool. These investigators promoted the concept that quantitative culture could discriminate between bladder bacteriuria and urine contamination during voiding. Significant bacteriuria has been defined as that quantity of bacteria in urine that reliably distinguishes true bacteriuria from such contamination. Kass (74) reported that 95% of 74 patients hospitalized with a clinical diagnosis of acute pyelonephritis had $\geq 10^5$ CFU of bacteria per ml, whereas only 6% of 337 asymptomatic outpatients had bacteriuria to this extent. The majority of asymptomatic patients had a degree of bacteriuria between 0 and $10^4$ CFU/ml. Eventually, it became accepted that $\geq 10^5$ CFU/ml defines significant bacteriuria in voided specimens.

Later studies evaluating adult women with symptoms of acute infection of the lower urinary tract found that only about 50% met the bacteriologic criteria that were established for acute pyelonephritis. The terms female "acute urethral syndrome," "frequency/dysuric syndrome," and "abacterial cystitis" were all applied to women with symptoms of acute onset of urinary frequency, urgency, and pain upon urination in the absence of the accepted level of significant bacteriuria. A variety of factors can lower the number of organisms cultured from a urinary specimen (Table 1). These factors were often invoked to explain the lowered bacterial counts whenever symptomatic patients presented with quantitative cultures of $<10^5$ CFU/ml (104, 168).

**TABLE 1** Causes of low-level bacterial counts

---
Colonization without infection
Dilution resulting from fluid loading of patient before collection
Urinary frequency
Use of cleansing agent with antibacterial activity during specimen collection
Concurrent use of antimicrobial agents
Infection by fastidious organisms
Presence of growth inhibitor
Antibacterial action of bladder mucosa
UTI acquired hematogenously and causing infection not contiguous with collection system
Ureteral obstruction distal to site of infection
Infection localized to urethra, possibly before establishment of bladder infection
Nonbacterial infection
Inflammation of urethra due to mechanical irritative or immune-mediated factors
---

In the past decade, the work of Stamm et al. (170) has brought about a change in conventional thinking. By comparing voided midstream specimens and suprapubic aspirates (SPA), Stamm and colleagues provided evidence for the significance of gram-negative bacilli with quantitative counts as low as $10^2$ CFU/ml in some symptomatic females (170). Stamm et al. documented that as many as half of women with symptoms of acute dysuric syndrome had infections caused not only by the same microorganisms generally associated with UTI (typically, coliforms) but also by bacterial counts as low as 100 CFU/ml. Furthermore, this degree of bacteriuria served as a better predictor of infection in this population than the $\geq 10^5$-CFU/ml threshold (91, 173). In a population of acutely dysuric young women, a criterion of $>10^2$ CFU/ml had a sensitivity of 95% and a specificity of 85% for the diagnosis of UTI. A criterion of $\geq 10^5$ CFU/ml would have failed to detect 50% of the symptomatic women (170). Stamm et al. (172) reported that women with $>10^2$ CFU/ml improved symptomatically after treatment with appropriate antimicrobial agents. Additional evidence continues to support these conclusions. Kunin and colleagues (88) found that 32.5% of symptomatic women had bacteriuria of $\geq 10^5$ CFU/ml and 45.8% had bacteriuria of $>10^2$ to $10^4$ CFU/ml; in comparison, only 3.1% of asymptomatic women had bacteriuria of $\geq 10^5$ CFU/ml, and 10.2% had $>10^2$ to $10^4$ CFU/ml. The odds ratio of an association between bacteriuria and urinary symptoms increased as the bacterial count increased, as it did for women who had urinary and vaginal symptoms (88).

Fihn et al. (35) also suggested that some patients with dysuria and low-count bacteriuria (associated typically with cystitis but sometimes with sterile SPA) may have an isolated urethritis. In these instances, an infection present in the urethra may not yet be established in the bladder.

Symptoms of acute dysuria may be due to other infectious and noninfectious etiologies. Among infectious causes of urethritis are *Neisseria gonorrhoeae*, *Chlamydia trachomatis* (especially when pyuria is present), herpesvirus, and *Ureaplasma urealyticum*. Fastidious organisms (even poorly growing coliforms) and organisms generally considered nonpathogens like *Lactobacillus* spp. and *Gardnerella vaginalis* have been suggested as occasional causes of UTIs (32, 103, 107), although these notions have remained controversial (see below) (17, 18). Despite increased understanding of the etiologies of infection, the acute dysuria syndrome in some patients lacks a definite cause.

The acceptance of this lower criterion for significant bacteriuria in voided specimens from symptomatic females has raised several concerns. The first concern is whether the reliable detection of bacteriuria at the $10^2$ CFU/ml level will be hopelessly confounded by the possibility of contaminated urine specimens. Certainly, acceptance of this criterion calls for very high standards of care in the collection of specimens (187). Another concern relates to the inclusion of patients with low-count bacteriuria in investigative research. As discussed by Kunin (86), clinical studies of UTIs should distinguish patients with low-count bacteriuria from those with higher counts.

Since the publication of Stamm's initial work (169), quantitative criteria for the definition of significant bacteriuria have been established by other investigators for a number of different patient populations.

Studies by Lipsky et al. (97) and Musher et al. (116) recommended that $>10^3$ CFU/ml be used to define significant bacteriuria in voided urine specimens from men.

Colony counts of $<10^5$ CFU/ml in asymptomatic women are rarely persistent. They suggest either contamination or transient bacteriuria. However, finding $\geq 10^5$ CFU/ml in repeated urine cultures suggests the persistence of bacteriuria. The prevalence of asymptomatic bacteriuria varies with patient population. Bacteriuria that is generally asymptomatic is seen in about 5% of school-age females and 0.5% of males. In young nonpregnant women, the prevalence is about 1 to 3% (146). The frequency of asymptomatic bacteriuria in pregnancy is 2 to 10% and rises with increasing age and parity (74, 75). In the elderly, the prevalence of bacteriuria approaches 20 to 50% in women (12) and 5 to 30% in men (11, 12, 97).

For asymptomatic patients, at least two urine cultures with significant counts of the same bacteria are necessary for establishing a diagnosis of bacteriuria (73). Screening for asymptomatic bacteriuria in children less than 5 years of age remains an unresolved issue (77). Random screening or culturing of urine for asymptomatic bacteriuria in populations other than pregnant females and patients undergoing urologic procedures is generally not recommended. When incidentally detected, however, bacteriuria in the noninstrumented male almost always warrants an evaluation. In the elderly male, asymptomatic bacteriuria is generally related to disease of the prostate (76, 124).

Although a relationship between asymptomatic bacteriuria and increased mortality in elderly patients has been reported (29), recent studies tend to discount such an association (126). For this reason, there is no need for urine screening or cultures in this population.

## Significant Bacteriuria in Catheterized Urine Specimens

Bacteriuria is found in almost all chronically catheterized patients. Bacteriuria associated with catheterization typically starts within days and tends to be asymptomatic. In short-term catheterization, most bacteriuria is derived from a single species. Polymicrobial bacteriuria becomes increasingly more prevalent with the chronicity of indwelling catheters. Stark and Maki (174) reported that the criterion of $>10^2$ CFU/ml was more reliable than that of $10^5$ CFU/ml for the detection of symptomatic infection in chronically catheterized patients. They also noted that initial bacterial counts of at least $10^2$ CFU/ml soon rise to exceed $10^5$ CFU/ml.

In a study of patients using intermittent catheterization, a comparison between SPA and catheterized urine with a criterion of $>10^2$ CFU/ml had a sensitivity of 91% and a specificity of 97% for the detection of bladder bacteriuria. Had the criterion for significance been $\geq 10^5$ CFU/ml for the catheterized specimens, then these specimens would have yielded sensitivities of only 65% for the detection of gram-negative organisms and 45% for the detection of gram-positive organisms in bladder bacteriuria.

## Significant Bacteriuria in Voided Urine Specimens in the Pediatric Population

In infants and children, voided urine with $>10^3$ CFU/ml is considered significant. It reflects bladder bacteriuria as determined by SPA (140, 141).

**TABLE 2** Methods used to collect urine specimens

| |
|---|
| Suprapubic aspiration |
| Midstream clean void |
| Midstream void |
| Uncleansed initial-void |
| In-and-out (or straight) catheterization |
| Use of indwelling catheter |
| Use of suprapubic catheter |
| Use of external collection device |
| Use of ileal conduit |
| Cystoscopy and/or surgery |

## SPECIMEN COLLECTION

Various methods may be used for the collection of urine specimens (Table 2). Routine specimens should be limited to one per 24-h period. Certain specimens are unacceptable for culture; among such unacceptable specimens are specimens obtained from urinals or bedpans, the tips of catheters (26), urine transported in broth media, grossly bloody specimens, diluted specimens, centrifuged sediment from clean-catch specimens, or anaerobic cultures of midstream or catheterized specimens. Pooled specimens and 24-h collections are not useful except for diagnosis of parasites (*Schistosoma haematobium*, *Trichomonas vaginalis* trophozoites in males, and *Onchocerca volvulus* microfilariae).

The volume of urine collected should vary depending on the suspected pathogens and the kind of processing necessary for isolation (196). When bacterial pathogens are suspected, 0.5 to 1 ml of urine is the minimum acceptable volume. However, if transport tubes containing a preservative are used (see below), at least 3 ml of urine must be collected. Larger volumes (1 to 10 ml) of specimen allow better mixing so that organisms in low-count specimens can be more reliably quantified. At least 1 ml of SPA urine should be submitted for the culture of anaerobes. Large volumes (at least 20 ml) of urine are recommended for the isolation of mycobacteria and fungi. To maximize the recovery of mycobacteria, three consecutive first-voided urine specimens are recommended. From 1 to 10 ml of urine may be submitted for the isolation of *C. trachomatis* from men. The detection of viruses requires from 10 to 50 ml of urine (65).

Once a urine specimen has been properly collected, proper labeling and transport ensure its utility. Labeling should include the patient's name and gender and identifying hospital numbers and location. On the laboratory requisition form, the method and time of collection should be clearly recorded. Pertinent clinical information, including the presence or absence of urinary symptoms or disease, the recent or current use of antimicrobial therapy, and whether or not female patients are pregnant, should be documented.

In the acutely ill patient and the patient with suspected upper urinary tract disease, concurrent blood cultures may be helpful in making a microbiologic diagnosis. A positive blood culture is more likely with hematogenously acquired infection resulting from pathogens such as *Staphylococcus aureus*, *Salmonella* spp., and *Candida* spp. Bacteremia is common in male neonates with UTI and neutropenic patients. Catheter-associated bacteremia occurs in 2 to 4% of catheterized patients (19). As a result of catheter use, UTI is the most frequent cause of bloodstream infection in the hospitalized patient (82, 185). The risk of bacteremia in patients with acute pyelonephritis is at least 15 to 20% (31, 66).

Depending on the method used, the collection of urine may be associated with various risks for contamination. To minimize contamination and false-negative results (Table 1), each method of collecting urine must be performed in a standardized manner. Whenever possible, the day's first void should be collected. If this is not possible, the time between collection and the last void should be maximized. Collections following administration of large volumes of fluid should be avoided.

## SPA

SPA is often considered the "gold standard" in the collection of urinary specimens. It is, however, an invasive procedure and for this reason is used only infrequently. Any bacterial count of a uropathogen cultured from SPA is considered significant. Contamination by skin flora is minimized by the use of careful aseptic technique. Growth of coagulase-negative staphylococci or diphtheroids may necessitate repetition of the collection procedure in order to confirm their role as uropathogens. SPA is contraindicated in patients with a coagulopathy. Otherwise, transient hematuria is uncommon after the procedure, and more serious consequences like bowel perforation are very rare.

SPA is generally reserved for (i) diagnosing bacteriuria in infants and small children, especially when other collection methods have not been useful; (ii) determining the significance of borderline or low counts of bacteria in repeat clean-voided midstream specimens, especially when catheterization is contraindicated or technically difficult; and (iii) determining the presence of anaerobic bacteriuria in such cases (a portion of the specimen should be inoculated into an anaerobic transport vial). Strict anaerobes are only rarely uropathogens (36, 158). In a large study, Segura et al. (158) reported that the overall incidence of anaerobic bacteriuria confirmed by SPA was 0.2% among all patients having urine cultures and 1.3% in patients with significant bacteriuria. When anaerobes are involved in UTIs, the organisms occur most frequently in association with abscess formation (either in the kidney or the prostate and often in association with a preexisting anatomic abnormality, a surgical procedure, or an indwelling catheter).

To perform an SPA, the patient is placed in a supine position. The bladder must be full and palpable above the symphysis pubis. The skin over the area should be shaved and disinfected. A local anesthetic is applied to the overlying skin. The bladder is percutaneously aspirated through the midline with a sterile 19-, 20-, or 22-gauge needle and syringe.

## Midstream Clean-Voided Specimen

For both males and females, the midstream clean-voided or clean-catch specimen is most often recommended. The procedures used are noninvasive and, with good instruction, yield an adequate specimen for microbiological examination. In some hospitals and clinics, specimens are obtained by a urine collection team or in a centralized station for outpatient urine specimen collection. Kunin (85) reported that for females, the accuracy of a single midstream clean-voided urine culture with $\geq 10^5$ CFU/ml is 80%. A second culture containing $\geq 10^5$ CFU/ml of the same organism provided 95% accuracy, and a third culture yielding the same organism provided approximately 100% accuracy. In males, a single clean-voided specimen with $\geq 10^5$ CFU/ml has close to a 100% reliability.

Adequate periurethral washing before sampling results in fewer positive cultures from female patients. Solutions of chlorhexidine or povidone-iodine have some residual antimicrobial effect on colony counts (144), so a 5% tincture of green soap is now recommended as the cleansing agent (26). Since the first-voided urine is contaminated by the flora of the distal urethra, it should be discarded. Stamey (167) reported that the initial 10 ml of voided urine may contain from $10^3$ to $10^4$ CFU/ml.

In preparation for collection of a clean-voided specimen, the patient (or nurse) should wash and dry her hands, and the nurse should wear sterile gloves. The patient should sit on the toilet with her knees widely separated for a patient-obtained specimen or in a semisitting position on a cystoscopy table with her legs in stirrups if a nurse is to assist.

After the labia are separated, the urethral meatus should be cleansed at least four times with green soap on gauze sponges with downward (front-to-back) strokes. The urethral meatus should then be rinsed with gauze sponges moistened with water, using front-to-back strokes. Keeping the labia spread, the patient should begin to void. The initial portion of the specimen (about 15 to 30 ml) should be discarded into the toilet or a separate container. Then, without any stopping of the urinary stream, the specimen should be collected in a sterile container.

The male patient should wash his hands. He should then retract the foreskin (if he is uncircumcised). The urethral meatus should be washed with soap and then rinsed with water, using wet gauze. The patient should then begin to void, discarding the initial flow into the toilet. Without interrupting the urinary stream, he should then aseptically collect a specimen in a sterile container.

## Uncleaned Initial-Voided Specimen

Lipsky et al. (96) studied the results of self-collected urine specimens from a group of unselected males and concluded that culture results were no different whether the specimen was an initial or a midstream specimen or whether the specimen was obtained after the cleansing of the urethral meatus (regardless of the patient's circumcision status). The contamination rate in initial-voided specimens was, however, higher than that of midstream specimens (13 versus 8.4%). A later study of men with heterogeneous genitourinary symptoms and disorders (97) found that in specimens with $\geq 10^3$ CFU/ml, the agreement between SPA and both supervised uncleansed first-voided specimens and clean-voided midstream specimens was excellent. Clean-voided midstream specimens had a 97% sensitivity and specificity. Uncleansed first-voided specimens had a 97% sensitivity with a somewhat diminished specificity of 92%. None of the clean-voided midstream specimens were contaminated (as defined by the presence of more than two microbial species). When bladder urine was sterile, clean-voided specimens had ≤$10^2$ CFU/ml.

The same study (97) found that quantitative leukocyte (WBC) counts were severalfold higher in the uncleansed first-voided specimens and only slightly higher in the clean-voided midstream specimens than in bladder specimens. Voided specimens with pyuria of >10 WBCs/mm$^3$ most accurately predicted bladder bacteriuria (positive predictive value [PPV] of 77% and negative predictive value [NPV] of 69% in clean-voided midstream specimens).

In the study by Lipsky et al. (96), specimen collection was supervised. In a study of unsupervised collections from presumably healthy young men, growth of $10^3$ to $10^5$ CFU/ml in 19% of midstream specimens was reported (181). As a consequence, Schaeffer (153) and Naber (118) contend that when men are symptomatic and lower degrees of bacteriuria may be significant, as in hospitalized male urological patients, the specimen should be a midstream clean catch.

## "In-and-Out" (Straight) Catheterization

"In-and-out" catheterization urine specimens are very similar but not identical to SPA. In-and-out catheterization is not routinely recommended because it is an invasive procedure and carries the risk of introducing bacteria into the bladder. After this procedure, bacteriuria develops in about 1 to 5% of patients. These risks are higher in diabetics, elderly or debilitated patients, and postpartum women. The straight-catheterization risk for bacteriuria has been reported to be as high as 20% in women hospitalized in a medical ward (178).

The procedure may be useful in the morbidly obese, elderly, actively vaginally bleeding patient, females with bladder incompetence, or patients who are acutely ill. This procedure is also used to accurately measure a patient's postvoid residual. In patients with strictures or obstruction of the urethra, catheterization may be difficult and traumatic. The procedure must be performed with aseptic technique.

## Chronic Indwelling Urethral Catheterization

Urine cultures obtained from chronic indwelling urethral catheters may not accurately reflect bladder pathogens. In a prospective study by Warren and colleagues (186) of patients with chronic indwelling urethral catheters, 98% of the catheters contained bacteria at high counts and 77% were polymicrobial. Only 22% of the specimens contained one organism; 35% contained two, 25% contained three, 14% contained four, and 2% contained five organisms. A subsequent study by Tenney and Warren (177) showed that bacterial counts obtained from a sterile replacement catheter were of a lower order of magnitude than those in the chronic indwelling urethral catheter prior to replacement; however, the rank order of organisms found in the urine obtained from the replacement catheter was essentially the same as in the prereplacement catheter.

Specimen collection requires strict adherence to aseptic techniques. The gloved examiner should clamp the catheter tubing above the sampling port to allow collection of freshly voided urine. The port should be disinfected with 70% alcohol, and the urine can then be collected by aspiration through the port with a sterile needle and syringe. The specimen is then transferred to a sterile container. If no port is provided, then the catheter should be disinfected at its junction with the drainage tube and aspirated at this location. The specimen should not be obtained from the collection bag or by disconnecting the catheter from the drainage bag.

## External Collection Devices

External collection devices are used most frequently in neonates and in males with urinary incompetence. These devices cannot be maintained in sterile condition because of their contact with the skin and urethra, which may have become colonized with uropathogens (34). Urine collected in this way is sometimes unreliable for determining bladder bacteriuria.

One study (128) evaluated the results of using external collection devices in elderly males suffering from genitourinary disease and urinary incontinence. Using new external condom catheters connected to closed drainage systems, Ouslander et al. (128) first cleansed the glans penis with a povidone-iodine solution and then collected the next voided specimen (from 30 to 120 min later). Subsequently, the patients underwent straight catheterization. Culture results from each method were the same in 22 (85%) of the 26 patients. Relative to those of straight catheterization, the overall sensitivity of the condom catheter method was 100%, and its specificity was 90%. This study has been criticized because it used only a small number of patients and because specimen collection was performed by a specialized research nurse. Furthermore, these studies were conducted on patients without acute illness.

A second small study assessed the results of urine specimens obtained from external collection devices but in this instance collected by ward nurses (125). For this study of 24 elderly incontinent men in a nursing home setting, three sequential specimens were analyzed. Two specimens were obtained using either an ethylene oxide-sterilized or a "clean" external collection device applied after the glans penis had been cleansed with soap and water. Subsequently, urine was obtained by straight catheterization. A significant level of bacteriuria was considered to be $\geq 10^5$ CFU/ml. Sterile and clean collection devices had PPVs of 86 and 93%, respectively, when the same organism was found in two consecutive collections. In this study, contamination rates showed no difference related to use of sterile and clean collection units, circumcision status, or length of time between device application and specimen collection. Most of the patients (20 of 24) had bladder bacteriuria detected by straight catheterization. Almost half of the patients with the clean or sterile collection devices had urine contamination. In 15% of sterile and 20% of clean collections from these patients, the extent of contamination exceeded $\geq 10^5$ CFU/ml. This study also emphasized the risks of straight catheterization; despite prophylactic antimicrobial therapy, 3 of the 20 bladder bacteriuric patients developed fever after catheterization, and 1 developed rigors. In this study, hemocytometer WBC counts of unspun urine were not significantly different regardless of which method of collection was used.

In the infant and young child, urine collection bags frequently must be used. A study by Edelmann and colleagues (30) showed that when a significant culture was considered to be one with $\geq 10^4$ CFU/ml, the bacterial contamination rate was 6% in full-term newborn infants and 37% in premature infants. The use of urine collection bags may lead to artifactually elevated WBC counts as a result of recent circumcision, vaginal reflux of urine, or confusion with round epithelial cells found in the urine in the neonatal period (117).

## Ileal Conduit-Urostomy Specimen

Specimens should be collected using strict aseptic technique. Urine should not be collected from the urostomy bag. The stomal opening should be cleansed with disinfectant, and a double-lumen catheter should be inserted through the stoma into the conduit to a depth beyond the fascial level to collect the specimen. For situations in which it is not possible to catheterize the stoma, contamination can be minimized by collecting urine into a fresh urostomy bag after the stoma has been carefully cleansed (14).

## Cystoscopy with Ureteral Sampling

Cystoscopy and bilateral ureteral sampling allow localization of an infection. This procedure, which was developed by Stamey (167), is described in the section on localization procedures. It also allows identification of an obstruction below which the urine may be sterile.

## SPECIMEN TRANSPORT

The proper handling and transport of urinary specimens are crucial to obtaining reliable information. Specimens transported without a preservative (see below) must be cultured within 1 to 2 h or else cooled immediately at 4°C. This refrigeration is necessary to prevent rapid logarithmic-phase growth, which can lead to a spurious increase in CFU per milliliter (56). If refrigerated, specimens should be stored for no more than 24 h. Although the number of CFU per milliliter may remain stable beyond this time, it is less stable (112). Refrigeration does not preserve WBCs very well. Frozen specimens are unacceptable for culture and should be rejected. Viral specimens should be transported on ice and not frozen. Rapid transport and culture are especially useful for specimens suspected of having a significant level of bacteriuria ($\leq 10^5$ CFU/ml) (62).

Unfortunately, adherence to these laboratory guidelines is poor. As reported by Doern and colleagues (28) in a recent study of eight hospitals, one-third of specimens were in transit for 2 h or more, and 11% remained at room temperature for 8 h or longer.

### Preservative-Containing Transport Devices

In the outpatient setting, it may not be possible to transport specimens rapidly or to refrigerate them. As a result, various transport devices with preservatives have been developed. Preservatives must be able to stabilize the number of CFU per milliliter. Furthermore, the preservative should not affect antimicrobial susceptibility testing. Two preservatives that have been used are sodium-chloride-polyvinylpyrrolidone and boric acid (189), both of which are available in liquid and lyophilized forms. Studies of boric acid preservative contained in the B-D Urine Collection Kit (Becton Dickinson Microbiology Systems, Cockeysville, Md.) and the Sage Products Urine Culture Tube (Sage Products, Inc., Cary, Ill.) showed them to be as effective as refrigeration in specimen preservation (44, 58, 92).

The use of boric acid as a preservative (139) requires that its final concentration in a transport kit not exceed that which would inhibit bacterial growth (105). The reliability of boric acid transport media has been questioned in some reports (48, 92, 133) because of its inhibitory effects on some uropathogens (133, 189). Hubbard and colleagues (58) found that the B-D Urine Collection Kit lowers the detection rates of bacteria after 24 h when the specimen is tested in the MS-2 system. Guenther and Washington (48) reported that one-third of the specimens containing bacteria at $10^4$ to $10^5$ CFU/ml in specimens cultured within 24 h yielded fewer than $10^4$ CFU/ml when culture was delayed beyond 24 h. The problem of bacterial inhibition has been especially evident in situations in which transport devices were underfilled (64, 121). For this reason, a urine specimen of 3 to 5 ml is recommended for filling these devices.

The FLORA-STAT Urine Transport System (Wasley Biosciences Corp./Lymphokine Partners Ltd., Dallas, Tex.) is a newly developed lyophilized transport system that seems to be able to stabilize microbial populations for 24 h at room temperature even in the presence of antibiotics (27). This transport system did not produce any precipitate that could interfere with urine screening based on filtration and staining (see below).

### Transport Culture Systems

In the outpatient setting, an alternative to the use of preservative-containing transport kits is direct inoculation of the urine specimen onto agar surfaces. These cultures and screening devices use several approaches, including filter paper, roll tube, and dipslide techniques. These systems are discussed below (see Bacterial Culture Methods below).

In addition, QUALTURE (Future Medical Technologies International, Inc., West Palm Beach, Fla.) is a detection and identification system that can be used for transport.

## MICROBIOLOGY OF UTI

The normal flora of the distal urethra consists of coagulase-negative staphylococci (excluding *Staphylococcus saprophyticus*), viridans and nonhemolytic streptococci, lactobacilli, diphtheroids (*Corynebacterium* spp.), nonpathogenic *Neisseria* spp., anaerobic cocci, *Propionibacterium* spp., anaerobic gram-negative bacilli, commensal *Mycobacterium* spp., and commensal *Mycoplasma* spp. (8). Also, coagulase-positive staphylococci, enterococci, *Acinetobacter calcoaceticus* (*baumanii*), *G. vaginalis*, and yeasts are occasionally found (60).

Urine is an excellent growth medium for many microorganisms. However, unfavorable environments for growth of bacteria in urine include the extremes of pH (<5.5 or >7.5), high tonicity of urea, and the presence of diet-derived weak organic acids. Glucose in urine is not a major limiting growth factor, nor is a high concentration of glucose an enhancing factor.

Most infections of the urinary tract are caused by a very limited group of organisms, and more than 95% of UTIs are attributed to a single bacterial species. True polymicrobial infections are much more likely in patients with underlying structural abnormalities, chronic indwelling catheters, or nosocomial infections. As many as one-third of elderly men with bacteriuria have more than one organism in urine cultures (124). Most bacteriuria found in patients with short-term catheterization is due to a single organism, but up to 15% of infections are mixed (6). In patients with chronic indwelling catheters, 95% have two to four species at $>10^5$ CFU/ml (186). Catheters may provide a unique niche for infection (177, 184). Patients with chronic indwelling catheters experience frequent new episodes of bacteriuria caused by various organisms (186).

Recurrent, complicated, and nosocomial infections of the urinary tract are also much more likely to be associated with a wider variety of pathogens that are often drug resistant. Such infections are due not only to *Escherichia coli* and *Klebsiella* spp. but also to *Enterobacter* spp., members of the tribe Proteeae, *Pseudomonas aeruginosa*, *Serratia marcescens*, *Acinetobacter baumannii*, coagulase-negative staphylococci (but not *S. saprophyticus*), enterococci, and yeasts (67, 87). Bacteriuria associated with indwelling-catheter use of less than 1 month is usually due to these organisms, whereas bacteriuria associated with chronic indwelling catheters is universal and tends to have an even more varied bacteriologic composition.

The complaints of dysuria, frequency, and urgency in a young woman may be due to vaginitis, the acute urethral syndrome if uropathogens show counts of $<10^5$ CFU/ml, or cystitis if counts are $\geq 10^5$ CFU/ml. As discussed previously, the acute urethral syndrome may also be a result of urethritis due to *N. gonorrhoeae*, *C. trachomatis*, herpes simplex virus, *T. vaginalis*, yeasts, *U. urealyticum*, or unknown causes. This syndrome is commonly caused by the same organisms, but in lower quantities, that can be isolated from patients with cystitis. About 70% of symptomatic UTIs in young women <40 years of age are due to uncomplicated cystitis or superficial infection of the bladder and urethra. Eighty percent of cases of acute uncomplicated cystitis in young women are due to *E. coli*, and 5 to 15% are due to *S. saprophyticus*. Occasionally, infection is caused by *Enterococcus* spp., *Klebsiella* spp., *Proteus mirabilis*, *Pseudomonas* spp., or other organisms. Infection with *S. saprophyticus* seems to occur more frequently in the late summer and fall for unknown reasons (71). The occurrence of this urease-producing uropathogen also appears to be age specific and rarely affects women older than 40 years of age (71). The reservoir for this organism is unclear, though the organism has been recovered from skin (102) and in small amounts from the rectum, urethra, and cervix in some women (148). Patients who have recurrent episodes of cystitis and who have received multiple courses of antimicrobial therapy may become colonized and may subsequently develop infection with progressively more resistant organisms (182).

A long-standing concept is that all UTIs in men represent complicated infections. Recently, it was found that some uropathogenic strains of *E. coli* can cause uncomplicated cystitis or urethritis in some men (94, 165).

At least 80% of cases of acute uncomplicated pyelonephritis in young women are caused by *E. coli*. Other uropathogens associated with pyelonephritis include *Proteus* spp., *P. aeruginosa*, and *Klebsiella* and *Enterobacter* species.

Complicated infections of the kidney tend to be due to a wider range of more resistant organism, predominantly gram-negative bacilli. Intrarenal and perinephric abscesses may be sequelae of complicated infection resulting from ascending infection or hematogenous spread. When due to ascending infection, they are generally caused by gram-negative bacilli, while those due to hematogenous spread are often caused by *S. aureus*.

Acute prostatitis is generally associated with UTI and is caused most commonly by gram-negative bacilli (*E. coli, Klebsiella* spp., and *Proteus* spp. among others). Acute prostatitis is associated with an increased number of WBCs per high-power field (HPF) (>10 to 20/HPF) in prostatic fluid. Gram-positive cocci, including *Enterococcus* spp. and *S. aureus*, are much less frequently associated with acute prostatitis. Prostatitis due to *S. aureus* is often the consequence of catheter use. Infection of the prostate may also occur with *N. gonorrhoeae, C. trachomatis, U. urealyticum, Mycoplasma* spp., or, rarely, trichomonads.

Chronic prostatitis can be associated with either relapsing UTI or the persistence of a pathogen within the prostate gland. When of nonbacterial origin, prostatitis is associated with increased numbers of inflammatory cells in prostatic fluid together with negative bacterial cultures. Nonbacterial prostatitis may occur with *Mycobacterium tuberculosis*, nontuberculous *Mycobacterium* spp., yeast or another deep-seated fungal infection, *C. trachomatis, U. urealyticum*, or, possibly, a viral infection.

UTI in the pediatric population is predominantly caused by gram-negative bacilli, most frequently *E. coli*, which causes 90% of acute infections and 70 to 80% of recurrent infections. Gram-positive bacteria other than enterococci are rare causes of infection in children, although infections due to coagulase-negative staphylococci have been reported (51).

The incubation times for media are generally selected for culture of common bacteria and will not support the growth of many fastidious organisms. Some of these fastidious organisms have been associated with UTIs, but for others, their pathogenic role in UTI is debatable (103). Among these fastidious organisms are *Lactobacillus* spp. (18, 104), microaerophilic streptococci, *G. vaginalis* (129, 131, 161) and cell wall-deficient protoplasts (32, 49). Other fastidious organisms, such as *U. urealyticum* (54, 129, 131, 137), *Mycoplasma hominis* (100, 179), or *Haemophilus influenzae* (40, 175), have rarely been found in complicated UTIs. *N. gonorrhoeae* grows poorly in urine but may be isolated from first-voided urine from infected males (26), especially when modified Thayer-Martin medium used.

Some bacteria now linked to UTIs would previously have been dismissed as contaminants. These include the coagulase-negative staphylococci (93), *Aerococcus urinae* (22, 23), *Oligella urethralis* (142), and corynebacteria (7, 95, 163, 176), including *Corynebacterium urealyticum* (formerly *Corynebacterium* sp. strain D2), *Corynebacterium pseudodiphtheriticum, Corynebacterium jeikium,* and "*Corynebacterium aquaticum*". Occasionally, enteric pathogens such as *Salmonella* spp. are isolated from urine (195).

## Uropathogenic Fungi

Yeasts associated with UTIs are discussed in detail elsewhere in this book (see chapter 5). The yeast genera associated with UTI include *Candida* (*Torulopsis*) and *Cryptococcus.* The dimorphic fungi *Histoplasma capsulatum, Coccidioides immitis, Blastomyces dermatitidis,* and rarely *Paracoccidioides brasiliensis* may be associated with UTI. On occasion, the yeast-like fungi, such as *Geotrichium* spp. (which may be found in the urine of normal individuals), *Sporothrix schenckii, Saccharomyces* spp., and *Rhodotorula* spp., are isolated from the urine.

*Candida* spp. are a part of the normal flora of the oropharynx, gastrointestinal tract, vagina, and skin. The presence of *Candida* spp. in the urinary tract in the absence of inflammation most frequently represents colonization of the bladder. The overall incidence of candiduria reported in various studies ranges from 0.2 to 4.8% (37). In a follow-up study of asymptomatic patients with candiduria, Schonebeck (156) found that the candiduria may be transient and can resolve spontaneously. Isolation of *Candida* spp. from an initially voided specimen should be followed by an attempt to culture the organism either from a clean-voided specimen or from a straight-catheterization specimen or SPA (if necessary) to rule out collection-related contamination and transient infection. *Candida albicans* is the most frequently isolated species, though *Candida glabrata, Candida tropicalis, Candida parapsilosis, Candida lusitaniae,* and *Candida guilliermondii* have all been isolated from urine. Species distribution varies by institution and over time.

All patients with confirmed candiduria should be evaluated for the possibility of a deep-seated infection by collection of fungal blood cultures. The isolation of the same yeast species at multiple body sites may indicate a systemic infection.

Unlike the situation with bacteriuria, there is no consensus on the utility of quantitative cultures in candiduria. Some authors suggest that counts of $>10^3$ to $10^4$ CFU/ml are correlated with significant candiuria and especially pyelonephritis (43), but others find the use of quantification criteria misleading (37).

The presence of any dimorphic fungus or *Cryptococcus neoformans* is pathologic and implies disseminated disease.

## Mycobacterial Infection of the Urinary Tract

*M. tuberculosis* and mycobacteria other than *M. tuberculosis,* including *Mycobacterium kansasii, Mycobacterium fortuitum,* and *Mycobacterium avium-Mycobacterium intracellulare* may infect the urinary tract (25). The presence of saprophytic mycobacteria in the anterior urethra may result in positive acid-fast smears. Three first-voided urinary samples should be collected for culture. Christensen (24) reported that with the use of several samples, cultures will be positive in 90% of patients with genitourinary *M. tuberculosis.* It is important to consider that infection with *M. tuberculosis* may be obscured by a coincident bacterial UTI.

Pooled 24-h urine collections are unacceptable for culture because of the frequency with which bacterial overgrowth of mycobacterial culture occurs.

## RAPID DETECTION OF UTI

### Gross Examination of Urine

Inspection of a urine sample may reveal a cloudiness, caused by the presence of crystals or WBCs, that may indicate infection. A foul odor to the urine can be the result of UTI or the excretion of dietary components.

## Rapid Urinary Screening Methods

Of the large number of urine specimens submitted daily to a hospital microbiology laboratory, only a small fraction yield significant growth in cultures. Urine cultures are frequently ordered, especially in the hospital, as part of the workup of a febrile patient, even in the absence of signs or symptoms of UTI (59). A variety of screening methods have been developed to hasten the detection of negative specimens and to lessen the workload associated with culturing large numbers of negative samples. Techniques currently available vary widely in their methodologies, simplicity, expense, turnaround times, level of automation, volume of urine required, and means of interpretation. Among the differences in methods are the indicators of infection detected and whether the techniques are growth dependent. Optimally, a screening paradigm should be 100% sensitive in detecting every sample that requires culture and 100% specific in rejecting every sample that is cultured unnecessarily. So far, no screen has achieved this goal. In addition to differences in sensitivities and specificities, screening procedures now in use vary in their PPV and NPV in detecting $\geq 10^5$ CFU/ml and low-count bacteriuria as well as fastidious organisms. Because the prevalence of infection is very low even in a hospital setting, it is possible for a screening method to have a high NPV but an absolute number of false negatives that is unacceptably high.

Other limitations on screening are the specimen characteristics. Specimens that are not usable include grossly bloody samples, specimens from neutropenic patients, and specimens in which low but significant colony counts might be expected. Certain specimens require culture regardless of screening test results; these specimens include those from renal transplant patients, SPAs, bladder washout specimens, prostatic massage specimens, or surgery and catheterization specimens from a pediatric urology or obstetrics-gynecology service that have been specifically labeled for culturing only. Some laboratories store screen-negative refrigerated specimens for a short time, thus allowing the physician to request a culture when one is clinically appropriate.

A positive screen may lead to culturing specimens that ultimately yield negative results either because of factors that limit specificity (e.g., a fastidious organism) or because of the persistence of indicators of infection following the initiation of antimicrobial therapy. In such instances, the screen may be a better predictor of infection than culture is (114).

## Microscopic Screening Methods

Microscopic analysis allows a direct identification of crystals, erythrocytes (RBCs), WBCs, casts, other cellular components, and bacterial morphology. The detection of squamous epithelial cells by the microscopic examination of urine suggests that the specimen has been poorly collected. Urinary RBCs may be seen in 40 to 60% of patients with acute cystitis but only rarely in association with other dysuric syndromes (173, 193). The finding of 1 or 2 RBCs/HPF is considered normal, however. Hematuria may also indicate renal mycobacterial infection with or without associated pyuria (159), or it may be due to noninfectious causes. Chemical determination methods used in routine analysis (e.g., dipsticks) detect both free hemoglobin and myoglobin, but positive results should be correlated with the presence of RBCs on microscopic examination. A highly alkaline urine or a urine with a very low specific gravity (<1.007) may cause lysis of the RBCs, revealing microscopically empty RBC membranes (ghosts). Hypertonic urine causes RBC crenation.

On occasion, yeasts in urine resemble RBCs and oxalate crystals. The presence of a doubly refractile wall, budding, hyphae, or pseudohyphae distinguishes yeasts from RBCs.

Wet mounts can be prepared by using 10% potassium hydroxide, which destroys background materials and makes discrimination of yeasts easier. Upon Gram staining, yeast elements stain gram positive. Fluorescent staining with calcofluor white is highly sensitive and allows rapid slide review. Yeast infections of the urinary tract may result in gross particulate matter, including RBCs and WBCs and other cellular material such as sloughed renal papillae, in the urine (38). Urinary casts of fungal elements, when detected, indicate upper urinary tract fungal disease.

The detection of oval fat bodies in the urine suggests an infective process, especially prostatitis. Rarely, a Gram stain shows sulfur-appearing granules in association with infection due to actinomycosis (183). *Mycobacterium* spp. may stain faintly gram positive or not at all. Acid-fast staining may be done either with a basic carbol fuchsin stain (either Ziehl-Nielsen or Kinyoun methods) or with an auramine-rhodamine fluorochrome stain. The numbers of organisms seen are generally small, and the reported sensitivities for detection of mycobacteria have therefore ranged from 20 to 70% (20).

**Microscopic Detection of Pyuria**
Normal urine can contain up to two WBCs/HPF. Significant pyuria is detected in 96% symptomatic patients with $\geq 10^5$ CFU/ml but in fewer than 1% of asymptomatic patients without bacteriuria (111); the absence of significant pyuria should raise doubts as to the diagnosis of infection (173). Therefore, with bacteriuria of $<10^5$ CFU/ml, the correlation with pyuria is less clear; however, Johnson and Stamm (67) found significant pyuria in 26 of 27 patients possessing $\geq 10^2$ CFU/ml in specimens collected by SPA or catheterization. Pyuria was also detected in patients with chlamydial infections (170). The presence of WBCs in the urine has a sensitivity of 80 to 90% for bacteriuria, though its specificity is only 50 to 70% (67).

Stamm and colleagues (170) found that pyuria together with bacteriuria of $>10^2$ CFU/ml provides a very sensitive indicator of UTI. These observations led Pezzlo and colleagues (132) to recognize that screening capable of detecting both bacteriuria and pyuria should be advantageous for identifying patients with UTIs, although such testing may decrease the specificity of screening. After the initiation of appropriate therapy for UTI, pyuria may persist for several days beyond the eradication of bacteriuria.

By itself, pyuria is less sensitive as an indicator of infection. Pyuria can be found in a variety of noninfectious situations, including appendicitis, pancreatitis, acute glomerulonephritis, renal calculi, lupus nephritis, nonbacterial gastroenteritis, respiratory infections, renal tubular acidosis, dehydration, stress, fever, and neoplasm. Other causes for pyuria include irritation to the ureter, bladder, or urethra (such as recent instrumentation or the presence of a foreign body). The concentration of WBCs in urine can also be affected by factors such as fluid loading of a patient or urinary frequency.

The stability of WBCs is limited, even if the specimen is refrigerated. Hence, delays can lead to false-negative results because of lysis (78). WBCs may also lyse when exposed to hypertonic or alkaline urine.

In dilute (specific gravity, $<1.019$) or hypotonic urine, granules within WBCs may demonstrate Brownian movement. Such WBCs are referred to as activated segmented neutrophils, or "glitter cells." Though the presence of these cells was once thought to be diagnostic of pyelonephritis, they are now recognized as an artifact of a hypotonic environment. WBC casts, when present, are highly suggestive of acute infection in the kidney (46). However, WBC casts can also be seen in noninfectious renal disorders, including interstitial nephritis, lupus nephritis, and glomerular disease.

The gold standard for detection of pyuria is the measurement of WBC excretion in the urine over a 24-h period (16). With infection, over 95% of patients excrete >400,000 WBC/h, a rate that only very rarely occurs in the absence of infection (98, 169). This method, however, is rarely used. A much more practical approach is to examine either an unstained preparation of centrifuged urine sediment or a hemocytometer chamber preparation.

In spun urine, the correlation between the number of WBCs and the hourly WBC excretion rate is not clear (169). A number of variables, including the volume of urine centrifuged, the force and duration of centrifugation, the volume in which sediment is suspended, and the volume to be examined, affect the procedure. When these factors are controlled by a standardized protocol, the microscopic examination of unstained urine sediment achieves some degree of reliability (1). If the urine is spun for 5 min at 2,000 rpm (400 × $g$) and suspended in 0.5 to 1.0 ml of supernatant, then each WBC seen under high power represents approximately 5 to 10 WBC/mm$^3$. Since 10 to 50 WBC/mm$^3$ is the upper limit of normal findings, then the observation in urinary sediment of 5 to 10 WBC/HPF can be regarded as normal (151).

A hemocytometer can give very accurate counts of the number of WBC per cubic millimeter. The presence of 8 to 10 WBC/mm$^3$ correlates closely with the excretion of >400,000 WBC/h (16) and >10$^5$ CFU/ml in patients with symptoms of UTI (98, 169). Kunin (87) suggested that this level of pyuria may be overly sensitive in detection of UTI, since he had previously reported (173) that midstream clean-voided specimens from 20% of healthy asymptomatic women had ≥20 WBC/mm$^3$ of vaginal origin. He suggested that a level of >100 WBC/mm$^3$ may be more appropriate for discriminating infection.

As a result of its accuracy and reproducibility in detecting pyuria, the counting chamber is recommended by the Infectious Disease Society of America (147). A less expensive alternative to the glass hemocytometer is a multitest plastic counting chamber, the KOVA slide (Hycor Biomedical, Inc., [formerly ICL Scientific], Irvine, Calif.) (149).

Unstained, uncentrifuged urine may be examined in a semiquantitative fashion by using either a microscope slide and coverslip or a microtiter tray examined with an inverted microscope.

## Microscopic Detection of Bacteriuria

Although not as reliable as quantitative culture in the detection of UTI, the microscopic examination of urine for the presence of bacteria can be very useful. However, <10$^4$ CFU of bacteria per ml in quantitative culture cannot be detected by microscopic screening. The bacterial count must be about 30,000 CFU/ml before bacteria can be detected in either stained or unstained, spun or unspun urine (84, 152).

The sensitivity of microscopy depends on whether the specimen is stained and whether it has been centrifuged.

The reported sensitivity and specificity of stained centrifuged urine range from 60 to 100% and 59 to 97%, respectively. In their review of this topic, Jenkins et al. (63) reported that the sensitivity and specificity of one organism or more per oil immersion field (OIF) in Gram-stained centrifuged urine were 95 and 74%, respectively, in the detection of ≥10$^5$ CFU/ml. They also found that detection of more than five organisms per OIF provided 95% specificity for detecting bacteriuria of ≥10$^5$ CFU/ml. Washington and colleagues (188) reported that the observation of one or more organisms per OIF (after examination of 20 fields) in Gram-stained smears of 10 µl of uncentrifuged urine correlated with $\geq 10^5$ CFU/ml with a sensitivity of 94% and a specificity of 90%.

Gram-stained preparations also assist in guiding antimicrobial therapy by making organism morphology visible. The slide centrifuge (cytospin) Gram stain technique appears to be nearly as sensitive as quantitative culture in detecting $\geq 10^5$ CFU/ml (45, 143). This technique makes use of a cytocentrifuge that deposits the specimen within a 0.25-in. (ca. 0.6-cm)-diameter spot on the slide. Well-mixed urine (0.2 ml) is spun at 2,000 rpm (400 × $g$) for 5 min in a capped chamber. The slides are then heat fixed and Gram stained. The slide is read by scanning 12 OIFs. The presence of the same organism (except gram-positive or gram-variable rods) in six or more fields is interpreted as being positive (45). In a 4,000-specimen study using this screen for detecting specimens with >$10^5$ CFU/ml (45), the cystospin Gram stain had 98% sensitivity, 90% specificity, an NPV of 99%, and a PPV of 65%. In detecting specimens with $\geq 10^4$ CFU/ml, the cytospin Gram stain had a sensitivity of 88%, a specificity of 95%, and NPV of 96%, and a PPV of 84%. False-positive cytospin slides have been attributed to fastidious organisms or growth inhibition due to antimicrobial agents. Despite its advantages, the cytospin method is more labor intensive than other available screening tests.

Other stains available for the detection of bacteriuria are methylene blue and acridine orange. Hoff and colleagues (57) examined stained unspun urine at ×200 magnification. One organism in any one of three fields was considered a positive. Epithelial cell and WBCs were also quantified. Positive fields were then examined further at ×400 to determine the number of organisms and their morphology. Though sensitivity was high (99%) for >$10^5$ CFU/ml, specificity was very low (58%) and neither the presence nor the absence of WBCs or epithelial cells correlated with clinically significant cultures.

An automated system of microscopy using acridine orange staining (Autotrak; Roche Ltd., Welwyn Garden, Hertfordshire, United Kingdom) has also been evaluated. The Autotrak is an epifluorescence microscope that automatically samples, heat fixes, and then stains specimens. Interpretation is done by a photomultiplier system. Unfortunately, the reported false-positive rate was 45% (162), and the equipment is costly to operate.

## ENZYMATIC METHODS OF SCREENING

Several commercially available dipsticks provide rapid chemical or enzymatic colorimetric analysis of urine specific gravity, pH, protein, glucose, ketones, blood, bilirubin, urobilinogen, nitrite, and WBC esterase. Urine discoloration by drugs and food pigments interferes with test interpretation. Grossly bloody specimens should not be tested by dipstick.

The tests should be done by dipping and immediately withdrawing the dipstick to prevent elution of the reagents into the urine. Excess urine is quickly blotted, and reactions are read with the strip in the horizontal position. Reactions are compared with those on an interpretive color chart.

The specific gravity reflects the hydration status of the patient. Fluid loading diminishes the number of CFU of organisms per milliliter and the number of WBCs per cubic millimeter. Normally, urine has an acid pH. Hence, an alkaline pH for a fresh urine sample (especially if the pH is >7.5) may indicate infection with a urea-splitting organism.

### WBC Esterase

For the WBC esterase test, the dipstick is impregnated with indoxyl carboxylic acid ester and a diazonium salt that, when exposed to WBC esterase, reacts chemically to form an indigo blue color. This reaction detects lysed as well as intact neutrophils.

The sensitivity of this test in detecting >10 WBC/HPF or $\geq 10^5$ CFU/ml is 75 to 96%, and its specificity is 94 to 98% (42, 80, 89, 136, 194). This test has a PPV of 50% and an NPV of 92% (171). In one study, the sensitivity of the WBC esterase dipstick decreased from 82 to 65% when it was used in detecting cultures with quantitative bacteriuria of $10^4$ CFU/ml (69). False positives may be caused by *Trichomonas* contamination, by large amounts of ascorbic acid in the urine, by detergents or preservatives, by certain drugs like nitrofurantoin and gentamicin, and by high concentrations ($\geq 300$ mg/dl) of albumin in the urine. False negatives are most common with a low number of WBCs (i.e., 5 to 10 cells per HPF) (81) or when urinary specific gravity is high.

## Nitrite Test (Griess Test)

Most uropathogens are members of the family *Enterobacteriaceae*, which reduce nitrate to nitrite. Normally, urine contains no nitrites but does contain nitrates from dietary sources. This dipstick test indirectly detects the reduction of nitrate by the *Enterobacteriaceae*. The nitrite product goes on to react with *p*-arsanilic acid, forming a diazonium compound that can couple with 1,2,3,4-tetrahydro-benzo-(h)quinolin-3-ol to produce a pink color. The test results can be read in about 30 s.

The test sensitivity has varied from 35 to 80%, but its specificity ranges from 92 to 100% (43, 127, 136). The generally low sensitivity may be caused by the organism's inability to reduce nitrate (e.g., enterococci, staphylococci, *Acinetobacter* spp., and some other nonfermenting gram-negative bacilli as well as yeasts). Incubation of the urine sample in the bladder (for <4 to 6 h) may have been insufficient to produce a detectable level of nitrite. The test is most accurate when performed on first-voided morning urine specimens (110).

Low concentrations of urinary nitrates, resulting from a vegetable-free diet or use of a diuretic, may lead to false-negative results. Interference with the test occurs with abnormal concentrations of urobilinogen and a urinary pH of <6.0 and with a daily dietary intake of vitamin C. Finally, if nitrites are further reduced to ammonia, the test will be falsely negative. Although the Griess test is highly specific, false positives occur rarely as a result of the presence of blood, a red dye, or drugs like phenazolyridine that cause a color reaction similar to that in a positive nitrite test.

## Combined WBC Esterase and Nitrite Testing

The combination of WBC esterase and nitrite has a reported sensitivity of 79 to 93% and a specificity of 82 to 98% in the detection of specimens with $\geq 10^5$ CFU/ml (69, 136, 160, 191). The sensitivity for lower levels of bacteriuria, however, is significantly less (69, 115). For example, one study that applied a standard of $\geq 10^4$ CFU/ml for significance reported a sensitivity of only 65% (69).

## Catalase Testing

The presence of catalase in bacteria (except in species of *Streptococcus, Enterococcus,* and *Aerococcus*) forms the basis of another rapid enzymatic test for detection of microorganisms. The test is also positive with somatic cells. Testing for catalase is performed by placing 2.0 ml of urine in a tube containing reagent powder, adding 4 drops of 10% hydrogen peroxide, and, after 2 min, looking for foam. A positive result is defined as production of enough foam to form a layer or ring above the surface of the urine. Such results are enhanced by the addition of a blue dye to the reagents.

The catalase test is considered more sensitive than dipstick tests for nitrite or erythrocyturia and similar in sensitivity to the dipstick test for WBC esterase. Comparisons of the Chemstrip LN (BioDynamics

Division, Boehringer Mannheim Diagnostics, Indianapolis, Ind.) and the URISCREEN catalase detection system (Analytab Products, Plainview, N.Y.) showed similarities between them in detecting probable pathogens at $\geq 10^5$ CFU/ml, whether or not pyuria was present (sensitivity, 93%). In specimens with pyuria, these tests could detect organisms at concentrations of $\geq 10^2$ CFU/ml. The URISCREEN was significantly more sensitive at detecting specimens with probable pathogens at $<10^5$ CFU/ml, especially *Candida* spp. Also, specimens containing WBCs (with or without pathogens) were detected more frequently, although with a higher false-positive rate (28 versus 13%) (132). In most instances, false-negative reactions with significant bacteriuria occurred in urine samples containing cells. False-negative reactions also occurred with *Enterococcus* spp. The specificity of the leukocyte nitrite components of another Chemstrip 9 (Behring, Inc., Somerville, N.J.) dipstick (98%) was reported to exceed that of the URISCREEN (21).

## FILTRATION-BASED METHODS OF RAPID SCREENING

The Filtracheck-UTI (Meridian Diagnostics, Inc., Cincinnati, Ohio) is a colorimetric-electrostatic filtration system for the detection of bacteria and WBCs. This disposable, manual apparatus uses a negatively charged filter that attracts bacteria electrostatically and retains them while staining them with safranin. Only 2 drops of urine are processed through the filter; for processing, the urine is combined with 6 drops of a dilute acid solution followed by 3 drops of safranin. A positive test is based on either conversion of the filter to a pink color or clogging of the filter after addition of the dye. To prevent false-positive test results due to rediffusion of the safranin from the periphery of the filter, the color of the filter must be interpreted within 30 s. False-positive rates are higher in specimens with higher WBC counts (143).

The Bac-T-Screen (Becton Dickinson; Vitek Systems, Inc., bioMerieux Vitek, Hazelwood, Mo.) is a semiautomated filtration screening device that detects bacteriuria and pyuria. A card for suction filtering is inserted into the instrument, and 1 ml of urine is added. The instrument then adds acetic acid (14.5%) to dilute the urine and lyse the nonmicrobial cells and then 3 ml of safranin to stain the remaining cellular elements on the filter. Finally, 3 ml of a 2.4% solution of acetic acid is added for decolorizing twice. The instrument provides a colorimetric reading. Specimens that clog the filter, which occurs with about 2% of specimens with the current model of the instrument, are considered positive (111). The results from this device may be uninterpretable because of chromogens in urine. The reported sensitivity ranges from 76 to 97% for detecting $10^5$ CFU/ml (135, 136, 138), with a 99% NPV (136, 138).

Comparative studies of the two filtration methods, Filtracheck-UTI and Bac-T-Screen, reported similar sensitivities in detecting $\geq 10^5$ CFU/ml ($>96\%$ in one report [114] and 85.8% in another [166]). Sensitivity drops significantly for detecting fewer CFU per milliliter (sensitivity of 21 to 79% at $10^4$ to $10^5$ CFU/ml [115, 135, 138]). As with the Filtracheck-UTI system, false-positive rates are high as a result of cellular elements (115), and specificity is low (64 to 84% at a threshold of $>10^5$ CFU/ml).

## BIOLUMINESCENCE SCREENING METHODS

The UTIscreen (CORAL Biomedical, Inc., San Diego, Calif.) is a semiautomated screen that uses a luciferin-luciferase reaction to detect ATP released from living bacterial cells. The ATP serves as an energy source for producing light as luciferin is oxidized. For this assay, 0.025 ml of urine is placed in a tube containing a dehydrated somatic-cell releasing agent and a detergent for a 20-min incubation to release and destroy ATP from cells other than bacteria. Luciferin and luciferase reagent and a bacterial releasing agent [formulated from 1,6-bis($N$-$p$-chlorophenyl-$N$G-diguanido)-helane salt and cationic surfactants] are added. If bacteria are present, their ATP facilitates light production as a correlate of luciferin oxidation. A device quantifies this light in terms of integrated light output; $\geq 5\%$ is considered positive (106, 134). At $\geq 10^5$ CFU/ml, this assay has a sensitivity for potential pathogens of 95% (106, 134, 143). At $\geq 10^4$ CFU/ml, the sensitivity decreases to 85%; specificities at $10^4$ and $10^5$ CFU/ml are 86 and 88%, respectively (143). At $\geq 10^5$ CFU/ml, the PPV is 53% and the NPV is 99% (143).

One limitation on the utility of the UTIScreen may be false-negative readings found with low numbers of organisms (i.e., $10^4$ CFU/ml). In such specimens, the concentration of ATP may be diminished because of a lag phase in the growth of contaminant organisms (79). Bloody specimens may result in false-positive results if the ATP contributed from RBCs has not been destroyed (10). False-positive test results have also been attributed to fastidious organisms and to nonviable bacteria (106). The UTIscreen can fail to detect some *Enterococcus* spp. (143, 180, 190). There has also been concern that some strains of bacteria and yeasts contain lower ATP levels in spite of high colony counts (180). Another problem is that the assay reagents may produce an incomplete lysis of gram-positive organisms (190).

Three bioluminescence screens are no longer available: Lumac (3M, St. Paul, Minn.), Monolight 500 (Analytical Luminescence Laboratory, Inc., San Diego, Calif.), and Amerlite Analyzer (Amersham International, UK).

### Electrical Conductance
The Malthus system (Malthus Ltd., Stoke on Trent, United Kingdom) detects the growth of bacteria by measuring changes in the flow of an electric current passing through a medium. This screening method is not useful when the specimen contains a preservative, because the preservative alters conductance. The incidence of false-positive readings has been high, and the long processing time limits the usefulness of this system as a screening method (162).

### Electrochemical Detection
The apparatus for electrochemical detection utilizes reference and platinum electrodes placed in the urine for detecting an increase of voltage caused by viable bacteria. Using this technique, Lamb et al. (90) had a 94% detection rate for specimens with $\geq 10^5$ CFU/ml. The false-positive rate was 10% because of contaminated media, and the false-negative rate was 6%.

## URINE CULTURE
In the treatment of uncomplicated cystitis, the recent trend has been to initiate empirical treatment without culture when pyuria is present (171). Several factors support this trend. One factor is that in uncomplicated cystitis, only a limited number of uropathogens with predictable antibiotic susceptibilities are involved. Another factor is that outcomes have been successful with 3-day and even single-dose regimens for this condition.

For guidance in the appropriate use of urine cultures, criteria were recently developed by the Connecticut Peer Review Organization (9). These guidelines, published by Bartlett (9), are expanded in Table 3 to include both outpatient and inpatient indicators. Although urine culture can be avoided in some situations, this procedure offers several advantages beyond those of screening, including detection of bacteriuria at lower counts, recognition of mixed

**TABLE 3** Criteria for urine cultures[a]

In a symptomatic patient, obtain urine for culture before therapy is initiated when a patient

- Is admitted to hospital or is acutely ill
- Develops symptoms of UTI after admission to hospital
- Has failed empiric course of antibiotic treatment given for suspected uncomplicated cystitis
- Remains symptomatic after 48 h of appropriate therapy directed by earlier culture
- Shows fever or sepsis with no source
- Shows symptoms of acute urethral syndrome, and screen has been negative
- Is suspected of low-count or fastidious organism, and urine collection is obtained by SPA or prostatic massage or during surgical procedure
- Provides a specimen not appropriate for laboratory's screening procedure
- Is less likely to be treated successfully by short course of therapy because of:
  (i) Suspected infection of a complicated nature
  (ii) Suspected infection of upper urinary tract
  (iii) Pregnancy
  (vi) Immunocompromised status
  (v) Neutropenia
  (vi) Persistent bacteriuria with episodes of recurrent infection
  (vii) Fever with Foley catheter in place
  (viii) Fever after manipulation of genitourinary tract

In an asymptomatic patient, obtain urine for culture

- When there has been asymptomatic bacteriuria during pregnancy
- When a child has evidence of bacteriuria on screening
- When there is pyuria, albuminuria, hematuria, or nitrates on screening
- When there is bacteriuria on screening prior to genitourinary procedure
- When short-term catheter has been removed
- After completion of therapy in complicated infections or infections with resistant organisms

[a] Adapted from Bartlett (9) and expanded by us.

infections suggesting contamination, and determination of susceptibilities in isolates.

# BACTERIAL CULTURE METHODS

## Quantitative Cultures: Pour Plate Method

A quantitative culture of urine can be obtained by the pour plate procedure, in which serial dilutions of a urine specimen are incorporated into 50°C agar, which is then mixed and poured into plates. The medium is allowed to solidify and incubate at 35°C for 24 h. This time-consuming process allows the enumeration of bacteria based on the dilution factor.

## Semiquantitative Cultures

### SURFACE STREAK PROCEDURE

Semiquantitative cultures are carried out in a standardized fashion by using the surface streak procedure for delivering a measured volume of well-mixed urine onto an agar surface. To ensure accuracy, a vertically held calibrated loop must be dipped quickly and without specimen carryover on the shank (53). The calibrated loop is used to streak a straight line down the middle of the agar surface. The agar surface is then cross-streaked for isolating colonies. When the plates are inoculated with an 0.001-ml loop, there must be at least $10^3$ CFU of organisms present per ml in order to detect growth. Inoculation with a 0.01-ml loop will permit detection of lower counts. To determine the number of CFU per milliliter in the original specimen, the number of CFUs detected after incubation is multiplied by 1,000 if a 0.001-ml loop was used or by 100 if a 0.01-ml loop was used.

Standardized loops are made of 95% platinum and 5% rhodium. The loop is calibrated by the gauge of the wire and the diameter of the loop. Quality control is achieved either by comparison with quantitative pour plate growth (which is cumbersome), by the Food and Drug Administration drill bit method, or by a colorimetric dye dilution protocol (26).

The media used are a standard combination of a nonselective and a selective agar for gram-negative bacilli. Most often, this combination is 5% sheep blood agar and MacConkey or eosin-methylene blue or, occasionally, tergitol (triphenyltetraolium chloride) agar. Selective media for gram-negative cocci include Columbia colistin-nalidixic acid agar and phenylethyl alcohol agar.

Cystine lactose electrolyte-deficient agar was developed specifically for use in urine cultures. It is a differential, nonselective medium that allows the detection of lactose-fermenting gram-negative bacilli but inhibits the swarming of *Proteus* spp.

For urine cultures, broth media are used only when the specimen has been collected either by SPA or during a surgical procedure. For SPAs, thioglycolate broth and agar media appropriate for anaerobic culture are also inoculated.

Agar plates are usually incubated at 35 to 37°C under aerobic conditions. Isolation of fastidious organisms may require different temperatures or atmospheric conditions, including anaerobic conditions for the isolation of anaerobes fron SPAs.

It is generally sufficient for plates to be incubated for 18 to 24 h. If no growth has occurred, reincubation is usually unnecessary. Murray and colleagues (113) reported that most significant pathogens were detectable after 16 h of growth. An additional day of incubation increased detection of isolates that were present in quantities of $<10^4$ CFU/ml at 24 h and of yeasts. In addition, some fastidious organisms and isolates from patients receiving antimicrobial therapy may require longer incubation (164), especially if Gram stain findings are positive. In such instances, it may be appropriate to incubate plates for 48 h.

## Semiquantitative, Miniaturized Culture Methods

As previously mentioned, methods for the direct inoculation of a urinary screen onto agar media have been developed. These methods are not useful for detecting $<10^4$ CFU/ml and should be used as screening cultures. Interpretation is usually based on a comparison of growth density with pictures supplied by the manufacturer.

### FILTER PAPER METHOD
A standard volume of freshly collected urine is absorbed into a filter paper strip. The strip is then inoculated onto a small agar surface for incubation overnight at room temperature. Quantification is done by comparing the density of colonies on the agar surface with pictures illustrating known quantities of colonies.

### ROLL TUBE METHOD
A specific volume of urine is poured into a plastic tube coated with agar. After the agar surface has been covered, the urine is discarded, and the tube is incubated overnight at room temperature. The density of colonies is compared with that in illustrations.

### DIPSLIDE
Several varieties of dipslides are available. Each consists of agar media attached to a paddle or spoon. The agar media used are generally both nonselective and selective. Inoculation is accomplished either by dipping the agar-coated surfaces into a sterile container containing the urine specimen or by holding the dipslide into the urinary stream. Incubation is then carried out overnight at room temperature. This method is simple and cost-effective. There have been some technical failures with dipslides because of detachment of the agar from the paddles or condensation on the container, which can interfere with evaluation. These devices have been limited in their usefulness when there is confluent growth at $\geq 10^6$ CFU/ml. A significant number of unreliable results have occurred with devices incubated at room temperature and transported to the laboratory (2, 4, 5).

## URINE CULTURES FOR FUNGI
*Candida* spp. usually grow well on the nonselective nutrient agar media used for bacterial culture. However, recovery may occasionally be delayed beyond the usual 24-h incubation period. Recovery of yeast cells may be improved with the incorporation of a colistin-nalidixic acid agar plate, Sabouraud's agar with dextrose, or media containing cycloheximide; however, not

all species of *Candida* will grow in the presence of cycloheximide. Media may be inoculated as with the surface streak method, or a 10-ml sample can be centrifuged and then 0.5 ml of the sediment can be inoculated onto media. Plates are incubated at 30°C in air. Incubation for 5 to 7 days may be necessary. Few, if any, studies have demonstrated any correlation between the level of candiduria and either bladder or invasive candidosis.

*Cryptococcus neoformans* will not grow on cycloheximide-containing media and is usually recovered in 3 to 10 days on blood-enriched and other fungal isolation media. In one study, only 6 of 15 patients with autopsy-proven renal cryptococcosis (40%) had the organism isolated from urine (150).

The slow growth of dimorphic fungi can require from 7 to at least 21 days of incubation at 30°C. Although *Coccidioides immitis* can be recovered in ≤5 days, the mold forms of other dimorphic fungi will grow more slowly at 25 to 30°C and require a humid environment. Some success has been derived from testing urine for the antigen of *H. capsulatum* (192).

## URINE CULTURES FOR THE RECOVERY OF *MYCOBACTERIUM* SPP.

First-voided urine specimens sent to the laboratory for the detection of *Mycobacterium* spp. must be concentrated and decontaminated before being cultured. Generally, three to five specimens are recommended. Infection with bacterial species may occur coincidentally with mycobacterial infections, and bacterial overgrowth may prevent recovery of mycobacteria. Digested and decontaminated material is inoculated on either egg- or agar-based media containing antifungal and antibacterial agents. Often, these cultures include inoculation of liquid media for use in the radiometric BACTEC system (Becton Dickinson, Sparks, Md.). BACTEC cultures offer the advantage of faster detection of mycobacteria than is possible on solid media.

The extremely long generation times of some mycobacterial species require that cultures be incubated for at least 8 weeks before they are reported as negative. Actual recovery times depend on the species present and the inoculum size. The optimal incubation temperature is species specific and may vary from 25 to 45°C.

Detection and identification of *M. tuberculosis*, *M. kansasii*, and *M. avium-M. intracellulare* has been expedited by use of the BACTEC system and of genetic probes specific for these species.

## ISOLATION AND IDENTIFICATION OF ORGANISMS

### Identification and Susceptibility Testing Guidelines

Guidelines have been established for the identification and susceptibility testing of urinary culture isolates (Table 4) (26). These guidelines are structured around the types of specimens cultured, the patient's sex, and the diagnosis (if available) for differentiation between significant bacteriuria and contaminants in various patient populations. In general, the isolation of one or two organisms at $\geq 10^4$ CFU/ml is considered significant. Whether or not each isolate is fully identified and its antimicrobial susceptibility is determined depends on its quantity (CFU per milliliter), the number of different species in the culture, and the types of organisms present in the culture.

### Microbial Identification

Initial recognition of a colony is based on its morphologic and growth characteristics on nonselective and selective media, microscopic morphology, and Gram reaction. When these criteria are used, some colonies consistent with a contaminant such as viridans streptococci, diphtheroids, or lactobacilli can be only superficially characterized and not otherwise identified.

The combination of characteristic colony morphology and rapid biochemical reactions (e.g., catalase, oxidase, coagulase, L-pyrrolidonyl-$\beta$-naphthylamide hydrolysis, spot indole, and germ tube) may allow a rapid identification of some organisms. A detailed description of rapid and other approaches to organism identification is not provided here but is discussed elsewhere (81).

## LOCALIZATION OF UTIs

Despite extensive descriptions of signs and symptoms distinguishing upper and lower UTIs, the characteristics are often not useful for reliably localizing UTIs. Invasive localization studies (discussed below) indicate that 30 to 50% of patients who present clinically with cystitis may also have subclinical upper urinary tract disease (145, 168). Johnson and Stamm (68) enumerated the characteristics associated with an increased likelihood of covert upper UTI (Table 5).

A number of methods have undergone investigation to determine if they might help in localizing bacterial infection within the urinary tract. The utility of these methods has been primarily in epidemiological studies and in determining which patients might need extended treatment and close follow-up in order to avoid renal parenchymal damage. These methods have been either indirect or invasive and direct. Unfortunately, the indirect methods of localization that have involved enzymatic or immunologic methods are insensitive and more of theoretical than of practical value.

### Renal Culture

Culture of renal tissue obtained via open biopsy is one means of determining the presence of infection in the upper urinary tract. However, this invasive procedure is only infrequently used. Because pyelonephritis is a focal pathology, percutaneous sampling of renal tissue may be unreliable.

### Stamey Test

Considered the gold standard, the invasive Stamey procedure allows lateralization in addition to localization in UTI (167). The Stamey test is highly sensitive and specific. False-negative results have been attributed to the intermittent shedding of uropathogens. False positives suggesting upper urinary tract disease can occur if the patient has a bladder infection and vesicoureteral reflux. The greater incidence of reflux in children makes this procedure less useful in them than in an older population.

In this procedure, a cystoscope with obturator is inserted into the bladder, and 5 to 10 ml of urine is collected and labeled CB. The bladder is then irrigated with a sterile bacteriostatic solution of physiological saline. Urethral catheters are then inserted through the cystoscope into the bladder, and the residual irrigation fluid is drained via both catheters and labeled washed bladder urine. The urethral catheters are then advanced into each midureter or renal pelvis. The initial 5 to 10 ml of urine is drained from each catheter, and four consecutive paired samples of 5 to 10 ml each are collected and labeled Left (LK) 1 through 4 and Right (RK) 1 through 4. All specimens are cultured quantitatively.

Bladder bacteriuria is present when specimen CB contains $\geq 10^5$ CFU/ml and specimens RK and LK contain no CFU. Upper UTI is documented by the growth of $\geq 10^2$ CFU/ml appearing in either the LK or RK samples or both.

### Fairley Washout Technique

Unlike the Stamey technique, the invasive Fairley washout localization procedure (33) does not allow lateralization of upper UTI. This test is less reliable in children than the Stamey procedure, because children have a high incidence of vesicoureteral reflux. The Fairley washout technique is also less reliable in patients with neurogenic bladders. It has been reported to be 90% sensitive in adults compared with the Stamey procedure (55).

**TABLE 4** Guidelines for specimen work-up and interpretation[a]

| No. of isolates from specimen | Density of isolate(s) (CFU/ml) | Type of specimen[b] | Significant clinical information influencing work-up |
|---|---|---|---|
| 1 | $>10^5$ | CC, FC, SC, IL, SP, CYS | None |
| 1 | $10^4$–$10^5$ | CC, FC, SC, IL, SP, CYS | None |
| 1 | $10^2$–$10^5$ | SP, CYS, SC | None |
| 1 | $10^3$–$10^4$ | CC, FC, SC, IL | Symptomatic female, or male with prostatitis, or WBCs present |
| 1 | $10^3$–$10^4$ | CC, FC, SC, IL | None available, or patient asymptomatic, or no WBCs |
| 1 | Any no. | CC, FC, SC, IL, SP, CYS | Physician specifies specific organism (*N. gonorrhoeae*) or syndrome (urethritis); or systemic disease (cryptococcosis) |
| 2 | Each $>10^3$ | SP, CYS, SC | None |
| 2 | $>10^5$ and $>10^5$, or $>10^5$ and $>10^4$, or $>10^4$ and $>10^4$ (if possible pathogens) | CC, IL, SC | None |
| 2 | As above | FC, IL | Patient with neurogenic bladder or indwelling catheter |
| 2 | One organism $>10^4$ and clearly predominant (i.e., at least 10-fold more than other) | CC, IL, FC, SC | None |
| 2 | Both $<10^4$, or one $10^4$–$10^5$ but not predominant | CC, IC, FC, SC | None |
| 2 or more | A possible pathogen such as *E. coli* or *S. saprophyticus* at $\geq 10^3$ and others at about the same level | CC, FC, SC, IL, SP, CYS | Symptomatic female, or male with prostatitis, or WBCs present |
| 3 or more | One organism at $>10^3$ and clearly predominant | SP, CYS | None |
| 3 or more | One organism at $>10^4$ and clearly predominant | CC, IC, FC, SC | None |
| 3 or more | Mix of any no. with none predominant | CC, IC, FC, SC | None |

*Continued on following page*

| Extent of identification[c] | Susceptibility testing | Example of report[d] | Reasonable laboratory interpretation |
|---|---|---|---|
| Definitive | Yes | >100,000 CFU/ml, genus, species | Probable UTI |
| Definitive | Yes | 50,000 CFU/ml, genus, species | Possible UTI; patient evaluation necessary |
| Definitive | Yes | 300 CFU/ml, genus, species | Probable UTI |
| Definitive (if gram-negative rod or possible *S. saprophyticus*) | Yes | 5,000 CFU/ml, genus, species | Probable UTI; patient evaluation necessary |
| Descriptive | No | 5,000 CFU/ml, GPC | No UTI |
| Definitive: specific organism if present | Yes | 100 CFU/ml, *N. gonorrhoeae*; or 1,000 CFU/ml, *H. influenzae*; or 3,000 CFU/ml, *Cryptococcus neoformans* | Possible UTI or evidence of disseminated infection |
| Definitive | Yes | >100,000 CFU/ml, genus, species; and 50,000 CFU/ml, genus, species | Probable UTI |
| Definitive | Yes | As above | Possible UTI; consider faulty collection, transportation, or colonization |
| Descriptive | No; hold plates (5–7 days) for tests in case patient becomes septic | >100,000 CFU/ml, NLF; and >100,000 CFU/ml, LF | Doubtful UTI; colonization likely |
| Definitive: predominant organism | Yes; predominant organism | >100,000 CFU/ml, genus, species; and 5,000 CFU/ml, GPC | Probable UTI caused by predominant species; the other is probably urethral or collection contaminant |
| Descriptive | No | 30,000 CFU/ml, GPR; and 40,000 CFU/ml, GPC | No UTI; consider urethral contamination |
| Definitive: possible pathogen(s) | Yes | 8,000 CFU/ml, *E. coli*, with 10,000 CFU/ml, GPR | Possible UTI; patient evaluation necessary |
| Definitive: predominant organism | Yes; predominant organism | 30,000 CFU/ml, genus, species; 1,000 CFU/ml, GPC; and 1,000 CFU/ml, GPR | Probable UTI |
| Definitive: predominant organism | Yes; predominant organism | As above | Probable UTI caused by predominant species; the rest is urethral or collection contamination |
| Descriptive | No | Mixed growth of >100,000 CFU/ml, GNR (3 kinds) | Faulty collection or transportation |

*Continued on following page*

**TABLE 4** *Continued*

| No. of isolates from specimen | Density of isolate(s) (CFU/ml) | Type of specimen[b] | Significant clinical information influencing work-up |
|---|---|---|---|
| 3 or more | Any combination of $>10^5$ or $>10^4$ | FC | Patient with neurogenic bladder or indwelling catheter |
| No growth | $<10^3$ if 0.001-ml loop used; $<10^2$ if 0.01-ml loop used | CC, IC, FC, SC, SP, CYS | None or asymptomatic |
| No growth | $<10^3$ if 0.001-ml loop used; $<10^2$ if 0.01-ml loop used | CC, IC, FC, SC, SP, CYS | Symptomatic |

[a] Reprinted from reference 26.
[b] CC, clean-catch (midstream) specimen; FC, specimen from indwelling catheter; SC, specimen from straight (in-and-out) catheter; IL, specimen from ileal conduit; SP, SPA; CYS, cystoscopy specimen.

For this test, a catheter is aseptically inserted into the bladder, and a urine sample is obtained for quantitative culture and Gram stain. The bladder is then instilled with a combination of normal saline, fibrinolysin, DNase, and an antimicrobial agent (neomycin), which is left in the bladder for 45 min and then drained. The bladder is then rinsed with 1 to 2 liters of saline given in 50- to 100-ml aliquots. While the last rinsing fluid is in the bladder, the patient receives furosemide intravenously. The remaining rinse solution is then drained, the catheter is clamped, and a specimen is collected for quantitative culture and labeled time 0. Subsequently, sequential specimens are obtained at 10, 20, 30, and 60 min after clamping. The volumes of the samples are recorded, and each sample is submitted independently for quantitative culture.

The bladder antimicrobial washout is considered adequate when the colony count at time 0 is <1% of that of the urine collected at the time of bladder catheterization. Upper urinary tract disease is present when subsequent samples (1 through 4) show a >10% increase in colony counts and when samples taken 20 to 30 min after washout have >3,000 CFU/ml.

**TABLE 5** Risk factors for covert upper UTI

Urban emergency room used for primary medical care
Lower socioeconomic status
Hospital-acquired infection
Pregnancy
Indwelling urinary catheter
Recent urinary tract instrumentation
Known urinary tract abnormality
Relapse
Infections occurring in children
History of acute pyelonephritis
More than 3 UTIs in past year
Symptoms lasting >7 days
Recent antibiotic use
Diabetes mellitus
Immunosuppression

### Detection of Urinary Antibody-Coated Bacteria

The premise behind the use of antibody-coated bacteria for localization is that an organism invading tissue (as occurs in upper but not lower urinary tract disease) provokes antibodies that should adhere to

| Extent of identification[c] | Susceptibility testing | Example of report[d] | Reasonable laboratory interpretation |
|---|---|---|---|
| Descriptive | Hold (5–7 days) for testing in case patient becomes septic | >100,000 CFU/ml, NLF (2 kinds); and >10,000 CFU/ml, GPC (2 kinds) | Colonization |
| | | No growth (<$10^3$ CFU/ml), or no growth (<$10^2$ CFU/ml) | No UTI |
| | | No growth (<$10^3$ CFU/ml), or no growth (<$10^2$ CFU/ml) | Patient on antibiotics: Unusual pathogen? Check Gram stain for pyuria; consider AFB, chlamydiae, mycoplasmas, viruses |

[c] Definitive, complete identification to species; Descriptive, identification as determined from plates or Gram stain, e.g., lactose fermenter or gram-positive cocci.

[d] GPC, gram-positive cocci; NLF, non-lactose-fermenting gram-negative rod; LF, lactose-fermenting gram-negative rod; GNR, gram-negative rod; AFB, acid-fast bacilli.

the organism that stimulated them (70). This antibody response can be detected by use of fluorescein-conjugated horse or goat immunoglobulin directed against human antibodies. The major limitation of the test is the lack of standardization of the percentage of fluorescent bacteria required for a positive test result (41).

The reported false-negative rate is 15% (41). Causes of false-negative test results include checking for antibody formation too early in the infection, before antibodies have formed; inability of antibody to adhere adequately to mucoid uropathogens (101); inconsistent antibody formation in children with pyelonephritis (99); and delays in specimen transport, which diminish the fraction of adherent antibody.

False-positive results have been related to infection due to gram-positive cocci, proteinuria, recent infection with antigenically similar organisms in women with recurrent bladder infections, contamination of the urine specimen with vaginal secretions, detection of antibody-coated bacteria of prostatic origin, interruption in the integrity of the bladder wall (e.g., by tumor, hemorrhagic cystitis, or ileal conduits), local antibody production in the bladder (e.g., the result of submucosal lymphoid follicles), and nonspecific fluorescence with *Candida* spp. and staphylococcal protein A.

### Segmental Urine Collection

Analysis of segmental collections of urine may allow localization of infection to the urethra or the prostate gland (108).

The diagnosis of urethritis may be established by separately collecting early-stream (the first ounce) and late-stream samples from a single voiding. Pyuria due to urethritis often clears early in voiding (154). Pyuria in urethritis is defined as an average of ≥5 WBCs per ×1,000 field after three fields have been examined (13, 157).

Infection can be localized to the prostate gland by comparing levels of pyuria in sequential specimens collected in association with prostatic massage. The segmented collections procedure includes (109) collection of the initial 5 to 8 ml of voided urine (urethral urine) (specimen VB1), collection of midstream urine (bladder urine) (VB2), performance of prostatic massage and collection of expressed prostatic secretions, and collection of first-voided 2 to 3 ml after prostatic massage (VB3).

If the level of pyuria in specimen VB3 is 10 times greater than that in specimen VB1, then bacterial prostatitis is likely. More than 15 WBC/HPF in the prostatic secretions is considered abnormal when the urethral and bladder WBC counts are within the normal range. The detection of oval fat droplets in macrophages within the prostatic fluid is evidence for bacterial prostatitis (107, 154). Note that immature sperm may look like WBCs. Increased WBC levels in prostatic fluid after ejaculation may also help to localize infection to the prostate (61).

## FUNGAL UTI

The unusual finding of fungal casts in the urine suggests upper urinary tract disease. Detection of a fungus ball or radiographic evidence for pyelonephritis may be a late manifestation of upper tract disease. Studies to apply the Fairley washout technique (39) and antibody-coated fungi (52) have been carried out, but reliable methods for localizing the source of candiuria are presently not available (38).

## ANTIMICROBIAL SUSCEPTIBILITY TESTING

Treatment is generally guided by the results of in vitro susceptibility testing when it is available. However, in selecting treatment, one needs to consider many variables that influence therapeutic outcome in addition to in vitro susceptibilities (such as antimicrobial pharmacodynamics, pharmacokinetics, and host characteristics). Even when these factors are considered, treatment with what appears to be appropriate antimicrobial therapy can fail. For example, in catheterized patients, biofilms composed of bacteria, bacterial glycocalyces, Tamm-Horsfall protein, and urinary salts (apatite and struvite) may shield bacteria from the action of antibiotics and result in treatment failure (122, 123).

## General Principles of Susceptibility Testing

Resistance to antimicrobial agents may be genetically intrinsic or acquired (3). Acquired resistance may be the result of chromosomally mediated mutations or of the transfer of genetic material encoding resistance. This genetic material may be a plasmid, which is transferable to other organisms of the same or different species. Alternatively, resistance can be acquired by a transposon (or "jumping gene"), which can integrate itself into the genetic material of many different species.

Plasmid-mediated resistance is common among gram-negative bacilli such as *E. coli* that are resistant to penicillins. Other examples of plasmid-mediated resistance are extended-spectrum cephalosporinases in *Klebsiella* species and aminoglycoside-modifying enzymes in the *Enterobacteriaceae* and in *P. aeruginosa*. Chromosomal mutations may affect outer membrane permeability and interfere, for example, with the entry of imipenem into *P. aeruginosa* or result in derepressed production of group I β-lactamase in *Enterobacter* spp., *Serratia marcescens*, or *P. aeruginosa*.

Antimicrobial susceptibility testing must be carried out with pure isolates. Several colonies should be selected from isolation plates to detect low-frequency mutations in a population of cells. A variety of antimicrobial agents have been recommended by the National Committee for Clinical Laboratory Standards (NCCLS) for testing against gram-positive and gram-negative isolates (119).

## Antimicrobial Susceptibility Testing Methods

### DISK DIFFUSION

In the disk diffusion method, a paper disk containing a specified amount of antimicrobial agent is applied to an agar surface that has been inoculated with a standardized density of bacteria. After overnight incubation, the resulting zone of inhibition is measured and interpreted as representing susceptibility, resistance, or an intermediate reading according to guidelines published by NCCLS (119).

This test is intended to be performed with an inoculum prepared from isolated colonies on a culture plate. Some success has been obtained with direct inoculation of plates with urine specimens; however, this direct approach requires initial microscopic examination of the urine to assess the number of bacteria present so that the specimen can be diluted to provide the correct inoculum, and it also requires the presence of only a single organism for accurate results to be obtained. It is generally recommended that direct tests be confirmed with the standard test with isolated colonies.

## DILUTION METHODS

Dilution susceptibility testing determines the lowest concentration of drug that inhibits the growth of the organism, i.e., the MIC, in micrograms per milliliter. Standardized procedures for this test have been developed by NCCLS (120). Dilution susceptibility testing may be performed on agar media or in broth by either macrodilution or microdilution techniques.

In this test, decreasing concentrations (on a $\log_2$ scale) of the drug to be tested in broth or agar are inoculated with a standardized bacterial inoculum (120).

The NCCLS publishes interpretative criteria for MICs that are based on recognized bacterial resistance mechanisms, pharmacokinetic properties of the antimicrobial agent, toxicity studies, and clinical cure and bacterial eradication data derived from premarket clinical trials with the antimicrobial agent. MICs are therefore interpreted as susceptible, intermediate, or resistant.

The designation "susceptible" implies that the organism that has been tested has no recognized resistance mechanism that is active against the antimicrobial agent, that the organism is inhibited in vitro by a concentration of the antimicrobial agent that is safely exceeded in serum by a factor of 2 to 4 with recommended doses of the antimicrobial agent, and that historical data from clinical trials of the agent strongly indicate that administration of the drug will result in clinical cure and eradication of the infection due to the organism. Conversely, the designation "resistant" suggests that a mechanism of resistance has been detected either directly (e.g., $\beta$-lactamase) or indirectly (based on the diameter of the inhibition zone in the disk diffusion test or on the MIC in the dilution test) and that these criteria and those derived from clinical trials indicate that clinical cure and bacterial eradication are unlikely to occur. The designation "intermediate" implies one of two things: first, that the organism might respond to higher doses of the drug if such doses can be safely given (e.g., as in the case of beta-lactams) or might respond in situations in which the drug is concentrated (e.g., in the urine) or, second, that the diameter of the inhibition zone or the MIC is in a buffer area that distinguishes between susceptibility and resistance to an antibiotic that cannot be safely given at a higher dose (e.g., as with an aminoglycoside).

The interpretative criteria that are applied to the diameters of zones of inhibition in the disk diffusion test are derived from the inverse linear relationship between these zone diameters and the MIC. This relationship is based initially on simultaneous disk diffusion testing and dilution testing of large numbers of organisms representing many species and including organisms with known resistance mechanisms that are active against the antimicrobial agent. Because of this relationship, both tests are generally equally accurate and clinically useful. From time to time, however, questions have been raised about the appropriateness of interpretative criteria that are based to a great extent on the pharmacokinetics of the drug in serum rather than in urine when the treatment of UTI is under consideration, especially for bladder infections in which tissue invasion is not a major problem. This argument has a long history; however, current interpretative criteria are based not only on pharmacokinetic studies in serum but also on the correlation between MICs and bacteriological eradication, which is readily assessed in the urinary tract.

Many laboratories use the disk diffusion test because of its ease of performance and flexibility. However, microdilution-based procedures that are semiautomated or fully automated and, in most cases, tested in conjunction with identification systems are also widely used. The choice of methods is multifactorial and beyond the scope of this chapter.

The selection of antimicrobial agents to be tested can be based on guidelines published by the NCCLS (119, 120) but generally includes a basic array of drugs such as ampicillin, cefazolin, tetracycline, gentamicin, and trimethoprim-sulfamethoxazole. This basic set is usually supplemented according to resistance patterns seen in isolates from a particular health care setting and according to deliberations by the formulary committee of the hospital. Antibiograms vary not only among hospitals but also within hospitals; therefore, susceptibility data from one institution should not be extrapolated to another. Numerous surveys of antimicrobial susceptibility trends that are of epidemiological interest but that have limited applicability within any given health care setting are currently under way. It is the microbiology laboratory's responsibility to provide the physicians within any group or health care setting with summaries of antimicrobial susceptibility data.

## CONCLUSIONS

Although the organisms causing infection in the urinary tract are few in number, the choices that need to be made for processing of urine specimens are not easy. Demands for more rapid results, greater cost-effectiveness, and improved accuracy of tests are increasing. The evolution of fully automated screening, identification, and susceptibility testing systems poses some risks of compromising accuracy. The pervasive issue of contamination in collection and the expanding definition of significant bacteriuria continue to pose challenges for the microbiology laboratory. The incidence of UTI and considerations of cost control dictate that routine screening and culture methods not have the aim of detecting either low-count bacteriuria or fastidious or rare pathogens in all specimens. This approach demands active communication between the clinician and the microbiologist as to circumstances when more than routine forms of testing need to be carried out.

The increasing development of resistance in uropathogens may have an influence in altering laboratory practices. The large number of specimens that are part of a laboratory's routine operations may dramatically increase if the therapy of even uncomplicated cystitis can no longer be chosen on an empirical basis because of an expanding challenge to detect resistance.

## REFERENCES

1. **Alwall, N.** 1973. Pyuria: deposit in high-power microscopic field—WBC/HPF versus WBC/mm$^3$ in counting chamber. Reappraisal of a valuable clinical routine method (urinary sediment). *Acta Med. Scand.* **194:**537–540.
2. **Alwall, N.** 1973. Factors affecting the reliability of screening tests for bacteriuria. II. Dipslide, false positive results following postal transport and false negatives owing to incubation at room temperature. *Acta Med. Scand.* **193:**505–509.

3. **Anonymous.** 1994. Emerging resistance in uropathogens. *PostGraduate Medicine,* Oct. 31, 1994, Consensus Conference, p. 1–24. McGraw Hill, Inc., Minneapolis.
4. **Arneil, G. C., T. A. McAllister, and P. Kay.** 1970. Detection of bacteriuria at room-temperature. *Lancet* **i:**119–121.
5. **Arneil, G. C., T. A. McAllister, and P. Kay.** 1973. Measurement of bacteriuria by plane dipslide culture. *Lancet* **i:**94–95.
6. **Asher, E. F., B. G. Oliver, and D. E. Fry.** 1988. Urinary tract infections in the surgical patient. *Am. Surg.* **54:**466–469.
7. **Bailey, R. R., and B. Harris.** 1994. Aerotolerant coryneforms as urinary tract pathogens. *N.Z. Med. J.* **107**(977)**:**179.
8. **Baron, E. J., L. Peterson, S. M. Finegold (ed.).** 1994. *Bailey & Scott's Diagnostic Microbiology,* 9th ed. The C. V. Mosby Co., St. Louis.
9. **Bartlett, R. C.** 1991. Quality assurance in the clinical microbiology laboratory, p. 36–43. *In* A. Balows, W. J. Hausler, Jr., K. L. Herrmann, H. D. Isenberg, and H. J. Shadomy (ed.), *Manual of Clinical Microbiology,* 5th ed. American Society for Microbiology, Washington, D.C.
10. **Bixler-Forell, E., M. A. Bertram, and D. A. Bruckner.** 1985. Clinical evaluation of three rapid methods for the detections of significant bacteriuria. *J. Clin. Microbiol.* **22:**62–67.
11. **Boscia, J. A., and D. Abrutyn Kaye.** 1987. Asymptomatic bacteriuria in elderly persons: treat or do not treat? *Ann. Intern. Med.* **106:**764–766.
12. **Boscia, J. A., and D. Kaye.** 1987. Asymptomatic bacteriuria in the elderly. *Infect. Dis. Clin. North Am.* **1:**893–905.
13. **Bowie, W. R.** 1978. Comparison of Gram stain and first-voided urine sediment in the diagnosis of urethritis. *Sex. Transm. Dis.* **5:**39–42.
14. **Breckman, B.** 1981. Urinary stomas and their management, p. 109. *In Stoma Care.* Beaconsfield Publishers, Beaconsfield, United Kingdom.
15. **Bronsema, D. A., J. R. Adams, R. Pallares, and R. P. Wenzel.** 1993. Secular trends in rates and etiology of nosocomial urinary tract infections at a university hospital. *J. Urol.* **150:**414–416.
16. **Brumfitt, W.** 1965. Urinary cell counts and their value. *J. Clin. Pathol.* **18:**550–555.
17. **Brumfitt, W., J. M. T. Hamilton-Miller, and W. A. Gillespie.** 1991. The mysterious "urethral Syndrome." *Br. Med. J.* **303:**1–2.
18. **Brumfitt, W., J. M. T. Hamilton-Miller, H. Ludham, and A. Gooding.** 1981. Lactobacilli do not cause frequency and dysuria syndrome. *Lancet* **ii:**393–396.
19. **Bryan, C., and K. Reynolds.** 1984. Hospital-acquired bacteremic urinary tract infection: epidemiology and outcome. *J. Urol.* **132:**494–498.
20. **Burdash, N. M., J. P. Manos, J. D. Ross, and E. R. Bannister.** 1976. Evaluation of the acid-fast smear. *J. Clin. Microbiol.* **4:**190–191.
21. **Carroll, K. C., D. C. Hale, D. H. Von Boerum, G. C. Reich, L. T. Hamilton, and J. M. Matsen.** 1994. Laboratory evaluation of urinary tract infections in an ambulatory clinic. *Am. J. Clin. Pathol.* **101:**100–103.
22. **Christensen, J. J., B. Korner, and H. Kjaegaard.** 1989. Aerococcus-like organism: an unnoticed urinary tract pathogen. *APMIS* **97:**539–546.
23. **Christensen, J. J., H. Vibits, J. Ursing, and B. Korner.** 1991. Aerococcus-like organism, a newly recognized potential urinary tract pathogen. *J. Clin. Microbiol.* **29:**1049–1053.
24. **Christensen, W. I.** 1974. Genito-urinary tuberculosis. Review of 102 cases. *Medicine* (Baltimore) **53:**377–390.
25. **Clark, R., L. Cardona, G. Valainis, and B. Hanna.** 1989. Genitourinary infections caused by mycobacteria other than *Mycobacterium tuberculosis. Tubercle* **70:**297–300.
26. **Clarridge, J. E., M. T. Pezzlo, and K. L. Vosti.** 1987. *Cumitech 2A, Laboratory Diagnosis of Urinary Tract Infections.* Coordinating ed., A. S. Weissfeld. American Society for Microbiology. Washington, D.C.
27. **Doern, G. L.** 1991. Microbial stabilization of antibiotics containing urine samples using the FLORA-STAT urine transport system. *J. Clin. Microbiol.* **29:**2169–2174.
28. **Doern, G. L., B. A. Brown, R. L. Cohen, J. A. Moore, J. F. Barlow, P. M. Southern, Jr., J. Ketchum, and J. S. Leonard.** 1989. Adherence to laboratory guidelines: a study on urine specimen transit time. *Diagn. Clin. Testing* **27:**28–31.
29. **Dontas, A. S., P. Kasviki-Charavati, P. C. Papanayiotou, and S. G. Marketos.** 1981. Bacteriuria and survival in old age. *N. Engl. J. Med.* **304:**939–943.
30. **Edelmann, C. M., Jr., J. E. Ogwo, B. P. Fine, and A. B. Martinez.** 1973. The prevalence of bacteriuria in full-term and premature newborn infants. *J. Pediatr.* **83:**125–132.

31. Esposito, A. L., R. A. Gleckman, S. Cram, L. Crowley, F. McCabe, and M. S. Drapkin. 1980. Community-acquired bacteremia in the elderly: analysis of one hundred consecutive episodes. *J. Am. Geriatr. Soc.* **28:**315–319.
32. Fairley, K. F., and D. F. Birch. 1983. Unconventional bacteria in urinary tract disease: *Gardnerella vaginalis. Kidney Int.* **23:**862–865.
33. Fairley, K. F., A. G. Bond, R. B. Brown, and P. Habersberger. 1967. Simple test to determine the site of urinary tract infection. *Lancet* **ii:**427–428.
34. Fierer, J., and N. Ehstrom. 1981. An outbreak of *Providencia stuartii* urinary tract infections: patients with condom catheters are a reservoir of the bacteria. *JAMA* **245:**1553–1555.
35. Fihn, S. D., C. Johnson, and W. E. Stamm. 1988. *Escherichia coli* urethritis in women with symptoms of acute urinary tract infection. *J. Infect. Dis.* **17:**196–199.
36. Finegold, S. M., L. G. Miller, S. L. Merrill, and D. J. Posnick. 1964. Significance of anaerobic and capnophilic bacteria isolated from the urinary tract, p. 159–178. *In* E. H. Kass (ed.), *Progress in Pyelonephritis*. FA Davis, Philadelphia.
37. Fisher, J. F., W. H. Chew, S. Shadomy, R. J. Duma, C. G. Mayhall, and W. C. House. 1982. Urinary tract infections due to *Candida albicans. Rev. Infect. Dis.* **4:**1107–1118.
38. Fisher, J. F., C. L. Newman, and J. D. Sobel. 1995. Yeast in the urine: solutions for a budding problem. *Clin. Infect. Dis.* **20:**183–189.
39. Fong, I. W., P. C. Cheng, and N. A. Hinton. 1991. Fungicidal effect of amphotericin B in urine: in vitro study to assess feasibility of bladder washout for localization of site of candiduria. *Antimicrob. Agents Chemother.* **35:**1856–1859.
40. Gabre-Kidan, T., B. A. Lipsky, and J. J. Plorde. 1984. *Haemophilus influenzae* as a cause of urinary tract infections in men. *Arch. Intern. Med.* **144:**1623–1627.
41. Gagan, R. A. W. Brumfitt, and J. M. T. Hamilton-Miller. 1983. Antibody-coated bacteria in urine: criterion for a positive test and its value in defining a higher risk of treatment failure. *Lancet* **ii:**704–706.
42. Gillenwater, J. Y. 1981. Detection of urinary leucocytes by Chemstrip-L. *J. Urol.* **125:**383–384.
43. Goldberg, P. K., P. J. Kozinin, G. J. Wise, N. Nouri, and R. B. Brooks. 1979. Incidence and significance of candiduria. *JAMA* **241:**582–584.
44. Goodman, L. J., R. K. Kaplan, W. Landau, E. Jung, J. E. Barrett, S. Levin, and A. A. Harris. 1985. A urine preservation system to maintain bacterial counts. *Clin. Pediatr.* **24:**383–386.
45. Goswitz, J. J., K. E. Willard, S. J. Eastep, T. Singleton, and L. R. Peterson. 1993. Utility of slide centrifuge Gram's stain versus quantitative culture for diagnosis of urinary tract infection. *Am. J. Clin. Pathol.* **99:**132–136.
46. Graff, L. 1983. Chemical examination, p. 21–67. *In A Handbook of Routine Urinalysis*. J. B. Lippincott Co., New York.
47. Gross, P. A., L. M. Harkavy, G. E. Barden, and M. Kerstin. 1974. Positive Foley catheter tip cultures—fact or fancy? *JAMA* **228:**72–73.
48. Guenther, K. L., and J. A. Washington II. 1981. Evaluation of the B-D urine culture kit. *J. Clin. Microbiol.* **14:**628–630.
49. Gutman, L. T., M. Turck, R. G. Petersdorf, and R. J. Wedgwood. 1965. Significance of bacterial variants in urine of patients with chronic bacteriuria. *J. Clin. Invest.* **44:**1945–1952.
50. Haley, R. W., D. H. Culver, J. W. White, W. M. Morgan, and T. G. Emori. 1985. The nation-wide nosocomial infection rate. A new need for vital statistics. *Am. J. Epidemiol.* **121:**159–167.
51. Hall, D. E., and J. A. Snitzer III. 1994. *Staphylococcus epidermidis* as a cause of urinary tract infections in children. *J. Pediatr.* **124:**437–438.
52. Hall, W. J. 1980. Study of antibody coated fungi in patients with funguria and suspected disseminated fungal infections in primary fungal pyelonephritis. *J. R. Soc. Med.* **73:**567–569.
53. Haugen, J., O. Strom, and B. Ostervold. 1968. Bacterial counts in urine. I. The reliability of the loop technique. *Acta Pathol. Microbiol. Scand.* **74:**391–396.
54. Hedelin, H., J. E. Brorson, L. Grenabo, and S. Pettersson. 1984. *Ureaplasma urealyticum* and upper urinary tract stones. *Br. J. Urol.* **56:**244–249.
55. Hellerstein, S., E. Duggan, E. Welchert, H. Grossman, and P. Sharma. 1981. Site of urinary tract infections with the bladder washout test. *J. Pediatr.* **98:**201–206.
56. Hindman, R., B. Tronic, and R. Bartlett. 1976. Effect of delay on culture of urine. *J. Clin. Microbiol.* **4:**102–103.

57. **Hoff, R. G., E. Newman, and J. L. Staneck.** 1985. Bacteriuria screening by use of acridine orange-stained smears. *J. Clin. Microbiol.* **21:**513–516.
58. **Hubbard, W. A., P. J. Shalis, and K. D. McClatchey.** 1983. Comparison of the B-D urine culture with a standard culture method and the MS-2. *J. Clin. Microbiol.* **17:**327–331.
59. **Hyams, K. C.** 1987. Inappropriate urine cultures in hospitalized patients receiving antibiotic therapy. *Arch. Intern. Med.* **147:**4–49.
60. **Isenberg, H. D., and R. F. D'Amato.** 1991. Indigenous and pathogenic microorganisms of humans, p. 2–14. *In* A. Balows, W. J. Hausler, Jr., K. L. Herrmann, H. D. Isenberg, and H. J. Shadomy (ed.), *Manual of Clinical Microbiology*, 5th ed. American Society for Microbiology, Washington, D.C.
61. **Jameson, R. M.** 1967. Sexual activity and the variations of the white blood cell content of the prostatic secretion. *Invest. Urol.* **5:**297–302.
62. **Jefferson, H., H. P. Dalton, M. R. Escobar, and M. J. Allison.** 1975. Transportation delay and the microbiological quality of clinical specimens. *Am. J. Clin. Pathol.* **64:**689–693.
63. **Jenkins, R. D., A. P. Fenn, and J. M. Matsen.** 1986. Review of urine microscopy for bacteriuria. *JAMA* **255:**3397–4003.
64. **Jewkes, F. E., D. J. McMaster, W. A. Napier, I. B. Houston, and R. J. Postlethwaite.** 1990. Home collection of urine specimens, boric acid or dipslides? *Arch. Dis. Child.* **65:**286–289.
65. **Johnson, F. B.** 1990. Transport of viral specimens. *Clin. Microbiol. Rev.* **3:**120–131.
66. **Johnson, J. R., M. F. Lyons II, W. Pearce, et al.** 1991. Therapy for women hospitalized with acute pyelonephritis: a randomized trial of ampicillin versus trimethoprim-sulfamethoxazole for 14 days. *J. Infect. Dis.* **163:**325–330.
67. **Johnson, J. R., and W. E. Stamm.** 1987. Diagnosis and treatment of acute urinary tract infections. *Infect. Dis. Clin. North Am.* **1:**773–791. (Erratum, **4:**xii, 1990.)
68. **Johnson, J. R., and W. E. Stamm.** 1989. Urinary tract infections in women: diagnosis and treatment. *Ann. Intern. Med.* **111:**906–917.
69. **Jones, C., D. W. MacPherson, and D. L. Stevens.** 1986. Inability of the Chemstrip LN compared with quantitative urine culture to predict significant bacteriuria. *J. Clin. Microbiol.* **23:**160–162.
70. **Jones, S. R., J. W. Smith, and J. P. Sanford.** 1974. Localization of urinary tract infection by detection of antibody coated bacteria in urine sediment. *N. Engl. J. Med.* **290:**591–593.
71. **Jordan, P. A., A. Iravani, G. A. Richard, and M. Baer.** 1980. Urinary tract infection caused by *Staphylococcus saprophyticus*. *J. Infect. Dis.* **142:**510–515.
72. **Kass, E. H.** 1957. Bacteriuria and the diagnosis of infections of the urinary tract. *Arch. Intern. Med.* **100:**709–714.
73. **Kass, E. H.** 1960. The role of asymptomatic bacteriuria in the pathogenesis of pyelonephritis, p. 399–412. *In* I. L. Quinn and E. H. Kass (ed.), *Biology of Pyelonephritis*. Churchill Livingstone, London.
74. **Kass, E. H.** 1960. Bacteriuria and pyelonephritis of pregnancy. *Arch. Intern. Med.* **105:**194–198.
75. **Kass, E. H., and M. Finland.** 1956. Asymptomatic infections of the urinary tract. *Trans. Assoc. Am. Physicians* **69:**56–64.
76. **Kaye, D.** 1980. Urinary tract infections in the elderly. *Bull. N.Y. Acad. Med.* **56:**209–220.
77. **Kemper, K. J.** 1992. The case against screening urinalyses for asymptomatic bacteriuria in children. *Am. J. Dis. Child.* **146:**343–346.
78. **Kierkegaard, H., U. Feldt-Rasmussen, M. Horder, H. J. Anderson, and P. J. Jorgensen.** 1980. Falsely negative urinary leucocyte counts due to delayed examination. *Scand. J. Clin. Lab. Invest.* **40:**259–261.
79. **Koenig, C., L. J. Tick, and B. A. Hanna.** 1992. Analyses of the FlashTrack DNA Probe and UTIscreen bioluminescence tests for bacteriuria. *J. Clin. Microbiol.* **30:**342–345.
80. **Komaroff, A. L.** 1986. Urinalysis and urine culture in women with dysuria. *Ann. Intern. Med.* **104:**212–218.
81. **Koneman, E. W., S. D. Allen, W. M. Janda, P. C. Schreckenberger, and W. C. Winn, Jr.** 1992. *Diagnostic Microbiology*, 4th ed. J. B. Lippincott & Co., Philadelphia.
82. **Krieger, J. N., D. L. Kaiser, and R. P. Wenzel.** 1983. Urinary tract etiology of bloodstream infections in hospitalized patients. *J. Infect. Dis.* **148:**57–62.
83. **Krieger, J. N., D. L. Kaiser, and R. P. Wenzel.** 1993. Nosocomial urinary tract infections: secular trends, treatment and economics in a university hospital. *J. Urol.* **130:**102–106.
84. **Kunin, C. M.** 1961. The quantitative significance of bacteria visualized in the unstained

urinary sediment. *N. Engl. J. Med.* **265:** 589–590.

85. **Kunin, C. M.** 1987. *Detection, Prevention and Management of Urinary Tract Infections*, 4th ed. Lea & Febiger, Philadelphia.

86. **Kunin, C. M.** 1994. Guidelines for urinary tract infections. Rationale for a separate strata for patients with "low-count" bacteriuria. *Infection* 22(Suppl. 1):S38–S41.

87. **Kunin, C. M.** 1994. Urinary tract infections in females. *Clin. Infect. Dis.* **18:**1–12.

88. **Kunin, C. M., L. VanArsdale, L. White, and H. H. Tong.** 1993. Reassessment of the importance of "low-count" bacteriuria in young women with acute urinary symptoms. *Ann. Intern. Med.* **119:**454–460.

89. **Kusumi, R. K., P. J. Grower, and C. M. Kunin.** 1981. Rapid detection of pyuria by leucocyte esterase activity. *JAMA* **245:** 1653–1655.

90. **Lamb, V. A., H. P. Dalton, and J. R. Wilkins.** 1976. Electrochemical method for the early detection of urinary tract infections. *Am. J. Clin. Pathol.* **66:**91–95.

91. **Latham, R. H., E. S. Wong, A. Larson, M. Coyle, and W. E. Stamm.** 1985. Laboratory diagnosis of urinary tract infections in ambulatory women. *JAMA* **254:**3333–3335.

92. **Lauer, B. A., L. B. Reller, and S. Mirrett.** 1979. Evaluation of preservative fluid for urine collected for culture. *J. Clin. Microbiol.* **10:**42–45.

93. **Leighton, P. M., and J. A. Little.** 1986. Identification of coagulase-negative staphylococci isolated from urinary tract infections. *Am. J. Clin. Pathol.* **85:**92–95.

94. **Lipsky, B. A.** 1989. Urinary tract infections in men: epidemiology, pathophysiology, diagnosis, and treatment. *Ann. Intern. Med.* **110:**138–150.

95. **Lipsky, B. A., A. C. Goldberger, L. S. Tomkins, and J. J. Plorde.** 1982. Infections caused by nondiphtheria corynebacteria. *Rev. Infect. Dis.* **4:**1220–1235.

96. **Lipsky, B. A., T. S. Inui, J. J. Plorde, and R. E. Berger.** 1984. Is the clean-catch midstream void procedure necessary for obtaining urine culture specimens from men? *Am. J. Med.* **76:**257–262.

97. **Lipsky, B. A., R. C. Ireton, S. D. Fihn, R. Hackett, and R. E. Berger.** 1987. Diagnosis of bacteriuria in men: specimen collection and culture interpretation. *J. Infect. Dis.* **155:**847–854.

98. **Little, P. J.** 1964. A comparison of urinary white cell concentration with the white cell excretion rare. *Br. J. Urol.* **36:**360–363.

99. **Lorentz, W. B., Jr., and M. I. Resnick.** 1979. Comparison of urinary lactic dehydrogenase with antibody-coated bacteria in the urine sediment as means of localizing the site of urinary tract infection. *Pediatrics* **64:** 672–677.

100. **Mardh, P. A., A. Lohi, and H. Fritz.** 1972. Mycoplasma in urine collected by suprapubic aspiration. *Acta Med. Scand.* **191:** 91–95.

101. **Marrie, T. J., G. K. M. Harding, A. R. Ronald, et al.** 1979. Influence of mucoid on antibody coating of *Pseudomonas aeruginosa*. *J. Infect. Dis.* **139:**357–361.

102. **Marrie, T. J., C. Kwam, M. A. Noble, A. West, and L. Duffield.** 1982. *Staphylococcus saprophyticus* as cause of urinary tract infections. *J. Clin. Microbiol.* **16:**427–431.

103. **Maskell, R.** 1986. Are fastidious organisms an important cause of dysuria and frequency? The case for, p. 1–18. *In* A. W. Asscher, and W. Brumfitt (ed.), *Microbial Diseases in Nephrology*. John Wiley & Sons, Chichester, England.

104. **Maskell, R., L. Pead, and J. Allen.** 1979. The puzzle of "urethral syndrome": a possible answer? *Lancet* **i:**1058–1059.

105. **Mathews, S. C. W.** 1987. An evaluation of a new commercial urine transport system. *Med. Lab. Sci.* **44:**341–344.

106. **McWalter, P. W., and C. A. Sharp.** 1982. Evaluation of a commercially available semiautomated bioluminescence system for bacteriuria screening. *Eur. J. Clin. Microbiol.* **1:** 22–27.

107. **Meares, E. M., Jr.** 1980. Prostatitis syndromes. New perspectives about old woes. *J. Urol.* **123:**141–147.

108. **Meares, E. M., Jr.** 1987. Acute and chronic prostatitis: diagnosis and treatment. *Infect. Dis. Clin. North Am.* **1:**855–873.

109. **Meares, E. M., and T. A. Stamey.** 1968. Bacteriologic localization patterns in bacterial prostatitis and urethritis. *Invest. Urol.* **5:** 492–518.

110. **Monte-Verde, D., and J. S. Nosanchuk.** 1981. The sensitivity and specificity of nitrite testing for bacteria. *Lab. Med.* **12:**755–757.

111. **Morgan, M. G., and H. McKenzie.** 1993. Controversies in the laboratory diagnosis of community-acquired urinary tract infection. *Eur. J. Clin. Microbiol. Infect. Dis.* **12:** 491–504.

112. **Mou, T. W., and H. A. Feldman.** 1961. The enumeration and preservation of bacteriuria in urine. *Am. J. Clin. Pathol.* **35:** 572–575.

113. **Murray, P., P. Traynor, and D. Hopson.** 1992. Evaluation of microbiological processing of urine specimens: comparison of overnight versus two-day incubation. *J. Clin. Microbiol.* **30:**1600–1601.
114. **Murray, P. R., A. C. Niles, R. L. Heeren, and F. Pikul.** 1988. Evaluation of the modified Bac-T-Screen and FiltraCheck-UTI urine screening systems for detection of clinically significant bacteriuria. *J. Clin. Microbiol.* **26:**2347–2350.
115. **Murray, P. R., R. V. Smith, and T. C. McKinney.** 1987. Clinical evaluation of three urine screening tests. *J. Clin. Microbiol.* **25:**467–470.
116. **Musher, D. M., S. B. Thorsteinsson, and V. M. Andriole.** 1976. Quantitative urinalysis: diagnosing urinary tract infection in men. *JAMA* **236:**2069–2072.
117. **Mustafa, M. M., and G. H. McCrackem, Jr.** 1992. Perinatal bacterial diseases, p. 891–924. *In* R. D. Feigan and J. D. Cherry (ed.), *Pediatric Infectious Diseases,* 3rd ed. The W.B. Saunders Co., Philadelphia.
118. **Naber, K. G.** 1990. The relevance of the urine sampling method on the amount of bacteriuria, p. 201–207. *In* M. Ohkoshi and Y. Kawada (ed.), *Clinical Evaluation of Drug Efficacy in UTI. Proceedings of the 1st International Symposium, Tokyo, Japan, 27–28 October 1989.* Excerpta Medica, Amsterdam.
119. **National Committee for Clinical Laboratory Standards.** 1993. *Performance Standards for Antimicrobial Disk Susceptibility Tests. Approved Standard.* NCCLS publication M2-A5. National Committee for Clinical Laboratory Standards, Villanova, Pa.
120. **National Committee for Clinical Laboratory Standards.** 1993. *Methods for Dilution Antimicrobial Susceptibility Tests for Bacteria That Grow Aerobically. Approved Standard.* NCCLS publication M7-A3. National Committee for Clinical Laboratory Standards, Villanova, Pa.
121. **Nickander, K. K., C. J. Shanholtzer, and L. R. Peterson.** 1982. Urine culture transport tubes: effect of sample volume on bacterial toxicity of the preservative. *J. Clin. Microbiol.* **15:**593–595.
122. **Nickel, J. C., A. G. Gristina, and J. W. Costerton.** 1985. Electron microscopic study of an infected Foley catheter. *Can. J. Surg.* **28(1):**50–51, 54.
123. **Nickel, J. C., I. Ruseska, J. B. Wright, and J. W. Costerton.** 1985. Tobramycin resistance of *Pseudomonas aeruginosa* cells growing as a biofilm on urinary catheter material. *Antimicrob. Agents Chemother.* **27:**619–624.
124. **Nicolle, L. E., J. Bjornson, G. K. M. Harding, and J. A. MacDonell.** 1983. Bacteriuria in elderly institutionalized men. *N. Engl. J. Med.* **309:**1420–1425.
125. **Nicolle, L. E., G. K. M. Harding, J. Kennedy, M. McIntyre, F. Aoki, and D. Murray.** 1988. Urine specimen collection with external devices for diagnosis of bacteriuria in elderly incontinent men. *J. Clin. Microbiol.* **26:**1115–1119.
126. **Nordenstam, G. R., C. A. Brandberg, A. S. Oden, C. M. Svanborg Eden, and A. Svanborg.** 1986. Bacteriuria and mortality in an elderly population. *N. Engl. J. Med.* **314:**1152–1156.
127. **Oneson, R., and D. H. Groschel.** 1985. Leukocyte esterase activity and nitrite test as a rapid screen for significant bacteriuria. *Am. J. Clin. Pathol.* **83:**84–87.
128. **Ouslander, J. G., B. A. Greengold, F. J. Silverblatt, and J. P. Garci.** 1987. An accurate method to obtain urine for culture in men with external catheters. *Arch. Intern. Med.* **147:**286–288.
129. **Patterson, T. F., and V. T. Andriole.** 1987. Bacteriuria in pregnancy. *Infect. Dis. Clin. North Am.* **1:**807–822.
130. **Patton, J. P., D. B. Nash, and E. Abrutyn.** 1991. Urinary tract infection: economic considerations. *Med. Clin. North Am.* **75:**495–513.
131. **Pedler Bint, A. J.** 1987. Management of bacteriuria in pregnancy. *Pract. Ther.* **33:**413–421.
132. **Pezzlo, M. T., D. Amsterdam, J. P. Anhalt, T. Lawrence, N. J. Stratton, E. A. Vetter, E. M. Peterson, and L. M. de la Maza.** 1992. Detection of bacteriuria and pyuria by URISCREEN, a rapid enzymatic screening test. *J. Clin. Microbiol.* **30:**680–684.
133. **Pezzlo, M. T., S. Conway, M. Jacobson, E. M. Peterson, and L. M. de la Maza.** 1984. Effect of the B-D urine culture kit on an automated bacteriuria screen. *J. Clin. Microbiol.* **20:**1207–1208.
134. **Pezzlo, M. T., V. Ige, A. P. Woolard, E. M. Peterson, and L. M. de la Maza.** 1989. Rapid bioluminescence method for bacteriuria screening. *J. Clin. Microbiol.* **27:**716–720.
135. **Pezzlo, M. T., M. A. Werkowski, E. M. Peterson, and L. M. de la Mazza.** 1983. Evaluation of a two-minute test for urine screening. *J. Clin. Microbiol.* **18:**697–701.
136. **Pfaler, M. A., and F. P. Koontz.** 1985. Laboratory evaluation of leukocyte esterase

and nitrite tests for detection of bacteriuria. *J. Clin. Microbiol.* **21**:840–842.
137. **Pickering, W. J., D. F. Birch, and P. Kincaid-Smith.** 1990. Biochemical and histologic findings in experimental pyelonephritis due to *Ureaplasma urealyticum*. *Infect. Immun.* **58**:3401–3406.
138. **Platt, M. L., W. D. Belville, C. Stones, and T. R. Oberhofer.** 1986. Rapid bacteriuria screening in a urological setting. *J. Urol.* **136**:1044–1046.
139. **Porter, I. A., and J. Brodie.** 1969. Boric acid preservation of urine samples. *Br. Med. J.* **ii**:353–355.
140. **Pryles, C. V., M. D. Atkin, T. S. Morse, and K. J. Welch.** 1959. Comparative bacteriologic study of urine obtained from children by percutaneous suprapubic aspiration of the bladder and by catheter. *Pediatrics* **24**:983–991.
141. **Pryles, C. V., D. Lüders, and M. K. Alkan.** 1961. A comparative study of bacterial cultures and colony counts in paired specimens of urine obtained by catheter versus voiding from normal infants and infants with urinary tract infection. *Pediatrics* **27**:17–28.
142. **Pugliese, A., B. Pacris, P. E. Schoch, and B. A. Cunha.** 1993. *Oligella urethralis* urosepsis. *Clin. Infect. Dis.* **17**:1069–1070. (Letter.)
143. **Rippin, K. P., W. C. Stinson, J. Eisenstadt, and J. A. Washington.** 1995. Clinical evaluation of the slide centrifuge (cytospin) Gram's stained smear for the detection of bacteriuria and comparison with the Filtracheck-UTI and UTIscreen. *Am. J. Clin. Pathol.* **103**:316–319.
144. **Roberts, A. P., R. E. Robinson, and R. W. Beard.** 1967. Some factors affecting bacterial colony counts in urinary infection. *Br. Med. J.* **i**:400–403.
145. **Ronald, A. R., P. Boutos, and H. Mourtada.** 1976. Bacteriuria localization and response to single-dose therapy in women. *JAMA* **235**:1854–1856.
146. **Ronald, A. R., and A. L. S. Patrillo.** 1991. The natural history of urinary infection in adults. *Med. Clin. North Am.* **75**:299–312.
147. **Rubin, R. H., E. D. Shapiro, V. T. Andriole, R. J. Davis, and W. E. Stamm.** 1992. Evaluation of new anti-infective drugs for the treatment of urinary tract infection. *Clin. Infect. Dis.* **15**:S216–S227.
148. **Rupp, M. E., D. E. Soper, and G. L. Archer.** 1992. Colonization of the female genital tract with *Staphylococcus saprophyticus*. *J. Clin. Microbiol.* **30**:2975–2979.
149. **Saito, A., and Y. Kawasa.** 1994. Reliability of pyuria detection method. *Infection* **22**(Suppl. 1):S36–S37.
150. **Salyer, W. R., and D. C. Slayer.** 1973. Involvement of the kidney and prostate in cryptococcosis. *J. Urol.* **109**:695–698.
151. **Sanford, J. P.** 1975. Urinary tract symptoms and infections. *Annu. Rev. Med.* **26**:485–498.
152. **Sanford, J. P., C. B. Favour, F. G. Mao, and J. H. Harrison.** 1956. Evaluation of the positive urine culture. *Am. J. Med.* **20**:88–93.
153. **Schaeffer, A. J.** 1994. Urinary tract infections in men-state of the art. Proceedings of the 3rd International Symposium on Clinical Evaluation of Drug Efficacy in UTI, Stockholm, Sweden 1993. *Infection* **22**(Suppl. 1):S19–S21.
154. **Schaeffer, A. J., E. F. Wendel, J. K. Dunn, et al.** 1981. Prevalence and significance of prostatic inflammation. *J. Urol.* **125**:215–219.
155. **Schappert, S. M.** 1992. National ambulatory medical care survey: 1990 summary. Advance data from vital and health statistics. no. 213, p. 1–12. National Center for Health Statistics, Hyattsville, Md.
156. **Schoenbeck, J.** 1972. Studies on *Candida* infection of the urinary tract and on the antimycotic drug 5-fluorocytosine. *Scand. J. Urol. Nephrol.* **11**(Suppl.):7–48.
157. **Schwartz, S. L., S. J. Kraus, K. L. Herrmann, M. D. Stargel, W. J. Brown, and D. S. Allen.** 1978. Diagnosis and etiology of nongonococcal urethritis. *J. Infect. Dis.* **138**:445–454.
158. **Segura, J. W., P. P. Kelalis, W. J. Martin, and L. H. Smith.** 1972. Anaerobic bacteria in the urinary tract. *Mayo Clin. Proc.* **47**:30–33.
159. **Simon, H. B., A. J. Weinstein, M. S. Pasternak, et al.** 1977. Genitourinary tuberculosis: clinical features in a general hospital population. *Am. J. Med.* **63**:410–420.
160. **Smalley, D. L., and M. E. Bradley.** 1984. Correlation of leukocyte esterase activity and bacterial isolation from body fluids. *J. Clin. Microbiol.* **18**:1256–1257.
161. **Smith, S. M., T. Ogbara, and R. H. K. Eng.** 1992. Involvement of *Gardnerella vaginalis* in urinary tract infections in men. *J. Clin. Microbiol.* **30**:1575–1577.
162. **Smith, T. K., A. J. Hudson, and R. C. Spencer.** 1988. Evaluation of six screening methods for detecting significant bacteriuria. *J. Clin. Pathol.* **41**:904–909.

163. **Soriano, F., J. M. Aguado, C. Ponte, R. Fernandez-Roblas, and J. L. Rodriquez-Tudela.** 1990. Urinary tract infection caused by *Corynebacterium* group D2: report of 82 cases and review. *Rev. Infect. Dis.* **12:** 1019–1034.
164. **Soriano, F., and C. Ponte.** 1992. Processing urine specimens: overnight versus two-day incubation. *J. Clin. Microbiol.* **30:** 3033–3034. (Letter.)
165. **Spach, D. H., A. E. Stapleton, and W. E. Stamm.** 1992. Lack of circumcision increases the risk of urinary tract infection in young men. *JAMA* **267:**679–681.
166. **Stager, C. E., and J. R. Davis.** 1990. Evaluation of the FiltraCheck-UTI for detection of bacteriuria. *Diagn. Microbiol. Infect. Dis.* **13:**289–295.
167. **Stamey, T. A.** 1980. *Pathogenesis and Treatment of Urinary Tract Infections*. The Williams & Wilkins Co., Baltimore.
168. **Stamey, T. A., and A. Pfau.** 1970. Urinary infections: a selective review and some observations. *Calif. Med.* **113:**16–35.
169. **Stamm, W. E.** 1983. Measurement of pyuria and its relation to bacteriuria. *Am. J. Med.* **75**(Suppl. 1B):53–58.
170. **Stamm, W. E., G. W. Counts, K. R. Runnings, S. Fihn, M. Turck, and K. K. Holmes.** 1982. Diagnosis of coliform infection in acutely dysuric women. *N. Engl. J. Med.* **307:**463–468.
171. **Stamm, W. E., and T. M. Hooton.** 1993. Management of urinary tract infections in adults. *N. Engl. J. Med.* **329:**1328–1334.
172. **Stamm, W. E., K. Running, G. W. McKevitt, G. W. Counts, M. Turck, and K. K. Holmes.** 1981. Treatment of the acute urethral syndrome. *N. Engl. J. Med.* **304:**956–958.
173. **Stamm, W. E., K. F. Wagner, E. Amsel, R. Alexander, M. Turck, G. W. Counts, and K. K. Holmes.** 1980. Causes of the acute urethral syndrome in women. *N. Engl. J. Med.* **303:**409–415.
174. **Stark, R. P., and D. G. Maki.** 1984. Bacteriuria in the catheterized patient: what quantitative level of bacteriuria is relevant? *N. Engl. J. Med.* **311:**560–564.
175. **Stegmayr, B., and A. S. Malmborg.** 1988. Urinary tract infection caused by *Haemophilus influenzae*. A case report. *Scand. J. Urol. Nephrol.* **22:**75–77.
176. **Tendler, C., and D. J. Bottone.** 1989. *Corynebacterium aquaticum* urinary tract infection in a neonate, and concepts regarding the role of the organism as a neonatal pathogen. *J. Clin. Microbiol.* **27:**343–345.
177. **Tenney, J. H., and J. W. Warren.** 1988. Bacteriuria in women with long-term catheters: paired comparison of indwelling and replacement catheters. *J. Infect. Dis.* **157:** 199–202.
178. **Thiael, G., and O. Spuhler.** 1965. Urinary tract infection by catheter and the so-called infectious (episomal) resistance. *Schweiz. Med. Wochenschr.* **95:**1155–1157.
179. **Thomsen, A. C.** 1978. Mycoplasmas in human pyelonephritis. Demonstration of antibodies in serum and urine. *J. Clin. Microbiol.* **18:**197–202.
180. **Thore, A. S., A. A. Lundin, and S. Bergmen.** 1975. Detection of bacteriuria by luciferase assay of adenosine triphosphate. *J. Clin. Microbiol.* **1:**1–8.
181. **Vijlsgaard, R.** 1965. Quantitative bacterial culture of urine (limit between contamination and significant bacteriuria), p. 468–477. *In* E. H. Kass (ed.), *Progress in Pyelonephritis*. F. A. Davis Publishing Co., Philadelphia.
182. **Vollaard, E. J., and H. A. L. Clasener.** 1994. Colonization resistance. *Antimicrob. Agents Chemother.* **38:**409–414.
183. **Wajaszczuk, C., T. Logan, A. W. Pasculle, and M. Ho.** 1984. Intra-abdominal actinomycosis presenting with sulfur granules in the urine. *Am. J. Med.* **77:**1126–1128.
184. **Warren, J. W.** 1986. *Providencia stuartii*: a common cause of antibiotic-resistant bacteriuria in patients with long-term indwelling catheters. *Rev. Infect. Dis.* **8:**61–67.
185. **Warren, J. W.** 1995. Nosocomial urinary tract infections, p. 2607–2616. *In* G. L. Mandell, R. G. Douglas, Jr., and J. E. Bennett (ed.), *Principles and Practice of Infectious Diseases*, 4th ed. Churchill Livingstone, New York.
186. **Warren, J. W., J. H. Tenney, J. N. Hoopes, H. L. Muncie, and W. C. Anthony.** 1982. Prospective microbiologic study of bacteriuria in patients with chronic indwelling urethral catheters. *J. Infect. Dis.* **146:**719–723.
187. **Washington, J. A., II.** 1990. Bacterial cultures for cystitis. *Ann. Intern. Med.* **112:** 387–388. (Letter.)
188. **Washington, J. A., II, C. M. White, M. Laganiere, and L. H. Smith.** 1981. Detection of significant bacteriuria by microscopic examination of urine. *Lab. Med.* **12:**294–296.
189. **Watson, P. G., and B. I. Duerden.** 1977. Laboratory assessment of physical and chemical methods of preserving urine specimens. *J. Clin. Pathol.* **30:**532–536.

190. **Welch, W. D., L. Thompson, M. Layman, and P. M. Southern, Jr.** 1984. Evaluation of two bioluminescence-measuring instruments, the Turner design and the Lumac systems, for the rapid screening of urine specimens. *J. Clin. Microbiol.* **20:**1165–1170.
191. **Wenk, R. E., D. Dutta, J. Rudert, Y. Kim, and C. Steinhager.** 1982. Sediment microscopy, microscopy, nitrituria and leukocyte esterasuria as predictors of significant bacteriuria. *J. Clin. Lab. Automation* **2:**117–121.
192. **Wheat, L. J., R. B. Kohler, and R. P. Tewari.** 1986. Diagnosis of disseminated histoplasmosis by detection of *Histoplasma capsulatum* antigen in serum and urine specimens. *N. Engl. J. Med.* **314:**83–88.
193. **Wigton, R. S., V. L. Hoellerich, J. P. Ornato, V. Lev, L. A. Mazzotta, and I. H. Cheng.** 1985. Use of clinical findings in the diagnosis of urinary tract infection in women. *Arch. Intern. Med.* **145:**2222–2227.
194. **Wilkins, E. G. L., J. G. Ratcliff, and C. Roberts.** 1985. Leucocyte esterase-nitrite screening methods for pyuria and bacteriuria. *J. Clin. Pathol.* **38:**1342–1345.
195. **Wilson, R., and R. A. Feldman.** 1982. *Salmonella* isolated from urine in the United States. *J. Infect. Dis.* **146:**293–296.
196. **Woods, G. L., and J. A. Washington II.** 1995. The clinician and the microbiology laboratory, p. 169–199. *In* G. L. Mandell, J. E. Bennett, and R. Dolin (ed.) *Principles and Practice of Infectious Disease,* 4th ed. Churchill Livingstone, New York.
197. **Woodwell, D. A.** 1993. *Office Visits to Urologists, United States. 1989–90.* National Center for Health Statistics, Centers for Disease Control, advance data no. 234. National Center for Health Statistics, Atlanta.

# THE VAGINAL FLORA AND URINARY TRACT INFECTIONS

*Thomas M. Hooton, M.D., and Walter E. Stamm, M.D.*

## BACKGROUND

Urinary tract infections (UTIs) in women develop when uropathogens, almost always from the reservoir of fecal flora, colonize the vaginal introitus, enter the urethra, ascend into the bladder, and stimulate a host response manifested by symptoms and, in most cases, pyuria. The increased incidence of UTI in women compared with that in men is likely to be at least partly related to the anatomic proximity of the distal urethra to the fecal flora as well as to the shortness of the urethra. Most uncomplicated UTIs in women cannot be explained by underlying functional or anatomic abnormalities of the urinary tract but instead appear to result from the interaction of infecting *Escherichia coli* strains with these patients' epithelial cells. Thus, the initial pathogenic event in the urinary tract occurs when the bacteria attach to the mucosa by interactions between bacterial surface ligands (adhesins) and complementary epithelial-cell structures (receptors) (42, 79, 167). It is likely that introital colonization with uropathogens merely provides a source of bacteria for entry into the bladder. Migration of the organisms from the introitus into the bladder is then facilitated by other factors such as sexual intercourse (18, 55, 96). Colonization of bladder epithelium by uropathogens gaining access to the bladder appears to be a necessary step in the pathogenesis of UTI, since in the healthy bladder, most unattached bacteria are eliminated with micturition (98). Certain bacterial virulence factors provide a selective advantage to those strains possessing them with regard to colonization and infection. However, such virulence determinants appear to be of less relevance in patients with anatomic or functional abnormalities of the genitourinary tract (65).

## VAGINAL FLORA IN HEALTHY WOMEN

Hormonally mediated events influence the vaginal microflora such that vaginal estrogen increases the glycogen content of vaginal epithelial cells, and this change results in a lower vaginal pH as the glycogen is being metabolized (112). In the prepubertal female, who has little vaginal estrogen, there are a correspondingly low glycogen content in the epithelium and a high vaginal pH of approximately 7.0. Acid-tolerant

---

*Thomas M. Hooton and Walter E. Stamm*, Department of Medicine, University of Washington School of Medicine, Harborview Medical Center, 325 Ninth Avenue, Seattle, Washington 98104.

bacteria do not have a selective advantage in such an environment. In postpubertal females, increased estrogen levels in the vagina lead to glycogen deposition in the epithelial cells and a consequent lowering of vaginal pH. This new environment selects for acid-tolerant and glycogen-metabolizing bacteria such as lactobacilli. In the postmenopausal female, hormonal changes again result in an increase in vaginal pH and profound alterations in the predominant microbial flora of the vagina, with a shift to an anaerobic flora (90). Administration of oral or topical estrogens to postmenopausal women results in a decrease in vaginal pH, an increase in the proportion of women with vaginal lactobacilli, and a decrease in the proportion with *E. coli* (95, 111). In contrast to these changes in the vaginal flora that occur with menarche and the menopause, microbial changes occurring during stages of the menstrual cycle are generally considered insignificant (112). Larsen and Galask, however, found a higher prevalence of several organisms during menstruation than was found several days after menstruation (75).

The microflora of the healthy vagina is made up of a large number of aerobic, facultative anaerobic, and obligate anaerobic species (5, 26, 43, 84, 90, 103, 112). The most prevalent organisms isolated, facultative members of the genus *Lactobacillus*, are isolated in 50 to 90% of women in mean quantities of $10^{7.2}$ to $10^{8.7}$ CFU/g or CFU/ml (112). However, the range among individuals is dramatic ($10^{3.7}$ to $10^{9.8}$ CFU/ml) (26). Obligate anaerobic lactobacilli are found in 29 to 60% of women in similar quantities (112). Aerobic gram-positive cocci, including *Staphylococcus epidermidis* and other *Staphylococcus* species, *Streptococcus* species, and *Enterococcus* species, are the second most frequently detected organisms, found in approximately 30 to 50% of women, generally in quantities 1 to 2 logs less than quantities of lactobacilli (112). Members of the family Enterobacteriaceae are found in approximately 10% of women at counts of $10^{5.1}$ to $10^{6.6}$ CFU/g or CFU/ml (112). Other predominant organisms often seen in the vaginas of healthy women include *Gardnerella vaginalis*, *Corynebacterium* species, *Bacteroides* species, *Fusobacterium* species, and *Veillonella* species (112). As determined by quantitative analysis, anaerobic bacteria are the predominant constituents of the vaginal flora, outnumbering aerobes overall by 10:1 (5).

The prevalence of vaginal colonization with *E. coli* has varied from 0 to 12% in studies of asymptomatic premenopausal women without UTI (5, 24, 84, 90). Marrie et al. found no aerobic gram-negative bacilli in 9 premenarchal girls or in 10 women of reproductive age, but such organisms were found in 5 of 10 postmenopausal women, although quantitatively these organisms represented only 1% of the total flora (90). Rates of *E. coli* vaginal colonization have been reported to be higher following vaginal hysterectomy (75%) (102). *E. coli* prevalence appears to be highest in the early part of the menstrual cycle (12, 24, 75).

## STUDIES OF ADHERENCE OF UROPATHOGENS TO VAGINAL AND UROEPITHELIAL CELLS

Colonization of the urinary tract arises from the interaction of infecting uropathogenic strains with patients' epithelial cells. Experimental studies have shown that persistence of strains in the kidney and bladder is associated with the ability of the strain to adhere to uroepithelial cells (42, 62). Likewise, in girls and women without underlying genitourinary defects but not in women with urological complications, there appears to be an association between adherence of *E. coli* strains to uroepithelial cells in vitro and the presence of and severity of UTI in vivo. Thus, *E. coli* strains from girls and women with acute pyelonephritis or acute cystitis adhere better to uroepithelial cells than do strains from individuals with asymptomatic bacteriuria or from fecal flora in nonbacteriuric subjects (163, 168, 170, 171). In these studies, almost all of the acute pyelonephritis strains, an intermediate number of the acute cystitis strains, and a minority of the asymptomatic bacteriuria and fecal strains attached to vaginal and uroepithelial cells, suggesting that the capacity to adhere is an important virulence factor for *E. coli* in the urinary tract. Schaeffer et al. demonstrated that vaginal strains with the same serotype as strains that later caused UTI adhered as well as urinary isolates, whereas vaginal isolates that did not cause bacteriuria adhered significantly less well (132).

Other investigators, however, have not demonstrated a difference between adhesive properties of bacterial strains from the fecal reservoir and properties of strains causing bacteriuria (36, 44, 132). Harber et al. found that freshly isolated uropathogens almost always had no fimbriae and did not adhere to uroepithelial cells (in contrast to incubated organisms, which generally developed fimbriae and demonstrated adherence) (44). This finding, however, has been challenged by others (108). Further, it has been demonstrated that 25% (44) to 40% (169) of urinary isolates of *E. coli* causing UTI do not adhere to uroepithelial cells, so questions about the importance of bacterial adherence in development of a UTI and about the validity of extrapolation from in vitro adherence data to what happens in vivo arise.

It is not clear, therefore, whether adherence is necessary for a UTI to occur. It does not appear to be necessary for persistence of bacteriuria. Thus, women with asymptomatic bacteriuria may be persistently colonized for years with the same *E. coli* strain that adheres poorly to uroepithelial cells. Women with a history of recurrent symptomatic UTIs refractory to conventional antibiotic therapy were deliberately colonized in the bladder with a mixture of nonvirulent *E. coli* (from a patient with asymptomatic bacteriuria) that lacked expressed adherence factors and transformed bacteria that express P and type 1 fimbriae, which facilitate adherence to epithelial cells (1). These women selectively eliminated the transformants rather than the nonvirulent strain, suggesting that the persistence of *E. coli* in the human urinary tract is determined by factors other than or in addition to adherence. Furthermore, strains causing symptomatic infections accompanied by a host response are likely to be rapidly eliminated, whereas strains that cause asymptomatic bacteriuria have a low frequency of other virulence factors that allow for a minimal host response and thus persistence (162). In another study of the association between bacterial attachment and bacteriuria, uroepithelial cells from healthy girls and women and from girls and women with asymptomatic bacteriuria and a history of recurrent UTI showed no difference in attachment of *E. coli,* but in the healthy subjects more of the attached bacteria were dead (137). In addition, uroepithelial cells from healthy donors suppressed growth of cocultivated *E. coli,* whereas cells obtained from asymptomatic bacteriuria patients did not exhibit any suppressive effect on the growth rate of *E. coli* (137). These data point to a host defect predisposing to asymptomatic bacteriuria, but such a defect has yet to be clearly defined.

The most important uroepithelial-cell receptor for attaching uropathogens appears to be the disaccharide Gal-Gal, which is commonly found in the globoseries glycolipids (66, 79). The importance of the globoseries of glycolipids in adherence of uropathogens is supported by several observations: the attachment of whole bacteria to uroepithelial cells can be inhibited by the globoseries of glycolipids as well as by isolated synthetic receptor oligosaccharides (80); bacteria with receptor specificity for the globoseries of glycolipids attach poorly to cells from individuals of blood group p, which lack this series of glycolipids (66, 79); binding of bacteria to inert surfaces can be induced by addition of the glycolipid receptor (7, 29); and there is a linear relationship between the proportion of bacteria attaching to Gal-Gal-containing receptors and the intensity of the inflammatory response in the urinary tract (167). The globoseries glycolipids, which are receptors for P fimbriae, are distributed in epithelial and nonepithelial tissues of the urinary tract and kidneys (79, 100). Receptors for P fimbriae are also expressed on human colonic epithelial cells (180), and P-fimbriated *E. coli* strains in the large intestines of children prone to UTI persist longer than do other *E. coli* strains (179). Attachment of uropathogens with receptors specific for the globoseries of glycolipids to uroepithelial cells is not inhibited by mannose (mannose resistant).

In humans, O'Hanley et al. found that 100% of *E. coli* strains from patients with pyelonephritis, 65% of strains from patients with cystitis, 17% of strains from patients with asymptomatic bacteriuria, and 29% of fecal strains from pregnant and nonpregnant controls demonstrated Gal-Gal binding (101). In other studies, *E. coli* strains expressing P fimbriae, with or without type 1 fimbriae, made up 76% of pyelonephritis strains, 32% of acute cystitis strains, and 17% of asymptomatic bacteriuria strains and normal fecal strains, whereas strains expressing type 1 fimbriae, with or without P fimbriae, made up 88% of pyelonephritis strains, 94% of cystitis strains, 69% of asymptomatic bacteriuria strains, and 94% of normal fecal strains (165). Likewise, Kallenius et al. demonstrated that 94% of pyelonephritogenic *E. coli* strains but only 7% of fecal *E. coli* strains from healthy controls had P fimbriae (67). The proportion of P-fimbriated strains among acute cystitis isolates (19%) and asymptomatic bacteriuria isolates (14%) was not significantly different from that among fecal isolates. The low prevalence of P-fimbriated strains in women with asymptomatic bacteriuria suggests that P fimbriae are not required for persistence of bacteria in the urinary tract.

Stapleton et al. found 41% of cystitis strains expressing the F adhesin, which is genetically related to the P-fimbria adhesin and also binds globoseries glycolipids, compared with 24% expressing P fimbriae; they also found that both types of fimbriae were more common among cystitis strains than among fecal isolates (154). Expression of P fimbriae alone was found in only 8% of the cystitis isolates. The relative importance of the roles of F and P adhesins in the pathogenesis of UTI has yet to be delineated.

Type 1 fimbriae with mannose-sensitive adhesins, which are blocked by mannose, are common among gram-negative bacteria, including the non-*E. coli* strains associated with UTI (30). Bacteria with mannose-sensitive adhesins generally bind poorly to human uroepithelial cells (121). Given that mannose residues or receptors are widely found in most tissue systems, including the uroepithelium, it is not clear why type 1-fimbriated *E. coli* strains adhere poorly in vitro to uroepithelial cells (121).

The relative importance of type 1-fimbriated *E. coli* strains in the pathogenesis of UTI in women has not been clearly determined. However, data from several studies suggest that type 1 fimbriae play an important role in vaginal colonization and cystitis. Schaeffer et al. evaluated adherence of fecal, vaginal, and bladder isolates of *E. coli* to vaginal epithelial cells from patients with documented recurrent UTI and found that D-mannose completely inhibited adherence of 42% of the 60 strains that had adhered, suggesting that for some strains, mannose-sensitive adhesins have an important role in *E. coli* colonization of the vaginal introitus (130). In addition, in the female green monkey, Roberts et al. demonstrated that an *E. coli* strain with both P and type 1 fimbriae caused vaginal colonization that was of no longer duration than that caused by a strain with only type

1 fimbriae, but the strain with P fimbriae was more likely to cause an ascending infection (125). Studies in the BALB/c mouse UTI model (BALB/c mice exhibit receptors for both type 1 and P fimbriae on their uroepithelial surfaces) demonstrated that whereas P fimbriae are important in development of pyelonephritis, type 1 fimbriae appear to be important in the production of cystitis (100, 135). Other experimental studies with mice have shown that mutant *E. coli* strains recognizing the Gal-Gal receptor have increased persistence in the kidneys compared with strains expressing the mannose-sensitive adhesin, whereas strains with the combination of adhesins with Gal-Gal and mannose specificity are optimal in the bladder (42). Other animal experiments also support the role of type 1 fimbriae in the pathogenesis of UTI (121).

Several studies have demonstrated that *E. coli* adheres to periurethral, vaginal, and/or uroepithelial cells from girls and women with recurrent UTI in much greater numbers than to cells from control patients (37, 68, 131, 132, 169). The underlying reason for this difference has not been established. However, the association with adherence appeared to be nonspecific in one study, prompting the authors to suggest that surface charge and hydrophobic properties may account for differences in adherence between UTI-prone and UTI-resistant individuals (68). Other studies, albeit small, did not show an association between UTI recurrence and adherence, suggesting that differences in adherence may not explain the difference in infection risk between UTI-prone and UTI-resistant women (105, 106).

## CLINICAL STUDIES OF VAGINAL COLONIZATION

### Temporal Association of Vaginal Colonization and UTI

It has been established that colonization of the vaginal introitus with *E. coli* precedes most episodes of asymptomatic bacteriuria or UTI caused by strains with the same serotype, although the preceding colonization may occur only intermittently weeks to months earlier (9, 73, 109, 143, 149). In studies of 16 women with recurrent UTIs, 25 (68%) of 37 episodes of bacteriuria were preceded by the establishment of the responsible pathogen on the vaginal introitus prior to entry of the pathogen into the bladder (143, 149). Eleven of the remaining 12 episodes occurred in patients in whom previous bacteriuria had been proved to be preceded by introital carriage of the responsible organism (143). Furthermore, more frequent culturing may well have allowed detection of preceding colonization prior to more episodes, as it was demonstrated that normal vaginal flora could revert to a "pathogenic one" only a few days before the bacteriuria (149). Bollgren and Winberg demonstrated that premenarchal girls with a history of recurrent UTIs who developed UTIs during a longitudinal study all had heavy colonization of the periurethral and urethral region preceding the bacteriuria, whereas girls who did not develop UTIs during the study period had no such colonization (9). However, in a study of 91 UTI episodes in women with recurrent UTI in which subjects were cultured only once within 12 weeks of the UTI, Brumfitt et al. detected no periurethral colonization in 31 episodes, the patients were colonized with the infective strain (by biotype and O serotype) in 31 episodes, and the patients were colonized only with heterologous strains in 29 episodes (17). In 9 (14%) of another 64 women with UTI, the infecting pathogen was not present in the periurethral flora at the time of diagnosis (17). Others have also shown the absence of introital colonization with the causative pathogen in as many as 32% of women with UTIs (4, 149). Stamey demonstrated the transient nature of colonization in some women who had significant vaginal colonization in cultures 2 days after a negative screening culture (143). Thus, persistent vaginal colonization may not be crucial in the pathogenesis of UTI. On the contrary, vaginally colonizing uropathogens, whether transient or persistent, can probably enter the bladder and cause infection either by spontaneous migration (39, 60) or when aided by mechanical factors such as sexual intercourse (18, 55, 96).

There is general agreement that *E. coli* strains causing UTI usually originate in the fecal flora of the individual. However, it is not entirely clear whether *E. coli* strains that cause UTI are selected because of their high prevalence in the fecal flora (the prevalence theory) or because of a selective advantage of the strain (the special pathogenicity theory) (40). The ability to detect causative strains in the fecal flora depends on the type of UTI (83). Thus, strains causing recurrent asymptomatic bacteriuria in girls appear to be a random sample of the fecal flora (supporting the prevalence theory), whereas strains from symptomatic infections do not appear to be a random sample of the fecal strains (supporting the special pathogenicity theory) (21, 83). Strains causing acute pyelonephritis in the healthy host are clearly a unique subsample of the fecal *E. coli* flora. These pyelonephritogenic strains of *E. coli* are efficient colonizers of the intestinal tract and are the dominating, resident fecal strain prior to onset of acute pyelonephritis (162). In contrast, strains causing pyelonephritis in girls with reflux are relatively more likely to be non-*E. coli* or less virulent *E. coli* (87). It thus appears that fecal strains with a greater capacity to adhere to receptors on vaginal epithelial cells and cells of the upper urinary tract are the strains most likely to cause UTI in normal individuals because their adherence capacity gives them a selective advantage over strains that do not adhere as well. Such strains are more likely to cause more persistent colonization. On the other hand, strains from the general fecal pool likely transiently colonize the vaginal introitus frequently and cause UTI generally only in the setting of a compromised host, such as one with vesicoureteral reflux.

Long-term prospective studies have demonstrated that *E. coli* strains causing UTI may, although appropriately treated and not found in repeated urine cultures in between, cause a new UTI up to 3 years later (14). It is not clear whether such strains persist in the fecal flora or are reacquired from another source. In a recent study of 23 women with recurrent UTI and 35 women with first-episode UTI, *E. coli* strains were evaluated by chromosomal restriction fragment length polymorphism (RFLP) analysis using pulsed-field gel electrophoresis (127). Thirty (68%) of 44 recurrent UTIs, including several that occurred several months apart, were caused by a strain previously identified in that individual, while 32 of the 35 strains from first-episode UTIs had unique RFLP profiles. The fecal flora was a reservoir for the strain reinfecting the urinary tract in a subset of patients analyzed, and it thus appeared that the strain responsible for a recurrent UTI in a given individual was usually eliminated from the urinary tract but persisted in the fecal flora, from which it subsequently recolonized the introitus and bladder and caused symptomatic disease.

## Vaginal Colonization in Women with and without Recurrent UTI

Stamey and others determined that premenopausal women with a history of recurrent UTI are more likely to carry *Enterobacteriaceae* and *Enterococcus faecalis* on the vaginal introital mucosa in greater numbers and for longer periods between infections than women without a history of recurrent UTI (35, 109, 136, 147, 149). These clinical observations corroborate the in vitro studies noted above, which demonstrated increased adherence of *E. coli* to uroepithelial cells in women with a history of recurrent UTI (37, 68, 131, 132, 169).

Stamey and Sexton demonstrated gram-negative bacilli in 56% of the vaginal cultures from 9 women with recurrent UTI but in only 24% of those from 20 women without a history of recurrent UTI ($P = 0.0003$) (147). Those with recurrent UTI had significantly higher prevalences of vaginal colonization with *E. coli, E. faecalis, Proteus mirabilis,* and *Klebsiella* spp. In women with recurrent UTI compared with controls, colonization with gram-negative bacilli was heavier ($\geq 10^4$ CFU/ml in 14.2 versus 0.5% of cultures, respectively) and lasted longer in terms of consecutive visits (mean duration of carriage, 7.9 versus 1.8 weeks, respectively). When bacteriuria developed, the causative organism was the same species of bacteria found on the introitus. The introital flora appears to return to normal in women with recurrent UTI who undergo long-term remission after successful antimicrobial therapy (143, 149).

Other investigators who compared women with and without histories of recurrent UTI generally demonstrated a high prevalence of vaginal colonization with uropathogens but less dramatic differences between the two groups (4, 17, 20, 27, 73). Differences between these various studies may have resulted from a number of factors. For example, some investigators did not culture the women with recurrent UTIs between UTI episodes. Stamey et al. demonstrated that some women with recurrent UTIs undergo long periods of remission, usually with normalization of their vaginal flora (149). In addition, methods of culture may be important, since higher concentrations of periurethral coliforms may characterize women with recurrent UTIs, and careful semiquantitative cultures may be needed to distinguish this state from low-grade colonization.

In a recent prospective study of 40 women (20 with and 20 without recurrent UTI), we, too, demonstrated that vaginal colonization with *E. coli* was common in both cohorts of women (median of 31% of visits in the recurrent-UTI cohort compared with 21% in the control cohort), with some women in both cohorts colonized at almost every visit (58). However, colonization with large quantities of vaginal *E. coli* was more common among women in the recurrent-UTI cohort (median of 29% of visits) than in the control cohort (median of 13% of visits). Although heavy vaginal colonization with *E. coli* was more common in women with recurrent UTI (twofold-greater risk in the recurrent-UTI cohort), the relative risk was considerably less than that for UTI (sixfold-greater risk in the recurrent-UTI cohort). Thus, an increase in colonization per se did not seem sufficient to completely explain the increased rate of infections in the recurrent-UTI cohort. It is possible that women with recurrent UTI have a greater propensity for being colonized with more virulent uropathogens or for colonization to eventuate in infection than women without a history of recurrent infection; this situation would explain the greater infection rates in women with recurrent UTI. Of note, women without recurrent UTI occasionally have heavy growth of introital *E. coli*, and some women with frequent recurrent UTI have no detectable growth of *E. coli* in their vaginas (58, 147).

Kunin et al. (73) argued that introital colonization is likely to be a "permissive" factor that only incompletely explains the pathogenesis of recurrent UTI. They further argued that the absence of a major difference in *E. coli* colonization prevalence between women with and without recurrent UTI makes it unlikely that most women with recurrent infection possess a local periurethral defect in host resistance (73). They believe instead that women with normal genitourinary tracts are likely to be at approximately the same risk for having a first UTI but that, once established, each infection sets the stage for the next episode.

## FACTORS THAT INFLUENCE VAGINAL COLONIZATION WITH UROPATHOGENS

### Host Factors

TYPE OF CELL

Transitional cells derived from the ureters and bladder and squamous cells derived from the urethra and outer genital area differ in their abilities to bind bacteria. Thus, pyelonephritogenic *E. coli* recognizing the globoseries glycolipid receptors attaches to both squamous and transitional cells, whereas *P. mirabilis* and *E. coli* with other receptor specificities bind only to squamous epithelial cells (85, 171). Such binding characteristics may partly explain the difference in frequency of UTI caused by *P. mirabilis* strains, which attach only to squamous cells and not to transitional cells, and UTI caused by uropathogenic *E. coli*, which attaches to both cell types, suggesting that *Proteus* spp. colonize the vaginal and periurethral area as efficiently as *E. coli* but are eliminated more easily from the bladder at voiding unless there are other predisposing factors (171).

SECRETOR STATUS

Several globoseries glycolipids on uroepithelial cells serve as receptors for *E. coli* expressing the P and F adhesins (79, 158). The carbohydrate compositions of globoseries and other cell surface glycolipids, such as the ABO, P, and Lewis antigens, are determined by the synthetic activities of genetically controlled glycosyltransferases (25). The secretor gene also encodes such a glycosyltransferase, and inheritance of this gene thus influences the cell surface glycolipid composition of tissues in which the gene is expressed (25). Women with a history of recurrent UTIs are two to four times more likely to be nonsecretors of histo-blood group antigens than are women without such a history (57, 69, 139). Children with febrile UTIs caused by *E. coli* also have a significantly higher prevalence of the nonsecretor phenotype than control subjects have (64). Further, uroepithelial cells from women who are nonsecretors show enhanced adherence of uropathogenic *E. coli* compared with cells from secretors (85). Recent studies suggest that the quantitative expression of blood group antigens on vaginal cells is a dynamic process and changes over time (133), but the clinical significance of this possibility is not known. It has not been determined whether nonsecretors are at greater risk for pyelonephritis.

In the prospective study of 20 women with and 20 women without recurrent UTI cited above (58), we evaluated 423 rectal and 159 vaginal *E. coli* isolates for P and/or F adhesins (153). P- and/or F-fimbriated *E. coli* strains were highly prevalent in the rectum (40%) and vagina (55%). Nonsecretors who developed UTI during the study period were significantly more likely to be colonized rectally with F-fimbriated *E. coli* than were the infected secretors (56 versus 27%; $P = 0.04$) or uninfected nonsecretors (56 versus 31%; $P = 0.05$). Persistent vaginal and rectal *E. coli* colonization with fimbriated organisms occurred commonly in the study patients but was not often temporally associated with the development of UTI. These results suggest that nonsecretors are more susceptible than secretors to colonization with F-adhesin-bearing *E. coli* isolates.

It has been hypothesized that the secretion of receptor substances in the vaginal fluids of secretors interferes with adhesion of *E. coli* to the vaginal epithelial cells of such women, thus explaining their lower risk of UTI (6, 85). However, more recent data suggest that the biochemical explanation for the increased adherence of *E. coli* to nonsecretors' uroepithelial cells and for the propensity of these patients to develop recurrent UTI may be the presence of unique globoseries glycolipid receptors that bind *E. coli* expressing the P and F adhesins. Through extraction of glycosphingolipids from vaginal epithelial cells collected from nonsecretors and secretors, it has been demonstrated that two extended globoseries glycosphingolipids are selectively expressed by the epithelial cells of nonsecretors but not by those of secretors, presumably as a result of sialylation of the Gal-globoside precursor glycolipid, which in secretors is fucosylated and processed to ABH antigens (155). The expression of these moieties in nonsecretors is not related to ABO status.

## OTHER HISTO-BLOOD GROUP AND HUMAN LEUKOCYTE ANTIGENS

The globoseries glycolipids of the P blood group system, P, $P_1$, and $P^k$, function as receptors for P fimbriae and mediate the adherence of P-fimbriated *E. coli* to colonic and uroepithelial cells (160). The expression of receptors varies with the P blood group. Approximately two-thirds of individuals have the $P_1$ phenotype and the three antigens P, $P_1$, and $P^k$ on their erythrocytes, whereas one-third of individuals have the $P_2$ phenotype, lack the $P_1$ antigen, and may have less of the $P^k$ antigen on their cells (34). Girls with recurrent pyelonephritis who do not have vesicoureteral reflux are more likely to possess the $P_1$ blood group phenotype than age-matched children without UTI or girls with recurrent pyelonephritis who have reflux (86). Thus, 35 (97%) of 36 girls with recurrent pyelonephritis without reflux had the $P_1$ phenotype compared with 63 (75%) of 84 healthy controls ($P < 0.01$) and 27 (84%) of 32 girls with recurrent pyelonephritis with reflux. In a Japanese population, the relative risk of having recurrent pyelonephritis among girls with the $P_1$ phenotype compared with those with the $P_2$ phenotype was 3.5 (174). The $P_1$ blood group phenotype is also overrepresented among women with recurrent pyelonephritis who have no known predisposing factor and underrepresented among girls and women prone to asymptomatic bacteriuria (88). The explanation for these epidemiologic observations remains to be determined. Some investigators have speculated that $P_1$ individuals may have more *E. coli*-binding glycolipids on their uroepithelial cells than $P_2$ individuals do, but Lomberg et al. found no difference in *E. coli* adherence to voided uroepithelial cells from $P_1$ and $P_2$ individuals (85). Others have speculated that perhaps the $P_1$ blood group phenotype influences the expression of Gal-Gal disaccharide-containing receptors in the large intestine and thus the carriage of pyelonephritogenic *E. coli* clones or that anti-$P_1$ antibodies found in individuals of blood group $P_2$ block bacterial binding to target cells and interfere with the infection process (174).

Epidemiologic studies have not shown an association between the ABO or P blood group phenotypes and the risk of cystitis in adult women (56, 139).

Schaeffer et al. found that 12 (34%) of 35 women with recurrent UTI but only 4 (8%) of 50 women without a history of recurrent UTI were positive for human leukocyte antigen A3 ($P = 0.08$), suggesting that recurrent UTIs in women are possibly associated with this antigen (134). None of the other human leukocyte antigens tested had a similar association with recurrent UTI.

## VAGINAL pH

Several studies have demonstrated an association between vaginal fluid pH and bactericidal activity of the vaginal fluid against uropathogens. In women without a history of recurrent UTI, normal vaginal fluid at pH 4.0 is bactericidal to *E. coli*, but as the pH is increased, increasing numbers of *E. coli* survive after inoculation into the vaginal fluid (145). *P. mirabilis* and *Pseudomonas aeruginosa* appear to be much more susceptible to low pH than are the serogroups of *E. coli* that commonly cause UTI (146). Perhaps this partly explains the low prevalence of *Proteus* and *Pseudomonas* spp. in healthy women with acute cystitis. In 169 women aged 18 to 81, colonization with *E. coli, P. mirabilis,* and *E. faecalis* was significantly heavier and more frequent in those with an introital pH greater than 4.4, but there was considerable variation among the women (148). Although a low vaginal pH in the premenopausal woman may have a direct protective effect against UTI, it seems most likely that a low vaginal pH simply reflects a normal vaginal microflora that likely exerts other protective effects against colonization with uropathogens besides pH per se. Interestingly, vaginal pH frequently does not correlate with the presence or absence of lactobacilli, and though most healthy women harbor lactobacilli in their vaginas, not all do (112).

## LOCAL CERVICOVAGINAL ANTIBODY

Data on the role of local vaginal antibody in modifying vaginal colonization are conflicting. Stamey and Howell, who used an agglutination technique, found no difference in local immunoglobulin G (IgG) or IgA concentrations in women with recurrent UTI compared with controls (144). However, in a later study with an indirect immunofluoresence technique using antibody-coated bacteria, only 26% of women with recurrent UTIs demonstrated cervicovaginal antibody production against colonizing introital *E. coli*. In contrast, 77% of women with no history of UTIs demonstrated antibody against their predominant fecal *E. coli* (150). Tuttle et al. demonstrated that children with recurrent UTIs had a lower mean concentration of vaginal IgA than those without a history of UTI (175). Kurdydyk et al. showed that only 3 (14%) of 22 women with recurrent UTI had cervicovaginal antibody directed against their introital *E. coli* but 10 (34%) of 29 control women had cervicovaginal antibody against their fecal *E. coli* ($P = 0.16$) (74). In addition, levels of secretory IgG and IgA as measured by radioimmunoassay were lower in women who had *E. coli* vaginal colonization than in those who did not, but none of these differences were statistically significant. These studies suggest that girls and women with recurrent UTI may have less cervicovaginal antibody than controls have, but the relative importance of this finding is not clear.

## Exposure to Exogenous Agents

### SPERMICIDAL COMPOUNDS

Both sexual intercourse (38, 96, 122, 157) and diaphragm-spermicide use (33, 38, 122, 157) predispose young women to acute UTI. Moreover, as noted above, vaginal colonization with *E. coli* precedes the development of *E. coli* UTI and is presumably an important predisposing event (9, 73, 109, 143, 149). However, the relationship between sexual intercourse with or without diaphragm-spermicide use and alterations in the vaginal flora that might predispose to UTI are less clear. Diaphragm-spermicide users have vaginal colonization with *E. coli* more frequently than oral contraceptive users do (33). We performed the studies described below in an attempt to elucidate the temporal effect of diaphragm-spermicide use and sexual intercourse on the vaginal microflora.

**Observational Study of College Women Using Different Contraceptive Measures before and after Intercourse.** We evaluated the effects of contraceptive method on the occurrence of bacteriuria and vaginal colonization with *E. coli* in 104 women who were evaluated prior to sexual intercourse, the morning after intercourse, and 24 h later (55). After intercourse, the prevalence of *E. coli* bacteriuria increased slightly in oral contraceptive users but dramatically both in spermicidal-foam-and-condom users and in diaphragm-spermicide users. Twenty-four hours later, the prevalence of bacteriuria remained significantly elevated only in the last two groups. Similarly, compared with baseline, vaginal colonization with *E. coli* increased in all three groups but was more dramatic in the diaphragm-spermicide users (26% at baseline versus 61% after diaphragm-spermicide use; $P = 0.0002$) than in foam-and-condom users (9 versus 41%; $P = 0.001$) and oral contraceptive users (15 versus 35%; $P = 0.03$). The effect on vaginal flora was more persistent in users of diaphragm-spermicide and of foam and condoms than in users of oral contraceptives. Vaginal colonization with lactobacilli was present in approximately 95% of women in each of the three groups at baseline and did not change significantly after intercourse in any of the groups. However, vaginal colonization with *Candida* species increased dramatically after intercourse in the group that used diaphragm-spermicide though not in the other two groups. Quantitative vaginal cultures done on a subset of the study population demonstrated no apparent effect on the concentration of lactobacilli or anaerobic species, but facultative bacteria other than lactobacilli, mainly enterococci and coagulase-negative staphylococci, increased 1,000-fold in the diaphragm-spermicide group.

This study demonstrated that bacteriuria and vaginal colonization with *E. coli* frequently follow sexual intercourse and that the effect is mild and transient in oral contraceptive users but much more dramatic and longer lasting in spermicidal-foam-and-condom users and especially in diaphragm-spermicide users.

**Prospective Study of College Women with and without Recurrent UTI.** We evaluated young, sexually active women prospectively over a 6-month period to determine the effects of sexual intercourse and diaphragm-spermicide use on the vaginal microflora (57). Two groups of young women (20 women with a history of recurrent UTI [three or more UTIs in the past year] and 20 women without such a history) were studied to determine whether sexual and contraceptive practices had different effects in women at different risks for UTI. After enrollment, each study patient maintained a daily diary and was seen and cultured at weekly intervals for 6 months to facilitate detailed temporal analysis between factors of interest and alterations in vaginal microflora. Overall, individuals were monitored for a median of 28 weeks and a total of 24.8 person-years.

To evaluate whether recent sexual intercourse alone or sexual intercourse with diaphragm-spermicide use was closely associated temporally with alterations in vaginal flora, visits preceded by no intercourse in the last 3 days were compared with visits preceded either by intercourse without diaphragm-spermicide use or intercourse with diaphragm-spermicide use. In comparing women seen at 414 visits preceded by no intercourse with women seen at 372 visits preceded by intercourse without diaphragm-spermicide use, the prevalences of women colonized vaginally with non-*E. coli* gram-negative uropathogens, group D streptococci, group B streptococci, *Candida* species, lactobacilli, and coagulase-negative staphylococci were nearly identical. *E. coli* was the only pathogen with significantly more common colonization in the postintercourse group ($P = 0.0004$). In contrast, at 192 visits at which sexual intercourse with diaphragm-spermicide use was reported in the 3 preceding days, the vaginal flora showed marked alterations from the status at visits preceded by no sex. Thus, the prevalences of colonization increased from 13 to 59% ($P < 0.0001$) for *E. coli,* from 4 to 20% ($P = 0.0045$) for other aerobic gram-negative uropathogens, from 17 to 33% ($P = 0.014$) for group D streptococci, from 7 to 27% ($P = 0.0015$) for group B streptococci, and from 7 to 40% ($P < 0.0001$) for *Candida* species. *Candida parapsilosis* prevalence increased from 0 to 35%, thus accounting for most of the *Candida* species isolated. Vaginal discharge and a positive wet mount for yeast cells were noted at 17% of the visits at which *C. parapsilosis* was isolated, 22% of the visits at which *Candida* species was isolated, and 0.6% of the visits at which no yeast species were isolated. In contrast to the effect of diaphragm-spermicide use on uropathogens and yeasts, the prevalence of lactobacilli decreased to 68% in association with recent diaphragm-spermicide use from 87% at visits preceded by no sex ($P < 0.0001$).

The effect of intercourse with and without diaphragm-spermicide use was similar in women with a history of recurrent UTI and without such a history except that those with recurrent UTI tended to have higher prevalences of these selected microorganisms, especially of *E. coli* and group D streptococci (57).

Forty-one study visits were preceded by intercourse with spermicide use but not diaphragm use (57). The effect on vaginal microflora after recent spermicide use was similar to that seen with recent diaphragm-spermicide use for some, but not all, of the organisms studied. Thus, the prevalence of colonization after spermicide use was 66% for *E. coli,* 44% for group D streptococci, 15% for coagulase-negative staphylococci, and 54% for lactobacilli but 2% for other gram-negative uropathogens, 7% for group B streptococci, and 2% for *Candida* species (no *C. parapsilosis* was isolated at visits recently preceded by spermicide use alone).

These prospectively collected data demonstrate a temporal relationship between diaphragm-spermicide use and striking alterations in vaginal flora. Sexual intercourse without use of the diaphragm-spermicide, on the other hand, had little effect on vaginal flora except for colonization with *E. coli.* Data from this study confirmed those collected in the previous observational study (55) by showing that under conditions of actual use, diaphragm-spermicide use markedly increases the prevalence of colonization with several different uropathogenic organisms and decreases the prevalence of lactobacillus colonization, whereas intercourse without spermicide or diaphragm-spermicide use is associated with little alteration in the vaginal flora. Although relatively few visits were preceded by recent spermicide use alone, the data available suggest that spermicide exposure itself has a major effect on vaginal ecology.

**In Vitro Studies of Nonoxynol-9.** We and others have performed in vitro studies with nonoxynol-9 to determine how the use of spermicides might result in altered vaginal flora. Nonoxynol-9 is a nonionic surfactant that is the active ingredient in most spermicidal compounds marketed in the United States. It has in vitro antibacterial activity against several sexually transmitted bacteria, viruses, and protozoans (3, 8, 52, 140).

McGroarty et al. (92) reported that the MIC of nonoxynol-9 for most of several uropathogenic bacterial species tested was ≥25%, whereas the MIC for 67% of the vaginal *Lactobacillus* strains tested was ≤1%. Likewise, we found that nonoxynol-9 was markedly less active against the 43 uropathogenic bacterial and yeast strains tested (MIC for 90% of strains [$MIC_{90}$], >32%) than against the 26 *G. vaginalis* strains ($MIC_{90}$, ≤0.015%) and the 53 *Lactobacillus* strains ($MIC_{90}$, 8%) tested (53). Hydrogen peroxide-producing *Lactobacillus* strains were more susceptible to nonoxynol-9 ($MIC_{90}$, 4%) than nonproducers were ($MIC_{90}$, 16%). *E. coli* strains that expressed type 1 fimbriae and vaginal strains of lactobacilli adhered in significantly higher numbers to vaginal epithelial cells preincubated with nonoxynol-9 than to control cells.

It has been hypothesized but not directly demonstrated that lactobacilli, the predominant vaginal organisms in normal women, protect the vagina by competitive exclusion of pathogenic bacteria (112). Hydrogen peroxide, produced by some vaginal *Lactobacillus* strains in almost all healthy women, may also be important in colonization resistance (31). Thus, vaginal colonization with uropathogens and subsequent UTI may be facilitated by alterations in the normal vaginal bacterial flora.

Judging from these in vitro and clinical studies, it seems likely that the differential antimicrobial activities of spermicides alter the vaginal ecosystem, provide an environment conducive to the growth of uropathogens, and thus predispose women who use these products to UTI. Spermicides may provide this selective advantage in colonizing the vagina with nonoxynol-9-resistant uropathogens via a reduction in vaginal lactobacilli (especially hydrogen peroxide-producing strains) and an enhancement of adherence of *E. coli* to epithelial cells. Uropathogens from the fecal reservoir that come into contact with the vaginal introitus during insertion of the diaphragm and during intercourse may be more likely to persist in the introitus in the presence of nonoxynol-9 because of a reduction in colonization resistance attributable to a reduction in vaginal lactobacilli (especially hydrogen peroxide-producing strains). In addition, increased adherence to epithelial cells would favor persistence of *E. coli*. Although lactobacilli also adhere better in the presence of nonoxynol-9, this effect may be negated by the antibacterial activity of the spermicide against many strains.

## ANTIMICROBIAL AGENTS

Antimicrobial prophylaxis is highly effective in reducing the risk of UTI in women with recurrent cystitis (97, 152). The comparative effectiveness of a wide variety of antimicrobial agents, some of which are very active against rectal and vaginal flora and some of which are not, used for prophylaxis in women with recurrent UTI suggests that the presence of an antimicrobial agent in the urine at the time of inoculation by susceptible uropathogens rather than simple eradication of uropathogens colonizing the vaginal or rectal flora accounts for the success of prophylaxis. An example of this is the experience with nitrofurantoin, which, although a highly effective prophylactic agent (97), appears to have little impact on introital colonization with enterobacteria (4). On the other hand, regimens that are more effective in eradicating *E. coli* from the vaginal flora appear to be more effective in reducing the risk of early recurrences following treatment (32), and prophylactic agents that eradicate fecal and vaginal coliforms (namely, trimethoprim-sulfamethoxazole [TMP-SMX] and fluoroquinolones) have generally been the most successful agents used for prophylaxis.

In addition to their antibacterial effects, some antimicrobial agents may reduce bacterial adherence to vaginal cells. Thus, vaginal cells from women with recurrent UTI who are given antimicrobial prophylaxis (with TMP-SMX or cinoxacin) are less receptive to *E. coli* than are vaginal cells of patients who are not given antimicrobial agents (131). If the antimicrobial agent is discontinued, the adherence characteristic returns to normal, and reinfection usually occurs. However, in another study of women on long-term prophylaxis with TMP-SMX, low levels of adherent bacteria were found on freshly voided uroepithelial cells of UTI patients, but the cells remained highly receptive to uropathogens in vitro (115). It thus appears unlikely that antibiotics alter the uroepithelial-cell surface receptors for uropathogens, at least in a major way, for an extended period.

Some antibiotics also appear to have an antiadherence effect on the uropathogen. *E. coli* that is still viable after treatment with subinhibitory amounts of ampicillin and amoxicillin (128, 172, 173) and other antimicrobial agents, including tetracycline, clindamycin, enoxacin, TMP, sulfadiazine, and SMX (19, 156, 176), adhered less well to epithelial cells. Subinhibitory concentrations of chloramphenicol and nitrofurantoin, on the other hand, did not affect the adherence of E. coli (128). In another study, sublethal concentrations of TMP decreased P-fimbria production and adherence of E. coli, but no such effect was found following exposure to fluoroquinolones (72). The mechanism for these effects is not known, but prophylactic antimicrobial agents may be effective in part because of effects other than bacterial killing.

Certain antimicrobial agents, on the other hand, particularly beta-lactams, can facilitate vaginal colonization with uropathogens in animals. In a study of adult female cynomolgus monkeys, who carry the Gal-Gal receptor for P fimbriae, persistent colonization with P-fimbriated E. coli could be obtained in only 4 (17%) of 24 experiments in which the vagina was washed with a suspension of the strain (47). However, when such colonization attempts were performed during intravaginal amoxicillin administration, a persistent and heavy colonization of the vagina occurred in five of five attempts. In a similar study of cynomolgus monkeys, previous exposure to intravaginal cephadroxil also promoted vaginal colonization with cephadroxil-susceptible P-fimbriated E. coli (178). The animals were also vaginally colonized with non-P-fimbriated E. coli strains from the rectum. The total number of indigenous vaginal anaerobic bacteria decreased markedly following cephadroxil exposure. Data from these studies and other amoxicillin studies (49, 51) suggest that facilitation of E. coli colonization by these antimicrobial agents may be due to alterations in the indigenous flora of the vagina and thus altered colonization resistance. Vaginal colonization with E. coli in monkeys could be eliminated by vaginal flushes with vaginal fluid from a healthy monkey, although the effect was not correlated with any increase in vaginal *Lactobacillus* growth (48). TMP and nitrofurantoin, which have much less effect on the periurethral anaerobic flora than amoxicillin does (82), did not result in enhanced vaginal colonization with E. coli in similar monkey experiments (50).

Whether certain antimicrobial agents facilitate susceptibility to UTI in humans has not been determined. It has been noted that the incidence of recurrent UTI among untreated patients with UTI who experience "spontaneous" cure is similar to that of patients cured by antimicrobial agents (89) and that the frequencies of reinfection before and after long-term prophylactic antimicrobial therapy are similar (151). However, ampicillin given to adult women with acute cystitis induces a profound reduction in the indigenous genital flora and a concomitant increase in genital E. coli colonization (116). Amoxicillin given to eight girls with respiratory tract infections resulted in a dramatic decrease in the periurethral anaerobic flora and a concomitant increase in the aerobic gram-negative periurethral flora, which normalized 3 weeks after therapy (81). In contrast, 10 girls given TMP-SMX had no major changes in their anaerobic or aerobic gram-negative microflora during or after therapy. Rosenstein et al. demonstrated that long-term prophylaxis with nitrofurantoin or TMP has no effect on the anaerobic flora of women with recurrent UTI (126). In one study, 119 women attending a family planning clinic who reported antibiotic use either currently or within the previous 4 weeks had a significantly higher prevalence of vaginal coliforms than 1,358 women who did not report recent antimicrobial therapy (24 versus 15%) (177). We found that women with E. coli cystitis who are treated with amoxicillin or cefadroxil are more likely to have persistent vaginal and urethral colonization with E. coli and more frequent recurrences of cystitis than women treated with TMP-SMX or fluoroquinolones (59). The superior efficacy of TMP-SMX and fluoroquinolones in treating cystitis as determined by a 4- to 6-week follow-up suggests that drugs that eradicate introital *E. coli* while maintaining anaerobic flora are associated with the best outcome.

## ESTROGEN

In vitro studies have demonstrated that adherence of *E. coli* (85, 113, 129, 138) and other uropathogens (11, 171, 182) to human vaginal or uroepithelial cells is highest for cells collected during the phase of the menstrual cycle when estrogen peaks. Animal studies have also shown a peak in adherence of bacteria to vaginal epithelial cells during the proestrus and estrus of rats (76, 77) that appeared to be related to estrogen levels (78). Sobel and Kaye demonstrated significantly increased attachment of *E. coli* to both vaginal and bladder epithelial cells in estrogenized rats compared with nonestrogenized rats (141). Moreover, several studies have shown that estrogen treatment facilitates experimental UTI in animals (28, 45, 123). Of note, some studies have not demonstrated any variation in adherence of uropathogens to vaginal epithelial cells during the menstrual cycle (171). Conflicting study results may be due to strain variability in estrogen-mediated alterations in adherence or to technical differences in the assays.

Human studies have shown that vaginal colonization with *E. coli* is most likely during and just after the menses (12, 24, 75). Botta demonstrated that oral contraception could completely abolish the observed cyclic changes in adherence of group B streptococci to human vaginal cells (11). Sharma et al. (138) showed that women administered oral contraceptives had increased adherence of *E. coli* to their uroepithelial cells compared with adherence before hormone administration. However, the cyclical variation in adherence, with the peak level just before the midcycle, was maintained after hormone administration, although the difference in the peak and trough adherence levels was less after hormone administration. Contraceptives possibly increased the risk of UTI in a general population of postmenopausal women (104), although these results were not controlled for possible increases in sexual activity in pill users. In premenopausal women, oral contraceptive use appears not to be associated with an increased risk of UTI (157).

In vitro experiments suggest that estrogens are more likely than progesterones to increase *E. coli* adherence. HeLa cells incubated with increasing concentrations of estrogens had progressively enhanced attachment of *E. coli*, staphylococci, and other bacteria, whereas other hormones, including progesterone, had no such effect (159).

To evaluate a possible association between UTI and the menstrual cycle in women, we studied 577 women enrolled in antimicrobial treatment trials for acute cystitis (58). Patients were administered a standardized questionnaire that asked for the date of onset of the last menstrual cycle. The menstrual cycle was divided into four intervals (days 0 to 7, 8 to 15, 16 to 23, and 24 to 31) for these analyses. Women were significantly more likely to present with UTI 8 to 15 days after the onset of their last menstrual period, which is generally the time of peak estrogen secretion, than at any other time of the cycle (41% presented during this interval) ($P < 0.001$). This association was true for women with UTI caused by *E. coli* (41% presented 8 to 15 days after onset of their cycle; $P < 0.001$) and for those with UTI caused by *S. saprophyticus* (47% presented 8 to 15 days after onset of their cycle; $P < 0.001$). These data demonstrate a strong association between the time at which women present with acute cystitis and the time from the onset of their last menstrual period. The menses-UTI association was independent of age, coital frequency in the previous month, and contraceptive method. We were not able to determine whether this association is due to a hormonal mechanism or to changes in sexual behavior in relation to the menstrual cycle (46, 63, 142).

Recent studies of postmenopausal women further support an association between hormonal status, vaginal flora, and UTI. Previous trials in postmenopausal women, mostly small, unblinded, and uncontrolled, suggested that estrogen replacement using either a topically applied vaginal cream or an orally administered agent lowers the vaginal pH and reduces the occurrence of UTI (13, 70, 107, 110). More recently, Raz and Stamm studied 93 postmenopausal women with a history of recurrent UTI in a randomized, double-blind, placebo-controlled trial of a topically applied intravaginal estriol cream; they evaluated these patients serially every month for 8 months (111). Vaginal cultures were obtained at entry and after 1 and 8 months. The incidence of UTI in the group given estriol was significantly less than that in the placebo group (0.5 versus 5.9 episodes per patient-year; $P < 0.001$). Lactobacilli were absent in all vaginal cultures before treatment and reappeared after 1 month in 61% of the 36 estriol-treated women but in none of 24 placebo recipients ($P < 0.001$). The prevalence of *Enterobacteriaceae* fell from 67 to 31% in estriol recipients but was virtually unchanged in placebo recipients ($P < 0.005$). Likewise, the vaginal pH fell dramatically in the estriol group (from a mean of 5.5 at entry to a mean of 3.6) but remained unchanged in the placebo group. There appeared to be a relation between UTI and vaginal colonization with lactobacilli in that 3 of 23 estriol-treated women who were colonized with lactobacilli after therapy developed UTI compared with 7 of 13 who were not colonized.

In summary, currently available data suggest that estrogens increase adherence of *E. coli* to vaginal and uroepithelial cells. It is possible, but not proven, that the increase in estrogen secretion in the early part of the menstrual cycle facilitates colonization with uropathogens and thus UTI in premenopausal women. In postmenopausal women, however, this effect may be overshadowed by estrogen's effect on restoration of indigenous lactobacilli to the vaginal environment and reduction of colonization and infection with uropathogens, perhaps by lowering pH, production of bactericidal substances, or competitive exclusion of uropathogens from uroepithelial cells.

## MODIFICATION OF THE VAGINAL FLORA TO PREVENT UTI

As noted above, multiple factors appear to influence the risk of vaginal colonization with uropathogens, and each factor offers a potential mechanism to prevent UTIs. The data are convincing that spermicides, especially when used in conjunction with a diaphragm, can alter the vaginal flora and facilitate both colonization with uropathogens and UTI. It is therefore advisable for women with frequent recurrences of UTI to consider changing to another contraceptive or another method of preventing sexually transmitted diseases to see whether there is a benefit in preventing UTIs. Studies have clearly shown that application of topical estrogen to the vagina in postmenopausal women with recurrent UTIs has a dramatic effect on normalization of vaginal flora and prevention of subsequent UTIs. Finally, it appears that TMP-SMX and fluoroquinolones minimally alter the perineal flora following therapy for UTI, while penicillins or cephalosporins may alter the flora such that the risk of recurrence is increased. In the section that follows, creative approaches to UTI prevention through alteration of vaginal colonization,

## Competitive Exclusion with Lactobacilli

Lactobacilli may protect the vagina from colonization by uropathogens through a variety of mechanisms. First, *Lactobacillus* whole cells and cell wall fragments block adherence of uropathogens to uroepithelial cells in vitro, perhaps by steric hindrance or by blocking potential sites of attachment (22, 23). *Lactobacillus* strains have different abilities to adhere to uroepithelial cells and different efficiencies in competitively excluding uropathogens from adhering to uroepithelial cells (120). Second, some *Lactobacillus* strains produce hydrogen peroxide, which may prevent vaginal colonization with uropathogens (31, 71). Third, lactobacilli may influence the vaginal flora through production of inhibitors of bacterial growth (93, 94). Finally, the maintenance of a low pH may be of direct importance, given early observations that introital colonization with *E. coli, P. mirabilis,* and *Enterococcus* spp. was significantly less at a mucosal pH of ≤4 than at a higher pH (148). In a study of 291 women who presented with acute urinary symptoms, we confirmed the association between a high vaginal-fluid pH and introital colonization with *E. coli* and also demonstrated an inverse association between vaginal *E. coli* colonization and vaginal *Lactobacillus* colonization, which suggests that the association of *E. coli* introital colonization with increased vaginal pH may simply reflect a decreased protective effect associated with the loss of lactobacilli (54). The relative importance of these factors in influencing vaginal colonization with uropathogens is unknown.

In 21 of 25 rats tested, *Lactobacillus casei* GR1 instilled into the bladder and swabbed onto the introitus prevented uropathogens subsequently introduced into the bladder from colonizing or stimulating an immune response (119). However, lactobacilli were recovered from the urinary tracts of only three of the animals after uropathogen challenge. To determine whether UTI could be prevented by recolonization of women with persistent UTI, Bruce and Reid conducted a small, uncontrolled study of five women, aged 13 to 56, with recurrent UTI who were given a *Lactobacillus* suspension intravaginally and on the perineum twice weekly for an unspecified period of time (15). The regimen was well tolerated, and Gram stains of vaginal epithelial cells demonstrated lactobacilli after treatment, but no culture results were presented, and no data on the persistence of colonization were provided. Patients appeared to have longer periods without recurrence of UTI than they had had with their previous prevention regimens. In another study, once- or twice-weekly intravaginal instillation of a *Lactobacillus* strain reduced the rate of recurrent UTIs in eight women over a 12-month period by 66% (16).

In a later study, Reid et al. attempted to prevent recurrent UTI in women who had been treated for acute cystitis with either norfloxacin or TMP-SMX (117). Following treatment with a 3-day regimen with these agents, patients were assigned in a blinded and randomized fashion to receive one capsule of a freeze-dried *Lactobacillus* strain or (as placebo) sterilized skim milk powder intravaginally twice weekly for 2 weeks and then at the end of each of the next 2 months. The lactobacilli incorporated into the capsules were selected for their adherence capacities and abilities to inhibit the growth and attachment of uropathogens (120). Three (21%) of 14 women who received lactobacilli and returned for follow-up had a recurrent UTI compared with 8 (47%) of 17 who received placebo ($P = 0.27$). Lactobacilli were absent from the vaginas of 50% of the patients upon entry into the study. Treatment with lactobacilli resulted in a "threefold increase in lactobacillus counts," but it was not stated whether the increase was in the species incorporated into the capsule (117). Some of the women given the placebo capsule had >10-fold increases in lactobacilli, and five of the eight placebo-treated patients who had recurrences had indigenous lactobacilli in their vaginas at the time of recurrence.

In summary, in vitro adherence studies provide convincing evidence that lactobacilli can competitively inhibit *E. coli* adherence to uroepithelial cells. However, although the clinical studies done to date are interesting, none provide convincing data that one can induce persistent colonization with exogenous lactobacilli and thus prevent UTI. Further research in this area is warranted. In this regard, note that lactobacilli isolated from clinical specimens adhere to vaginal epithelial cells in significantly larger amounts than do lactobacilli isolated from yogurt douches (181). In addition, commercial preparations of lactobacilli touted for restoration of vaginal flora often have contaminants and often do not contain the *Lactobacillus* species advertised (61). Genetically engineered lactobacilli that maximize adherence and production of other beneficial characteristics (e.g., $H_2O_2$ production) may offer advantages over wild-type strains.

## Competitive Exclusion with Nonpathogenic *E. coli*

*E. coli* strains with few virulence markers instilled intravesically in women with recurrent UTI colonize the mucosa and apparently interfere with the onset of symptomatic infection, raising the possibility that a genetically engineered avirulent strain could prove useful in high-risk patients who continually fail to respond to conventional prophylaxis measures (41). Considerable additional work would be needed to move this approach from the theoretical to the practical sphere.

## Other Competitive Inhibitors of Bacterial Attachment

### IN VITRO

Several studies have shown that the in vitro attachment of *E. coli* to human or mouse epithelial cells can be inhibited by competitive inhibition with receptor analogs. Thus, the attachment of *E. coli* to human uroepithelial cells in vitro is inhibited by glycolipids of the globoseries as well as by the corresponding isolated oligosaccharides, including the simple disaccharide Gal-Gal (161). The efficiency of the intact glycolipids in reducing attachment of bacteria is greater than that of the isolated sugars on a molar basis. Inhibition of attachment of bacteria to epithelial cells has also been demonstrated with synthetic oligosaccharides that serve as soluble false receptors (80) and mannose or mannose-like sugars (99). In the mouse, in vitro attachment of *E. coli* to epithelial cells was abolished after incubation of the strain with globotetraose (164).

### IN VIVO

Studies with mice have demonstrated that receptor analogs instilled into the vagina or bladder can prevent bacteriuria with *E. coli*. When a mouse UTI model in which bacteria were injected through a urethral catheter was used, *E. coli* preincubated with globotetraose was recovered from both the kidneys and the bladder in significantly reduced numbers compared with levels in controls (164). Use of methyl-$\alpha$-D-mannopyranoside also protected mice from experimental UTI (2).

These studies suggest a possible approach to prophylaxis and treatment of infections occurring on mucous membranes. Compounds mimicking the host receptors may competitively bind to bacterial surface ligands, which might decrease the number of bacteria attaching to the mucosa sufficiently to alter the delicate balance of host-parasite interaction in favor of the host

(164). However, considerable additional work is needed to ascertain whether such approaches are actually feasible from the pharmacologic viewpoint. For example, can the inhibitor be given orally and still be absorbed and delivered to the bladder mucosa in sufficiently high concentrations to be effective? Topically applied inhibitors aimed at preventing vaginal colonization may be more practical.

**Vaccines**
The important topic of vaccines is covered in chapter 15.

**SUMMARY**
Vaginal colonization with *E. coli* appears to be an important determinant of UTI in women. Nevertheless, such colonization may be transient and not detectable in some women, even when they present with UTI. Compared with healthy controls, girls and women with a history of recurrent UTI have greater attachment of *E. coli* to their uroepithelial and vaginal epithelial cells and are more likely to be colonized with *E. coli* in the vagina between recurrences. The reasons for this predilection for greater adherence and colonization among women with recurrent UTI are not clear. In some women, the predilection appears to be genetically determined. In this regard, the nonsecretor phenotype and the $P_1$ phenotype are overrepresented among girls and women with recurrent UTI and recurrent pyelonephritis, respectively. In other women, however, the exogenous factors outlined below may predispose to recurrences. Some data suggest that cervicovaginal antibody may be deficient in women with recurrent UTI.

*E. coli* strains vary in their abilities to adhere to uroepithelial and vaginal epithelial cells. Strains causing cystitis and especially pyelonephritis are more often P fimbriated than are strains causing asymptomatic bacteriuria or strains appearing in the feces of healthy individuals. These fimbriae demonstrate receptor specificity for the Gal-Gal disaccharide in globoseries glycolipids, which constitute a portion of the cell surface of epithelial cells in the urinary and gastrointestinal tracts. Thus, individuals harboring P-fimbriated strains in their feces are presumably at much greater risk for UTI, especially pyelonephritis, than are those not harboring such strains. However, specific factors that predispose to such colonization have not been elucidated.

Several exogenous factors influence the adherence of *E. coli* to uroepithelial and vaginal epithelial cells and vaginal colonization with *E. coli*. Thus, use of spermicide-containing products dramatically affects the vaginal flora, decreasing colonization with lactobacilli and increasing *E. coli* colonization. Such alterations in vaginal flora are thought to at least partly explain the increased risk of UTI among diaphragm-spermicide users. Antimicrobial agents are highly effective in the treatment and prevention of UTI, but studies with primates and humans clearly show that certain antimicrobial agents, particularly amoxicillin and narrow-spectrum cephalosporins, facilitate vaginal colonization and/or UTI with *E. coli,* probably because they adversely affect anaerobic vaginal flora more than other commonly used anti-UTI agents do. In addition, estrogen appears to facilitate *E. coli* adherence and colonization in premenopausal women, but whether it predisposes to UTI in this group is not yet known. Conversely, in postmenopausal women, replacement topical estrogen clearly normalizes the vaginal flora and greatly reduces the risk of UTI.

Several strategies can be used to decrease the risk of UTI by reducing vaginal colonization with uropathogens. A decrease or elimination of the usage of spermicide-containing products would be expected to improve vaginal flora. Likewise, treatment with or prophylactic use of antimicrobial agents that have less impact on the anaerobic vaginal and rectal flora, such as TMP-SMX, nitrofurantoin, or fluoroquinolones, is likely to result in a lower risk of subsequent UTI than use of amoxicillin or a narrow-spectrum cephalosporin. The competitive exclusion of uropathogens with lactobacilli or receptor analogs holds promise, but much more work remains to be done to bring such strategies to the clinical setting. Similarly, although studies of vaccines for the prevention of recurrent UTI in humans have been conducted, a much more detailed understanding of the immune events associated with recurrent UTI is needed before a rational vaccine strategy can be developed.

## REFERENCES

1. **Andersson, P., I. Engberg, G. Lidin-Janson, K. Lincoln, R. Hull, S. Hull, and C. Svanborg.** 1991. Persistence of *Escherichia coli* bacteriuria is not determined by bacterial adherence. *Infect. Immun.* **59:**2915–2921.
2. **Aronson, M., O. Medalia, L. Schori, D. Mirelman, N. Sharon, and I. Ofek.** 1979. Prevention of colonization of the urinary tract of mice with *Escherichia coli* by blocking of bacterial adherence with methyl alpha-D-mannopyranoside. *J. Infect. Dis.* **139:**329–332.
3. **Asculai, S. S., M. T. Weis, M. W. Rancourt, and A. B. Kupferberg.** 1978. Inactivation of herpes simplex virus by nonionic surfactants. *Antimicrob. Agents Chemother.* **13:**686–690.
4. **Bailey, R. R., A. P. Roberts, P. E. Gower, and G. Stacey.** 1973. Urinary-tract infection in non-pregnant women. *Lancet* **ii:**275–277.
5. **Bartlett, J. G., A. B. Onderdonk, E. Drude, C. Goldstein, M. Anderka, S. Alpert, and W. M. McCormack.** 1977. Quantitative bacteriology of the vaginal flora. *J. Infect. Dis.* **136:**271–277.
6. **Blackwell, C. C.** 1989. The role of ABO blood groups and secretor status in host defences. *FEMS Microbiol. Immunol.* **47:**341–350.
7. **Bock, K., M. E. Breimer, A. Brignole, G. C. Hansson, K.-A. Karlsson, G. Larson, H. Leffler, B. E. Samuelsson, N. Stromberg, C. Svanborg Eden, and J. Thursin.** 1985. Specificity of binding of a strain of uropathogenic *Escherichia coli* to Gal$\alpha$1-4Gal-containing glycosphingolipids. *J. Biol. Chem.* **260:**8545–8551.
8. **Bolch, O. H., and J. C. Warren.** 1973. In vitro effects of Emko on *Neisseria gonorrhoeae* and *Trichomonas vaginalis*. *Am. J. Obstet. Gynecol.* **115:**1145–1148.
9. **Bollgren, I., and J. Winberg.** 1976. The periurethral aerobic flora in girls highly susceptible to urinary infections. *Acta Paediatr. Scand.* **65:**81–87.
10. **Bollgren, I.** 1979. Periurethral anaerobic microflora of healthy girls. *J. Clin. Microbiol.* **10:**419–424.
11. **Botta, G. A.** 1979. Hormonal and type-dependent adhesion of group B streptococci to human vaginal cells. *Infect. Immun.* **25:**1084–1086.
12. **Botta, G. A., D. Pedulla, G. Melioli, S. Madoff, and L. Minuto.** 1981. Absence of fluctuation in vaginal colonization by Enterobacteriaceae during their menstrual cycle in patients with recurrent cystitis. *Lancet* **ii:**1116–1117.
13. **Brandberg, A., D. Mellstrom, and G. Samsioe.** 1987. Low dose oral estriol treatment in elderly women with urogenital infections. *Acta Obstet. Gynecol. Scand. Suppl.* **140:**33–38.
14. **Brauner, A., S. H. Jacobson, and I. Kuhn.** 1992. Urinary *Escherichia coli* causing recurrent infections—a prospective follow-up of biochemical phenotypes. *Clin. Nephrol.* **38:**318–323.
15. **Bruce, A. W., and G. Reid.** 1988. Intravaginal instillation of lactobacilli for prevention of recurrent urinary tract infections. *Can. J. Microbiol.* **34:**339–343.
16. **Bruce, A. W., G. Reid, J. A. McGroarty, M. Taylor, and C. Preston.** 1992. Preliminary study on the prevention of recurrent urinary tract infection in adult women using intravaginal lactobacilli. *Int. Urogynecol. J.* **3:**22–25.
17. **Brumfitt, W., R. A. Gargan, and J. M. T. Hamilton-Miller.** 1987. Periurethral enterobacterial carriage preceding urinary infection. *Lancet* **i:**824–826.
18. **Buckley, R. M., M. McGuckin, and R. R. MacGregor.** 1978. Urine bacterial counts after sexual intercourse. *N. Engl. J. Med.* **298:**321–324.
19. **Burnham, J. C.** 1988. Mediation by enoxacin of adherence of *Escherichia coli* to uroepithelial cells. *Rev. Infect. Dis.* **10:**S175.
20. **Cattell, W. R., M. A. McSherry, A. Northeast, E. Powell, H. J. L. Brooks,**

and F. O'Grady. 1974. Periurethral enterobacterial carriage in pathogenesis of recurrent urinary infection. *Br. Med. J.* **2:** 136–139.
21. **Caugant, D. A., B. R. Levin, G. Lidin-Janson, T. S. Whittam, C. Svanborg Eden, and R. K. Selander.** 1983. Genetic diversity and relationships among strains of *Escherichia coli* in the intestine and those causing urinary tract infections. *Prog. Allergy* **33:** 203–227.
22. **Chan, R. C. Y., A. W. Bruce, and G. Reid.** 1984. Adherence of cervical, vaginal and distal urethral normal microbial flora to human uroepithelial cells and the inhibition of adherence of gram-negative uropathogens by competitive exclusion. *J. Urol.* **131:** 596–601.
23. **Chan, R. C. Y., G. Reid, R. T. Irwin, A. W. Bruce, and J. W. Costerton.** 1985. Competitive exclusion of uropathogens from human uroepithelial cells by *Lactobacillus* whole cells and cell wall fragments. *Infect. Immun.* **47:**84–89.
24. **Chow, A. W., R. Percival-Smith, K. H. Bartlett, A. M. Goldring, and B. J. Morrison.** 1986. Vaginal colonization with *Escherichia coli* in healthy women: determination of relative risks by quantitative culture and multivariate statistical analysis. *Am. J. Obstet. Gynecol.* **154:**120–126.
25. **Clausen, H., and S. I. Hakomori.** 1989. ABO and related histo-blood group antigens: immunochemical differences in carrier isotypes and their distribution. *Vox Sang* **56:** 1–20.
26. **Cook, R., G. Tannock, and R. Meech.** 1984. The normal microflora of the vagina. *Proc. Univ. Otago Med. School* **62:**72–74.
27. **Cooper, J., W. Brumfitt, J. M. T. Hamilton-Miller, and A. V. Reynolds.** 1980. The role of periurethral colonization in the aetiology of recurrent urinary infection in women. *Br. J. Obstet. Gynaecol.* **87:** 1145–1151.
28. **Corriere, J. N., Jr., and J. J. Murphy.** 1968. The effect of oestrogen upon ascending urinary tract infection in rats. *Br. J. Urol.* **40:**306–314.
29. **de Man, P., B. Cedergren, S. Enerbäck, A.-C. Larsson, H. Leffler, A.-L. Lundell, B. Nilsson, and C. Svanborg-Edén.** 1987. Receptor-specific agglutination tests for detection of bacteria that bind globoseries glycolipids. *J. Clin. Microbiol.* **25:** 401–406.
30. **Duguid, J. P., and D. C. Old.** 1980. Adhesive properties of enterobacteriaceae, p. 187–217. *In* E. H. Beachey (ed.), *Bacterial Adherence*. Chapman & Hall Ltd., London.
31. **Eschenbach, D. A., P. R. Davick, B. L. Williams, S. J. Klebanoff, K. Young-Smith, C. M. Critchlow, and K. K. Holmes.** 1989. Prevalence of hydrogen peroxide-producing *Lactobacillus* species in normal women and women with bacterial vaginosis. *J. Clin. Microbiol.* **27:**251–256.
32. **Fihn, S. D., C. Johnson, P. L. Roberts, K. Running, and W. E. Stamm.** 1988. Trimethoprim-sulfamethoxazole for acute dysuria in women: a single-dose or 10-day course. *Ann. Intern. Med.* **108:**350–357.
33. **Fihn, S. D., R. H. Latham, P. Roberts, K. Running, and W. E. Stamm.** 1985. Association between diaphragm use and urinary tract infection. *JAMA* **254:**240–245.
34. **Fletcher, K. S., E. G. Bremer, and G. A. Schwarting.** 1979. P blood group regulation of glycosphingolipid levels in human erythrocytes. *J. Biol. Chem.* **254:** 11196–11198.
35. **Fowler, J. E., R. Latta, and T. A. Stamey.** 1977. Studies of introital colonization in women with recurrent urinary infections. VIII. The role of bacterial interference. *J. Urol.* **118:**296–298.
36. **Fowler, J. E., and T. A. Stamey.** 1978. Studies of introital colonization in women with recurrent urinary infections. X. Adhesive properties of *Escherichia coli* and *Proteus mirabilis*: lack of correlation with urinary pathogenicity. *J. Urol.* **120:**315–318.
37. **Fowler, J. E., Jr., and T. A. Stamey.** 1977. Studies of introital colonization in women with recurrent urinary infections. VII. The role of bacterial adherence. *J. Urol.* **117:**472–476.
38. **Foxman, B., and R. R. Frerichs.** 1985. Epidemiology of urinary tract infection. I. Diaphragm use and sexual intercourse. *Am. J. Public Health* **75:**1308–1313.
39. **Furtado, D., and D. Garrison.** 1967. The distribution of *Aerobacter aerogenes* in the urinary tract of guinea pigs following ascending routes of inoculation. *J. Urol.* **98:**267–273.
40. **Gruneberg, R. N., D. A. Leigh, and W. Brumfitt.** 1968. *Escherichia coli* serotypes in urinary tract infection: studies in domiciliary, antenatal and hospital practice, p. 68–79. *In* F. O'Grady and W. Brumfitt (ed.), *Urinary Tract Infection. Proceedings of the First National Symposium, London, April 1968.* Oxford University Press, Oxford.
41. **Hagberg, L., A. W. Bruce, G. Reid, C. Svanborg Eden, K. Lincoln, and G.**

Lidin-Janson. 1989. Colonization of the urinary tract with bacteria from the normal fecal and urethral flora in patients with recurrent urinary tract infections, p. 194–197. *In* E. H. Kass and C. Svanborg Eden (ed.), *Host-Parasite Interactions in Urinary Tract Infections*. University of Chicago Press, Chicago.

42. Hagberg, L., R. Hull, S. Hull, S. Falkow, R. Freter, and C. Svanborg. 1983. Contribution of adhesion to bacterial persistence in the mouse urinary tract. *Infect. Immun.* **40**:265–272.

43. Hammill, H. A. 1989. Normal vaginal flora in relation to vaginitis. *Obstet. Gynecol. Clin. North Am.* **16**:329–336.

44. Harber, M. J., R. Mackenzie, S. Chick, and A. W. Asscher. 1982. Lack of adherence to epithelial cells by freshly isolated urinary pathogens. *Lancet* **ii**:586–588.

45. Harle, E. M. J., J. J. Bullen, and D. A. Thomson. 1975. Influence of oestrogen on experimental pyelonephritis caused by *Escherichia coli*. *Lancet* **ii**:283–286.

46. Hedricks, C., L. J. Piccinino, J. R. Udry, and T. H. Chimbira. 1987. Peak coital rate coincides with onset of leuteinizing hormone surge. *Fertil. Steril.* **48**:234–238.

47. Herthelius, B. M., K. G. Hedstrom, R. Möllby, C. E. Nord, L. Pettersson, and J. Winberg. 1988. Pathogenesis of urinary tract infections—amoxicillin induces genital *Escherichia coli* colonization. *Infection* **16**:263–266.

48. Herthelius, M., S. L. Gorbach, R. Möllby, C. E. Nord, L. Pettersson, and J. Winberg. 1989. Elimination of vaginal colonization with *Escherichia coli* by administration of indigenous flora. *Infect. Immun.* **57**:2447–2451.

49. Herthelius, M., R. Möllby, C. E. Nord, and J. Winberg. 1989. Amoxicillin promotes vaginal colonization with adhering *Escherichia coli* present in faeces. *Paediatr. Nephrol.* **3**:443–447.

50. Herthelius-Elman, M., R. Mollby, C. E. Nord, and J. Winberg. 1992. Lack of effect of trimethoprim and nitrofurantoin on colonization resistance in the vagina of monkeys. *Infection* **20**:105–110.

51. Herthelius-Elman, M., R. Mollby, C. E. Nord, and J. Winberg. 1992. The effect of amoxycillin on vaginal colonization resistance and normal vaginal flora in monkeys. *J. Antimicrob. Chemother.* **29**:329–340.

52. Hicks, D. R., L. S. Martin, J. P. Getchell, J. L. Heath, D. P. Francis, J. S. McDougal, J. W. Curran, and B. Voeller. 1985. Inactivation of HTLV-III/LAV-infected cultures of normal human lymphocytes by nonoxynol-9 in vitro. *Lancet* **ii**:1422–1423.

53. Hooton, T. M., C. L. Fennell, A. M. Clark, and W. E. Stamm. 1991. Nonoxynol-9: differential antibacterial activity and enhancement of bacterial adherence to vaginal epithelial cells. *J. Infect. Dis.* **164**:1216–1219.

54. Hooton, T. M., S. D. Fihn, C. Johnson, P. L. Roberts, and W. E. Stamm. 1989. Association between bacterial vaginosis and acute cystitis in women using diaphragms. *Arch. Intern. Med.* **149**:1932–1936.

55. Hooton, T. M., S. Hillier, C. Johnson, P. L. Roberts, and W. E. Stamm. 1991. *Escherichia coli* bacteriuria and contraceptive method. *JAMA* **265**:64–69.

56. Hooton, T. M., C. Johnson, P. L. Roberts, and W. E. Stamm. 1989. The association of sex, with or without diaphragm and spermicide use, with UTI, abstr. 8, p. 102. *Program Abstr. 29th Intersci. Conf. Antimicrob. Agents. Chemother. Am. Soc. Microbiol.*

57. Hooton, T. M., P. L. Roberts, and W. E. Stamm. 1994. Effects of recent sexual activity and use of a diaphragm on the vaginal microflora. *Clin. Infect. Dis.* **19**:274–278.

58. Hooton, T. M., and W. E. Stamm. Unpublished data.

59. Hooton, T. M., C. Winter, F. Tiu, and W. E. Stamm. 1995. Randomized comparative trial and cost analysis of 3-day antimicrobial regimens for treatment of acute cystitis in women. *JAMA* **273**:41–45.

60. Hopkins, W. J., J. A. Hall, B. P. Conway, and D. T. Uehling. 1995. Induction of urinary tract infection by intraurethral inoculation with *Escherichia coli*: refining the murine model. *J. Infect. Dis.* **171**:462–465.

61. Hughes, V. L., and S. L. Hillier. 1990. Microbiologic characteristics of *Lactobacillus* products used for colonization of the vagina. *Obstet. Gynecol.* **75**:244–248.

62. Iwahi, T., Y. Abe, M. Nakao, A. Imada, and K. Tsuchiya. 1983. Role of type 1 fimbriae in the pathogenesis of ascending urinary tract infection induced by *Escherichia coli* in mice. *Infect. Immun.* **39**:1307–1315.

63. James, W. H. 1971. The distribution of coitus within the human intermenstruum. *J. Biosoc. Sci.* **3**:159–171.

64. Jantausch, B. A., V. R. Criss, R. O'Donnell, B. L. Wiedermann, M. Majd, H. G. Rushton, R. S. Shirey, and N. L. C. Luban. 1994. Association of Lewis blood group phenotypes with urinary tract infection in children. *J. Pediatr.* **124**:863–868.

65. Johnson, J. R. 1991. Virulence factors in *Escherichia coli* urinary tract infection. *Clin. Microbiol. Rev.* **4**:80–128.
66. Kallenius, G., R. Mollby, S. B. Svenson, J. Winberg, A. Lundblad, S. Svensson, and B. Cedergren. 1980. The p$^k$ antigen as receptor for the haemagglutinin of pyelonephritic *Escherichia coli*. *FEMS Microbiol. Lett.* **7**:297–302.
67. Kallenius, G., S. B. Svenson, H. Hultberg, R. Mollby, I. Helin, B. Cedergren, and J. Winberg. 1981. Occurrence of P-fimbriated *Escherichia coli* in urinary tract infections. *Lancet* **ii**:1369–1372.
68. Kallenius, G., and J. Winberg. 1978. Bacterial adherence to periurethral epithelial cells in girls prone to urinary-tract infections. *Lancet* **ii**:540–543.
69. Kinane, D. F., C. C. Blackwell, R. P. Brettle, D. M. Weir, F. P. Winstanley, and R. A. Elton. 1982. ABO blood group, secretor state, and susceptibility to recurrent urinary tract infection in women. *Br. Med. J.* **285**:7–9.
70. Kirkengen, A. L., P. Andersen, E. Gjersoe, G. R. Johannessen, N. Johnsen, and E. Bodd. 1992. Oestriol in the prophylactic treatment of recurrent urinary tract infections in postmenopausal women. *Scand. J. Primary Health Care* **10**:139–142.
71. Klebanoff, S. J., S. L. Hillier, D. A. Eschenbach, and A. M. Waltersdorph. 1991. Control of the microbial flora of the vagina by $H_2O_2$-generating lactobacilli. *J. Infect. Dis.* **164**:94–100.
72. Kovarik, J. M., I. M. Hoepelman, and J. Verhoef. 1989. Influence of fluoroquinolones on expression and function of P fimbriae in uropathogenic *Escherichia coli*. *Antimicrob. Agents Chemother.* **33**:684–688.
73. Kunin, C. M., F. Polyak, and E. Postel. 1980. Periurethral bacterial flora in women. Prolonged intermittent colonization with *Escherichia coli*. *JAMA* **243**:134–139.
74. Kurdydyk, L. M., K. Kelly, G. K. M. Harding, P. Mirwaldt, L. Thompson, F. J. Buckwold, and A. R. Ronald. 1980. Role of cervicovaginal antibody in the pathogenesis of recurrent urinary tract infection in women. *Infect. Immun.* **29**:76–82.
75. Larsen, B., and R. P. Galask. 1982. Vaginal microbial flora: composition and influences of host physiology. *Ann. Intern. Med.* **96**:926–930.
76. Larsen, B., A. J. Markovetz, and R. P. Galask. 1976. Quantitative alterations in the genital microflora of female rats in relation to the estrous cycle. *J. Infect. Dis.* **134**:486–489.
77. Larsen, B., A. J. Markovetz, and R. P. Galask. 1977. Relationship of vaginal cytology to alterations of the vaginal microflora of rats during the estrous cycle. *Appl. Environ. Microbiol.* **33**:556–562.
78. Larsen, B., A. J. Markovetz, and R. P. Galask. 1977. Role of estrogen in controlling the genital microflora of female rats. *Appl. Environ. Microbiol.* **34**:534–540.
79. Leffler, H., and C. Svanborg Eden. 1980. Chemical identification of a glycosphingolipid receptor for *Escherichia coli* attaching to human urinary tract cells and agglutinating human erythrocytes. *FEMS Microbiol. Lett.* **8**:127–134.
80. Leffler, H., and C. Svanborg-Eden. 1986. Glycolipids as receptors for *Escherichia coli* lectins or adhesins, p. 83–111. *In* D. Mirelman (ed.), *Microbial Lectins*. John Wiley & Sons, Inc., New York.
81. Lidefelt, K. J., I. Bollgren, and C. E. Nord. 1991. Changes in periurethral microflora after antimicrobial drugs. *Arch. Dis. Child.* **66**:683–685.
82. Lidefelt, K. J., I. Bollgren, A. Wiman, and C. E. Nord. 1990. Antibiotic susceptibility of periurethral anaerobic microflora in healthy girls. *Drugs Exp. Clin. Res.* **16**:417–422.
83. Lidin-Janson, G., L. A. Hanson, B. Kaijser, K. Lincoln, U. Lindberg, S. Olling, and H. Wedel. 1977. Comparison of *Escherichia coli* from bacteriuric patients with those from feces of healthy school-children. *J. Infect. Dis.* **136**:346–353.
84. Lindner, J. G. E. M., F. H. F. Plantema, and J. A. A. Hoogkamp-Korstanje. 1978. Quantitative studies of the vaginal flora of healthy women and of obstetric and gynaecological patients. *J. Med. Microbiol.* **11**:233–241.
85. Lomberg, H., B. Cedergren, H. Leffler, B. Nilsson, A. S. Carlstrom, and C. Svanborg-Eden. 1986. Influence of blood group on the availability of receptors for attachment of uropathogenic *Escherichia coli*. *Infect. Immun.* **51**:919–926.
86. Lomberg, H., L. A. Hanson, B. Jacobsson, U. Jodal, H. Leffler, and C. Svanborg Eden. 1983. Correlation of P glood group, vesicoureteral reflux, and bacterial attachment in patients with recurrent pyelonephritis. *N. Engl. J. Med.* **308**:1189–1192.
87. Lomberg, H., M. Hellstrom, U. Jodal, H. Leffler, K. Lincoln, and C. Svanborg

Eden. 1984. Virulence-associated traits in *Escherichia coli* causing first and recurrent episodes of urinary tract infection in children with or without vesicoureteral reflux. *J. Infect. Dis.* **150**:561–569.

88. Lomberg, H., and C. Svanborg Eden. 1989. Influence of P blood group phenotype on susceptibility to urinary tract infection. *FEMS Microbiol. Immun.* **47**:363–370.

89. Mabeck, C. E. 1972. Treatment of uncomplicated urinary tract infection in non-pregnant women. *Postgrad. Med. J.* **48**:69–75.

90. Marrie, T. J., C. A. Swantee, and M. Hartlen. 1980. Aerobic and anaerobic urethral flora of healthy females in various physiological age groups and of females with urinary tract infections. *J. Clin. Microbiol.* **11**:654–659.

91. Marsh, E. P., M. Murray, and P. Panchamia. 1972. The relationship between bacterial cultures of the vaginal introitus and urinary infection. *Br. J. Urol.* **44**:368–375.

92. McGroarty, J. A., S. Chong, G. Reid, and A. W. Bruce. 1990. Influence of the spermicidal compound nonoxynol-9 on the growth and adhesion of urogenital bacteria in vitro. *Curr. Microbiol.* **21**:219–223.

93. McGroarty, J. A., and G. Reid. 1988. Detection of a lactobacillus substance that inhibits *Escherichia coli*. *Can. J. Microbiol.* **34**:974–978.

94. McGroarty, J. A., and G. Reid. 1988. Inhibition of enterococci by *Lactobacillus* species in vitro. *Microb. Ecol. Health Dis.* **1**:215–219.

95. Molander, U., I. Milsom, P. Ekelund, D. Mellstrom, and O. Eriksson. 1990. Effect of oral oestriol on vaginal flora and cytology and urogenital symptoms in the post-menopause. *Maturitas* **12**:113–120.

96. Nicolle, L. E., G. K. M. Harding, J. Preikasaitis, and A. R. Ronald. 1982. The association of urinary tract infection with sexual intercourse. *J. Infect. Dis.* **146**:579–583.

97. Nicolle, L. E., and A. R. Ronald. 1987. Recurrent urinary tract infection in adult women: diagnosis and treatment. *Infect. Dis. Clin. North Am.* **1**:793–806.

98. Norden, C. W., G. M. Green, and E. H. Kass. 1968. Antibacterial mechanisms of the urinary bladder. *J. Clin. Invest.* **47**:2689–2700.

99. Ofek, I., D. Mirelman, and N. Sharon. 1977. Adherence of *Escherichia coli* to human mucosal cells mediated by mannose receptors. *Nature* (London) **265**:623–625.

100. O'Hanley, P., D. Lark, S. Falkow, and G. Schoolnik. 1985. Molecular basis of *Escherichia coli* colonization of the upper urinary tract in BALB/c mice. *J. Clin. Invest.* **75**:347–360.

101. O'Hanley, P., D. Low, I. Romero, D. Lark, K. Vosti, S. Falkow, and G. Schoolnik. 1985. Gal-Gal binding and hemolysin phenotypes and genotypes associated with uropathogenic *Escherichia coli*. *N. Engl. J. Med.* **313**:414–420.

102. Ohm, M. J., and R. P. Galask. 1975. The effect of antibiotic prophylaxis on patients undergoing vaginal operations. II. Alterations of microbial flora. *Am. J. Obstet. Gynecol.* **123**:597–604.

103. Onderdonk, A. B., B. F. Polk, N. E. Moon, B. Goren, and J. G. Bartlett. 1977. Methods for quantitative vaginal flora studies. *Am. J. Obstet. Gynecol.* **128**:777–781.

104. Orlander, J. D., S. S. Jick, A. D. Dean, and H. Jick. 1992. Urinary tract infections and estrogen use in older women. *J. Am. Geriatr. Soc.* **40**:817–820.

105. Parsons, C. L., H. Anwar, C. Stauffer, and J. D. Schmidt. 1979. In vitro adherence of radioactively labeled *Escherichia coli* in normal and cystitis-prone females. *Infect. Immun.* **26**:453–457.

106. Parsons, C. L., and J. D. Schmidt. 1980. In vitro bacterial adherence to vaginal cells of normal and cystitis-prone women. *J. Urol.* **123**:184–186.

107. Parsons, C. L., and J. D. Schmidt. 1982. Control of recurrent lower urinary tract infection in the postmenopausal woman. *J. Urol.* **128**:1224–1226.

108. Pere, A., B. Nowicki, H. Saxen, A. Siitonen, and T. K. Korhonen. 1987. Expression of P, type-1, and type-1C fimbriae of *Escherichia coli* in the urine of patients with acute urinary tract infection. *J. Infect. Dis.* **156**:567–574.

109. Pfau, A., and T. Sacks. 1981. The bacterial flora of the vaginal vestibule, urethra and vagina in premenopausal women with recurrent urinary tract infections. *J. Urol.* **126**:630–634.

110. Privette, M., R. Cade, J. Peterson, and D. Mars. 1988. Prevention of recurrent urinary tract infections in postmenopausal women. *Nephron* **50**:24–27.

111. Raz, R., and W. E. Stamm. 1993. A controlled trial of intravaginal estriol in postmenopausal women with recurrent urinary tract infections. *N. Engl. J. Med.* **329**:753–756.

112. Redondo-Lopez, V., R. L. Cook, and J. D. Sobel. 1990. Emerging role of lactobacilli in the control and maintenance of the

vaginal bacterial microflora. *Rev. Infect. Dis.* **12**:856–872.

113. **Reid, G., J. L. Brooks, and D. F. Bacon.** 1983. In vitro attachment of *Escherichia coli* to human uroepithelial cells: variation in receptivity during the menstrual cycle and pregnancy. *J. Infect. Dis.* **148**:412–420.

114. **Reid, G., and A. W. Bruce.** 1991. Development of lactobacilli therapy to prevent recurrent urinary tract infections in females. *Int. Urogynecol. J.* **2**:40–43.

115. **Reid, G., A. W. Bruce, and M. Beheshti.** 1988. Effect of antibiotic treatment on receptivity of uroepithelial cells to uropathogens. *Can. J. Microbiol.* **34**:327–331.

116. **Reid, G., A. W. Bruce, R. L. Cook, and M. Llano.** 1990. Effect on urogenital flora of antibiotic therapy for urinary tract infection. *Scand. J. Infect. Dis.* **22**:43–47.

117. **Reid, G., A. W. Bruce, and M. Taylor.** 1992. Influence of three-day antimicrobial therapy and lactobacillus vaginal suppositories on recurrence of urinary tract infections. *Clin. Ther.* **14**:11–16.

118. **Reid, G., A. W. Bruce, and D. T. Uehling.** 1991. Vaginal flora and urinary tract infections. *Curr. Opin. Infect. Dis.* **4**:37–41.

119. **Reid, G., R. C. Y. Chan, A. W. Bruce, and J. W. Costerton.** 1985. Prevention of urinary tract infection in rats with an indigenous *Lactobacillus casei* strain. *Infect. Immun.* **49**:320–324.

120. **Reid, G., R. L. Cook, and A. W. Bruce.** 1987. Examination of strains of lactobacilli for properties which may influence bacterial interference in the urinary tract. *J. Urol.* **138**:330–335.

121. **Reid, G., and J. D. Sobel.** 1987. Bacterial adherence in the pathogenesis of urinary tract infection: a review. *Rev. Infect. Dis.* **9**:470–487.

122. **Remis, R. S., M. J. Gurwith, D. Gurwith, N. T. Hargrett-Bean, and P. M. Layde.** 1987. Risk factors for urinary tract infection. *Am. J. Epidemiol.* **126**:685–694.

123. **Riedasch, G., K. Setzis, W. Bersch, and E. Ritz.** 1983. Estrogens influence antibody coating in experimental urinary tract infection. *Klin. Wochenschr.* **61**:529–531.

124. **Roberts, A. P., and R. Phillips.** 1979. Bacteria causing symptomatic urinary tract infection or asymptomatic bacteriuria. *J. Clin. Pathol.* **32**:492–496.

125. **Roberts, J. A., M. B. Kaack, and E. N. Fussell.** 1989. Bacterial adherence in urinary tract infections: preliminary studies in a primate model. *Infection* **17**:401–404.

126. **Rosenstein, I. J., H. Ludlam, J. M. T. Hamilton-Miller, and W. Brumfitt.** 1980. Anaerobic periurethral flora of healthy women and women susceptible to urinary-tract infection. *J. Med. Microbiol.* **15**:565–568.

127. **Russo, T. A., A. Stapleton, S. Wenderoth, T. M. Hooton, and W. E. Stamm.** 1995. Chromosomal restriction fragment length polymorphism analysis of *Escherichia coli* strains causing recurrent urinary tract infections in young women. *J. Infect. Dis.*, **172**:440–445.

128. **Sandberg, T., K. Stenqvist, and C. Svanborg-Eden.** 1979. Effects of subminimal inhibitory concentrations of ampicillin, chloramphenicol, and nitrofurantoin on the attachment of *Escherichia coli* to human uroepithelial cells in vitro. *Rev. Infect. Dis.* **1**:838–844.

129. **Schaeffer, A. J., S. K. Amundsen, and L. N. Schmidt.** 1979. Adherence of *Escherichia coli* to human urinary tract epithelial cells. *Infect. Immun.* **24**:753–759.

130. **Schaeffer, A. J., J. S. Chmiel, J. L. Duncan, and W. S. Falkowski.** 1984. Mannose-sensitive adherence of *Escherichia coli* to epithelial cells from women with recurrent urinary tract infections. *J. Urol.* **131**:906–910.

131. **Schaeffer, A. J., J. M. Jones, and J. K. Dunn.** 1981. Association of in vitro *Escherichia coli* adherence to vaginal and buccal epithelial cells with susceptibility of women to recurrent urinary-tract infections. *N. Engl. J. Med.* **304**:1062–1066.

132. **Schaeffer, A. J., J. M. Jones, W. S. Falkowski, J. L. Duncan, J. S. Chmiel, and B. J. Plotkin.** 1982. Variable adherence of uropathogenic *Escherichia coli* to epithelial cells from women with recurrent urinary tract infection. *J. Urol.* **128**:1227–1230.

133. **Schaeffer, A. J., E. L. Navas, M. F. Venegas, B. E. Anderson, C. Kanerva, J. S. Chmiel, and J. L. Duncan.** 1994. Variation of blood group antigen expression on vaginal cells and mucus in secretor and nonsecretor women. *J. Urol.* **152**:859–864.

134. **Schaeffer, A. J., R. M. Radvany, and J. S. Chmiel.** 1983. Human leukocyte antigens in women with recurrent urinary tract infections. *J. Infect. Dis.* **148**:604.

135. **Schaeffer, A. J., W. R. Schwan, S. J. Hultgren, and J. L. Duncan.** 1987. Relationship of type 1 pilus expression in *Escherichia coli* to ascending urinary tract infections in mice. *Infect. Immun.* **55**:373–380.

136. **Schaeffer, A. J., and T. A. Stamey.** 1977. Studies of introital colonization in women

with recurrent urinary infections. IX. The role of antimicrobial therapy. *J. Urol.* **118**:221–224.
137. **Schulte-Wissermann, H., W. Mannhardt, J. Schwarz, F. Zepp, and D. Bitter-Suermann.** 1985. Comparison of the antibacterial effect of uroepithelial cells from healthy donors and children with asymptomatic bacteriuria. *Eur. J. Pediatr.* **144**:230–233.
138. **Sharma, S., B. S. Madhur, R. Singh, and B. K. Sharma.** 1987. Effect of contraceptives on the adhesion of *Escherichia coli* to uroepithelial cells. *J. Infect. Dis.* **156**:490–494.
139. **Sheinfeld, J., A. J. Schaeffer, C. Cordon-Cardo, A. Rogatko, and W. R. Fair.** 1989. Association of the Lewis blood-group phenotype with recurrent urinary tract infections in women. *N. Engl. J. Med.* **320**:773–777.
140. **Singh, B., and J. C. Cutler.** 1982. Demonstration of a spirochetal effect of chemical contraceptives on *Treponema pallidum*. *Bull. Pan Am. Health Org.* **16**:59–64.
141. **Sobel, J. D., and D. Kaye.** 1986. Enhancement of *Escherichia coli* adherence to epithelial cells derived from estrogen-stimulated rats. *Infect. Immun.* **53**:53–56.
142. **Spitz, C. J., A. R. Gold, and D. B. Adams.** 1975. Cognitive and hormonal factors affecting coital frequency. *Arch. Sex Behavior* **4**:249–263.
143. **Stamey, T. A.** 1973. The role of introital enterobacteria in recurrent urinary infections. *J. Urol.* **109**:467–472.
144. **Stamey, T. A., and J. J. Howell.** 1976. Studies of introital colonization in women with recurrent urinary infections. IV. The role of local vaginal antibodies. *J. Urol.* **115**:413–415.
145. **Stamey, T. A., and M. F. Kaufman.** 1975. Studies of introital colonization in women with recurrent urinary infections. II. A comparison of growth in normal vaginal fluid of common versus uncommon serogroups of *Escherichia coli*. *J. Urol.* **114**:264–267.
146. **Stamey, T. A., and G. Mihara.** 1976. Studies of introital colonization in women with recurrent urinary infections. V. The inhibitory activity of normal vaginal fluid on *Proteus mirabilis* and *Pseudomonas aeruginosa*. *J. Urol.* **115**:416–417.
147. **Stamey, T. A., and C. C. Sexton.** 1975. The role of vaginal colonization with Enterobacteriaceae in recurrent urinary tract infections. *J. Urol.* **113**:214–217.
148. **Stamey, T. A., and M. M. Timothy.** 1975. Studies of introital colonization in women with recurrent urinary infection. I. The role of vaginal pH. *J. Urol.* **114**:261–263.
149. **Stamey, T. A., M. Timothy, M. Millar, and G. Mihara.** 1971. Recurrent urinary infections in adult women. The role of introital enterobacteria. *Calif. Med.* **115**:1–19.
150. **Stamey, T. A., N. Wehner, G. Mihara, and M. Condy.** 1978. The immunologic basis of recurrent bacteriuria: role of cervicovaginal antibody in enterobacterial colonization of the introital mucosa. *Medicine* **57**:47–56.
151. **Stamm, W. E., G. W. Counts, K. F. Wagner, D. Martin, D. Gregory, M. McKevitt, M. Turck, and K. K. Holmes.** 1980. Antimicrobial prophylaxis of recurrent urinary tract infections: a double-blind, placebo-controlled trial. *Ann. Intern. Med.* **92**:770–775.
152. **Stamm, W. E., and T. M. Hooton.** 1993. Management of urinary tract infections in adults. *N. Engl. J. Med.* **329**:1328–1334.
153. **Stapleton, A., T. M. Hooton, C. Fennell, P. L. Roberts, and W. E. Stamm.** 1995. Effect of secretor status on vaginal and rectal colonization with fimbriated *Escherichia coli* in women with and without recurrent urinary tract infection. *J. Infect. Dis.* **171**:717–720.
154. **Stapleton, A., S. Moseley, and W. E. Stamm.** 1991. Urovirulence determinants in *Escherichia coli* isolates causing first-episode and recurrent cystitis in women. *J. Infect. Dis.* **163**:773–779.
155. **Stapleton, A., E. Nudelman, H. Clausen, S. Hakomori, and W. E. Stamm.** 1992. Binding of uropathogenic *Escherichia coli* R45 to glycolipids extracted from vaginal epithelial cells is dependent on histo-blood group secretor status. *J. Clin. Invest.* **90**:965–972.
156. **Stenqvist, K., T. Sandberg, S. Ahlstedt, T. K. Korhonen, and C. Svanborg-Eden.** 1982. Effects of subinhibitory concentrations of antibiotics and antibodies on the adherence of *Escherichia coli* to human uroepithelial cells in vitro. *Scand. J. Infect. Dis.* **33**(Suppl.):104–107.
157. **Strom, B. L., M. Collins, S. L. West, J. Kreisberg, and S. Weller.** 1987. Sexual activity, contraceptive use, and other risk factors for symptomatic and asymptomatic bacteriuria. A case-control study. *Ann. Intern. Med.* **107**:816–823.

158. Stromberg, N., B.-I. Marklund, B. Lund, D. Ilver, A. Hamers, W. Gaastra, K.-A. Karlsson, and S. Normark. 1990. Host-specificity of uropathogenic *Escherichia coli* depends on differences in binding specificity to Galα1-4 Gal-containing isoreceptors. *EMBO J.* **9:**2001–2010.
159. Sugarman, B., and L. R. Epps. 1982. Effect of estrogens on bacterial adherence to HeLa cells. *Infect. Immun.* **35:**633–638.
160. Svanborg, C. 1993. Resistance to urinary tract infection. *N. Engl. J. Med.* **329:**802–803.
161. Svanborg Eden, C., B. Andersson, L. Hagberg, L. A. Hanson, H. Leffler, G. Magnusson, G. Noori, J. Dahmen, and T. Soderstrom. 1983. Receptor analogues and anti-pili antibodies as inhibitors of bacterial attachment in vivo and in vitro. *Ann. N.Y. Acad. Sci.* **409:**580–591.
162. Svanborg Eden, C., and P. de Man. 1987. Bacterial virulence in urinary tract infection. *Infect. Dis. Clin. North Am.* **1:**731–750.
163. Svanborg Eden, C., B. Eriksson, L. A. Hanson, U. Jodal, B. Kaijser, G. Lidin-Janson, U. Lindberg, and S. Olling. 1978. Adhesion to normal human uroepithelial cells of *Escherichia coli* from children with various forms of urinary tract infection. *J. Pediatr.* **93:**398–403.
164. Svanborg-Eden, C., R. Freter, L. Hagberg, R. Hull, S. Hull, H. Leffler, and G. Schoolnik. 1982. Inhibition of experimental ascending urinary tract infection by an epithelial cell-surface receptor analogue. *Nature* (London) **298:**560–562.
165. Svanborg-Eden, C., L. Hagberg, L. A. Hanson, T. Korhonen, H. Leffler, and S. Olling. 1981. Adhesion of *Escherichia coli* in urinary tract infection. *Ciba Found. Symp.* **80:**161–187.
166. Svanborg-Eden, C., and L. A. Hanson. 1978. *Escherichia coli* pili as possible mediators of attachment to human urinary tract epithelial cells. *Infect. Immun.* **21:**229–237.
167. Svanborg Eden, C., S. Hausson, U. Jodal, G. Lidin-Janson, K. Lincoln, H. Linder, H. Lomberg, P. de Man, S. Marild, J. Martinell, K. Plos, T. Sandberg, and K. Stenqvist. 1988. Host-parasite interaction in the urinary tract. *J. Infect. Dis.* **157:**421–426.
168. Svanborg Eden, C., G. L. Janson, and U. Lindberg. 1979. Adhesiveness to urinary tract epithelial cells of fecal and urinary *Escherichia coli* isolates from patients with symptomatic urinary tract infections or asymptomatic bacteriuria of varying duration. *J. Urol.* **122:**185–188.
169. Svanborg-Eden, C., and U. Jodal. 1979. Attachment of *Escherichia coli* to urinary sediment epithelial cells from urinary tract infection-prone and healthy children. *Infect. Immun.* **26:**837–840.
170. Svanborg-Eden, C., U. Jodal, L. A. Hanson, U. Lindberg, and A. S. Akerlund. 1976. Variable adherence to normal human urinary-tract epithelial cells of *Escherichia coli* associated with various forms of urinary-tract infection. *Lancet* **ii:**490–492.
171. Svanborg Eden, C., P. Larsson, and H. Lomberg. 1980. Attachment of *Proteus mirabilis* to human urinary sediment epithelial cells in vitro is different from that for *Escherichia coli*. *Infect. Immun.* **28:**804–807.
172. Svanborg-Eden, C., T. Sandberg, K. Stenqvist, and S. Ahlstedt. 1978. Decrease in adhesion of *Escherichia coli* to human urinary tract epithelial cells in vitro by subinhibitory concentrations of ampicillin: a preliminary study. *Infection* **6**(Suppl. 1):121–123.
173. Svanborg-Eden, C., T. Sandberg, K. Stenqvist, and S. Ahlstedt. 1979. Effects of subinhibitory amounts of ampicillin, amoxycillin and mecillinam on the adhesion of *Escherichia coli* bacteria to human urinary tract epithelial cells: a preliminary study. *Infection* **7**(Suppl.):452–455.
174. Tomisawa, S., T. Kogure, T. Kuroume, H. Leffler, H. Lomberg, N. Shimabukoro, K. Terao, and C. Svanborg Eden. 1989. P blood group and proneness to urinary tract infection in Japanese children. *Scand. J. Infect. Dis.* **21:**403–408.
175. Tuttle, J. P., H. Sarvas, and J. Koistinen. 1978. The role of vaginal immunoglobulin A in girls with recurrent urinary tract infections. *J. Urol.* **120:**742–744.
176. Vosbeck, K., H. Handschin, E. B. Menge, and O. Zak. 1979. Effects of subminimal inhibitory concentrations of antibiotics on adhesiveness of *Escherichia coli* in vitro. *Rev. Infect. Dis.* **1:**845–851.
177. Watt, B., M. J. Goldacre, N. Loudon, D. J. Annat, R. I. Harris, and M. P. Vessey. 1981. Prevalence of bacteria in the vagina of normal young women. *Br. J. Obstet. Gynaecol.* **88:**588–595.
178. Winberg, J., L. Gezelius, L. Guldevall, and R. Mollby. 1993. Cephadroxil promotes vaginal colonization with *Escherichia coli*. *Infection* **21:**201–205.
179. Wold, A. E., D. A. Caugant, G. Lidin-

Janson, P. de Man, and C. Svanborg. 1992. Resident colonic *Escherichia coli* strains frequently display uropathogenic characteristics. *J. Infect. Dis.* **165:**46–52.

180. Wold, A. E., M. Thorssen, S. Hull, and C. Svanborg Eden. 1988. Attachment of *Escherichia coli* via mannose- or Gal$\alpha$1-4Gal$\beta$-containing receptors to human colonic epithelial cells. *Infect. Immun.* **56:**2531–2537.

181. Wood, J. R., R. L. Sweet, A. Catena, W. K. Hadley, and M. Robbie. 1985. In vitro adherence of *Lactobacillus* species to vaginal epithelial cells. *Am. J. Obstet. Gynecol.* **153:**740–743.

182. Zawaneh, S. M., E. M. Ayoub, H. Baer, A. C. Cruz, and W. N. Spellacy. 1981. Cyclic variation in the adherence of group B streptococci to human vaginal epithelial cells. *Am. J. Obstet. Gynecol.* **140:**381.

# TREATMENT AND PREVENTION OF URINARY TRACT INFECTIONS

*James R. Johnson, M.D.*

# 4

Treatment of urinary tract infection (UTI) is often a gratifying undertaking for the physician because of the prompt and dramatic symptomatic relief many patients experience after beginning antimicrobial therapy (61). On the other hand, UTI can also be a vexing challenge, either failing to respond to therapy or recurring repeatedly after seemingly successful treatment. To achieve maximal therapeutic efficacy while keeping costs and drug-related adverse effects to a minimum, physicians must be able to tailor UTI therapy to the patient's particular clinical situation. This undertaking requires delineation of each patient's UTI syndrome and underlying host status, familiarity with the antimicrobial agents commonly used to treat UTI and with current practice guidelines, and awareness of local antimicrobial susceptibility patterns. This chapter reviews general principles of UTI therapy and provides practical guidelines for both treatment and prevention of UTI in specific clinical settings.

---

*James R. Johnson,* Division of Infectious Diseases, University of Minnesota School of Medicine, 420 Delaware Street, S.E., Minneapolis, Minnesota 55455.

## FUNDAMENTAL CONSIDERATIONS IN UTI THERAPY

### Defining the Problem

The term "urinary tract infection" embraces a wide range of clinical entities, each with its own particular requirements for diagnostic evaluation (as discussed in chapter 2) and antimicrobial therapy. Management strategies must be individualized on the basis of the specific clinical syndrome present in a given patient, the patient's underlying host status, and the results of relevant laboratory tests, including (in many cases) the identity and antimicrobial susceptibility pattern of the urinary organism (53).

### CLINICAL SYNDROME

A rational approach to the treatment of UTI requires that the patient's clinical UTI syndrome be assigned to one of several standard categories for which treatment guidelines are available (53). The primary distinction to be made is between asymptomatic UTI, symptomatic infection of the lower urinary tract (cystitis), and infection of the upper urinary tract (pyelonephritis) or invasive (febrile) UTI. In asymptomatic infections (asymptomatic bacteriuria [ABU]), there is culture evidence of UTI in the absence of associated signs or symptoms. In contrast, the clinical syndrome of cystitis is defined by the presence of symptoms localized to the bladder and urethra (e.g., frequency, dysuria, suprapubic pain) but the absence of evidence of renal or systemic involvement. Pyelonephritis and invasive or febrile UTI can be considered together in terms of their therapeutic implications. These syndromes are defined by indicators of renal involvement (e.g., flank pain or tenderness), evidence of a systemic inflammatory response (e.g., fever, malaise, or leukocytosis), or a combination of these. In pyelonephritis and invasive or febrile UTI, local symptoms of bladder involvement may or may not be present (50).

It must be recognized that the anatomic distinctions implied by this three-way stratification of UTI syndromes are artificial, since even asymptomatic infections or episodes of clinical cystitis in many cases can be shown through specialized tests to involve the upper urinary tract as well (53) and since some patients can develop frank urosepsis from an invasive infection of the lower urinary tract in the absence of renal involvement (51). Nonetheless, this schema is useful in helping select a treatment regimen for a patient with UTI. The underlying principle is that the importance of treating at all and the intensity and duration of therapy required increase in proportion to the severity of the clinical syndrome, from ABU to cystitis to pyelonephritis and invasive or febrile UTI. For selection of the appropriate antimicrobial agent and duration of therapy, knowledge of the precise anatomical locus of infection is probably less important than awareness of the severity of the patient's UTI syndrome (57).

## HOST STATUS

Devising an optimal treatment regimen for UTI requires not only delineation of the patient's particular UTI syndrome but also consideration of the underlying host status. Such factors as older age, male gender, underlying illnesses, underlying anatomic or functional abnormalities of the urinary tract, and pregnancy are associated with less-susceptible pathogens, lower cure rates, higher recurrence rates, and greater severity of illness and hence influence the preferred treatment of different UTI syndromes (53, 100). For example, acute cystitis is much more responsive to therapy and so can be cured with less aggressive therapy when it occurs in a young, healthy, nonpregnant woman than when it occurs in an elderly nursing home resident with diabetes and an indwelling catheter. When UTI occurs in the setting of any of the complicating factors just listed, the term "complicated UTI" is applied, and a modified approach to therapy must be adopted (100).

## LABORATORY EVALUATION

Treatment of UTI has traditionally been based on results of quantitative urine cultures, with antimicrobial susceptibility patterns determined for all significant isolates (53). This approach is still appropriate in most clinical contexts, e.g., invasive or febrile UTI, complicated UTI, and UTI in patients recently treated with an antimicrobial agent (53, 65). It allows precisely targeted antimicrobial therapy based on the known urine organism(s). However, because of the predictability of the flora and their associated susceptibility patterns in uncomplicated cystitis occurring in healthy young women (Table 1), many authorities now recommend that pretherapy cultures be dispensed with in this context in favor of less expensive rapid tests, such as urine dipstick testing or microscopic examination of urine for pyuria (as discussed in chapter 2), to support the diagnosis of UTI. In these cases, antimicrobial agents can be selected empirically on the basis of their known spectra of activity in comparison with the likely therapeutic requirements of the expected urine organism(s). In all other clinical circumstances, culture and susceptibility testing should be done, and therapy should be tailored to the organism(s) isolated (53).

In some situations (e.g., pyelonephritis or febrile UTI), it is desirable not only to obtain a pretherapy urine culture but also to begin therapy immediately, before culture and susceptibility test results are available. In such a case, the clinical context should dictate the choice of initial (empirical) therapy (Table 1). The therapeutic regimen can be modified later when culture and susceptibility results are known.

## Antimicrobial Agents in UTI Therapy

### FACTORS INFLUENCING THE CHOICE OF ANTIMICROBIAL AGENT

Among the dozens of currently available antimicrobial agents, certain compounds have emerged as preferred choices for the treatment of UTI because of specific features that make them well-suited for this clinical role (Table 2) (76, 138). Pharmacological considerations such as oral bioavailability, achievement of high concentrations in urine, and prolonged half-life (which allows infrequent dosing) are useful attributes for UTI therapy (76). Activity in vitro against bacterial agents of UTI is required of successful UTI agents. For example, increasing bacterial resistance to traditional agents such as ampicillin has eroded the usefulness of these compounds for empirical monotherapy of UTI (53). In certain locales, even trimethoprim-sulfamethoxazole encounters sufficient resistance among uropathogens to render it unreliable for empirical therapy (75, 132). In contrast, newer agents such as the fluoroquinolones, which have broader activity and lower MICs for gram-negative bacilli, have emerged as the agents of choice for complicated UTI, in which resistant pathogens are the rule (108, 126).

Pharmacokinetic profiles and in vitro activity notwithstanding, the ultimate measure of the efficacy of antimicrobial agents in UTI therapy is performance in clinical trials. Preference should be given to agents with the most extensive and most favorable track record in the relevant clinical context.

Adverse drug effects are often a determining factor in drug selection. The known frequency and pattern of likely adverse effects with a particular drug in the population at large influence the drug's suitability for use in UTI therapy. In addition, a history of drug intolerance for a specific agent may eliminate this drug (and congeners) from consideration for use with an individual patient.

Cost is an increasingly important consideration in the selection of all medical interventions, including antimicrobial agents (76). In general, older agents tend to be less costly than newer ones. In some instances, the increased cost of a newer agent is warranted because of specific advantages it offers, such as better efficacy or better patient tolerance. If side effects can be avoided or relapse prevented, the savings may more than balance the drug's higher cost. However, when other factors are balanced for two agents, the less expensive agent should be used.

### SPECIFIC AGENTS (TABLE 1)

Antimicrobial agents of special relevance to the treatment of UTI are shown in Table 1. Ampicillin and amoxicillin, for many years the cornerstone of UTI therapy, are no longer preferred for empirical therapy of any UTI syndrome because of the high prevalence of resistance even among community-acquired infections and the availability of more effective alternative agents (53). These drugs still have a role in selected patients, such as pregnant women and others with susceptible organisms who are intolerant of first-line agents. The addition of a $\beta$-lactamase inhibitor extends the spectra and efficacies of these agents, but because of their higher cost, the combination drugs should be reserved for special

**TABLE 1** Antimicrobial agents useful in treatment or prevention of UTI[a]

| Agent(s) | Route(s) | Pharmacokinetics | Spectrum and activity | Frequency (type) of adverse effects |
|---|---|---|---|---|
| Ampicillin, amoxicillin | p.o., i.v. | High levels in urine but rapid elimination | Increasing resistance among GNRs; active against enterococci | Moderate (GI, rash) |
| Amoxicillin-clavulanate, ampicillin-sulbactam | p.o., i.v. | High levels in urine but rapid elimination | Good for most GNRs and gram-positive bacteria; many nosocomial GNRs resistant | Moderate (GI, rash) |
| Trimethoprim-sulfamethoxazole | p.o., i.v. | High levels in urine, long half-life | Good for most GNRs (depends on locale); many nosocomial GNRs resistant | Low if ≤3 days of therapy; moderate to high with ≥5 days of therapy (GI, rash, vaginitis) |
| Trimethoprim | p.o. | High levels in urine, long half-life | Good for most GNRs (depends on locale); many nosocomial GNRs resistant | Low to moderate (GI, rash, vaginitis) |
| Narrow-spectrum cephalosporins | p.o., i.v. | High levels in urine but rapid elimination | Many GNRs resistant; no enterococcal activity | Low |
| Broad- and extended-spectrum cephalosporins; ticarcillin-clavulanate, piperacillin-tazobactam; aztreonam; imipenem-cilastatin | p.o. (cephalosporins), i.v. (all) | High levels in urine; half-life depends on agent | Broader GNR activity; inadequate enterococcal activity with cephalosporins and aztreonam | Low to moderate (rash with penicillins; rarely, seizures with imipenem-cilastatin) |
| Aminoglycosides | i.v., (i.m.) | High levels in urine, prolonged excretion, once-daily dosing possible | Almost all GNRs, including resistant nosocomial organisms | Low with short-term use; nephro- and ototoxicities with prolonged use |
| FQs | p.o. (all), i.v. (ciprofloxacin and ofloxacin) | High levels in urine, long half-life | Excellent against most GNRs including resistant nosocomial organisms; weaker for *Staphylococcus saprophyticus* and enterococci | Low (GI, neuro) |
| Nitrofurantoin | p.o. | Adequate levels in urine only, rapid elimination | Most agents of uncomplicated UTI | Low (GI, neuro; risk of pulmonary and hepatic toxicities with prolonged use) |

[a] FQ, fluoroquinolone; p.o., peroral; i.v., intravenous; i.m., intramuscular; GNR, gram-negative rod; GI, gastrointestinal; neuro, neurological; TMP-SMX, trimethoprim-sulfamethoxazole.

| Safety during pregnancy and in children | Relative cost | Clinical efficacy | Uses |
|---|---|---|---|
| Pregnancy: safe<br>Children: safe | Inexpensive | Long track record; inferior to TMP-SMZ and FQs; avoid for SDT | ABU or cystitis in pregnancy; alternative for uncomplicated UTI |
| Pregnancy: safe<br>Children: safe | Expensive | Limited experience: probably similar to TMP-SMZ and FQs | Pyelonephritis (including pregnancy); resistant organisms |
| Pregnancy: caution in first trimester; kernicterus at term (sulfamethoxazole)<br>Children: safe | Inexpensive | Long track record; high efficacy in uncomplicated UTI | Preferred agent for uncomplicated UTI; alternative for complicated UTI if organism is susceptible; chronic prophylaxis |
| Pregnancy: caution in first trimester<br>Children: safe | Inexpensive | Probably as effective as TMP-SMZ in uncomplicated UTI | Preferred agent for uncomplicated cystitis; chronic prophylaxis |
| Pregnancy: safe<br>Children: safe | Expensive | p.o. inferior to alternatives; little experience with i.v. | Lower UTI in pregnancy |
| Pregnancy: safe<br>Children: safe | Expensive | Little experience; probably comparable to TMP-SMZ and FQs for uncomplicated UTI | p.o.: complicated UTI, resistant organism, or intolerance to less expensive alternatives; i.v.: initial therapy of pyelonephritis or serious complicated UTI |
| Pregnancy: caution<br>Children: safe (short-term) | Inexpensive (gentamicin); expensive (tobramycin and amikacin) | Long track record with pyelonephritis and serious UTI | Initial therapy of pyelonephritis or serious complicated UTI (± added ampicillin) |
| Pregnancy: avoid<br>Children: avoid | Expensive (but oral FQs less expensive than alternative i.v. agents with comparable efficacy) | High efficacy in all UTI syndromes | Preferred agent for complicated UTI unless organism is susceptible to less expensive agent; alternative for uncomplicated UTI |
| Pregnancy: caution<br>Children: safe | Variable | Good for uncomplicated lower UTI | Alternative for acute cystitis; chronic prophylaxis |

**TABLE 2** Treatment regimens for bacterial UTIs[a]

| Condition | Characteristic pathogens | Mitigating circumstances | Recommended empirical treatment[b] |
|---|---|---|---|
| Acute uncomplicated cystitis in women | Escherichia coli, Staphylococcus saprophyticus, Proteus mirabilis, Klebsiella pneumoniae | None | 3-day regimens: oral trimethoprim-sulfamethoxazole, trimethoprim, norfloxacin, ciprofloxacin, ofloxacin, lomefloxacin, or enoxacin[c] |
| | | Diabetes, symptoms for >7 days, recent UTI, use of diaphragm, age >65 yr | Consider 7-day regimen: oral trimethoprim-sulfamethoxazole, trimethoprim, norfloxacin, ciprofloxacin, ofloxacin, lomefloxacin, or enoxacin[c] |
| | | Pregnancy | Consider 7-day regimen: oral amoxicillin, macrocrystalline nitrofurantoin, cefpodoxime proxetil, cefixime, or trimethoprim-sulfamethoxazole[c] |
| Acute uncomplicated pyelonephritis in women | E. coli, P. mirabilis, K. pneumoniae, S. saprophyticus | Mild-to-moderate illness, no nausea or vomiting: outpatient therapy acceptable | Oral[d] trimethoprim-sulfamethoxazole, norfloxacin, ciprofloxacin, ofloxacin, lomefloxacin, or enoxacin for 10–14 days |
| | | Severe illness or possible urosepsis: hospitalization required | Parenteral[e] trimethoprim-sulfamethoxazole, ceftriaxone, ciprofloxacin, gentamicin (with or without ampicillin), or ampicillin-sulbactam until fever is better; then oral[d] trimethoprim-sulfamethoxazole, norfloxacin, ciprofloxacin, ofloxacin, lomefloxacin, or enoxacin to complete 14-day therapy |
| | | Pregnancy: hospitalization recommended | Parenteral[e] ceftriaxone, gentamicin (with or without ampicillin), aztreonam, ampicillin-sulbactam, or trimethoprim-sulfamethoxazole until fever is gone; then oral[d] amoxicillin, amoxicillin-clavulanate, a cephalosporin, or trimethoprim-sulfamethoxazole for 14 days |
| Complicated UTI | E. coli; Proteus, Klebsiella, Pseudomonas, and Serratia species; enterococci; staphylococci | Mild-to-moderate illness, no nausea or vomiting: outpatient therapy acceptable | Oral[d] norfloxacin, ciprofloxacin, ofloxacin, lomefloxacin, or enoxacin for 10–14 days |
| | | Severe illness or possible urosepsis: hospitalization required | Parenteral[e] ampicillin and gentamicin, ciprofloxacin, ofloxacin, ceftriaxone, aztreonam, ticarcillin-clavulanate, piperacillin-tazobactam, or imipenem-cilastatin until fever is gone; then oral[d] trimethoprim-sulfamethoxazole, norfloxacin, ciprofloxacin, ofloxacin, lomefloxacin, or enoxacin for 14–21 days |

*Footnotes on following page*

**TABLE 2** *Continued*

$^a$ Adapted from reference 126. Reprinted by permission of the New England Journal of Medicine (Vol. 329; 1328–1334, 1993).

$^b$ Treatments listed are those to be prescribed before the etiologic agent is known (Gram staining can be helpful); they can be modified once the agent has been identified. The recommendations are the author's and are limited to drugs currently approved by the Food and Drug Administration, although not all the regimens listed are approved for these indications. Fluoroquinolones should not be used in pregnancy. Trimethoprim-sulfamethoxazole, although not approved for use in pregnancy, has been widely used. Gentamicin should be used with caution in pregnancy because of its possible toxicity to eighth-nerve development in the fetus.

$^c$ Multiday oral regimens for cystitis are as follows: trimethoprim-sulfamethoxazole, 160 plus 800 mg every 12 h; trimethoprim, 100 mg every 12 h; norfloxacin, 400 mg every 12 h; ciprofloxacin, 250 mg every 12 h; ofloxacin, 200 mg every 12 h; lomefloxacin, 400 mg every day; enoxacin, 400 mg every 12 h; macrocrystalline nitrofurantoin, 100 mg four times a day; amoxicillin, 250 mg every 8 h; cefpodoxime proxetil, 100 mg every 12 h; and cefixime, 400 mg every day.

$^d$ Oral regimens for pyelonephritis and complicated UTI are as follows: trimethoprim-sulfamethoxazole, 160 plus 800 mg every 12 h; norfloxacin, 400 mg every 12 h; ciprofloxacin, 500 mg every 12 h; ofloxacin, 200 plus 300 mg every 12 h; lomefloxacin, 400 mg every day; enoxacin, 400 mg every 12 h; amoxicillin 500 mg every 8 h; cefpodoxime proxetil, 200 mg every 12 h; and cefixime, 400 mg every day.

$^e$ Parenteral regimens are as follows: trimethoprim-sulfamethoxazole, 160 plus 800 mg every 12 h; ciprofloxacin, 200 to 400 mg every 12 h; ofloxacin, 200 to 400 mg every 12 h; gentamicin, 1 mg/kg of body weight every 8 h or 3 to 5 mg/kg every 24 h; ceftriaxone, 1 to 2 g every day; ampicillin, 1 g every 6 h; imipenem-cilastatin, 250 to 500 mg every 6 to 8 h; ampicillin-sulbactam, 1.5 g every 6 h; ticarcillin-clavulanate, 3.2 g every 6 to 8 h; piperacillin-tazobactam, 3.375 g every 6 to 8 h; and aztreonam, 1 g every 8 to 12 h.

circumstances, such as acute pyelonephritis or the presence of a known resistant pathogen (Table 2).

Trimethoprim and trimethoprim-sulfamethoxazole (Table 1) are considered by many to be the drugs of first choice for uncomplicated UTI (and for complicated UTI as well when the pathogen is susceptible) because of their low cost and well-established efficacy (126) and their "quinolone-sparing" effect (i.e., allowing fluoroquinolones to be reserved for special circumstances, which should help delay the emergence of fluoroquinolone-resistant uropathogens) (42). They currently are the standard against which new antimicrobial agents for the treatment of UTI should be compared. Adverse effects are less frequent with trimethoprim alone (61) and with shorter courses of therapy ($\leq 3$ days) (36, 87).

Oral narrow-spectrum cephalosporins (Table 2) have not performed well in UTI therapy (53), but the newer oral broad- and expanded-spectrum agents appear to do better (76, 103), although experience with them is limited. These agents and their intravenous counterparts as well as the extended-spectrum $\beta$-lactamase inhibitor combination agents, aztreonam, and imipenem-cilastatin are relatively nontoxic and are safe in pregnancy, but they are expensive (Table 1). They offer activity against many resistant gram-negative bacilli and are thus attractive for the empirical therapy of complicated UTI. For patients initially treated intravenously with one of these agents, prompt conversion to oral therapy with a fluoroquinolone, trimethoprim-sulfamethoxazole, or an oral advanced cephalosporin can reduce costs once the urine organism's susceptibility pattern is known.

Aminoglycosides (Table 1) are traditional agents of established efficacy in the treatment of infections due to gram-negative bacilli, including UTI (50). Their potential nephro- and ototoxicities should usually limit their use to the initial phase of treatment for acute pyelonephritis or serious complicated UTI. In exceptional cases, the presence of a resistant organism may require that these agents be used for more extended treatment, in which case once-daily dosing can be used to facilitate home intravenous therapy (67). Caution is advised in pregnancy because of possible fetal toxicity (55).

Fluoroquinolone agents (Table 1) represent a significant advance in antimicrobial therapy for UTI (53). Their cost and the importance of limiting their use to prevent the emergence of antimicrobial resistance exclude them from first-line therapy of uncomplicated UTI (42, 126), but their excellent spectra of activity (particularly against resistant gram-negative uropathogens), their favorable adverse-effect profiles, and their oral bioavailability make them the preferred drug class for therapy of complicated UTI (108).

Nitrofurantoin (Table 1) is a traditional favorite for chronic low-dose prophylactic therapy (20). It achieves high levels in the urine but negligible levels in serum and so is not used for treating invasive infections (e.g., pyelonephritis or bacteremia).

## Duration of Therapy

Having selected an antimicrobial agent appropriate for a patient's UTI syndrome and underlying host status, the physician must then decide how long to treat. Considerable energy has been devoted to defining the optimal duration of therapy for various UTI syndromes that balances efficacy, cost, and adverse effects. In principle, the more invasive the UTI syndrome, the greater the severity of illness, and the more compromised the host, the longer therapy should be continued; the more active the antimicrobial regimen is against the pathogen, the briefer therapy can be. In practice, duration of therapy usually is determined empirically on the basis of clinical experience. The successive introduction in recent years of increasingly effective antimicrobial agents, the ongoing revision of classification schemes for UTI syndromes, and the accumulating results from multiple treatment trials have necessitated repeated re-examinations of traditionally recommended durations of therapy for UTI. Areas of recent active debate include acute uncomplicated cystitis and pyelonephritis in adult women, as described below.

## THERAPY OF UTI IN SPECIFIC CLINICAL SETTINGS

## Adult Women with Uncomplicated UTI

### ABU

ABU has no documented serious adverse sequelae in otherwise healthy nonpregnant women and need not be treated except during pregnancy (53). Treatment of ABU may prevent some women from subsequently developing symptomatic infection (18). However, whether in the aggregate this small benefit is worth the cost, risk of adverse effects, and increased antimicrobial selection pressure that treatment of all episodes of ABU would entail is doubtful, especially when it is considered that symptomatic episodes can usually be treated quite readily when they occur.

### CYSTITIS

In contrast to ABU, symptomatic lower UTI (acute cystitis) should be treated, both to relieve symptoms and to forestall possible progression to pyelonephritis (Table 2). Therapy for acute uncomplicated cystitis has received considerable attention in the past decade, and a new consensus favoring 3-day therapy with one of several highly active oral agents has emerged.

**SDT.** In the 1970s, enthusiasm for single-dose therapy (SDT) for women with uncomplicated cystitis was high, since SDT gave cure rates almost as high as those of traditional 7- to 10-day courses of therapy but with lower costs and fewer side effects (125). More recently, the pendulum has swung away from SDT because of a growing recognition that although adverse effects are indeed impressively less frequent, efficacy rates are slightly but significantly lower as well (8, 66, 92, 123, 125, 126).

The apparent lower cost of SDT may be illusory if the savings per initial treatment course are offset by the added cost of retreating individuals who fail therapy (125). The lower efficacy of SDT compared with that of traditional treatment courses may be due in part to SDT's lesser ability to eradicate colonization of the intestine or vagina by the pathogenic strain, thereby allowing early reinfection from a persisting extraurinary reservoir (27, 125, 126).

In the past, the propensity of ampicillin SDT for cystitis to fail in patients with occult upper urinary tract infection was considered a possible advantage, in that relapse after SDT could be used to identify such patients for more intensive therapy or for urological investigation (106). However, this concept has fallen by the wayside with the realization that such patients usually can be cured by a single dose of a more effective agent or by longer initial therapy, making it unnecessary to differentiate them from similar patients in whom infection is confined to the bladder (53, 125). Today, most authorities suggest that if SDT is used, it should be reserved for uncomplicated acute cystitis in nonpregnant young adult women who have had symptoms for <3 days, in which setting experience with SDT is most extensive and success rates are the highest (43, 126).

**Three-Day Therapy.** As enthusiasm for SDT has waned, the concept has emerged that 3-day treatment regimens for uncomplicated cystitis deliver the chief benefits of SDT, i.e., reduced costs and adverse effects, while largely preserving the higher success rates of traditional longer treatment courses (3, 5, 23, 32, 42, 53, 87, 102, 119, 125, 126, 131). The balance of evidence from the multiple studies available suggests that with trimethoprim-sulfamethoxazole, 3-day treatment courses achieve near-maximal efficacy without the increased adverse effects seen with ≥5-day courses. In contrast, beta-lactam agents require more extended courses of therapy for their maximal efficacy (which is still lower than that achievable with trimethoprim-sulfamethoxazole), with correspondingly greater adverse effects. Fluoroquinolones give high cure rates regardless of treatment duration (23, 56), but outcomes are slightly better with multidose treatment (23, 45), leading some to recommend 3-day therapy over SDT with these agents as well (126).

A recent randomized comparative trial of 3-day therapy for cystitis found that trimethoprim-sulfamethoxazole is the most effective of the traditional UTI agents (compared with nitrofurantoin, cefadroxil, and amoxicillin), with a cure rate of 82% compared with 61 to 67% for the other agents (42). Trimethoprim-sulfamethoxazole was associated with a slightly higher frequency of recurrent UTI and vaginitis than was ofloxacin, resulting in a net cost per treated patient of $114, which is similar to that for ofloxacin ($115) despite ofloxacin's higher cost per dose (42). Thus, cost, adverse effects, and efficacy appear to be well balanced between trimethoprim-sulfamethoxazole and the fluoroquinolones for uncomplicated cystitis in women. Trimethoprim and trimethoprim-sulfamethoxazole are preferable because of the desirability of limiting the exposure of the microbial flora to fluoroquinolones (42, 126). Since the sulfonamide component of trimethoprim-sulfamethoxazole may contribute to adverse effects but not efficacy against cystitis, some recommend trimethoprim alone (61). Fluoroquinolones are best reserved for when patients have recurrent infections, when therapy with first-line agents cannot be tolerated or fails, or when known resistant organisms are present (126).

## PYELONEPHRITIS

An important development in the management of acute uncomplicated pyelonephritis in women is the growing recognition that oral therapy on an ambulatory basis is acceptable for selected patients (1, 98, 109, 127, 132). Since severity of illness is the main determinant of the need for hospital admission and parenteral therapy, it is unlikely that a randomized trial comparing intravenous therapy in the hospital with oral therapy in the outpatient setting will ever be done. However, the available evidence suggests that outcomes with oral therapy for selected ambulatory patients who are clinically stable and able to take oral medications are comparable to those obtained with sicker patients given traditional in-hospital parenteral therapy and show a considerable cost savings (98, 109).

Mildly ill women with pyelonephritis can be started on an oral antimicrobial regimen (Table 2) and sent home after close follow-up has been arranged. More severely ill patients who are not sick enough to require hospitalization can be hydrated, given an initial parenteral dose of antibiotic in the clinic or emergency department, and observed for several hours before discharge. If their condition fails to improve sufficiently during the observation period, they can then be admitted to the hospital for continued parenteral therapy, whereas if they improve, they can be discharged with oral medication, again with close follow-up arranged (1).

Initial oral therapy for uncomplicated pyelonephritis should cover the usual expected pathogens (Table 2); knowledge of local resistance patterns may be important (132). Hospitalized patients should be started on a regimen broadly active against gram-negative bacilli (including ampicillin-resistant strains) and possibly gram-positive uropathogens as well (43, 53). Gentamicin (with or without ampicillin), an extended-spectrum cephalosporin, trimethoprim-sulfamethoxazole, or a β-lactamase inhibitor combination agent has been suggested for this role (53, 61, 126). In one study, decision analysis suggested that a traditional ampicillin-gentamicin regimen is better for initial therapy of pyelonephritis than regimens consisting of ampicillin, cefazolin, cefuroxime, gentamicin, or trimethoprim-sulfamethoxazole alone or cefazolin and gentamicin combined (24). In a recent clinical trial, the efficacies of an ampicillin-plus-gentamicin regimen and a trimethoprim-sulfamethoxazole-plus-gentamicin regimen were similar, with no difference in adverse effects. Costs were lower and administration was simpler with the trimethoprim-sulfamethoxazole regimen because of decreased dosing frequency, and more patients were able to complete therapy with the corresponding oral agent in the trimethoprim-sulfamethoxazole group because of the high prevalence of ampicillin resistance but the absence of trimethoprim-sulfamethoxazole resistance (50).

Failure of a patient's clinical status to improve after 48 to 72 h of treatment should suggest a complicating factor, missed diagnosis, or inappropriate therapy and should prompt detailed clinical reassessment, reevaluation of the laboratory data and treatment regimen, and consideration of urinary tract imaging studies. For patients who respond to initial intravenous therapy, a single oral agent active against the urine isolate can be substituted once susceptibility results are known and the patient can tolerate oral medication (126).

In the past, therapy for up to 6 weeks has been recommended for uncomplicated acute pyelonephritis in women (50). However, recent trials have shown that shorter treatment courses with highly effective agents are predictably curative (34, 50, 107, 127). For mild pyelonephritis, treatment with oral trimethoprim-sulfamethoxazole for 14 days was as effective as treatment for 6 weeks, whereas treatment with oral ampicillin for 14 days was actually superior to treatment for 6 weeks, largely because of reinfections with ampicillin-resistant organisms in the 6-week group (127). In another study involving hospitalized patients, 14 days of therapy with regimens that initially included gentamicin was sufficient to eradicate the initial infection in all subjects (50).

Some patients are cured of pyelonephritis by courses of therapy even shorter than the 14-day benchmark established in the trials discussed above; treatment for as little as 5 days has been advocated (12, 61). However, acceptable success rates with such short treatment courses are probably limited to certain highly effective antimicrobial agents (e.g., amino-glycosides, expanded-spectrum cephalosporins, trimethoprim-sulfamethoxazole, and fluoroquinolones), since treatment with beta-lactam agents for less than 14 days has given unacceptably high failure rates (46, 91).

## Adults with Complicated UTI
ABU
There is no clear indication for therapy of ABU in men or in anyone with complicating factors (i.e., functional or anatomic urinary tract abnormalities, urinary tract instrumentation, or significant medical illnesses). Furthermore, in this context, treatment of ABU is often ineffective and can be harmful, as in a recent treatment trial for ABU in patients with spinal cord injury (136) in which therapy for 7 to 14 days with follow-up treatment for 28 days in those with persistence or relapse showed little success but promoted the emergence of resistant organisms (136). However, ABU should be treated in patients at particular risk for severe consequences (e.g., neutropenic patients) should they develop symptomatic UTI and in patients scheduled for invasive urinary tract procedures, where the risk of bacteremia is substantial in the presence of infected urine (80).

CYSTITIS AND PYELONEPHRITIS
UTIs in men and in patients with underlying urinary tract abnormalities or significant systemic illnesses respond less well to therapy and more often involve resistant pathogens than do uncomplicated UTIs in otherwise healthy young women (53, 68, 100). Consequently, the duration of therapy must be extended, and empiric antibiotic selection must take into consideration resistant gram-negative bacilli and enterococci (Table 2).

Treatment for a minimum of 7 to 10 days is recommended for UTIs in men even in the absence of signs of renal or systemic involvement (13, 68, 77, 126). Similar courses are used for patients with other complicating factors (53, 84). Extended treatment courses of up to 3 months have been recommended for selected subgroups of patients with complicated UTI (16, 61).

For initial intravenous therapy of seriously ill patients with complicated UTI, a combination regimen such as ampicillin-gentamicin or imipenem-cilastatin will provide activity not only against gram-negative bacilli but also against most strains of enterococci (126). Less ill patients with complicated UTI can be treated empirically with one of the oral fluoroquinolones, which have emerged as the drugs of choice for empiric therapy of complicated UTI because of their excellent activity against many multiresistant gram-negative bacteria and their satisfactory performance in clinical trials compared with that of traditional intravenous regimens (84, 108, 126). Subsequent therapy in either situation can be guided by the results of urine culture and susceptibility tests (53).

For patients with serious complicated UTI, a high level of suspicion for the possibility of an anatomical complication, such as obstruction to urine flow, that might require mechanical intervention must be maintained. Appropriate diagnostic tests and urological consultation (53) should be pursued if the response to therapy is delayed, if the patient's condition deteriorates despite presumably appropriate medical therapy, or if other evidence suggests the presence of an anatomical complication.

## The Elderly
Bacteriuria is highly prevalent among the elderly, in whom it often occurs in the setting of other complicating factors. Because

of the special attention UTI in the elderly has received, this topic is discussed separately from complicated UTI, of which it may be considered a subset.

## ABU

Early observations associating ABU with increased mortality in the elderly raised the concern that ABU may contribute to mortality (25, 26, 122). However, numerous subsequent studies have failed to find a causal connection (or in some cases, even an association) between ABU and mortality in the elderly (2, 18, 80, 81, 85, 86). Furthermore, these studies have documented the inability of antimicrobial therapy for ABU to produce lasting urinary tract sterility or to reduce mortality in elderly subjects (80, 81, 83, 85, 122). On the contrary, treatment of ABU in the elderly is associated with increased adverse effects, selects for resistant organisms, and possibly increases mortality (80, 81, 85, 122). Thus, most authorities recommend against treatment of ABU in elderly individuals, particularly the institutionalized elderly (43, 71, 77, 80). Some reduction in subsequent infectious morbidity may result from treating ABU in less-impaired elderly individuals (18), but this finding has not been interpreted as justifying treatment of ABU in such patients (17).

## CYSTITIS

Symptomatic UTI in the elderly responds poorly to short-course therapy (54) and generally should be treated with longer courses of therapy, much as other types of complicated UTI are treated (43, 77). For functionally intact women, short-course (3-day) therapy may be worth a trial (13, 77), with retreatment for a longer period (e.g., 14 days) if relapse occurs (13).

Prostatism may predispose to UTI and should be considered when an older man presents with syptomatic UTI (80). Relapsing UTI in elderly men suggests prostatitis, which is best treated with prolonged courses, i.e., 6 to 12 weeks (80). Prostatic massage, with a "four-cup test" to confirm prostatic localization of infection, is of uncertain benefit; presumptive therapy may be preferable when prostatic involvement is suspected (68, 121).

As in UTI complicated by other underlying host factors, UTI in the elderly often involves mixed or resistant organisms, so narrow-spectrum therapy (e.g., with amoxicillin) should be avoided until culture and sensitivity results are known (71). A fluoroquinolone, trimethoprim-sulfamethoxazole (depending on local susceptibility patterns), or a broad- or extended-spectrum oral cephalosporin is preferable (71).

## PYELONEPHRITIS

Pyelonephritis in the elderly can cause diagnostic confusion, with clinical manifestations sometimes suggesting pulmonary or gastrointestinal disorders (13). Bacteremia appears to be more common in elderly patients with pyelonephritis than in younger patients (35, 49, 93, 111), and acute renal failure may complicate management (88, 145). Treatment considerations are similar to those described above for pyelonephritis in patients with other complicating factors (13, 80).

## Pregnant Women

### ABU

Pregnant women with ABU are at increased risk of developing pyelonephritis, which during pregnancy can be a devastating illness (39). Identification and treatment of ABU prevent the development of pyelonephritis and are widely recommended as parts of routine prenatal care if for this reason only, independent of the possible impact of ABU on prematurity or low birth weight (6, 43, 147).

The optimal strategy for surveillance for ABU during pregnancy remains somewhat controversial, as does the best approach to treatment (6, 43, 147). Despite clinical trials demonstrating the efficacy of SDT for ABU in pregnancy (147) and the theoretical desirability of limiting fetal exposure to antibiotics by using short-course therapy (147), many authorities recommend a more cautious 3- to 10-day treatment course (43). Antibiotic selection must take into consideration not only all the usual parameters but also potential toxicity to the fetus (55) (Table 1).

## CYSTITIS AND PYELONEPHRITIS

Symptomatic UTI during pregnancy should be treated much as it is treated in nonpregnant women. Important differences are that SDT for cystitis is even less favored for pregnant women than for nonpregnant women and that the choice of agents is constrained by the need to avoid fetal toxicity (6, 43, 55). Three-day short-course therapy for cystitis in pregnant women is accepted by many authorities (23, 43). However, regardless of the duration of therapy used, careful follow-up is required to identify relapse or reinfection (6, 53). Pyelonephritis, because of its potential for fulminating during pregnancy and because of the potential hazard to the fetus, is best treated initially in the hospital for close monitoring of mother and fetus and intravenous antimicrobial therapy (39), although precedent for oral therapy does exist (7).

### Children

The treatment of ABU in children is considered unnecessary except in the setting of vesicoureteral reflux, where silent UTI can lead to renal scarring and chronic renal damage (118, 140). For acute symptomatic UTI in children, experience with short-course regimens (SDT or 3-day therapy) is limited; most authorities recommend against short-course therapy in favor of traditional 7- to 10-day treatment courses (23, 43, 118) with one of the agents indicated in Table 2. Given the difficulty of administering antibiotics to children and the desirability of reducing overall antibiotic use, further studies of short-course regimens in children (e.g., such as that described in reference 32) would be useful. Febrile UTI and pyelonephritis in children are treated much as they are treated in adults (see below) (118).

Urinary tract imaging is commonly recommended for children who have had one or more episodes of symptomatic UTI in order to identify those with underlying anatomic abnormalities that may predispose to recurrent infection and renal damage (33, 118). Opinion varies regarding the optimal approach to such an investigation (33, 118).

### Catheter-Associated UTI

Catheter-associated UTI does not require treatment in the absence of symptoms (43, 77, 126). For catheterized patients with UTI and signs suggestive of sepsis, treatment can be given as for complicated pyelonephritis (see above), generally with intravenous antimicrobial agents in doses adequate to treat bacteremia, if present (126, 137). Less ill patients can be treated with an oral regimen. A fluoroquinolone alone is a reasonable choice for initial empirical therapy of a mildly ill patient with catheter-associated UTI if the urine Gram stain shows gram-negative bacilli. The optimal duration of therapy for catheter-associated UTI is undefined and is probably best tailored to the patient's severity of illness.

### Fungal UTI

Fungal (yeast) UTI most often occurs in patients with indwelling bladder catheters who are receiving systemic antimicrobial therapy, a common scenario in the acute care hospital (52). Bladder infection, which is the most common form of fungal UTI, is thought to be usually acquired via a retrograde (ascending) route, whereas renal parenchymal infection is thought to arise from hematogenous seeding during a prior episode of fungemia (28, 73).

The natural history and clinical significance of asymptomatic fungal UTI in catheterized patients are unknown (48, 114), but the available evidence suggests that fungal UTI is usually a benign, self-limited condition (144). The best management approach to asymptomatic fungal UTI may thus be watchful waiting (48, 114, 144), with removal of predisposing factors such as the catheter and antibacterial therapy where possible (28, 114, 144).

For symptomatic patients, the optimal therapy for fungal UTI is undefined. Various regimens for bladder irrigation with amphotericin B have been proposed, but which regimen provides the best balance of efficacy, toxicity, and cost is controversial (90, 94, 113, 144). Single intravenous doses of amphotericin B (0.3 mg/kg of body weight) have cleared candiduria (29), a result that argues against the need for supplemental therapy directed specifically toward the urinary tract in patients also receiving systemic amphotericin B (63). Fluconazole gives high levels in urine, is active against most *Candida* species, is well absorbed via the oral route, and has a favorable adverse-effect profile. This relatively new addition to the antifungal armamentarium is probably the most appropriate treatment for symptomatic fungal UTI today (129).

When funguria persists even after removal of an indwelling catheter, some authorities advocate an aggressive diagnostic evaluation to look for occult disseminated fungal infection and obstruction (74). Whether this aggressive approach is preferable to a simple trial of oral fluconazole (for symptomatic patients) or expectant observation (for asymptomatic patients) is unknown. Catheter-associated funguria that persists despite therapy is an adverse prognostic sign (72).

## PREVENTION OF UTI

Symptomatic UTI can often be prevented by the judicious use of antimicrobial agents or other specific interventions. As with treatment of established UTI, an optimal regimen must be tailored to the patient's individual clinical circumstances.

## Specific Clinical Settings

RECURRENT CYSTITIS IN WOMEN
One of the greatest challenges for UTI therapy is recurrent UTI in adult women, because although any one episode can be readily eliminated, it is rapidly followed by another that is often due to a different organism (61). Most women with recurrent UTI do not have a predisposing anatomical abnormality amenable to surgical therapy or warranting radiological or urological investigation (33, 53). On the contrary, in most cases, recurrent UTI is attributable either to an underlying biological predisposition to infection or to UTI-promoting behaviors.

At present, no interventions directly address the underlying biological tendency some women have toward vaginal and perineal colonization with uropathogenic *Escherichia coli,* which predisposes them to UTI (117, 126). In contrast, spermicide-diaphragm use is a potentially reversible risk factor for perineal colonization with coliform bacteria and symptomatic UTI (41, 79). Although not yet demonstrated in a clinical trial, changing to an alternative method of contraception should be advantageous for diaphragm-using women with recurrent UTI. However, women may be reluctant to abandon a contraceptive method with which they are comfortable and which they have selected on the basis of other important criteria from among the limited available alternatives. Similarly, although sexual intercourse per se is associated with UTI in both women and men (14, 40, 64, 82, 143) and also could be considered a potentially reversible risk factor for coitus-associated UTI, forgoing intercourse to prevent UTI is probably an alternative few sexually active persons would accept.

**TABLE 3** Oral regimens for daily prophylaxis of UTI

| Agent | Daily dose (mg) |
|---|---|
| Trimethoprim[a] | 100 |
| Trimethoprim-sulfamethoxazole[a] | 40-200[b] |
| Nitrofurantoin[a] | 50 |
| Nitrofurantoin macrocrystals[a] | 100 |
| Cephalexin, cephradine, or cefaclor | 250 |
| Norfloxacin | 200 |

[a] Preferred agent.
[b] Also effective as 40-200 mg three times weekly.

A variety of medical interventions are available to assist sufferers of recurrent UTI (79). Twice-daily perineal cleansing with a disinfectant is partially protective (21). More commonly used is oral antimicrobial therapy, either as chronic prophylaxis, postcoital prophylaxis, or intermittent self-administered therapy for symptomatic recurrences.

Numerous trials have shown that chronic prophylaxis (daily or thrice weekly) with low doses of any of several antimicrobial agents (Table 3) reduces the frequency of recurrences among women with frequent UTI from two to three episodes per year to approximately 0.2 episodes per year (4, 11, 20, 78, 79, 89). Prophylaxis is commonly continued for 6 months to 1 year and then interrupted to see if the previous pattern of recurrent UTI has "burned itself out" or will resume. Surprisingly, emergence of resistant strains has not been a problem in studies of chronic prophylaxis in otherwise healthy young women (79).

For women with coitus-associated UTI, a small dose of an antimicrobial agent after intercourse can provide effective prophylaxis (96, 97, 128, 135). For individuals with infrequent sexual activity, such treatment may allow the use of considerably fewer antibiotic doses than daily prophylaxis would require.

Some women with recurrent UTI are highly accurate in identifying when they are developing a recurrence, and such accuracy permits early self-initiated treatment from a supply of antibiotic kept at home (4, 142). On balance, such intermittent self-administered therapy involves the consumption of less drug than does daily prophylaxis, but it costs about the same (142). It may be preferred by women who have infrequent recurrences or who are willing to occasionally experience the beginning symptoms of a UTI episode in exchange for not having to take daily drug therapy (142).

Thus, for women with frequent (more than two or three per year) recurrences of UTI, alternative management options include chronic prophylactic antibiotic therapy, postcoital antibiotics, and intermittent self-administered antibiotics. Frequency of recurrences, association of recurrences with intercourse, and patient preferences will determine which approach is best suited for an individual patient. Finally, for the few women who have repeated bouts of UTI with the same organism (suggesting relapse from a persisting internal focus) or who have breakthrough UTI despite prophylactic therapy, the possibility of an underlying anatomical or functional abnormality of the urinary tract that might warrant further investigation and therapy should be considered (33).

## COMPLICATED UTI AND UTI IN THE ELDERLY

In contrast to the information available about healthy young women, publications discussing UTI prevention efforts for adults with complicating conditions that predispose to UTI are comparatively few. Several recent reports document success with prophylyactic antimicrobial therapy in compromised adults and with nonantibiotic measures in the elderly.

**Spinal Cord Injury.** For patients with spinal cord injury, UTI is a major cause of morbidity and mortality (15).

Chronic prophylactic systemic antibiotics appear to be effective (15), as they are in urologically intact women with recurrent UTI (78, 79). In a recent trial, low-dose daily ciprofloxacin prevented bacteriuria in spinal cord injury patients without increasing the prevalence of resistant bacteria (15). The risk-benefit ratio for such long-term prophylaxis (considering cost, adverse effects, and induction of resistance) remains to be conclusively assessed.

**Renal Transplant Recipients.** Renal transplant recipients are at high risk for renal infection both for mechanical reasons and because of the immunosuppressive therapy used to prevent graft rejection (30). Chronic prophylactic antibiotic therapy with trimethoprim-sulfamethoxazole is commonly used in this context, at least in the early post-transplant period; such therapy additionally provides protection against nocardiosis, toxoplasmosis, and pneumocystosis, for which these patients also are at risk (30). The efficacy of chronic prophylaxis with trimethoprim-sulfamethoxazole therapy in preventing UTI and bacteremia in kidney transplant recipients was documented in a recent trial for both a standard-dose (160 plus 800 mg daily) and a higher-dose (320 plus 1600 mg daily) regimen (30). Emergence of resistance was not observed (30).

**Estrogen Replacement Therapy for Elderly Women.** The normal premenopausal vaginal microenvironment exhibits a low pH (<4.5) and a bacterial flora characterized by an abundance of lactobacilli and anaerobes and a paucity of gram-negative bacilli (104). In contrast, the postmenopausal vaginal microenvironment exhibits an elevated pH, absence of lactobacilli, and abundant coliform bacilli (104). Similar conditions are seen among premenopausal women who use spermicide-diaphragm contraception, in whom these conditions are thought to contribute to the increased risk of UTI in this population by establishing vaginal colonization with potentially uropathogenic bacteria (41). Oral (19, 101) or topical (95, 101, 104) estrogen replacement therapy in postmenopausal women reduces the frequency of bacteriuria in these women, possibly because of the effectiveness of such therapy in restoring a premenopausal vaginal microenvironment and diminishing vaginal colonization with coliform bacilli (104).

**Cranberry Juice for the Elderly.** Daily consumption of cranberry juice cocktail (in comparison with an indistinguishable placebo beverage) for 6 months significantly decreased the prevalence of bacteriuria among elderly residents of a seniors' home in a recent clinical trial (9). On a monthly basis, cranberry cocktail recipients with bacteriuria were more likely to become abacteriuric and those without bacteriuria were more likely to remain abacteriuric than were the corresponding placebo recipients (9). Most of the episodes of bacteriuria were asymptomatic, so the clinical value of the observed preventive effect could be questioned. However, there were trends toward decreased antibiotic use and fewer symptomatic UTI episodes in the treatment group (9), evidence suggesting that the intervention may have provided a meaningful benefit.

The mechanism of action of cranberry cocktail in this trial probably was not related to cranberry juice's hippurate content (38), because the placebo had a similar hippurate concentration (10). The mechanism of action may have involved inhibitors of *E. coli* adherence that are present in cranberry juice (9, 146).

## PREGNANT WOMEN
UTI in pregnant women who have been treated for ABU or an episode of symptomatic UTI can be prevented either by daily oral antibiotic prophylaxis for the duration of pregnancy (43) or by close monitoring with prompt treatment of any

newly detected bacteriuria (43). Close monitoring for bacteriuria without daily prophylaxis minimizes fetal exposure to antimicrobial agents. Daily prophylaxis may be especially appropriate following an episode of pyelonephritis (110, 139).

## CHILDREN

**Recurrent UTI in Girls.** Girls without underlying anatomical urinary tract abnormalities who suffer from frequent episodes of recurrent symptomatic UTI can be protected by the use of chronic prophylactic antibiotic therapy much like that used for adult women with recurrent UTI (see above). Antibiotics in combination, e.g., nitrofurantoin and trimethoprim, offer an advantage over monotherapy in these cases (120).

**Children with Vesicoureteral Reflux.** Vesicoureteral reflux puts children at increased risk for renal scarring and chronic renal impairment with repeated infection episodes (140). Neither antireflux surgery nor the casual use of prophylactic antibiotic therapy can adequately protect such children from recurrent UTI (140). Optimal care for these patients requires, in addition to prophylactic antibiotic therapy, close monitoring, a coordinated team approach, and enlistment of the patient and parents as cooperative partners in the management plan (140).

## Catheter-Associated UTI

The best way to prevent catheter-associated UTI is to avoid the use of indwelling catheters altogether and to keep the duration of use to an absolute minimum when catheters cannot be avoided (137). Other than the use of a closed catheter system (62, 99), few of the many interventions that have been explored as ways to reduce the risk of UTI in patients who must have a catheter, including meatal care, coated catheters, drainage bag additives, bladder-irrigation, and special antireflux drainage bags, have proved clearly effective (52, 58, 60, 124, 137).

Prophylactic systemic antimicrobial therapy (22) has received increased attention recently as a way to prevent catheter-associated UTI in patients with short-term catheter use (112). The traditional view has been that antibiotic prophylaxis should be avoided in catheterized patients because of the likelihood of selecting for resistant organisms. However, observational data from numerous studies demonstrate a significant protective effect of antibiotic use during the first 2 weeks of catheterization without apparent ill effects (44, 124). Furthermore, prospective trials have shown benefits with prophylactic norfloxacin (134), amoxicillin (69), and ciprofloxacin (133) for patients with indwelling catheters in the acute care setting. In contrast, cephalexin was of no apparent benefit among patients catheterized for only 72 h in another study (70), but the absence of UTI even in the control group precluded firm conclusions.

Thus, the risk of UTI may be small enough during periods of catheterization shorter than 3 days to preclude any benefit from antibiotic prophylaxis. Similarly, the likelihood of UTI in patients with long-term catheter use may be so great that chronic prophylactic therapy could only be expected to select for resistant organisms (137). However, patients with short-term catheter use for more than several days who otherwise would not be receiving antimicrobial agents might benefit from prophylactic antimicrobial therapy. A cost-benefit analysis that takes into account the adverse effects and the increased antimicrobial resistance that might result from such prophylaxis is needed.

## Unestablished Preventive Modalities

### LACTOBACILLUS THERAPY

Despite some evidence that ingestion or topical application of live preparations of lactobacilli provides protection against gastrointestinal infections, vaginitis, and UTI (as reviewed in reference 105), no lactobacillus-based regimen for UTI prevention has achieved general acceptance. The absence of convincing evidence of the efficacy of lactobacillus therapy may indicate that alterations in the vaginal flora other than lactobacillus depletion account for the increased vaginal colonization with coliform bacteria associated with antibiotic administration (141), spermicide-diaphragm use (41), and the postmenopausal state (104). Alternatively, it may be that most of the lactobacillus trials done to date have not used the proper type(s) of lactobacilli or optimal delivery strategies (105).

## IMMUNOBIOTHERAPY

Although a vaccine to prevent UTI by interfering with specific bacterial virulence properties is envisioned by some (115), it faces many practical and theoretical obstacles (47, 59). However, a less specifically targeted UTI vaccine has already undergone several clinical trials (31, 37, 116, 130). Compared with placebo, daily oral administration of a vaccine consisting of a hydrolysate of several *E. coli* strains significantly reduced the frequency of bacteriuria during a 3-month treatment period and a subsequent 3-month observation period among subjects with a history of recurrent UTI (116, 130). Abnormal urinalysis findings and dysuria were less consistently improved (116, 130). Interestingly, in the most recent of these studies, UTI with organisms other than gram-negative bacilli as well as with *E. coli* was reduced (116). These provocative findings suggest a need for further study of this or similar products.

## SUMMARY

Current approaches to the treatment of UTI require delineation of the patient's clinical syndrome and consideration of the underlying host status followed by selection of an antimicrobial agent and a duration of therapy appropriate to the clinical situation. Antimicrobial agents with demonstrated efficacy in UTI therapy are selected on the basis their spectra of activity (in comparison with the known or predicted susceptibility pattern of the urine organism), their pharmacokinetic properties, adverse effect profile, cost, convenience, and track record in specific clinical syndromes. The optimal duration of therapy with today's agents is fairly well defined for women with uncomplicated cystitis, for whom short treatment courses ($\leq 3$ days) with first-line agents are highly effective and inexpensive and are associated with an acceptably low frequency of adverse effects. In other clinical situations, treatment usually must be extended, success rates often are lower, and adverse effects are more frequent. Urine cultures should be used to guide therapy in all circumstances other than acute cystitis in healthy young adult women.

ABU requires treatment only during pregnancy and in a few other uncommon situations. Urological investigation is warranted for patients who do not respond to therapy for UTI, in whom obstruction is suspected, or who have relapsing infections due to the same strain; for children who have symptomatic UTI; but not for the great majority of women with recurrent UTI.

Prevention of UTI relies mainly on judicious use of antimicrobial agents either for chronic prophylaxis, postcoital prophylaxis, or intermittent self-administered therapy. Avoidance of indwelling catheters is the best way to prevent catheter-associated UTI. Several nonantibiotic preventive measures, including estrogen replacement in postmenopausal women, may be useful for selected patients with recurrent UTI.

## ACKNOWLEDGMENT

Jodi A. Aasmundrud helped with manuscript preparation.

## REFERENCES

1. **Abraham, E., and L. J. Baraff.** 1982. Oral versus parenteral therapy of pyelonephritis. *Curr. Ther. Res. Clin. Exp.* **31:**536–542.
2. **Abrutyn, E., J. Mossey, J. A. Berlin, J. Boscia, M. Levison, P. Pitsakis, and D. Kaye.** 1994. Does asymptomatic bacteriuria predict mortality and does antimicrobial treatment reduce mortality in elderly ambulatory women? *Ann. Intern. Med.* **120:**827–833.
3. **Ahlmén, J., J. Frisén, and G. Ekbladh.** 1982. Experience of three-day trimethoprim therapy for dysuria-frequency in primary health care. *Scand. J. Infect. Dis.* **14:**213–216.
4. **Andriole, V. T.** 1992. Discussion of L. E. Nicolle's presentation. *Infection* **20**(Suppl. 3):S210.
5. **Andriole, V. T.** 1992. Urinary tract infections in the 90s: pathogenesis and management. *Infection* **20**(Suppl. 4):S251–S256.
6. **Andriole, V. T., and T. F. Patterson.** 1991. Epidemiology, natural history, and management of urinary tract infections in pregnancy. *Med. Clin. North Am.* **75:**359–373.
7. **Angel, J. L., W. F. O'Brien, M. A. Finan, W. J. Morales, M. Lake, and R. A. Knuppel.** 1990. Acute pyelonephritis in pregnancy: a prospective study of oral versus intravenous antibiotic therapy. *Obstet. Gynecol.* **76:**28–32.
8. **Arav-Boger, R., L. Leibovici, and Y. L. Danon.** 1994. Urinary tract infections with low and high colony counts in young women. Spontaneous remission and single-dose vs. multiple-day treatment. *Arch. Intern. Med.* **154:**300–304.
9. **Avorn, J., M. Monane, J. H. Gurwitz, R. J. Glynn, I. Choodnovskiy, and L. A. Lipsitz.** 1994. Reduction of bacteriuria and pyuria after ingestion of cranberry juice. *JAMA* **271:**751–754.
10. **Avorn, J., M. Monane, J. H. Gurwitz, R. J. Glynn, I. Choodnovskiy, and L. A. Lipsitz.** 1994. Reduction of bacteriuria and pyuria using cranberry juice. *JAMA* **272:**589–590. (Letter.)
11. **Bailey, R. R.** 1992. Discussion of L. E. Nicolle's presentation. *Infection* **20**(Suppl. 3):S206–S207.
12. **Bailey, R. R., and B. A. Peddie.** 1987. Treatment of acute urinary tract infection in women. *Ann. Intern. Med.* **107:**430.
13. **Baldassarre, J. S., and D. Kaye.** 1991. Special problems of urinary tract infection in the elderly. *Med. Clin. North Am.* **75:**375–390.
14. **Barnes, R. C., R. Daifuku, R. E. Roddy, and W. E. Stamm.** 1986. Urinary-tract infection in sexually active homosexual men. *Lancet* **i:**171–173.
15. **Biering-Sorensen, F., N. Hoiby, A. Nordenbo, M. Ravnborg, B. Bruun, and V. Rahm.** 1994. Ciprofloxacin as prophylaxis for urinary tract infection: prospective, randomized, cross-over, placebo controlled study in patients with spinal cord lesion. *J. Urol.* **151:**105–108.
16. **Boerema, J. B. J., and K. F. Van Saene.** 1986. Norfloxacin treatment in complicated urinary tract infection. *Scand. J. Infect. Dis.* **Supplement 48:**20–26.
17. **Boscia, J. A., E. Abrutyn, and D. Kaye.** 1987. Asymptomatic bacteriuria in elderly persons: treat or do not treat? *Ann. Intern. Med.* **106:**764–766.
18. **Boscia, J. A., W. D. Kobasa, R. A. Knight, E. Abrutyn, M. E. Levison, and D. Kaye.** 1987. Therapy vs no therapy for bacteriuria in elderly ambulatory nonhospitalized women. *JAMA* **257:**1067–1071.
19. **Brandenberg, A., D. Mellstrom, and G. Samsioe.** 1973. Low dose oral estriol treatment in elderly women with urogenital infections. *Acta Obstet. Gynecol. Scand.* **52:**257–264.
20. **Brumfitt, W., and J. M. T. Hamilton-Miller.** 1990. Prophylactic antibiotics for recurrent urinary tract infections. *J. Antimicrob. Chemother.* **25:**505–512.
21. **Brumfitt, W., J. M. T. Hamilton-Miller, R. A. Gargan, J. Cooper, and G. W. Smith.** 1983. Long-term prophylaxis of urinary infections in women: comparative trial of trimethoprim, methenamine hippurate and topical povidone-iodine. *J. Urol.* **130:**1110–1114.
22. **Butler, H. K., and C. M. Kunin.** 1968. Evaluation of specific systemic antimicrobial therapy in patients while on closed catheter drainage. *J. Urol.* **100:**567–572.
23. **Caron, F., and G. Humbert.** 1992. Short-term treatment of urinary tract infections: the French concept. *Infection* **20**(Suppl. 4):S286–S290.
24. **Dolan, J. G.** 1989. Medical decision making using the analytic hierarchy process: choice

25. **Dontas, A. S., P. Kasviki-Charvati, P. C. Papanayiotou, and S. G. Marketos.** 1981. Bacteriuria and survival in old age. *N. Engl. J. Med.* **304:**939–943.
26. **Evans, D. A., E. H. Kass, C. H. Hennekens, B. Rosner, L. Miao, M. I. Kendrick, W. E. Miall, and K. L. Stuart.** 1982. Bacteriuria and subsequent mortality in women. *Lancet* **i:**156–158.
27. **Fihn, S. D., C. Johnson, P. L. Roberts, K. Running, and W. E. Stamm.** 1988. Trimethoprim-sulfamethoxazole for acute dysuria in women: a single-dose or 10-day course. A double-blind, randomized trial. *Ann. Intern. Med.* **108:**350–357.
28. **Fisher, J. F., W. H. Chew, S. Shadomy, R. J. Duma, C. G. Mayhall, and W. C. House.** 1982. Urinary tract infections due to *Candida albicans*. *Rev. Infect. Dis.* **4:**1107–1118.
29. **Fisher, J. F., B. C. Hicks, J. T. Dipiro, J. Venable, and R.-M. E. Fincher.** 1987. Efficacy of a single intravenous dose of amphotericin B in urinary tract infections caused by *Candida*. *J. Infect. Dis.* **156:**685.
30. **Fox, B. C., H. W. Sollinger, F. O. Belzer, and D. G. Maki.** 1990. A prospective, randomized, double-blind study of trimethoprim-sulfamethoxazole for prophylaxis of infection in renal transplantation: clinical efficacy, absorption of trimethoprim-sulfamethoxazole, effects on the microflora, and the cost-benefit of prophylaxis. *Am. J. Med.* **89:**255–274.
31. **Frey, C., W. Obolensky, and H. Wyss.** 1986. Treatment of recurrent urinary tract infections: efficacy of an orally administered biological response modifier. *Urol. Int.* **41:**444–446.
32. **Gaudreault, P., M. Beland, J. B. Girodias, and R. L. Thivierge.** 1992. Single daily doses of trimethoprim/sulphadiazine for three or 10 days in urinary tract infections. *Acta Paediatr.* **81:**695–697.
33. **Gillenwater, J. Y.** 1991. The role of the urologist in urinary tract infection. *Med. Clin. North Am.* **75:**471–479.
34. **Gleckman, R., P. Bradley, R. Roth, D. Hibert, and C. Pelletier.** 1985. Therapy of symptomatic pyelonephritis in women. *J. Urol.* **133:**176–178.
35. **Gleckman, R. A., P. J. Bradley, R. M. Roth, and D. M. Hibert.** 1985. Bacteremia urosepsis: a phenomenon unique to elderly women. *J. Urol.* **133:**174–175.
36. **Grubbs, N. C., H. J. Schultz, N. K. Henry, D. M. Ilstrup, S. M. Muller, and W. R. Wilson.** 1992. Ciprofloxacin versus trimethoprim-sulfamethoxazole: treatment of community-acquired urinary tract infections in a prospective, controlled, double-blind comparison. *Mayo Clin. Proc.* **67:**1163–1168.
37. **Hachen, H. J.** 1990. Oral immunotherapy in paraplegic patients with chronic urinary tract infections: a double-blind, placebo-controlled trial. *J. Urol.* **143:**759–762.
38. **Hamilton-Miller, J. M. T.** 1994. Reduction of bacteriuria and pyuria using cranberry juice. *JAMA* **272:**588–589.
39. **Hankins, G. D. V., and P. J. Whalley.** 1985. Acute urinary tract infections in pregnancy. *Clin. Obstet. Gynecol.* **28:**266–278.
40. **Hebelka, M., K. Lincoln, and T. Sandberg.** 1993. Sexual acquisition of acute pyelonephritis in a man. *Scand. J. Infect. Dis.* **25:**141–143.
41. **Hooton, T. M., S. Hillier, C. Johnson, P. L. Roberts, and W. E. Stamm.** 1991. *Escherichia coli* bacteriuria and contraceptive method. *JAMA* **265:**64–69.
42. **Hooton, T. M., C. Winter, F. Tiu, and W. E. Stamm.** 1995. Randomized comparative trial and cost analysis of 3-day antimicrobial regimens for treatment of acute cystitis in women. *JAMA* **273:**41–45.
43. **Humbert, G.** 1992. French consensus on antibiotherapy of urinary tract infections. *Infection* **20**(Suppl. 3)**:**S171–S172.
44. **Hustinx, W. N. M., A. J. Mintges-de Groot, R. P. Verkooyen, and H. A. Verbrugh.** 1991. Impact of concurrent antimicrobial therapy on catheter-associated urinary tract infection. *J. Hosp. Infect.* **18:**45–56.
45. **Inter-Nordic Urinary Tract Infection Study Group.** 1988. Double-blind comparison of 3-day versus 7-day treatment with norfloxacin in symptomatic urinary tract infections. *Scand. J. Infect. Dis.* **20:**619–624.
46. **Jernelius, H., J. Zbornik, and C.-A. Bauer.** 1988. One or three weeks' treatment of acute pyelonephritis? A double-blind comparison, using a fixed combination of pivampicillin plus pivmecillinam. *Acta Med. Scand.* **223:**469–477.
47. **Johnson, J. R.** 1991. Virulence factors in *Escherichia coli* urinary tract infection. *Clin. Microbiol. Rev.* **4:**80–128.
48. **Johnson, J. R.** 1993. Should all catheterized patients with candiduria be treated? *Clin. Infect. Dis.* **17:**814.

49. **Johnson, J. R.** 1994. Pathogenesis of bacteremia during pyelonephritis. *Clin. Infect. Dis.* **18:**1014–1015. (Letters.)
50. **Johnson, J. R., M. F. Lyons II, W. Pearce, P. Gorman, P. L. Roberts, N. White, P. Brust, R. Olsen, J. W. Gnann, Jr., and W. E. Stamm.** 1991. Therapy for women hospitalized with acute pyelonephritis: a randomized trial of ampicillin versus trimethoprim-sulfamethoxazole for 14 days. *J. Infect. Dis.* **163:**325–330.
51. **Johnson, J. R., P. Roberts, and W. E. Stamm.** 1987. P fimbriae and other virulence factors in *Escherichia coli* urosepsis: association with patients' characteristics. *J. Infect. Dis.* **156:**225–229.
52. **Johnson, J. R., P. L. Roberts, R. J. Olsen, K. A. Moyer, and W. E. Stamm.** 1990. Prevention of catheter-associated urinary tract infection with a silver oxide-coated urinary catheter: clinical and microbiological correlates. *J. Infect. Dis.* **162:**1145–1150.
53. **Johnson, J. R., and W. E. Stamm.** 1989. Urinary tract infections in women: diagnosis and treatment. *Ann. Intern. Med.* **111:**906–917.
54. **Kozinn, W. P., R. L. Holmes, and A. Mulrooney.** 1990. Emergence of ciprofloxacin resistance in bacterial isolates from nursing home patients, abstr. 49. *Program Abstr. 30th Intersci. Conf. Antimicrob. Agents Chemother.*
55. **Krieger, J. N.** 1986. Complications and treatment of urinary tract infections during pregnancy. *Urol. Clin. North Am.* **13:**685–693.
56. **Kromann-Andersen, B., and K. Kroyer Nielsen.** 1990. Ofloxacin in urinary tract infections. *Scand. J. Infect. Dis.* **Suppl. 68:**35–40.
57. **Kunin, C. M.** 1985. Use of antimicrobial agents in treating urinary tract infection. *Adv. Nephrol.* **14:**39–65.
58. **Kunin, C. M.** 1985. The drainage bag additive saga. *Infect. Control.* **6:**261–262.
59. **Kunin, C. M.** 1986. The prospects for a vaccine to prevent pyelonephritis. *N. Engl. J. Med.* **314:**514.
60. **Kunin, C. M.** 1988. Can we build a better urinary catheter? *N. Engl. J. Med.* **319:**365–366.
61. **Kunin, C. M.** 1994. Urinary tract infections in females. *Clin. Infect. Dis.* **18:**1–12.
62. **Kunin, C. M., and R. C. McCormack.** 1966. Prevention of catheter-induced urinary-tract infections by sterile closed drainage. *N. Engl. J. Med.* **274:**1155–1162.
63. **Lapierre, G., and R. S. Porter.** 1983. Concomitant systemic and local amphotericin B for fungal cystitis. *Clin. Pharm.* **2:**396–399.
64. **Leibovici, L., G. Alpert, A. Laor, O. Kalter-Leibovivi, and Y. L. Danon.** 1987. Urinary tract infections and sexual activity in young women. *Arch. Intern. Med.* **147:**345–347.
65. **Leibovici, L., S. Greenshtain, O. Cohen, and A. J. Wysenbeek.** 1992. Toward improved empiric management of moderate to severe urinary tract infections. *Arch. Intern. Med.* **152:**2481–2486.
66. **Leibovici, L., and A. J. Wysenbeek.** 1991. Single-dose antibiotic treatment for symptomatic urinary tract infections in women: a meta-analysis of randomized trials. *Q. J. Med.* **78:**43–57.
67. **Levison, M. E.** 1992. New dosing regimens for aminoglycoside antibiotics. *Ann. Intern. Med.* **117:**693–694.
68. **Lipsky, B. A.** 1989. Urinary tract infections in men. *Ann. Intern. Med.* **110:**138–150.
69. **Little, P. J., S. Pearson, B. A. Peddie, N. F. Greenslade, and W. L. F. Utley.** 1974. Amoxicillin in the prevention of catheter-induced urinary infection. *J. Infect. Dis.* **129:**241–242.
70. **Malek, R. S., W. H. Boyce, and R. M. Wilkiemeyer.** 1973. Urinary tract sterility and indwelling catheters. *J. Urol.* **100:**84–85.
71. **McCue, J. D.** 1993. Urinary tract infections in the elderly. *Pharmacotherapy* **13:**51S–53S.
72. **McDonald, C. L., K. M. Ramsey, K. Roveda, C. J. Hoff, and K. Chapin.** 1993. Relationship of severity of illness and microbiologic outcome of funguria in hospitalized patients. *Clin. Res.* **41:**767A.
73. **Michigan, S.** 1976. Genitourinary fungal infections. *J. Urol.* **116:**390–397.
74. **Moyer, D. V., and J. E. Edwards, Jr.** 1992. Postcatheterization candiduria: issues—and answers. *J. Crit. Illness* **7:**1024.
75. **Murray, B. E., T. Alvarado, K.-H. Kim, M. Vorachit, P. Jayanetra, M. M. Levine, I. Prenzel, M. Fling, L. Elwell, G. H. McCracken, G. Madrigal, C. Odio, and L. R. Trabulsi.** 1985. Increasing resistance to trimethoprim-sulfamethoxazole among isolates of *Escherichia coli* in developing countries. *J. Infect. Dis.* **152:**1107–1113.
76. **Neu, H. C.** 1992. Optimal characteristics of agents to treat uncomplicated urinary tract infections. *Infection* **20**(Suppl. 4)**:**S266–S271.
77. **Nickel, J. C., and R. Pidutti.** 1992. A rational approach to urinary tract infections in older patients. *Geriatrics* **47:**49–55.

78. Nicolle, L. E. 1990. The optimal management of lower urinary tract infections. *Infection* **18**(Suppl. 2):S50–S52.
79. Nicolle, L. E. 1992. Prophylaxis: recurrent urinary tract infection in women. *Infection* **20**(Suppl. 3):S203–S205.
80. Nicolle, L. E. 1992. Urinary tract infection in the elderly. How to treat and when? *Infection* **20**(Suppl. 4):S261–S265.
81. Nicolle, L. E., J. Bjornson, G. K. M. Harding, and J. A. MacDonell. 1983. Bacteriuria in elderly institutionalized men. *N. Engl. J. Med.* **309**:1420–1425.
82. Nicolle, L. E., G. K. M. Harding, J. Preiksaitis, and A. R. Ronald. 1982. The association of urinary tract infection with sexual intercourse. *J. Infect. Dis.* **146**:579–583.
83. Nicolle, L. E., E. Henderson, J. Bjornson, M. McIntyre, G. K. M. Harding, and J. A. MacDonell. 1987. The association of bacteriuria with resident characteristics and survival in elderly institutionalized men. *Ann. Intern. Med.* **106**:682–686.
84. Nicolle, L. E., T. J. Louie, J. Dubois, A. Martel, G. K. Harding, and C. P. Sinave. 1994. Treatment of complicated urinary tract infections with lomefloxacin compared with that with trimethoprim-sulfamethoxazole. *Antimicrob. Agents Chemother.* **38**:1368–1373.
85. Nicolle, L. E., W. J. Mayhew, and L. Bryan. 1987. Prospective randomized comparison of therapy and no therapy for asymptomatic bacteriuria in institutionalized elderly women. *Am. J. Med.* **83**:27–33.
86. Nordenstam, G. R., C. A. Brandberg, A. S. Odén, C. M. Svanborg Edén, and A. Svanborg. 1986. Bacteriuria and mortality in an elderly population. *N. Engl. J. Med.* **314**:1152–1156.
87. Norrby, S. R. 1990. Short-term treatment of uncomplicated lower urinary tract infections in women. *Rev. Infect. Dis.* **12**:458–467.
88. Nunez, J. E., E. Perez, S. Gunasekaran, J. Narvarte, and G. Ramirez. 1992. Acute renal failure secondary to acute bacterial pyelonephritis. *Nephron* **62**:240–241.
89. Nuñez, U., and Z. Solís. 1990. Macrocrystalline nitrofurantoin versus norfloxacin as treatment and prophylaxis in uncomplicated recurrent urinary tract infection. *Curr. Ther. Res. Clin. Exp.* **48**:234–245.
90. Occhipinti, D. J., L. L. Schoonover, and L. H. Danziger. 1993. Bladder irrigation with amphotericin B for treatment of patients with candiduria. *Clin. Infect. Dis.* **17**:812–813.
91. Ode, B., M. Bröms, M. Walder, and S. Cronberg. 1980. Failure of excessive doses of ampicillin to prevent bacterial relapse in the treatment of acute pyelonephritis. *Acta Med. Scand.* **207**:305–307.
92. Österberg, E., H. Aberg, H. O. Hallander, A. Kallner, and A. Lundin. 1990. Efficacy of single-dose versus seven-day trimethoprim treatment of cystitis in women: a randomized double-blind study. *J. Infect. Dis.* **161**:942–947.
93. Otto, G., T. Sandberg, B.-I. Marklund, P. Ulleryd, and C. Svanborg. 1993. Virulence factors and *pap* genotype in *Escherichia coli* isolates from women with acute pyelonephritis, with or without bacteremia. *Clin. Infect. Dis.* **17**:448–456.
94. Paladino, J. A., and R. E. Crass. 1982. Amphotericin B and flucytosine in the treatment of candidal cystitis. *Clin. Pharm.* **1**:349–352.
95. Parsons, C. L., and J. D. Schmidt. 1982. Control of recurrent lower UTI in the postmenopausal woman. *J. Urol.* **128**:1224–1226.
96. Pfau, A. 1991. Sex and recurrent UTI in young women. *Med. Aspects Hum. Sex.* **25**(6):34–39.
97. Pfau, A. 1992. Discussion of L. E. Nicolle's presentation. *Infection* **20**(Suppl. 3):S208–S209.
98. Pinson, A. G., J. T. Philbrick, G. H. Lindbeck, and J. B. Schorling. 1992. Oral antibiotic therapy for acute pyelonephritis. *J. Gen. Intern. Med.* **7**:544–553.
99. Platt, R., B. Murdock, B. F. Polk, and b. Rosner. 1983. Reduction of mortality associated with nosocomial urinary tract infection. *Lancet* **i**:893–897.
100. Preheim, L. C. 1985. Complicated urinary tract infections. *Am. J. Med.* **79**:62–66.
101. Privette, M., R. Cade, and J. Peterson. 1988. Prevention of recurrent UTI in postmenopausal women. *Nephron* **50**:24–27.
102. Raz, R., E. Rottensterich, S. Boger, and I. Potasman. 1991. Comparison of single-dose administration and three-day course of amoxicillin with those of clavulanic acid for treatment of uncomplicated urinary tract infection in women. *Antimicrob. Agents Chemother.* **35**:1688–1690.
103. Raz, R., E. Rottensterich, Y. Leshem, and H. Tabenkin. 1994. Double-blind study comparing regimens of cefixime and ofloxacin in treatment of uncomplicated urinary tract infections in women. *Antimicrob. Agents Chemother.* **38**:1176–1177.

104. **Raz, R., and W. E. Stamm.** 1993. A controlled trial of intravaginal estriol in postmenopausal women with recurrent urinary tract infections. *N. Engl. J. Med.* **329:**753–756.
105. **Reid, G., A. W. Bruce, J. A. McGroarty, K.-J. Cheng, and J. W. Costerton.** 1990. Is there a role for lactobacilli in prevention of urogenital and intestinal infections? *Clin. Microbiol. Rev.* **3:**335–344.
106. **Ronald, A., L. E. Nicolle, and G. Harding.** 1992. Single dose treatment failure in women with acute cystitis. *Infection* **20**(Suppl. 4)**:**S276–S279.
107. **Ronald, A. R.** 1987. Optimal duration of treatment for kidney infection. *Ann. Intern. Med.* **106:**467–468.
108. **Sable, C. A., and W. M. Scheld.** 1993. Fluoroquinolones: how to use (but not overuse) these antibiotics. *Geriatrics* **48:**41–51.
109. **Safrin, S., D. Siegel, and D. Black.** 1988. Pyelonephritis in adult women: inpatient versus outpatient therapy. *Am. J. Med.* **85:**793–798.
110. **Sandberg, T., and J. E. Brorson.** 1991. Efficacy of long-term antimicrobial prophylaxis after acute pyelonephritis in pregnancy. *Scand. J. Infect. Dis.* **23:**221–223.
111. **Sandberg, T., G. Otto, and C. Svanborg.** 1994. Pathogenesis of bacteremia during pyelonephritis. *Clin. Infect. Dis.* **18:**1015. (Letter.)
112. **Sanderson, P. J.** 1991. Prophylaxis for catheter related urinary tract infection. *J. Hosp. Infect.* **18:**1–3.
113. **Sanford, J. P.** 1993. The enigma of candiduria: evolution of bladder irrigation with amphotericin B for management—from anecdote to dogma and a lesson from Machiavelli. *Clin. Infect. Dis.* **16:**145–147.
114. **Sanford, J. P.** 1993. Should all catheterized patients with candiduria be treated? *Clin. Infect. Dis.* **17:**814.
115. **Schoolnik, G. K., and P. O'Hanley.** 1986. The prospects for a vaccine to prevent pyelonephritis. *N. Engl. J. Med.* **314:**515.
116. **Schulman, C. C., A. Corbusier, H. Michiels, and H. J. Taenzer.** 1993. Oral immunotherapy of recurrent urinary tract infections: a double-blind placebo-controlled multicenter study. *J. Urol.* **150:**917–921.
117. **Sheinfeld, J., A. J. Schaeffer, C. Cordon-Cardo, A. Rogatko, and W. R. Fair.** 1989. Association of the Lewis blood-group phenotype with recurrent urinary tract infections in women. *N. Engl. J. Med.* **320:**773–777.
118. **Sherbotie, J. R., and D. Cornfeld.** 1991. Management of urinary tract infections in children. *Med. Clin. North Am.* **75:**327–338.
119. **Sigurdsson, J. A., J. Ahlmen, and L. Berglund.** 1983. Three-day treatment of acute lower urinary tract infections in women. *Acta Med. Scand.* **213:**55–60.
120. **Smith, E. M., and J. S. Elder.** 1994. Double antimicrobial prophylaxis in girls with breakthrough urinary tract infections. *Urology* **43:**708–712.
121. **Smith, J. W., and M. Segal.** 1994. Urinary tract infection in men—an internist's viewpoint. *Infection* **22**(Suppl. 1)**:**S31–S34.
122. **Sourander, L. B., and A. Kasanen.** 1972. A 5-year follow-up of bacteriuria in the aged. *Gerontol. Clin.* **14:**274–281.
123. **Stamm, W. E.** 1989. Urinary tract infections. *Curr. Opin. Infect. Dis.* **2:**210–212.
124. **Stamm, W. E.** 1991. Catheter-associated urinary tract infections: epidemiology, pathogenesis, and prevention. *Am. J. Med.* **91**(Suppl. 3B)**:**65S–71S.
125. **Stamm, W. E.** 1992. Controversies in single dose therapy of acute uncomplicated urinary tract infections in women. *Infection* **20**(Suppl. 4)**:**S272–S275.
126. **Stamm, W. E., and T. M. Hooton.** 1993. Management of urinary tract infections in adults. *N. Engl. J. Med.* **329:**1328–1334.
127. **Stamm, W. E., M. McKevitt, and G. W. Counts.** 1987. Acute renal infection in women: treatment with trimethoprim-sulfamethoxazole or ampicillin for two or six weeks. *Ann. Intern. Med.* **106:**341–345.
128. **Stapleton, A., R. H. Latham, C. Johnson, and W. E. Stamm.** 1990. Postcoital antimicrobial prophylaxis for recurrent urinary tract infection: a randomized, double-blind, placebo-controlled trial. *JAMA* **264:**703–706.
129. **Tacker, J. R.** 1992. Successful use of fluconazole for treatment of urinary tract fungal infections. *J. Urol.* **148:**1917–1918.
130. **Tammen, H. J., and The German Urinary Tract Infection Study Group.** 1990. Immunobiotherapy with Uro-Vaxom in recurrent urinary tract infection. *Br. J. Urol.* **65:**6–9.
131. **Trienekens, T., E. E. Stofferingh, R. Winkens, and A. W. Houben.** 1989. Different lengths of treatment with co-trimoxazole for acute uncomplicated urinary tract infections in women. *Br. Med. J.* **299:**1319–1322.
132. **Tungsanga, K., A. Chongthaleong, N. Udomsantisuk, O.-A. Petcharabutr, V.

Sitprija, and E. C. K. Wong. 1988. Norfloxacin versus co-trimoxazole for the treatment of upper urinary tract infections: a double blind trial. *Scand. J. Infect. Dis.* **Suppl. 56:**28–34.
133. van der Wall, E. 1992. Prophylactic ciprofloxacin for catheter-associated urinary-tract infection. *Lancet* **339:**946–951.
134. Verbrugh, H. A., A. J. Mintjes-de Groot, R. Andriesse, K. Hamersma, and A. van Dijk. 1988. Postoperative prophylaxis with norfloxacin in patients requiring bladder catheters. *Eur. J. Clin. Microbiol. Infect. Dis.* **7:**490–494.
135. Vosti, K. L. 1975. Recurrent urinary tract infections. Prevention of prophylactic antibiotics after sexual intercourse. *JAMA* **231:**934–940.
136. Waites, K. B., K. C. Canupp, and M. J. DeVivo. 1993. Eradication of urinary tract infection following spinal cord injury. *Paraplegia* **31:**645–652.
137. Warren, J. W. 1991. The catheter and urinary tract infection. *Med. Clin. North Am.* **75:**481–493.
138. Wilhelm, M. P., and R. S. Edson. 1987. Antimicrobial agents in urinary tract infections. *Mayo Clin. Proc.* **62:**1025–1032.
139. Wilkie, M. E., M. K. Almond, and F. P. Marsh. 1992. Diagnosis and management of urinary tract infection in adults. *Br. Med. J.* **305:**1137–1141.
140. Winberg, J. 1994. Management of primary vesico-uretric reflux in children—operation ineffective in preventing progressive renal damage. *Infection* **22**(Suppl. 1)**:**S4–S7.
141. Winberg, J., M. Herthelius-Elman, R. Mollby, and C. E. Nord. 1993. Pathogenesis of urinary tract infection: experimental studies of vaginal resistance to colonization. *Pediatr. Nephrol.* **7:**509–514.
142. Wong, E. S., M. McKevitt, K. Running, G. W. Counts, M. Turck, and W. E. Stamm. 1985. Management of recurrent urinary tract infections with patient-administered single-dose therapy. *Ann. Intern. Med.* **102:**302–307.
143. Wong, E. S., and W. E. Stamm. 1983. Sexual acquisition of urinary tract infection in a man. *JAMA* **250:**3087–3088.
144. Wong-Berigner, A., R. A. Jacobs, and J. Guglielmo. 1992. Treatment of funguria. *JAMA* **267:**2780–2785.
145. Woodrow, G., S. Patel, P. Berman, A. G. Morgan, and R. P. Burden. 1993. Asymptomatic acute pyelonephritis as a cause of acute renal failure in the elderly. *Postgrad. Med. J.* **69:**211–213.
146. Zafriri, D., I. Ofek, R. Adar, M. Pocino, and N. Sharon. 1989. Inhibitory activity of cranberry juice on adherence of type 1- and type P-fimbriated *Escherichia coli* to eucaryotic cells. *Antimicrob. Agents Chemother.* **33:**92–98.
147. Zinner, S. H. 1992. Management of urinary tract infections in pregnancy: a review with comments on single dose therapy. *Infection* **20**(Suppl. 4)**:**S280–S285.

# URINARY TRACT INFECTIONS DUE TO *CANDIDA* SPECIES

Jack D. Sobel, M.D., and Jose A. Vazquez, M.D.

## 5

*Candida* species are responsible for the overwhelming majority of fungal infections involving the urinary tract (6, 12, 14, 32). Although bladder infection is almost always the result of ascending infection, renal invasion by fungi is usually the result of hematogenous spread. Regardless of the site of infection, candiduria is inevitably the consequence of *Candida* urinary tract infection. Table 1 lists risk factors for *Candida* urinary tract infections. Fungal prostatitis is not the subject of this chapter.

## MICROBIOLOGY

*Candida* species are ubiquitous in nature. More than 80 species of *Candida* have been identified, but only a minority are important human pathogens: *Candida albicans, C. (Torulopsis) glabrata, C. tropicalis, C. parapsilosis, C. stellatoidea, C. kefyr, C. guilliermondii, C. krusei,* and *C. lusitaniae*. Although *C. albicans* is the commonest species isolated from the urine, non-*C. albicans* species account for almost half the *Candida* urinary isolates (27, 48). *C. glabrata* accounts for 25 to 35% of infections, and other *Candida* species account for 8 to 28% (15). Unusual species are especially common in hospitalized patients, especially diabetics with chronic indwelling bladder catheters. In addition, catheter specimens of urine often reveal simultaneous or coexistent infection with two or more species of *Candida*. *Candida* yeast cells, often called blastospores, reproduce by budding and under favorable conditions produce pseudohyphae and hyphae, which represent a more virulent and invasive phase of this dimorphic fungus. Recently introduced DNA-typing systems have revealed enormous genetic diversity among the multiple strains of *C. albicans* so far differentiated (45). These molecular epidemiological techniques have not been applied to urinary *Candida* isolates to correlate virulence with strain type or to further our knowledge of the pathogenesis of candiduria.

## EPIDEMIOLOGY

Although *Candida* microorganisms can exist as saprophytes on the external genitalia or urethra, yeast cells in any amount are found in <1% of clean-voided urine specimens (41). Of urine cultures obtained from patients in community hospitals,

---

*Jack D. Sobel and Jose A. Vazquez,* Division of Infectious Diseases, Department of Internal Medicine, Wayne State University School of Medicine, Detroit Medical Center, Detroit, Michigan 48201.

**TABLE 1** Risk factors for *Candida* urinary tract infection

| Type of infection | Route of infection | Risk factors |
|---|---|---|
| Renal candidiasis | Hematogenous | Neutropenia (prolonged), intravascular catheter, i.v. drug use, burns, recent surgery (abdominal, thoracic), systemic infection |
| *Candida* lower urinary tract | Ascending | Urinary catheter, female gender, extremes of age, instrumentation, diabetes mellitus, obstruction or stasis, recent antibacterial therapy, recent bacterial urinary tract infection, urinary stent, nephrostomy tube, renal transplantation |
| *Candida* pyelonephritis | Ascending | Diabetes, obstruction or stasis, instrumentation, postoperative status, nephrostomy tube, ureteral stent, nephrolithiasis |

5% yield *Candida* spp., and in tertiary care centers, *Candida* spp. account for approximately 10% of all urinary isolates (48). In contrast, the overall frequency of *Candida* infections in hospitalized subjects has increased by 200 to 300% in the 1980s (21). Indeed, most episodes of candiduria are nosocomial in origin, and Platt et al. determined that 26% of nosocomial catheter-associated urinary infections are caused by fungi (36). Even within the hospital environment, the incidence and prevalence of candiduria vary by unit, reaching 25 to 60% in high-risk patients in intensive care units (9, 14, 21, 32, 39, 48), thus emphasizing that candiduria is a marker of severe underlying disease. Moreover, Hsu and Ukleja found that 25% of hospitalized nursing home patients with indwelling urethral catheters had *Candida* spp. present in their urine (22).

Most positive cultures are isolated or transient findings of little significance and represent colonization rather than true infection. Less than 10% of candidemias are the consequence of candiduria (1), but even so, *Candida* urinary tract infections have emerged as important nosocomial infections (21, 36, 46).

**Renal Candidiasis**
Since renal candidiasis is most frequently the consequence of hematogenous spread, the epidemiology of renal candidiasis resembles that of candidemia and systemic candidiasis, with infection originating predominantly from endogenous sites, especially the gastrointestinal tract (GIT) in hospitalized patients (30). At highest risk are immunocompromised patients, particularly those with lymphohematological malignancies or profound granulocytopenia and/or those receiving corticosteroid and other immunosuppressive therapies. *Candida* colonization of the GIT occurs rapidly following hospitalization, and yeast counts increase following administration of antineoplastic chemotherapy and antimicrobial agents (45). Most candidemias and hence most renal involvement originate from asymptomatic GIT invasion by *Candida* organisms.

Another major nosocomial source of candidemia, particularly in nononcologic patients in medical and surgical intensive care units, is the indwelling intravascular catheter (37). Different *Candida* species appear to be uniquely associated with different portals of entry: *C. tropicalis* in some institutions has surpassed *C. albicans* as the commonest species causing candidemia in patients with hematological malignancies. Candidemia is now also a frequent complication of intravascular catheter use in premature infants. In patients with serious burns, candidemia follows prolonged intravenous (i.v.) catheter use and also frequently results from invasion of burn wounds. Following surgery, patients who have recently undergone abdominal operations, especially for neoplasia, and complicated cardiovascular patients are at highest risk.

## Lower Urinary Tract Infection

Lower urinary tract infection with *Candida* spp. occurs mainly as a result of urinary catheters. *Candida* cystitis occurs more frequently in women and may relate to the concomitant presence of *Candida* vaginitis; however, proof of this relationship is lacking. The factors that predispose to bladder infection by bacteria in catheterized patients have been delineated, but less information is available regarding *Candida* infections. In general, most catheter-related fungal infections follow bacteriuria and antibiotic therapy; however, *Candida* infection also frequently occurs simultaneously. Presumably, catheter colonization with *Candida* spp. originates from the fecal flora and perineal fecal contamination and colonization, with the vagina functioning as an additional reservoir. Nurses handling catheters may also contaminate catheters. *Candida* infection of the bladder in diabetics is also likely to be the result of an ascending infection.

Local mechanical factors other than the urinary catheter that increase susceptibility to *Candida* infection include congenital urinary tract anomalies, calculi, trauma, foreign bodies, and recent genitourinary surgery. Ureteral stents and nephrostomy tubes constitute major risk factors for the acquisition of candiduria, especially in diabetics (25). Renal transplantation is an additional high-risk situation for ascending *Candida* infection because of the presence of indwelling catheters, stents, antibiotics, anastomotic leaks, obstruction, and immunosuppressive therapy.

## PATHOGENESIS

See Table 2 for a listing of virulence factors important in the pathogenesis of *Candida* urinary tract infections.

**TABLE 2** *Candida* virulence factors in the pathogenesis of *Candida* urinary tract infections

| |
|---|
| Adherence to: |
|    Endothelial cells (renal candidiasis) |
|    Uroepithelial cells (ascending infections) |
|    Foreign surfaces (catheters) |
| Dimorphism capacity with formation of hyphae |
| Protease elaboration |
| Phospholipid secretion |
| Phenotype switching |
| Iron-binding capacity |
| Resistance to phagocytosis |
| Complement receptor (CR2, CR3) expression |

## Renal Candidiasis

*Candida* species gain access to the bloodstream from the heavily colonized GIT, especially postoperatively and in the presence of mucosal ulceration secondary to antineoplastic chemotherapy. Additional access can be by intravascular lines (especially in the setting of hyperalimentation), by venipuncture in heroin addicts, and by surgical sites, burns, and peritonitis. Hematogenous renal candidiasis has been fairly well studied in numerous animal models (29, 44). Not all *Candida* species have the same virulence capacity in hematogenous renal candidiasis. *C. albicans* and *C. tropicalis* demonstrate the greatest propensity to produce widespread metastatic disease, including renal involvement. The capacity of these species to invade the kidney reflects numerous virulence factors, in particular their enhanced capacities to adhere to capillary endothelial cells in the renal glomeruli and peritubular capillary network (7, 8, 19, 31). The propensity of *Candida* strains to produce germ tubes and hyphae also appears to be important in the invasion of renal parenchyma and the formation of abscesses (40). It is not entirely understood why the kidney is so susceptible to *Candida* metastatic infection, but this susceptibility may reflect the extensive vascular endothelial surface available. In the animal model, extrarenal lesions frequently heal spontaneously, but renal disease rarely does so.

With renal disease, renal invasion and penetration into the renal parenchyma associated with hyphal formation are progressive. In the renal cortex, mico- and macroabscesses may develop, but they rarely lead to perinephric abscess formation. Involvement of the renal vasculature by fungal elements may predispose to infarction and papillary necrosis (44). Not infrequently, *Candida* spp. may penetrate into the renal tubules, creating multiple sites of tubular obstruction. Extensive intraluminal pseudomycelial formation occurs, resulting in larger aggregates of fungi within the collecting system (11). The ensuing larger aggregates may form fungus balls, or bezoars, within the renal pelvis and ureters and not infrequently result in obstruction and hydronephrosis. In the animal model, corticosteroids and urinary obstruction facilitate progressive renal invasion. *C. glabrata,* which is incapable of producing pseudohyphae and hyphae but capable of causing renal infection, rarely produces fungal masses within the renal pelvis (15), thus emphasizing the importance of yeast virulence factors.

Within the kidneys, the dominant host defense mechanism is the inflammatory response by phagocytic polymorphonuclear leukocytes, monocytes, and tissue macrophages (26). Although cell-mediated immunity in the form of T-lymphocyte function is critical at the mucosal surfaces, defective cell-mediated immunity does not predispose to candidemia and renal candidiasis, as is evidenced in AIDS patients. Phagocytic cells possess fungistatic and fungicidal mechanisms, including oxidative and nonoxidative activities, against both *Candida* blastospores and hyphae. Germinated organisms are too large to be ingested by single phagocytic cells. Although phagocytosis and killing of *Candida* spp. are facilitated in vitro by complement and antibodies, there is no evidence that humoral deficiencies predispose to life-threatening *Candida* infections.

## Lower Urinary Tract Infection

Even less is known about the pathogenesis of lower urinary tract fungal infections, since few experimental animal studies have been done (20). Clinical observations indicate that *Candida* cystitis is rare in the absence of prior urologic abnormality, urine stasis, diabetes, recent antibacterial therapy, or, most important, bladder catheterization or instrumentation. The occasional development of bladder colonization and infection with *Candida* spp. in noncatheterized and noninstrumented adults, especially diabetics, is poorly understood. Ascending urethral infection is more likely to occur in women; however, given the marked prevalence of *Candida* vulvovaginitis, the rarity of urethral and bladder involvement has not been explained.

Levison and Pitsakis confirmed that the animal bladder is markedly resistant to experimental *Candida* infections even after the injection of a large inoculum into the bladder in association with alloxan-induced diabetes (28). It appears that the nonobstructed bladder with normal mucosal lining is resistant to *Candida* adherence and hence colonization. Parkash et al. required the presence of intravesical glass beads to establish *Candida* cystitis (34). Their studies did, however, reveal that upper urinary tract infection occurs in a subset of animals with severe *Candida* cystitis and bladder outlet obstruction. Even in the absence of good experimental data, clinicians recognize the possibility of retrograde ascending infection of the kidney from the bladder, especially in the presence of obstruction or internal foreign bodies.

Following colonization of both the luminal and the external surfaces of the urinary catheter, *Candida* blastospores achieve colonization of bladder mucosa, possibly facilitated by the erosive effect of the catheter, which results in denuded bladder areas. Thereafter, the yeast cells increase in number and form hyphae, which facilitate more extensive bladder colonization. The antifungal activity of urine, if any, has not been investigated, but secretions from the prostate in males and from the periurethral glands in females have been reported to be fungistatic (16). The association of bacterial cystitis and candiduria, possibly independent of the use of antibiotics, may be explained by the observation of Centeno et al. that certain fimbriated strains of *Escherichia coli* may act as a bridge between *Candida* spp. and epithelial cells, facilitating attachment and invasion (4).

## CLINICAL MANIFESTATIONS

### Asymptomatic Candiduria

Most catheterized patients with persistent candiduria are asymptomatic, as noncatheterized subjects may be. The majority of noncatheterized patients have easily identifiable predisposing factors, including diabetes mellitus, obstruction of the urinary tract, nephrostomy tubes, or ureteral stents. A history of recent or concurrent antibacterial therapy is usually present. Unexplained candiduria should prompt evaluation for upper or lower urinary tract structural abnormalities. Asymptomatic candiduria is sometimes observed in patients with ileal conduits and after ureterosigmoidostomy. Finally, asymptomatic candiduria has been described in up to 30% of renal transplant patients.

### Urethritis

Whether *Candida* species are capable of causing symptomatic urethritis remains a controversial issue. In the usual clinical setting, a symptomatic male patient with antibiotic-resistant nongonococcal urethritis may well have a urine or semen ejaculate culture positive for a *Candida* sp. Since such urinary findings may also be true of asymptomatic males, the clinician faces the dilemma of attributing the symptoms to *Candida* spp. The clinical picture attributed to *Candida* urethritis is that of mild urethral itching, discomfort or burning on micturition, and a scant mucosal or watery discharge. If the entity exists, the diagnosis should be considered for males only when all other causes of urethritis have been excluded. Given the frequency of *Candida* vulvovaginitis, *Candida* urethritis is rare in women, and although burning on micturition and dysuria are common, these symptoms are usually the result of the urinary stream coming into contact with inflamed, edematous periurethral tissue. *C. albicans* prostatitis has only infrequently been reported in diabetic patients, usually following instrumentation.

### Cystitis

Although the majority of catheterized subjects with candiduria are asymptomatic, bladder mucosal invasion by *Candida* spp. may result in frequency, urgency, dysuria, and suprapubic pain. Hematuria is fairly common, and in poorly controlled diabetics, pneumaturia and emphysematous cystitis are described. Symptoms are often chronic or recurrent. *Candida* cystitis as visualized by cystoscopy resembles oral thrush, with scattered soft, white, slightly elevated patches adhering firmly to the mucosa and bleeding following attempts at plaque removal. Other features include diffuse erythema and petechial hemorrhage. Scrapings of plaque reveal a meshwork of yeast and filamentous elements.

A complication of cystitis is the development of a fungus ball, or bezoar, within the bladder lumen (11). These hard or gelatinous masses may be single or multiple and may develop in the bladder or originate in the upper urinary tract. Fungus balls may further obstruct the urethral orifice. Smaller bezoars may be voided spontaneously, giving rise to symptoms during their passage. Ascending *Candida* pyelonephritis may occur, but this event is uncommon and rarely follows symptomatic cystitis in the absence of severe obstruction or foreign bodies. Usually, upper urinary tract candidiasis is assumed to arise from the lower urinary tract when lower tract predisposing factors exist and when there is no evidence of hematogenous dissemination to the kidney.

## Ascending Pyelonephritis

The growing use of nephrostomy tubes and other permanent indwelling devices and stents has been a major factor in predisposing patients to ascending *Candida* renal infection or true pyelonephritis, which may in turn lead to fungemia and septic shock. A feature of ascending infection is the prominence of fungus ball elements in the ureter and renal pelvis. These fungal masses are frequently associated with hematuria and cause urinary obstruction. Renal papillary necrosis has been reported under these circumstances. Bilateral obstruction with progressive anuria and azotemia may occur. Occasionally, the obstruction is intermittent. Less commonly, renal *Candida* infection is followed by intrarenal and perinephric *Candida* abscess formation, with diabetics at highest risk for these serious infections. Passage of the fungus balls in the urine may result in renal or ureteral colic and is characterized by ureteral scalloping on excretory urography (11).

## Renal Candidiasis

Most patients with hematogenous renal involvement lack symptoms referable to the kidney (30). The only clues are fever, candiduria, and unexplained deteriorating renal function (33). Although renal involvement occurs at the time of the responsible candidemia, symptomatic renal involvement may be recognized only long after the candidemia has resolved. Renal lesions include multiple cortical and medullary abscesses with prominent tubular involvement and occasionally papillary necrosis.

## DIAGNOSIS

### Significant Candiduria

In contrast to our understanding of bacteriuria, our uncertainty as to what quantitative levels of candiduria reflect true *Candida* urinary tract infection rather than catheter colonization or contamination of a urine specimen is considerable (6). Since *Candida* spp. often colonize contiguous perineal mucosal surfaces in women, especially in the presence of *Candida* vaginitis, diabetes, or recent antibiotic therapy, contamination of urine specimens is common and may be associated with high *Candida* culture colony counts. Accordingly, no decision should be made on the strength of a single specimen, especially with catheterized patients, and a second specimen should be submitted after careful collection with the risks of contamination minimized.

Schonebeck and Ansehn concluded that for noncatheterized patients, samples collected by the midstream clean-catch technique are adequate for demonstrating candiduria in males but not females (41). Nevertheless, even when steps to reduce contamination are taken, the critical concentration of candiduria that indicates the presence of urinary tract infection in noncatheterized patients remains controversial. Kozinn et al. concluded that renal candidiasis (ascending or hematogenous) is almost invariably associated with $>10^4$ CFU/ml, and lower counts thus militate against renal involvement (27). Bladder involvement in the absence of catheterization frequently results in low *Candida* counts, e.g., $10^2$ to $10^4$ CFU/ml.

It is generally agreed that in the presence of a urinary catheter, stent, or nephrostomy tube, quantitative data are unreliable in differentiating between colonization of the catheter and true infection. Catheter-associated candiduria, reflecting colonization that occasionally resolves upon removal of the catheter, may be associated with $>10^5$ CFU/mm$^3$ of urine; i.e., high counts are compatible with heavy colonization, but low counts, e.g., $<10^3$ CFU/mm$^3$, are more likely to represent colonization only. Similarly, quantification of candiduria in the catheterized patient is of no value in localizing *Candida* infection to the upper or lower urinary tract (27). The finding of hyphae in the urine has no diagnostic significance.

Although most *Candida* urinary tract infections are associated with and accompanied by pyuria, the absence of pyuria should not exclude a diagnosis of fungal infection, especially in the granulocytopenic host. Pyuria has no localizing value in terms of the site of *Candida* infection.

## Localization of the Site of *Candida* Infection

No reliable method of localizing the site of *Candida* infection in the urinary tract exists, since quantification of candiduria is of limited value, particularly in the catheterized host. Similarly, the presence of filamentous forms lacks localizing value. When *Candida* casts are observed as cylinders of fungi within a homogeneous matrix during urine examination, which occurs infrequently, the observation strongly suggests renal involvement (2). The presence of papillary necrosis as revealed by i.v. pyelography or computed tomographic scan, although suggesting renal candidiasis, is more frequently associated with conditions that predispose to renal candidiasis, i.e., diabetes and obstructive uropathy. In contrast to testing bacterial pathogens, testing fresh urinary fungal isolates for antibody coating lacks diagnostic usefulness in localizing the site of infection.

Serodiagnosis in localizing the site of infection is unsatisfactory. Many tests have been used, although only a few are standardized; immunocompromised subjects may be unable to produce an adequate serological response. Tests for *Candida* enolase antigen are of limited value in diagnosing renal candidiasis.

The diagnosis of *Candida* cystitis is usually made in high-risk patients in the presence of symptoms of bladder inflammation or irritation and candiduria. Less frequently, the passage of fungus-derived extraneous matter is observed. In doubtful cases in noncatheterized patients, the diagnosis of *Candida* cystitis is verified by cystoscopy. When the diagnosis is suggested, an ultrasound examination of the bladder is advisable to exclude predisposing factors such as bladder malignancy or urethral obstruction and to exclude the presence of bladder fungus balls. Under these circumstances, it is also advisable to extend the ultrasound examination to the upper urinary tract to exclude obstructive uropathy and additional bezoars. In the catheterized patient with candiduria, clearing of the urine with several days of local amphotericin B therapy indicates that the candiduria originates from the bladder and not the upper urinary tract (47). A rare exception to this dictum is invasive bladder disease. More recently, Fong et al. demonstrated the feasibility of a 2-h amphotericin B irrigation as a rapid diagnostic test, which requires verification in the clinical setting (13).

The diagnosis of ascending renal candidiasis is suggested by the presence of fever, declining renal function, candiduria of $\geq 10^5$ CFU/ml, and, occasionally, papillary necrosis and the passage of fungus balls. Fungus-positive blood cultures may also ensue if obstruction persists. Investigation of such patients should include careful anatomical delineation of the entire urinary drainage system. This usually requires an i.v. pyelogram, although this examination fails to identify ureteric fungus balls in approximately one-third of patients shown by retrograde pyelogram to have anomalies. Retrograde pyelography, although invasive, avoids the administration of intravenous dye to diabetics with renal insufficiency. Percutaneous anterograde and nephrostomy tube studies are similarly useful in identifying the site of obstruction.

Renal candidiasis secondary to hematogenous dissemination is suggested by the presence of antibiotic-resistant fever, candiduria of $\geq 10^5$ CFU/ml, and unexplained declining renal function in the hospitalized patient at risk of disseminated candidiasis (33). For catheterized patients with renal involvement, a course of daily amphotericin B bladder irrigation is followed by persistent candiduria. Blood cultures for *Candida* spp. are frequently negative by the time candiduria is detected and may never have been positive. Occasionally, patients with renal candidiasis have clinical manifestations of dissemination to other sites such as the central nervous system, skin, retina, liver, and spleen. Although renal function frequently declines because of metastatic renal candidiasis, renal failure rarely results unless complicating postrenal obstruction ensues.

## TREATMENT OF *CANDIDA* URINARY TRACT INFECTION

As with bacterial urinary tract infections, management of *Candida* urinary tract infection depends on several critical factors (Table 3) (38, 50). These factors include presence or absence of symptoms (local and systemic), localization of site of infection, presence or absence of catheter and other foreign bodies (e.g., stent, nephrostomy tube), local complications (fungus ball), underlying predisposing factors (e.g., congenital or acquired obstruction), renal function, and susceptibility of the yeast pathogen. Accordingly, following the confirmation of candiduria in a second urine specimen, the clinical significance of candiduria must be determined on a case-by-case basis. In general, the more gravely ill the patient, the more ominous the finding (9, 33). More important than selecting an antifungal agent is identifying the need for treatment and the appropriate therapeutic modality (Table 4).

### Antimycotic Agents

Amphotericin B has been the dominant agent used in the treatment of urinary tract fungal infections. This polyene is fungicidal and continues to have the broadest

**TABLE 3** Considerations in the management of candiduria

Host factors
  Asymptomatic or symptomatic infection (local or systemic)
  Localization of site of infection in urinary tract
  Presence or absence of catheter or other foreign body (stent)
  Local complication (fungus ball)
  Evidence of systemic candidiasis
  Underlying predisposing factors (obstruction, reflux)
  Renal failure (excretion of antifungal in urine)
Fungal factor
  Susceptibility to antifungal agents
Drug factors
  Activity against offending pathogen
  Excretion into urine
  Safety, side effect, and toxicity profiles

**TABLE 4** Suggested indications for treatment of candiduria

| Indications for treatment | Therapeutic modalities[a] |
|---|---|
| Symptomatic patient with definite or probable (? possible) systemic candidiasis (hence renal candidiasis) | Systemic antifungal agents i.v. AMB i.v. fluconazole |
| Symptomatic UTI | |
| Pyelonephritis | Systemic antifungal agents i.v. or oral fluconazole i.v. AMB |
| Lower tract | Systemic antifungal agent Oral fluconazole i.v. single-dose AMB Local AMB irrigation |
| Nonlocalized | Systemic antifungal agent |
| Complicated | Systemic antifungal agent and drainage, change, or irrigation of nephrostomy tubes |
| Asymptomatic candiduria (rare)[b] | Systemic antifungal agent |

[a] AMB, amphotericin B.
[b] Treatment is rarely indicated except following renal transplant, with preoperative urology, or with neutropenia. Consider treatment (?) in the presence of upper tract obstruction.

spectrum of any antifungal agent available. Most strains of *C. albicans* are susceptible to amphotericin B at concentrations ranging from 0.05 to 1.0 µg/ml (38, 50). Amphotericin binds to ergosterol in fungal cell membranes, creating leaks in membranes; it is also a cell membrane oxidant. The pharmacokinetics of amphotericin B remain incompletely understood. Renal excretion accounts for only about 3% of total elimination (5). Levels in serum seldom exceed 1.5 to 2.0 µg/ml, with no accumulation in the presence of renal failure. Amphotericin B does not appear to be metabolized in vivo, and the drug is not dialyzable. Although only low concentrations are found, amphotericin B can be detected in urine for several weeks following cessation of therapy (5). It appears that sufficient amphotericin B is concentrated in the kidney and excreted in the urine that even single-dose i.v. therapy may cure uncomplicated cases of candiduria (10). In dogs, concentrations in urine exceeded MICs reported for most candidal strains for days to weeks following a single dose of 1 mg/kg of body weight (50).

The side effects of amphotericin B include fever, chills, headaches, gastrointestinal upsets, anemia, and nephrotoxicity. Renal effects include hypokalemia, renal tubular acidosis, and azotemia. Azotemia continues to be a major limiting factor for amphotericin therapy, especially in patients with preexisting renal failure. Decreased glomerular filtration is thought to be the result of arteriolar spasm.

The antimetabolite flucytosine (5-fluorocytosine) has a useful role as a single agent in urinary tract candidiasis because it is excreted unchanged in the urine, achieving high concentrations therein (42). Accordingly, flucytosine has been successful in eradicating *Candida* species and *C. glabrata* from the urinary tract except in patients with renal failure or an indwelling drainage catheter (49). Its role is limited by the frequency of both intrinsic and acquired resistance and by its toxicity, which includes myelosuppression, hepatotoxicity, and gastrointestinal upset. It can be administered orally or intravenously at a dose of approximately 150 mg/kg/day. Since flucytosine is excreted by the kidneys and accumulates in patients with renal failure, dosage adjustments are required, and levels in serum should be monitored. In general, toxicity correlates with levels in excess of 100 µg/ml in serum.

Of the newer orally absorbed systemic azole derivatives, the imidazole ketoconazole has a limited role, since only 15% of absorbed ketoconazole is excreted in an active form in the urine (18). Accordingly, inconsistent results have been obtained with it in the therapy of lower urinary tract *Candida* infections (18). The newer triazole itraconazole, although more potent and less toxic than ketoconazole, similarly achieves low concentrations in urine and hence is unlikely to be useful (35).

In contrast, fluconazole, being water soluble, enjoys superior absorption and penetration and is excreted unchanged in high concentrations in the urine, making this relatively unstudied agent of great potential importance in the treatment of *Candida* urinary tract infections. Fluconazole is highly active against the vast majority of strains of *C. albicans,* showing MICs of 0.8 µg/ml or less (23). Although non-*C. albicans* species, including *C. glabrata,* are less predictably susceptible, limited clinical experience suggests that non-*C. albicans* candiduria may also be eradicated with fluconazole (3, 43) because of the high fluconazole concentrations achievable in urine and renal tissue (17). Walsh et al. found levels in renal tissue threefold higher than those in simultaneously collected serum samples, confirming fluconazole renal accumulation (46). Concentrations of fluconazole in urine in excess of 100 µg/ml have been reported (17). Clinical experience is currently limited, and little has been published on this topic (3, 43). However, most reports indicate great success (70 to 90%) with an efficiency of eradication of candiduria comparable to that of the less convenient, labor-intensive amphotericin irrigation. Fluconazole failures often relate to failure to change urinary catheters and remove internal stents, nephrostomy tubes, and fungus balls. Other causes of failure include presence of non-*C. albicans* species and coexistent end-stage renal failure with inadequate urinary concentrations of fluconazole being achieved. Alkalinization of the urine has no role in therapy.

## Asymptomatic Candiduria

Management of asymptomatic candiduria depends primarily on the presence or absence of an indwelling urinary catheter. When a catheter is present, candiduria occasionally resolves with change of the catheter in the absence of antifungal therapy (approximately 20 to 25% of patients). Because of the high incidence of persistent candiduria and rare complications in patients with chronic indwelling catheters, most clinicians believe that asymptomatic candiduria should not be treated. This conclusion is based on the widespread clinical impression (but not natural history studies) that asymptomatic candiduria infrequently leads to complications (39, 41). It is, however, prudent to eradicate or suppress candiduria in catheterized patients before invasive urological surgery or instrumentation is performed. This is particularly important with patients with obstructed upper urinary tract disease, in whom the risk of pyelonephritis or candidemia is greatest (1). Regrettably, there are no other known clinical or laboratory criteria or clues that could help in deciding which asymptomatic subjects should be treated. Asymptomatic candiduria should also be treated in patients following renal transplantation, regardless of the presence or absence of a catheter. Similarly, asymptomatic candiduria in a neutropenic patient is worthy of investigation to define the source and decide on the therapy. In general, for all candiduria patients, every effort should be made to identify the source of the candiduria and where possible to eliminate predisposing causes, e.g., to remove catheters and stents. Control of asymptomatic candiduria in noncatheterized subjects includes ultrasound to rule out obstruction and urinary tract bezoars. Given the availability of multiple antimycotic agents today, it appears reasonable to attempt at least one course of oral therapy with flucytosine or fluconazole for lower urinary tract fungal infection.

## *Candida* Urethritis

If *Candida* urethritis exists, a trial of flucytosine or fluconazole therapy may be of value. In the past, urethritis was treated with urethral instillation of amphotericin B.

## *Candida* Cystitis

Symptomatic cystitis in noncatheterized patients should be treated with 200 mg of oral fluconazole or 50 to 150 mg of flucytosine per kg per day in divided doses for 1 to 4 weeks. However, excellent results have been obtained with a single i.v. dose of amphotericin B (0.3 mg/kg) (10). Such patients require full urological investigation of their lower urinary tracts.

Although catheterized patients with candiduria are usually asymptomatic, when symptoms do occur, local amphotericin B or miconazole irrigation done in addition to the systemic amphotericin B therapy described above is highly efficacious. In the presence of permanent indwelling catheters, oral flucytosine and fluconazole may reduce the funguria, but they rarely eradicate it. Local bladder irrigation utilizes 50 mg of amphotericin B diluted in 1 liter of sterile water and infused by slow continuous flow (40 ml/h) via a three-way indwelling catheter or via a two-way catheter with intermittent clamping (24, 47, 50).

## Renal Candidiasis

Regardless of the route of infection, renal involvement requires systemic antifungal therapy. When renal infection follows hematogenous spread, systemic therapy is also aimed at eliminating other extrarenal metastatic *Candida* foci. The total dose of amphotericin B should be 1 to 2 g administered over 4 to 6 weeks. The daily dose of amphotericin B is 0.5 to 0.7 mg/kg. This does not mean that one cannot eradicate candiduria with much lower doses (250 to 500 mg) of amphotericin B, but the other simultaneously infected focal sites of infection, e.g., as in endophthalmitis, necessitate the higher dose. Similarly, ascending infections require therapy with at least 1.0 g of amphotericin B. Under these circumstances, investigation of the entire urinary tract is necessary to identify obstructive mechanisms. Occasionally, persistent ureteric obstruction and candiduria mandate surgical removal of the bezoar (11). Similarly, when renal infection is associated with infected nephrostomy catheters, local irrigation with amphotericin B (50 mg/liter) is indicated in addition to systemic therapy. Recent comparative studies indicate that fluconazole at 400 mg/day i.v. or orally is as effective as i.v. amphotericin for candidemia and systemic *Candida* infection (37).

## REFERENCES

1. **Ang, B. S. P., A. Telenti, B. King, J. M. Steckelberg, and W. D. Wilson.** 1993. Candidemia from a urinary tract source: microbial and clinical significance. *Clin. Infect. Dis.* **17:**662–666.
2. **Argyle, C., G. B. Schumann, L. Genack, and M. Gregory.** 1984. Identification of fungal casts in a patient with renal candidiasis. *Hum. Pathol.* **15:**480–481.
3. **Bren, A., A. Kandus, J. Lindic, and J. Varl.** 1992. Fluconazole in the treatment of fungal infections in kidney-transplanted patients. *Transplant. Proc.* **24:**2765–2766.
4. **Centeno, A., C. P. David, M. S. Cohen, and M. M. Warren.** 1983. Modulation of *Candida albicans* attachment to human epithelial cells by bacteria and carbohydrates. *Infect. Immun.* **39:**1354–1360.
5. **Craven, P. C., T. M. Ludden, D. J. Drutz, W. Rogers, K. A. Haegele, and H. B. Skrdlant.** 1979. Excretion pathways of amphotericin B. *J. Infect. Dis.* **140:**329–341.
6. **Drutz, D. J., and R. Fetchik.** 1988. Fungal infections of the kidney and urinary tract, p. 1015–1047. *In* J. Y. Gillenwater, J. T. Grayhack, S. S. Howards, and J. W. Duckeh (ed.), *Adult and Pediatric Urology*. Year Book Medical Publishers, St. Louis, Mo.
7. **Edwards, J. E., Jr., T. A. Gaither, J. J. O'Shea, D. Rotrosen, T. J. Lawley, S. A. Wright, M. M. Frank, and I. Green.** 1986. Expression of specific binding sites on *Candida* with functional and antigenic characteristics of human complement receptors. *J. Immunol.* **137:**3577–3583.
8. **Edwards, J. E., Jr., C. L. Mayer, S. G. Filler, E. Wadsworth, and R. A. Calderone.** 1992. Cell extracts of *Candida albicans* block adherence of the organisms to endothelial cells. *Infect. Immun.* **60:**3087–3091.
9. **Fisher, J. F., W. H. Chew, S. Shadomy, R. J. Duma, C. G. Maygall, and W. C. House.** 1982. Urinary tract infections due to *Candida albicans*. *Rev. Infect. Dis.* **4:**1107–1117.
10. **Fisher, J. F., B. C. Hicks, J. T. Dipiro, J. Venable, and R. M. E. Fincher.** 1987. Efficacy of a single intravenous dose of amphotericin B in urinary tract infections caused by *Candida*. *J. Infect. Dis.* **156:**685.
11. **Fisher, J. F., C. G. Mayhall, R. J. Duma, S. Shadomy, H. J. Shadomy, and C. Watlington.** 1979. Fungus balls of the urinary tract. *South. Med. J.* **72:**1281–1284.
12. **Flechner, S. M., and J. W. McAninch.** 1981. Aspergillosis of the urinary tract: ascending route of infection and evolving patterns of disease. *J. Urol.* **125:**598–601.
13. **Fong, I. W., P. C. Cheng, and N. A. Hinton.** 1991. Fungicidal effect of amphotericin B in urine: in vitro study to assess feasibility of bladder washout for localization of site of candiduria. *Antimicrob. Agents Chemother.* **35:**1856–1859.
14. **Frangos, D. N., and L. M. Nyberg, Jr.** 1988. Genitourinary fungal infections. *South. Med. J.* **79:**455–459.
15. **Frye, K. R., J. M. Donovan, and G. W. Drach.** 1988. *Torulopsis glabrata* urinary infections: a review. *J. Urol.* **139:**1245–1249.
16. **Gip, L., and L. Molin.** 1978. On the inhibitory activity of human prostatic fluid on *Candida albicans*. *Mykosen* **13:**61–63.
17. **Grant, S. M., and S. P. Clissold.** 1990. Fluconazole: a review of its pharmacodynamic and pharmacokinetic properties and therapeutic potential in superficial and systemic mycoses. *Drugs 1990* **39:**877–916.
18. **Graybill, J. R., J. N. Galgiani, J. H. Jorgensen, and D. A. Strandberg.** 1983. Ketoconazole therapy for fungal urinary tract infections. *J. Urol.* **129:**68–70.

19. Gustafson, K. S., G. M. Vercellotti, C. M. Bendel, and M. K. Hostetter. 1991. Molecular mimicry in *Candida albicans*. Role of an integrin analogue in adhesin of the yeast to human endothelium. *J. Clin. Invest.* **87:** 1896–1902.
20. Haley, L. D. 1965. Yeast infection of the lower urinary tract. In vitro studies of the tissue phase of *Candida albicans*. *Sabouraudia* **4:** 98–105.
21. Hamory, B. H., and R. P. Wenzel. 1978. Hospital-associated candiduria: predisposing factors and review of the literature. *J. Urol.* **120:**444–448.
22. Hsu, C. C. S., and B. Ukleja. 1990. Clearance of *Candida* colonizing the urinary bladder by a two-day amphotericin B irrigation. *Infection* **18:**280–282.
23. Hughes, C. E., R. L. Bennett, I. C. Tuna, and W. H. Beggs. 1988. Activities of fluconazole (UK 49,858) and ketoconazole against ketoconazole-susceptible and -resistant *Candida albicans*. *Antimicrob. Agents Chemother.* **32:** 209–212.
24. Jacobs, L. G., E. A. Skidmore, L. A. Cardosa, and F. Ziv. 1994. Bladder irrigation with amphotericin B for treatment of fungal urinary tract infections. *Clin. Infect. Dis.* **18:** 313–318.
25. Klotz, S. A., D. J. Drutz, and J. E. Zajic. 1985. Factors governing adherence of *Candida* species to plastic surfaces. *Infect. Immun.* **50:** 97–101.
26. Kolotila, M. D., and R. D. Diamond. 1990. Effects of neutrophils and in vitro oxidants on survival and phenotypic switching of *Candida albicans* WO-1. *Infect. Immun.* **58:** 1174–1179.
27. Kozinn, P. J., C. L. Taschdjian, P. K. Goldberg, G. J. Wise, E. F. Toni, and M. S. Seelig. 1978. Advances in the diagnosis of renal candidiasis. *J. Urol.* **119:**184–187.
28. Levison, M. E., and P. P. Pitsakis. 1987. Susceptibility to experimental *Candida albicans* urinary tract infection in the rat. *J. Infect. Dis.* **155:**841–844.
29. Louria, D. B., R. G. Brayton, and G. Finkel. 1963. Studies on the pathogenesis of experimental *Candida albicans* infections in mice. *Sabouraudia* **2:**217–283.
30. Louria, D. B., D. P. Stiff, and B. Bennett. 1962. Disseminated moniliasis in the adult. *Medicine* **41:**307–337.
31. McCourtie, J., and L. J. Douglas. 1984. Relationship between cell surface composition, adherence, and virulence of *Candida albicans*. *Infect. Immun.* **45:**6–12.
32. Michigan, S. 1976. Genitourinary fungal infections. *J. Urol.* **116:**390–402.
33. Nassoura, Z., R. R. Ivatury, R. J. Simon, M. Jabbour, and W. M. Stahl. 1993. Candiduria as an early marker of disseminated infection in critically ill surgical patients: the role of fluconazole therapy. *J. Trauma* **35:** 290–295.
34. Parkash, C., T. D. Chugh, S. P. Supta, and K. D. Thanik. 1970. Candida infection of the urinary tract—an experimental study. *J. Assoc. Physicians India* **18:**497–505.
35. Perfect, J. R., D. V. Savani, and D. T. Durack. 1986. Comparison of itraconazole and *Candida* pyelonephritis in rabbits. *Antimicrob. Agents Chemother.* **29:**579–583.
36. Platt, R., B. F. Polk, B. Murdock, et al. 1986. Risk factors for nosocomial urinary tract infection. *Am. J. Epidemiol.* **124:** 977–985.
37. Rex, J. H., J. E. Bennett, A. M. Sugar, et al. 1994. A randomized trial comparing fluconazole with amphotericin B for the treatment of candidemia in patients without neutropenia. *N. Engl. J. Med.* **331:**1325–1330.
38. Rippon, J. W. 1982. Antimycotic agents, p. 726–730. *In* J. W. Rippon (ed.), *Medical Mycology*, 2nd ed. The W. B. Saunders Co., Philadelphia.
39. Rivett, A. F., J. A. Perry, and J. Cohen. 1986. Urinary candidiasis: a prospective study in hospitalized patients. *Urol. Res.* **12:** 183–186.
40. Ryley, J. F., and N. G. Ryley. 1990. *Candida albicans*—do mycelia matter? *J. Med. Vet. Mycol.* **28:**225–239.
41. Schonebeck, J., and S. Ansehn. 1972. The occurrence of yeast-like fungi in the urine under normal conditions and in various types of urinary tract pathology. *Scand. J. Urol. Nephrol.* **6:**123–129.
42. Schonebeck, J., A. Polak, M. Fernex, and H. J. Scholer. 1973. Pharmacokinetic studies on the oral antimycotic agent 5-fluorocytosine in individuals with normal and impaired kidney function. *Chemotherapy* **18:**321–336.
43. Tacker, J. R. 1992. Successful use of fluconazole for treatment of urinary tract fungal infections. *J. Urol.* **148:**1917–1918.
44. Tomashefski, J. F., and C. R. Abramowsky. 1981. *Candida*-associated papillary necrosis. *Am. J. Clin. Pathol.* **75:**190–194.
45. Vazquez, J. A., C. Dmuchowski, L. Dembry, V. Sanchez, J. D. Sobel, and M. J. Zervos. 1993. Nosocomial acquisition of *Candida albicans*: an epidemiologic study. *J. Infect. Dis.* **168:**195–201.
46. Walsh, T. J., G. Foulds, and P. A. Pizzo. 1989. Pharmacokinetics and tissue penetration of fluconazole in rabbits. *Antimicrob. Agents Chemother.* **33:**467–469.

47. **Wise, G. J., P. J. Kozinn, and P. Goldberg.** 1982. Amphotericin B as a urological irrigant in the management of non-invasive candiduria. *J. Urol.* **128:**82–84.
48. **Wise, G. J., and D. A. Silver.** 1993. Fungal infections of the genitourinary system. *J. Urol.* **149:**1377–1388.
49. **Wise, G. J., S. Wainstein, P. Goldberg, and P. J. Kozinn.** 1974. Flucytosine in urinary *Candida* infections. *Urology* **3:**708–711.
50. **Wong-Beringer, A., R. A. Jacobs, and B. J. Guglielmo.** 1992. Treatment of funguria: a critical review. *JAMA* **267:**2780–2785.

# MOLECULAR MECHANISMS OF BACTERIAL PATHOGENESIS IN URINARY TRACT INFECTIONS

II

# VIRULENCE DETERMINANTS OF UROPATHOGENIC *ESCHERICHIA COLI*

*Michael S. Donnenberg, M.D., and Rodney A. Welch*

## 6

## INTRODUCTION

In this review we discuss the relative importance of *Escherichia coli* as a human pathogen causing disease outside of the intestinal tract, its specific occurrence as a uropathogen, and the chromosomal linkage of genes that encode virulence factors for uropathogenic *E. coli,* and we provide an in-depth review of the epidemiology of these pathogenic determinants and their apparent role in disease within the urinary tract.

## Significance of *E. coli* Extraintestinal Diseases

*E. coli* is a remarkable pathogen because of its nearly singular potential among bacteria to cause diverse diseases in animals. Humans alone are affected by at least five different enteric *E. coli* pathogens, and if extraintestinal diseases are considered, strains clearly fall into two group: those that cause infections in neonates (neonatal septicemia or meningitis), children, and adults and those that are commonly associated with urinary tract and bloodstream infections. It is unarguable that *E. coli* is one of the principal causes of morbidity and mortality from community- and hospital-acquired extraintestinal infections. The most common infections involve the urinary tract. Between 40 and 50% of adult women will probably have a urinary tract infection (UTI) in their lifetimes (120). It is estimated that as many as 90% of all community-acquired UTIs and more than 30% of nosocomially acquired UTIs are caused by *E. coli* (76). *E. coli* and *Staphylococcus aureus* account for 30% of the estimated 2 million patients per year in the United States who are affected by nosocomial infections (reviewed in reference 245). It is estimated that 25,000 to 100,000 deaths per year are attributable to nosocomial infections; most of these deaths are due to bloodstream infections. The total cost of these hospital-acquired infections is estimated to be more than \$7,000,000,000/year in the United States. We have no figures that show directly how many deaths or how much of the cost is due solely to *E. coli,* but overall, considering all types of infections in hospitals, *E. coli* is probably the most common

---

*Michael S. Donnenberg,* Division of Infectious Diseases, University of Maryland School of Medicine, 10 South Pine Street, MSTF 900, Baltimore, Maryland 21201.  *Rodney A. Welch,* Department of Microbiology and Immunology, University of Wisconsin School of Medicine, 1300 University Avenue, Madison, Wisconsin 53706.

pathogen. In hospitalized individuals, UTIs are the leading cause of bloodstream infection with gram-negative bacteria (245).

## Epidemiology of *E. coli* Involved in Extraintestinal Diseases

There is little argument that a small group of *E. coli* clones is responsible for neonatal infections (201). On the other hand, whether specific clones of *E. coli* cause disease in the urinary tract and whether specific virulence factors are responsible for UTIs are subjects of controversy (93, 95, 97, 126, 161, 163, 164, 173, 222, 247). The controversy stems from various problems in epidemiological analyses because of a failure to always take into account such variables as patient age and sex, presence of underlying diseases and anatomical complications, specific diagnosis criteria, method of maintenance and storage of the isolated *E. coli* strains, and genotypic versus phenotypic identification of putative virulence factors. What is clear is that there are distinct types of infections based on sex, age, and presence or absence of anatomical problems and underlying diseases. Other problems with these epidemiological-type studies have less to do with experimental variables and more to do with bacteriology and genetic principles. Some workers apparently find it difficult to entertain the possibility that *E. coli* strains with distinct virulence gene genotypes can cause the same disease (126). Candidate virulence genes are dismissed as being insignificant because they cannot be found in all strains that apparently cause the same disease. The prevailing hypothesis is that well-defined bacterial clones cause well-defined diseases. The question becomes, how do we identify a clone? The present candidates for virulence genes among uropathogenic *E. coli* appear to have inconsistent gene linkage relationships within different clonal populations. A new hypothesis is that the different clones share, in some yet to be recognized way, fundamental virulence gene blocks (linkages). So, despite the fact these uropathogenic clones are not recognizable as a homogeneous group on the basis of multilocus electrophoretic profiles or O:K:H serotype groupings, they share virulence gene blocks that are genotypically missing from other *E. coli*. The possible overuse of the clonal concept for analysis of *E. coli* uropathogens may have trivialized the influence of horizontal transfer events that introduce virulence factors and directed attention away from potentially important virulence factors because they do not fit consistently within an ordained, homogenized pathogenic clone. The best case for uropathogenic *E. coli* clones and a specific virulence factor is cases of pyelonephritis in women without underlying complications, in whom strains with specific O serotypes (O1, O2, O4, O6, O7, O18, and O75) usually harbor at least one of the P-fimbrial type of adhesins (96, 163, 165, 166, 247). These strains are less common than those that occur in surveys of the *E. coli* strains most commonly isolated from the feces of randomly chosen healthy individuals (see our statistical analyses below). What lends strength to the argument that these *E. coli* strains are extraordinary is that they are also the strains that most commonly invade the bloodstream from the urinary tract (urosepsis) (94–97). Other putative urovirulence factors such as hemolysin and aerobactin are less frequently identified within the uroseptic clones than the P-fimbrial determinants yet are two to three times more common among these uroseptic isolates than among common fecal strains. The hypothesis being tested in one of our laboratories (R.A.W.) is that uropathogenic and bacteremic *E. coli* strains have common genetic elements that distinguish them from other *E. coli* strains (normal fecal strains as well as enteric pathogens of humans and other pathogenic *E. coli* such as the neonatal pathogens). These elements vary in virulence gene composition but contain recognizable patterns of genetic organization.

**Virulence Genes Are Often Linked**
The addition of large, multiple-gene-encoding elements has occurred frequently during the evolution of bacterial genomes. This observation with *Pseudomonas* spp. led Holloway to propose that a significant aspect of genomic evolution occurs by what he calls an accretion process (78). Among members of the family *Enterobacteriaceae*, the genetic maps of *Salmonella typhimurium* and *E. coli* are similar, but they differ significantly because of large insertions, deletions, and inversions (190). The alignment of their genetic maps creates 14 loops in the *E. coli* map and 15 in *S. typhimurium* (a loop is created when the genetic distance between corresponding genes exceeds 0.6 map units [1 map unit is approximately 45 kb]). Therefore, many of the differences in the pathogenesis and biology of the two bacteria are likely to result from the genes within the chromosomal rearrangements as well as from the contributions of different extrachomosomal elements. An accretion-like process appears to have led to novel genotypes among the different disease-causing *E. coli*. For *E. coli* associated with extraintestinal diseases such as pyelonephritis and sepsis, the known or putative virulence factors that are not shared with common fecal *E. coli* strains are different adhesins, hemolysin, cytotoxic necrotizing factor 1 (CNF1), and aerobactin production. The close linkage of genes encoding pyelonephritis-associated pili and hemolysin was recognized by Low et al., who found cosmid clones containing both the P fimbriae and the hemolysin genes in cosmid libraries of genomic DNA from uropathogenic *E. coli* strains (132). Welch et al. (242) and Low et al. (132) found outside of the operons encoding these two factors a continuation of DNA sequences that are unique to the virulent strains and are not found in fecal *E. coli* isolates. Hacker et al. demonstrated that the P-fimbrial and hemolysin determinants can be lost from different uropathogenic isolates by large, spontaneous chromosomal deletions that are up to 200 kb long (71, 73). All of the deleted DNA proves to be unique to the uropathogenic strains and missing from the K-12 laboratory strain of *E. coli* (71). The presence of multiple P-fimbrial and P-fimbrial-like operons along with hemolysin genes within the unique insertions led Hacker and his colleagues to label these chromosomal elements pathogenicity-associated islands (PAI) (71). The best studied PAIs are present within the chromosome of strain 536 (O6:K15:H31). In addition to the factors mentioned above, the loss of the islands is associated with loss of serum resistance and with loss of mouse lethality (114). A cosmid library of a UTI *E. coli* strain was recently found to have single clones encoding both hemolysin and CNF1 (51). The genes encoding the synthesis of the iron chelator aerobactin are known to occur on plasmids such as ColV as well as at chromosomal loci (226). The locations of the chromosomal genes responsible for aerobactin and their possible linkages to other genes are unknown.

Recently, enteropathogenic *E. coli* and enterohemorrhagic *E. coli* were found to have virulence-associated genes located within unique inserts of their chromosomes (139). McDaniel et al. found that the genes encoding the attaching and effacing phenotype of enteropathogenic *E. coli* are present within a 35-kb insert (locus of enterocyte effacement [LEE]) that has at its termini some sequences in common with the PAIs from uropathogenic strain 536 described by Hacker et al. (139). The *E. coli* PAIs and LEEs are just two examples among pathogenic bacteria of virulence genes that appear to be linked. In *Listeria monocytogenes* is a well-described chromosomal locus at which the genes encoding at least five virulence factors and several operons are located (reviewed in reference 185). Another example occurs in *Vibrio cholerae,* in which three chromosomal genes encoding toxins (Ctx, Ace, and Zot) are found together (218). In *Salmonella* and *Yersinia* species, blocks of cellular-invasion-associated genes are found together in the chromosome (49, 57, 63, 125).

PAIs and LEEs from different types of pathogenic *E. coli* strains have some interesting genetic similarities. Hacker's laboratory determined that the apparent endpoints of PAIs in strain 536 are at tRNA genes. PAI I is 70 kb and is located at min 82 in the K-12 chromosome, 16 bp downstream of *selC,* and PAI II is 190 kb and resides at min 97 within *leuX* (19). McDaniel et al. found that the 35-kb LEE is located at *selC* in an insertion site identical to that for what Hacker's group calls PAI I. McDaniel and colleagues found that the LEE-specific DNA sequences just inside the insert junction share 68% identity with PAI I over a 94-bp stretch but that the identity between the two inserts then disappears and, judging from Southern blotting with internal probes of LEE, no sequences are shared between the enteropathogenic *E. coli* LEE and either of the PAIs of strain 536 (139). The insertion of genetic elements at the *selC* site has also been observed with the retronphage $\phi$R173, which is a reverse transcriptase-encoding derivative of the temperate phage P4 (86, 212). In preliminary data from one of our laboratories, the two PAIs of uropathogenic *E. coli* strain J96 are two new sites: *pheV* (64 min) and *pheU* (94 min) (214). In addition, DNA sequence analysis of the J96 PAIs reveals DNA sequences similar to those of the P4 phage present in both PAIs (214). So why is there a predilection for apparent integration sites at tRNA loci for these genetic elements? Reiter et al. speculate that the sequences common to the ends of these genetic elements are similar to the generally conserved sequences within the 3' termini of tRNA genes and serve as sites for site-specific recombination (187). They hypothesize that genetic elements capable of horizontal transmission between different bacteria may have used the generally conserved tRNA genes as sites of recombination into the chromosome.

## FIMBRIAE AND OTHER ADHESINS

### Importance of Adherence in UTIs

With the exception of the distal urethra, the urinary tract is normally sterile. In women, infection of the urinary tract by *E. coli* is often preceded by colonization of the periurethral and vaginal mucosae (207). UTI ensues when organisms ascend to colonize the unoccupied niches of the proximal urethra and bladder mucosae. The migration of bacteria into these and more proximal sites within the urinary tract requires that the organisms travel "upstream" and resist being carried away by the flow of urine. A multilayered (stratified) squamous epithelium lines the vagina and distal urethra. The proximal urethral epithelium is considered transitional; that is, the number of layers and the shapes of cells vary with distention. Similar cells line the bladder, ureters, and renal pelvis. In contrast, the epithelium lining the renal tubules is composed of a single layer of highly specialized epithelial cells that actively secrete and absorb water, ions, and other substances from the urine (31). The microenvironment of these disparate anatomical sites displays considerable variation in surface structures, pH, osmolarity, and pressure. Colonization of these varied surfaces is neither accidental nor inevitable but requires binding of specific ligands (adhesins) on the surfaces of the bacteria to appropriate receptors on the surfaces of the epithelial cells. This interaction requires a precise molecular fit between sites on receptor and adhesin to overcome the electrostatic repulsive forces generated by the negative surface charges of both cell and bacteria.

The adhesins that function in one environment may not be functional or even expressed at another site, and the receptors for particular adhesins may be restricted anatomically.

Strong evidence to support the importance of adherence in the pathogenesis of UTI was provided by the studies of Svanborg Eden et al., who showed that *E. coli* from children with pyelonephritis binds to exfoliated human urothelial cells in greater numbers than do control *E. coli* strains from the feces of healthy volunteers (46). Soon, this ability to adhere to cells was shown to persist in the presence of mannose and thus to be distinct from adherence due to common type 1 fimbriae. It was also shown to correlate with the ability to agglutinate human erythrocytes in the presence of mannose (75). Thus, the ability to bring about mannose-resistant hemagglutination (MRHA) was recognized as an attribute of pyelonephritis-associated *E. coli*, and this ability has been the subject of intensive research.

It is now appreciated that the MRHA phenotype is associated with several different adhesins. A plethora of adherence factors have been identified in *E. coli* isolated from patients with UTIs. Many of these factors may play important roles in the pathogenesis of such infections. The factors described include both fimbriae and afimbrial adhesins. Fimbriae, also known as pili, are composed of repeating protein subunits arranged in a tightly packed helical array to form appendages that extend from the bacterial surface (174). Fimbriae, which may be rigid or flexible, range from 5 to 10 nm in diameter and up to several micrometers in length. In contrast, fibrillae, also composed of repeating subunits, are thinner (2 to 5 $\mu$m) and wiry rather than elongated. In addition, a variety of outer membrane proteins and capsular materials function as afimbrial adhesins.

Individual bacteria may be capable of expressing multiple different adhesins. The expression of these adhesins is often subject to phase variation, a process by which organisms that stably express the property give rise at low frequency to organisms that lack the property (47, 228). These organisms in turn give rise at low frequency to descendants that once again express the property. This capacity for phase variation endows the pathogen with a plasticity that enables it to react to different environmental conditions. Thus, organisms that begin to express an adhesin at a site where receptors for that adhesin are found may have a selective advantage over those that do not and may outcompete them for the niche. On the other hand, when expressing the adhesin is detrimental to the organism, for example, because of an increasing immune response to the antigens associated with the adhesin, then phase variants lacking the adhesin may be selected.

## P FIMBRIAE

The best-studied adhesin of *E. coli* strains that cause UTIs, indeed, perhaps the best-studied bacterial adhesin of all, is the P fimbria (for P blood group antigen, which contains the minimal binding site of the adhesin). Chapter 7 in this volume is devoted to the genetics, biogenesis, and molecular structures of these organelles. In this chapter, we focus on the epidemiological association of P fimbriae with infection and discuss the role of these adhesins in infection.

**Epidemiology of P Fimbriae in Pyelonephritis.** A great many studies have confirmed that *E. coli* strains isolated from patients with pyelonephritis more commonly produce or have the genes for P fimbriae than do strains isolated from the feces of healthy individuals. The large number of studies published permits the analysis of P-fimbrial expression in strains from many subgroups of patients. Pooled results from many studies (7, 30, 38, 40, 43, 48, 50, 85, 90, 96, 103, 124, 129, 130, 131, 159, 173,

196, 197, 215, 221, 223, 247) indicate that among *E. coli* strains from patients with pyelonephritis who lack underlying medical or anatomical conditions associated with increased risk of infection, 80.8% (95% confidence interval [CI], 78.8 to 83.0%) possess P fimbriae. A review of controlled studies that compared the prevalence of P fimbriae among strains from patients with uncomplicated pyelonephritis to the prevalence in fecal *E. coli* strains indicates that strains from patients with pyelonephritis are 6.1 times as likely (95% CI, 4.7 to 7.9) to possess P fimbriae (Fig. 1) (48, 50, 90, 103, 159).

The prevalence of P fimbriae varies directly with the severity of the infection and inversely with the degree of host compromise. Arguably, pyelonephritis complicated by bacteremia is the most severe UTI. Results pooled from five studies indicate that P fimbriae are found in 88.9% (95% CI, 81.9 to 96.5%) of strains from normal patients with pyelonephritis complicated by bacteremia (85, 96, 108, 173, 219). Results from the two studies that compared patients with and without bacteremia indicate that strains from patients with bacteremia are significantly more likely to have P fimbriae (relative risk, 1.32; 95% CI, 1.11 to 1.57) (85, 173). On the other hand, P fimbriae are found in only 33.8% (95% CI, 30.7 to 37.1%) of strains isolated from patients with pyelonephritis complicated by compromising host factors such as diabetes mellitus, corticosteroid use, other immunosuppressive conditions, pregnancy, vesicoureteral reflux, urinary tract anatomical abnormalities, nephrolithiasis, and recent urinary tract instrumentation (7, 10, 30, 38, 40, 43, 48, 85, 96, 129–131, 173, 196, 197, 209). In comparison to *E. coli* from these compromised patients, strains from normal hosts with pyelonephritis are significantly more likely to produce P fimbriae (relative risk, 2.11; 95% CI, 1.92 to 2.33) (7, 30, 38, 40, 43, 48, 85, 96, 129–131, 173, 196, 197).

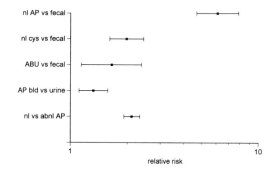

**FIGURE 1** Relative risk of P fimbriae in *E. coli* strains from various clinical sources. Shown are the relative risks (closed boxes) and the 95% CI of these risks (horizontal lines) of having P fimbriae in *E. coli* cultured from the urine of normal hosts with acute pyelonephritis and the feces of normal volunteers (nl AP vs fecal), the urine of normal hosts with cystitis and the feces of normal volunteers (nl cys vs fecal), the urine of patients with asymptomatic bacteriuria and the feces of normal volunteers (ABU vs fecal), the blood of normal hosts with acute pyelonephritis and the urine of similar patients (AP bld vs urine), and the urine of normal hosts with acute pyelonephritis and the urine of patients with acute pyelonephritis complicated by conditions that increase the risk of UTIs (nl vs abnl AP). Data were pooled from multiple primary studies that consisted of concurrent comparisons of the prevalence of P fimbriae in strains from different groups. Studies were excluded if they failed to specify whether patients had underlying factors that increase the risk of infection, if they failed to distinguish between clinical syndromes, or if they included data published in previous reports. The definitions of acute pyelonephritis, cystitis, and asymptomatic bacteriuria, of complicated and uncomplicated infections, and of compromised and uncompromised hosts and the methods used to test for P fimbriae varied among studies. Bacteremia concurrent with bacteriuria was assumed to represent pyelonephritis.

P fimbriae are also commonly found in strains isolated from normal hosts with cystitis. Pooled data indicate that 31.1% (95% CI, 28.7 to 33.6%) of such strains produce P fimbriae (7, 38, 43, 50, 83, 103, 127, 130, 159, 197, 208, 215), a proportion that significantly exceeds that of fecal isolates that produce these pili (relative risk from studies with concurrent controls, 1.98; 95% CI, 1.61 to 2.44) (7, 50, 103, 159, 208).

P fimbriae are often found in combination with other potential virulence factors such as other fimbriae, hemolysin, and certain O serogroups (see below). Strains of *E. coli* may possess two or more copies of operons encoding P fimbriae (77, 144, 183). Often termed P-related fimbriae, these may represent serologically distinct variants of the major structural subunit protein PapA and/or fimbriae with slight differences in the binding specificity of the tip adhesin PapG (92, 167). As mentioned above, operons that encode P-related fimbriae have been detected within PAIs, providing an explanation for the linkage to other virulence factors encoded therein (19). While studies that use multivariate analysis demonstrate a significant association of P fimbriae with pyelonephritis that is independent of other known potential virulence factors (221), it remains possible that as yet unknown factors linked to P fimbriae are responsible for the association of these pili with disease.

Immunofluorescence studies of *E. coli* in fresh urine specimens demonstrate that P fimbriae are expressed in vivo in the majority of patients with UTIs caused by strains that can produce the pili (113, 181). Additional evidence that the fimbriae are produced in vivo is provided by the demonstration that patients with pyelonephritis mount antibody responses to these pili (41).

**Role of P Fimbriae in the Pathogenesis of UTIs.** The strong epidemiological association between P fimbriae and pyelonephritis has led many investigators to propose that these organelles play an important role in the pathogenesis of the disease. Evidence to support such a role is provided by studies that indicate that the receptors for P fimbriae are present in the human urinary tract, by studies of the effect of cloned P-fimbrial determinants in experimental models of pyelonephritis, and by studies of isogenic mutants in animal models. The evidence that P fimbriae are involved in cystitis is much weaker.

*(i) Receptors.* Details about receptors for P fimbriae are presented in chapter 7 of this volume. A short review is included here to support the role of the pili in pyelonephritis. Three classes of P fimbriae are distinguished on the basis of the receptor specificity of the PapG adhesin protein (92, 211). All three classes bind to $\alpha$-linked digalactoside [Gal$\alpha$(1-4)Gal], the minimal receptor moiety present within the globoseries of glycolipids to which the adhesins bind (20, 104–106). The classes differ in the context of the digalactoside moiety favored, with preferences for globotriosylceramide, globotetraosylceramide, and Forssman antigen (92, 211). Of these glycolipids, globotriosylceramide and globotetraosylceramide are found in epithelial cells of the human kidney (210). Purified P fimbriae bind to structures in fixed human kidneys, including the apical aspects of proximal and distal tubule cells, vascular endothelium, and parietal epithelium of the glomeruli (117). The pili bind poorly, however, to the epithelium of the bladder, although they do bind to endothelium in the bladder wall. There is some evidence that different classes of P fimbriae bind to different locations in the kidney (109). In vitro, binding of P-fimbriated *E. coli* to primary human renal tubular epithelial cells is inhibited by antiserum directed at P fimbriae and by an antidigalactoside monoclonal antibody (217). When mice are challenged with a mixed urethral inoculum of a strain producing P fimbriae and a strain lacking P fimbriae, recovery of the strain producing the fimbriae can be inhibited by including globotriosylceramide in the inoculum (45). Human neutrophils lack receptors for P fimbriae, and P-fimbriated

bacteria do not bind to and are not killed by neutrophils unless the bacteria are opsonized, perhaps because of the net negative charge of the PapG tip adhesin protein (216). The abilities of strains expressing P fimbriae to resist phagocytosis may contribute to virulence and may account for the high proportion of P-fimbriated strains among urosepsis isolates (85, 96, 108, 173, 219).

*(ii) Effect of Cloned P-Fimbrial Determinants.* Hagberg et al. performed comparative studies of a fecal strain of *E. coli* transformed with a plasmid containing the P-fimbrial operon and the same strain transformed with vector alone (74). The strain transformed with the P-fimbrial operon adhered to uroepithelial cells from several species, including humans and mice. Furthermore, transformants containing the P-fimbrial operon outcompeted the strain containing vector alone for kidney colonization when the two strains were coinoculated in a murine ascending model of pyelonephritis. On the other hand, a pyelonephritis strain containing the P-fimbrial operon colonized the kidney better than the fecal strain containing the cloned operon, even though the operon would presumably be better expressed from the plasmid, where it is present in higher copy number. This result is consistent with the hypothesis that wild-type *E. coli* strains associated with pyelonephritis possess alternative mechanisms for kidney colonization in addition to P fimbriae. Similar results were obtained by O'Hanley et al., who compared a nonpathogenic minicell-producing strain of *E. coli* transformed with a plasmid containing the P-fimbrial operon to the same strain containing no plasmid in a murine ascending model of pyelonephritis (158). The strain carrying the P-fimbrial operon was able to colonize the kidneys of all 10 mice inoculated, while the strain lacking the plasmid colonized no kidneys, even in higher doses. However, the strain containing the cloned determinants on a plasmid was unable to invade the renal parenchyma, as assessed by light microscopy, while the wild-type pyelonephritis strain from which the determinants were cloned was able to invade all kidneys tested, which suggests that determinants in addition to P fimbriae are required for invasion.

Although these studies indicate that P fimbriae expressed in artificially high copy number in nonpathogenic strains are capable of allowing colonization of the kidney in a mouse model of pyelonephritis, the studies do not prove that these organelles are responsible for this function when the organelles are present on the chromosome of pathogenic strains in natural infection. P fimbriae are sufficient to allow renal colonization in these models, but are they necessary?

*(iii) Isogenic Mutants.* According to the molecular Koch's postulates as espoused by Falkow (53), for a genetic determinant to be considered a virulence factor, the determinant must be associated with pathogenic clones, specific inactivation of the determinant must result in a loss of pathogenicity, and restoration of the determinant must be associated with restored pathogenicity. These criteria, when fulfilled, ensure that the determinant under investigation is a necessary part of the pathogenic strategy of the organism under study. Genes that play a role in pathogenesis but are backed up by redundant systems may not meet these stringent criteria for virulence factors. There is no doubt, given the epidemiological data summarized above, that P fimbriae are more commonly found in uropathogenic clones of *E. coli,* and therefore, these organelles satisfy the first criterion for consideration as virulence factors. However, few studies have adequately addressed the second criterion, and none, to our knowledge, has satisfied the third.

Hagberg et al. were the first to test a mutant incapable of producing P fimbriae in an animal model (74). They found that the mutant was significantly outcompeted by the parent strain when the two strains were coinoculated in mice. However, this mutant was produced by chemical means, making it highly likely that the mutant had any mutations other than those responsible for loss of P fimbriae and making it impossible to conclude that the loss of P fimbriae was responsible for the colonization defect.

Mobley et al. used allelic exchange mutagenesis to create a precise deletion of the *papEFG* genes of a clinical pyelonephritis isolate (144). This type of mutagenesis is designed to produce a strain identical to wild type except for the mutation of the specific genes targeted. The *papEFG* genes encode the fibrillum tip structural protein, the tip adaptor, and the tip adhesin, respectively, of the fimbria (see chapter 7). Since the strain Mobley et al. chose possessed two copies of the operon encoding P fimbriae, the investigators had to use two rounds of mutagenesis to inactivate both copies of these genes. As expected, loss of either copy of the genes had no effect on the ability of the strain to agglutinate latex beads coated with the digalactoside fimbrial receptor. Also as expected, the mutant that had lost both copies of the genes still made fimbriae, as assessed by electron microscopy (since the genes required for pilus biosynthesis and the *papA* gene encoding the structural subunit of the fimbrial shaft were still intact). However, loss of both copies led to loss of the ability to agglutinate the receptor-coated beads. Nevertheless, no difference in the abilities of the double mutant and the wild-type strain from which it was derived to colonize the urine, bladders, or kidneys of mice at a variety of inoculum concentrations could be detected. Furthermore, no difference in the kidney pathology scores of the mutant and wild-type strains was detected. Thus, Mobley et al. were unable to confirm that P fimbriae are required for pathogenesis of pyelonephritis or cystitis.

Roberts et al. used allelic exchange to replace the *papG* gene of a pyelonephritis outbreak-associated strain with a *papG* allele that has a single base pair deletion that leads to a truncated adhesin (194). As expected, the resulting mutant still produced P fimbriae but did not react with a PapG-specific monoclonal antibody. The mutant failed to bind to tissue sections of cynomolgus monkey kidney. The mutant was compared to the wild-type strain from which it was derived in a primate model of pyelonephritis that involved direct inoculation into the ureters. Both strains were able to colonize and cause pyelonephritis, but the wild-type strain was able to persist significantly longer. Furthermore, the mutant caused much less extensive and less severe pathological damage to the kidney. Thus, this is the first study to demonstrate a role for P fimbriae in the pathogenesis of pyelonephritis by using isogenic wild-type bacteria. However, the third tenet of the molecular Koch's postulates, that virulence is restored by reintroduction of the mutated gene, has yet to be demonstrated.

The disparate results obtained by two groups using similar molecular approaches to inactivate the P-fimbrial adhesin may be explained by differences in the strains and models tested. The strain used by Mobley et al. contained, in addition to two copies of the *pap* operon, a member of the S-fimbrial family (see below), subsequently shown to be F1C fimbria (107). This fimbria, or other adhesins not yet identified, could serve as a backup to allow kidney colonization in the absence of P fimbriae. The strain used by Roberts et al. lacks the genes for the S-fimbrial adhesin and afimbrial adhesin I (AFA-I). An alternative explanation for the disparate results could be that P fimbriae are required for pyelonephritis in monkeys but are dispensable in mice, though both species have the receptors for these adhesins (158, 192).

*(iv) P-Fimbrial Vaccines.* In a mouse model of ascending pyelonephritis, purified P fimbriae inoculated parenterally provided 87 and 91% protection against renal colonization and invasion, respectively, upon challenge 2 weeks later with a P-fimbriated clinical isolate (158). In a follow-up study, immunizations with P fimbriae from three different strains each afforded significant protection against renal colonization and histologic damage upon challenge with the homologous strains and upon challenge with some, but not all, heterologous strains (178). In monkeys, after multiple intravenous and intramuscular injections with P fimbriae, a high-titer serum immunoglobulin G response was produced in 8 of 12 animals (191). Upon intraureteral challenge with the homologous strain, there was no difference in histologic damage between monkeys with low-titer antibody and controls, but animals with high-titer responses had significantly less renal involvement both at 48 h and at 4 weeks postinfection than did nonimmunized controls. Partial protection was also seen in monkeys immunized with one P-fimbriated strain and challenged with another (193).

*(v) Volunteer Studies.* Andersson et al. tested the effect of cloned P-fimbrial determinants on persistent bladder colonization in women with a history of recurrent UTI (3). The strain they used was a wild-type isolate that caused asymptomatic colonization of a girl for 3 years and that lacked the genes for P fimbriae. This strain was coinoculated with the same strain transformed with a low-copy-number plasmid containing the *pap* operon into 8 patients on 11 occasions by urethral catheter. The strain containing the plasmid-encoded P determinants was rapidly cleared from the urine of all volunteers, while the strain lacking the plasmid colonized the patients, all but one of whom was asymptomatic, for a mean of 88 days. Andersson et al. concluded that adherence did not promote colonization of the urinary tract in their volunteers. Among the possible reasons for failure of the strains containing the cloned determinants to colonize was a growth disadvantage conferred by the plasmid. This disadvantage was documented but thought not to fully account for the results.

In conclusion, several lines of evidence provide strong support for the notion that P fimbriae are important for the pathogenesis of pyelonephritis. The evidence in favor of a role in cystitis is less persuasive. P fimbriae are strongly associated with *E. coli* strains that cause pyelonephritis, and the strength of this association is directly related to the severity of the disease and inversely related to the degree of host impairment. Receptors for P fimbriae are present throughout the urinary tract, making a role for these organelles in infection plausible. Several experimental approaches have yielded similar results that are consistent with P fimbriae performing their predicted role in allowing adherence of *E. coli* to kidney tissue to facilitate parenchymal infection. Finally, immunization with P fimbriae can protect against pyelonephritis. On the other hand, the association with pyelonephritis could be due to linkage to other, perhaps undescribed virulence genes within the PAIs on which the operons encoding these pili reside. No studies have fulfilled the molecular Koch's postulates to prove a role in virulence, and some studies have suggested that P fimbriae are dispensable under certain circumstances. The lack of definitive proof that P fimbriae are required for UTIs points out the complexity of the pathogenesis of these diseases and provides an illustration of the difficulty ahead in defining the roles of other traits less closely linked to strains causing these infections.

## THE S FAMILY OF FIMBRIAE

The S-fimbrial family consists of S fimbria, encoded by the *sfa* operon (200); F1C fimbria, encoded by the *foc* operon (189); and S/F1C-related fimbria, encoded by the *sfr* operon (176). S fimbriae come in two varieties, which are encoded by the *sfaI* operon cloned from a urinary tract isolate and the *sfaII* operon from a meningitis isolate and which differ principally in the sequence of the major structural subunit (72). All members of the S-fimbrial family are highly similar, with similar physical maps and high degrees of sequence identity among many of the predicted protein products of the genes (72, 171, 172). Gene probes derived from the *sfaI* operon hybridize with the *sfaII* operon (176), the *sfr* operon (176), and the *foc* operon (172), and genes from the *foc* cluster are able to complement mutations in the *sfaI* cluster (172). Furthermore, antiserum raised against S fimbria reacts against the major structural subunits of S/F1C-related fimbria and F1C fimbria. However, antisera raised against S/F1C-related fimbria and F1C fimbria react neither with each other nor with S fimbria (176). A monoclonal antibody that reacts with SfaSI, the adhesin encoded by the *sfaI* operon, cross-reacts with the virtually identical SfaSII protein, but a monoclonal antibody specific for SfaAI, the major structural subunit of SfaI, does not react with SfaAII (72).

The epidemiology of UTI with *E. coli* strains that produce fimbriae of the S family is not well described. Few or no reported studies compare the prevalence of such strains in normal versus abnormal hosts, patients with upper versus lower UTI, or patients with pyelonephritis complicated by bacteremia versus those for whom the organism was isolated only from urine. S fimbriae are commonly found in *E. coli* isolates from neonates with meningitis and less commonly found in urinary tract isolates (116). When tested

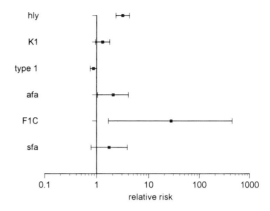

**FIGURE 2** Relative risk of expressing various putative virulence factors in *E. coli* strains from patients with acute pyelonephritis compared with strains from the feces of normal volunteers. Shown are the relative risks (closed boxes) and the 95% CI of these risks (horizontal lines) for possession of the genes for or expression of hemolysin (hly), possession of K1 capsule (K1), expression of type 1 fimbriae in vitro (type 1), possession of genes from the *afa* operon encoding members of the Dr family of adhesins (afa), expression of F1C fimbriae (F1C), and possession of genes from the *sfa* operon encoding members of the S family of fimbria (sfa). Data were pooled from multiple primary studies that consisted of concurrent comparisons of the prevalence of these factors in strains from patients with acute pyelonephritis and in fecal controls. Studies were excluded if they failed to distinguish between clinical syndromes or if they included data published in previous reports. Patients were included regardless of the presence or absence of factors that increase the risk of UTIs. The definition of acute pyelonephritis varied among studies. Bacteremia concurrent with bacteriuria was assumed to represent pyelonephritis.

with DNA probes that cross-react with all members of the family, 22.8% of *E. coli* isolates from patients with pyelonephritis show positive reactions regardless of host status (95% CI, 16.4 to 31.5%) (4, 37). Probe-positive strains are no more common among blood isolates from patients with pyelonephritis than among isolates from the feces of normal controls (relative risk, 1.73; 95% CI, 0.78 to 3.82) (Fig. 2)

(4). Moreover, it seems that few of these probe-positive strains produce S fimbriae. Of 102 strains from children and adults with pyelonephritis complicated by bacteremia, 23 contained sequences that hybridized with an *sfa*-derived probe that recognizes all members of the family, but only 3 displayed the hemagglutination pattern characteristic of S fimbriae (5). Similarly, only 4 of 12 *sfa*-positive strains from another study of patients with a variety of UTIs displayed such hemagglutination (37). Many of these *sfa*-probe-positive, S-fimbria-negative strains are likely to produce F1C fimbriae. F1C fimbriae have been detected by immunological methods in 22.3% (95% CI, 17.6 to 28.4%) of strains from patients with pyelonephritis (data pooled from references 85, 180, 205, and 247). In comparison, F1C fimbriae are detected in only 6.2% (95% CI, 4.1 to 9.4%) of samples from the feces of healthy controls (data from references 180 and 204). The one study with concurrent controls found that F1C fimbriae are significantly more common among strains from children with pyelonephritis than among controls (180). F1C-positive strains are also common among *E. coli* strains isolated from patients with cystitis, constituting 13.9% (95% CI, 11.4 to 17.0%) of such strains (83, 180, 205, 247). However, these *sfa*-probe-positive strains usually contain sequences coding for P or P-related fimbriae as well (4, 5, 37, 144). Indeed, the *foc* operon may be present in multiple copies (18) and may be located in proximity to P-related operons in some strains (77). Even when they are not physically linked, S-fimbrial expression may depend on the presence of PAIs that encode regulatory factors from the P-related fimbrial operons (146). Therefore, it should come as no surprise that production of F1C fimbriae is not independently associated with virulence but is linked to production of P fimbriae and to certain serogroups and capsules (205). The S/F1C-related fimbria has yet to be described in strains other than the one in which it was identified.

S fimbriae mediate hemagglutination of bovine erythrocytes that can be inhibited by sialyloligosaccharides or by pretreatment of erythrocytes with neuraminidase. The erythrocyte receptors for S fimbriae have been identified as derivatives of the membrane protein glycophorin A that contain $N$-acetylneuraminic acid-$(\alpha 2$-$3)$-galactose-$(\beta 1$-$3)$-$N$-acetyl-$D$-galactosamine (175). Purified S fimbriae bind to tissue sections from human kidneys, particularly to tubular epithelial cells, endothelial cells, and the glomerular epithelium (115). In addition, S fimbriae bind in vitro to laminin, a component of the extracellular matrix (229). The binding specificity of F1C fimbriae is unknown. F1C fimbriae do not mediate hemagglutination, which may account for the relatively slow progress in identifying their receptor. However, studies using inhibitors and tissue culture cells suggest that the binding specificity of F1C fimbriae may be similar to that of S fimbriae (137). F1C fimbriae have been reported to bind to epithelial cells in the distal tubules and collecting ducts as well as to endothelial cells of human kidneys and bladders (118).

The role of members of the S fimbrial family in pathogenesis has yet to be established. In one study, strains producing F1C fimbriae were detected in 4 of 20 patients with assorted UTIs. Immunofluorescence of urinary sediment from patient samples showed that two of these four strains were producing F1C fimbriae in vivo (181). The first evidence of the role of S fimbriae in the pathogenesis of pyelonephritis was provided by a study involving a spontaneous mutant, now appreciated to have suffered deletion of two PAIs, that is unable to produce S fimbriae despite the presence of the structural genes (146). When inoculated into rats by the transurethral route, this mutant colonized the kidneys at levels 2,000-fold lower than those of wild type. When the mutant was complemented with the cloned *sfa* gene cluster (which, though present, was not transcriptionally active in the mutant), colonization increased 20-fold, though it remained much lower than colonization by wild type (136). When a coinfection experiment was performed with the same PAI-deficient mutant containing either a plasmid encoding S fimbriae or one encoding type 1 fimbriae, the mutant encoding S fimbriae colonized the kidney in higher numbers (135). However, while compelling, these studies can hardly be deemed definitive. Studies using true isogenic mutants to evaluate the roles of these fimbriae in pathogenesis are lacking.

## THE Dr FAMILY OF ADHESINS

Members of the Dr family of adhesins include the Dr hemagglutinin (formerly known as the O75X adhesin), AFA-I, AFA-III, and the F1845 fimbria (152). The members of this family share considerable deduced amino acid sequence homology (213) or cross-react with DNA probes from other members of the family (122). Functional homology between genes from two members of the family has also been demonstrated (213). Members of this family also share a common receptor, the Dr blood group antigen component of the decay-accelerating factor, a membrane glycoprotein that protects host tissues from damage due to complement activation (150). Interestingly, the various members of the family bind to similar but functionally distinct sites on the decay-accelerating factor molecule (150, 152). The F1845 fimbria has a typical morphology when visualized by electron microscopy (13), while the Dr hemagglutinin has a relaxed coiled structure more consistent with fibrillae (149, 224). In contrast, no ultrastructural features have been detected in strains expressing AFA-I (123).

Very little that links members of the Dr adhesin family to UTIs has been published. A few studies have used DNA probes that recognize the genes encoding AFA-I, AFA-II, AFA-III, and AFA-IV to investigate the prevalence of strains containing these genes in UTIs. Pooled results from several studies indicate that positive signals are found in 16.0% (95% CI, 11.6 to 22.3%) of strains from patients with pyelonephritis, usually in association with P fimbriae (4, 7, 37, 122). Although individual studies showed no significant differences between the prevalence of *afa* genes in strains from patients with pyelonephritis and that in fecal control strains, pooled data indicate that pyelonephritis strains are 2.05 times as likely (95% CI, 1.05 to 4.01) to have these genes (4, 7, 122) (Fig. 2). The prevalence of the Dr adhesin, assessed by using a DNA probe that may cross-react with other members of the family, was not significantly different in strains from patients with pyelonephritis and in fecal control strains (154). A variety of probes that cross-react with all members of the family have been tested on isolates from patients with cystitis. Of cystitis strains, 19.2% (95% CI, 15.6 to 23.5%) hybridize with these probes (4, 7, 37, 122, 154, 208). Studies with concurrent controls show that these sequences are 2.33 (95% CI, 1.55 to 3.51) times more common among cystitis than among fecal strains (Fig. 3) (4, 7, 122, 154, 208). The F1845 fimbrial genes were originally cloned from an *E. coli* strain isolated from a patient with diarrhea (13) and have been epidemiologically associated with diarrheal illness (65). No association of F1845 genes with UTI has been reported.

*E. coli* strains bearing the Dr hemagglutinin have been reported to bind to basement membranes of the glomerulus and tubules within the human kidney, sites that are distinct from those recognized by P fimbriae (118, 151). In addition, recombinant clones expressing Dr hemagglutinin and purified adhesin bind to these same sites (153). The identity of the molecular

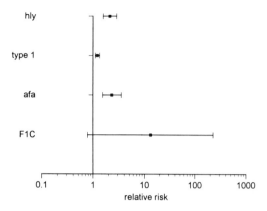

**FIGURE 3** Relative risk of expressing various putative virulence factors in *E. coli* strains from patients with cystitis compared with strains from the feces of normal volunteers. Shown are the relative risks (closed boxes) and the 95% CI of these risks (horizontal lines) for possession of the genes for or expression of hemolysin (hly), expression of type 1 fimbriae in vitro (type 1), possession of genes from the *afa* operon encoding members of the Dr family of adhesins (afa), and expression of F1C fimbriae (F1C). Data were pooled from multiple primary studies that consisted of concurrent comparisons of the prevalence of these factors in strains from patients with cystitis and in fecal controls. Studies were excluded if they failed to distinguish between clinical syndromes or if they included data published in previous reports. Patients were included regardless of the presence or absence of factors that increase the risk of UTIs. The definition of cystitis varied among studies.

receptor of the Dr hemagglutinin in human kidneys is not yet clear. The decay-accelerating factor seems to be responsible for the hemagglutination properties of the adhesin (153) and can serve as a receptor when transfected into Chinese hamster ovary cells (150). However, type IV collagen also binds specifically to the adhesin and seems to be a plausible candidate for the receptor in tissues (246). *E. coli* strains bearing the Dr hemagglutinin also bind to human neutrophils, but in contrast to *E. coli* expressing type 1 fimbriae, this binding does not lead to bacterial killing (98).

A recent study with mice examined the contribution of the Dr hemagglutinin to chronic pyelonephritis. In this model, a wild-type *E. coli* strain from a patient with pyelonephritis caused persistent infection and severe chronic pyelonephritis in 14 of 28 mice, while an isogenic mutant with an insertional inactivation of the genes encoding the Dr hemagglutinin colonized at much lower concentrations, caused mild pyelitis in only 3 of 25 mice, and did not cause chronic pyelonephritis (69). Attempts to fulfill the molecular Koch's postulates by testing for restoration of pathogenicity to the mutant by the cloned determinants have not yet been reported, nor have pathogenicity studies of other members of the family been reported.

## OTHER ADHESINS CONFERRING MRHA

In several studies, the ability to agglutinate erythrocytes lacking the P blood group antigen was more common in strains isolated from patients with pyelonephritis and cystitis than in fecal strains (48, 83, 87, 158, 225). Indeed, in multivariate analysis, non-P MRHA is independently associated with virulence (205, 221). These so-called X adhesins imparting MRHA no doubt include members of the S and Dr families of fimbriae and afimbrial adhesins, since these were not specifically sought in most of the studies cited above. However, additional known and as yet undiscovered adhesins may account for the bulk of these strains. Among the former is nonfimbrial adhesin I, originally identified from an O83:K1:H4 strain isolated from a patient with bacteremic pyelonephritis (68) and subsequently cloned (2). Nonfimbrial adhesin I is localized to the outer surfaces of bacteria by immunoelectron microscopy, and the DNA sequence predicts a structural protein with similarities to a protein involved in the assembly of a fibrillum of enterotoxigenic *E. coli* (2). A serologically similar adhesin has been identified in another strain (67). Other factors conferring non-P MRHA include the M-specific hemagglutinin, which mediates agglutination of erythrocytes bearing the M blood group antigen (188), and G fimbriae, which agglutinate erythrocytes treated to expose N-acetyl-D-glucosamine residues (188). None of these putative adhesins has been epidemiologically associated with UTIs or has been assigned a role in virulence in animal models.

## TYPE 1 FIMBRIAE AND MANNOSE-SENSITIVE HEMAGGLUTINATION

Type 1 fimbriae are ubiquitous adhesion pili that are found in many species within the enterobacterial family. The genes that direct synthesis of type 1 fimbriae are arranged in an operon at 98 min on the *E. coli* chromosome (reviewed in reference 162) and are present in the vast majority of *E. coli* strains regardless of their source (97, 144). Synthesis of type 1 fimbriae is subject to phase variation at a rate of approximately $10^{-3}$ to $10^{-4}$ per cell per generation and involves an invertible element that places the promoter in either the same or the opposite orientation relative to the operon (1, 47). The proportion of *E. coli* strains that produce type 1 fimbriae varies with culture conditions, since fimbriated phase variants have a selective advantage in static liquid media as opposed to agar plates. These factors weigh heavily in studies that seek to determine the role of type 1 fimbriae in UTIs. Since almost all strains have the operon for these pili, production must be sought phenotypically. However, since biogenesis of the pili varies with culture conditions, studies that seek production of pili may yield different results depending on how the bacteria are grown prior to testing.

**Epidemiology of Type 1 Fimbriae in UTIs.** As expected, the results of studies that investigated the prevalence of type 1 fimbriae in *E. coli* strains from patients with various clinical syndromes vary widely. Results pooled from many studies indicate that such pili are expressed by about half (47.2%; 95% CI, 43.3 to 51.5%) of strains from patients with pyelonephritis (7, 30, 38, 48, 50, 64, 97, 124, 159, 203, 247) and the majority (64.1%; 95% CI, 61.4 to 67.0%) of strains from patients with cystitis (7, 30, 38, 48, 50, 64, 75, 124, 159, 203, 247). Pooled results from studies with concurrent fecal control isolates indicate that these pili are significantly more common in isolates from patients with cystitis than in control isolates from the feces of healthy individuals (odds ratio, 1.22; 95% CI, 1.11 to 1.35) (Fig. 3) (48, 50, 64, 75, 124, 159, 203, 247). On the other hand, type 1 fimbriae are no more common in isolates from patients with pyelonephritis than in isolates from controls (odds ratio, 0.87; 95% CI, 0.75 to 1.01) (Fig. 2) (48, 50, 64, 75, 124, 159, 203, 247). Among isolates from patients with indwelling urinary tract catheters, strains persisting for more than 1 week are more likely to express type 1 fimbriae than strains from episodes lasting less than 1 week (142).

**Receptors and In Vivo Expression of Type 1 Fimbriae.** Type 1 fimbriae confer mannose-sensitive agglutination of erythrocytes and mannose-sensitive adherence to epithelial cells (155). Proposed receptors for these pili include a variety of mannose-containing surface structures. Bacteria expressing type 1 fimbriae adhere to human ureteral mucosal tissue (61), the proximal tubules of kidney, and the muscular layer but apparently not to the epithelium of the bladder (118). In addition, bacteria bearing type 1 fimbriae bind to, are internalized by, and are killed by neutrophils in the absence of opsonins in a manner that can be inhibited by mannose (reviewed in reference 156). Immunofluorescence studies of *E. coli* in voided urine from patients with cystitis indicate that bacteria expressing type 1 pili can be found in the majority of patients, though the proportion of bacteria from each patient expressing the fimbriae varies (113). Interestingly, many of the bacteria producing pili were found adhering to exfoliated urothelial cells and neutrophils. Similarly, in another study, one-half of 18 strains that were isolated from patients with either cystitis or pyelonephritis and that produced type 1 fimbriae in vitro expressed the fimbriae in freshly voided urine (181).

**Role of Type 1 Fimbriae in the Pathogenesis of UTIs.** The role of type 1 fimbriae in experimental UTI has been evaluated in a variety of animal models and in volunteer studies. In a murine model in which organisms were introduced via intravesical injection, suspensions of *E. coli* in α-methyl mannoside (an inhibitor of type 1 fimbrial adhesion) colonized less well than suspensions in sodium chloride (6). In a murine model of ascending infection, mutants produced by chemical means (nonisogenic) that did not express type 1 fimbriae were outcompeted for bladder colonization but not kidney colonization by strains that produce these pili (74). Similarly, wild-type strains transformed with plasmids causing expression of type 1 fimbriae outcompete strains transformed with vector alone. Hultgren et al. reported a series of experiments with phase variants of clinical cystitis *E. coli* isolates that were grown to express or not express type 1 fimbriae (82). They found that strains expressing type 1 fimbriae colonize the mouse bladder in significantly higher numbers than do phase variants lacking fimbriae. Furthermore, when phase variants expressing type 1 fimbriae are inoculated into the mouse bladder, they adhere to the bladder walls and continue to express type 1 fimbriae while giving rise to nonpiliated progeny that are expelled in the urine. In addition, when nonpiliated variants inoculated into the bladder do establish colonization, they have undergone variation to the piliated phase. In another study, a heavily type 1-piliated clinical *E. coli* isolate was passaged on agar to produce progressively less piliated progeny. The degree of piliation was directly related to the number of organisms recovered from the murine bladder after intraurethral inoculation (199). Interestingly, organisms colonizing the bladder remained heavily piliated over time, while those recovered from the kidneys rapidly lost the ability to bring about mannose-sensitive hemagglutination. In one study using isogenic mutants of a clinical pyelonephritis isolate, both an insertion in the pilus structural subunit (which may have been polar on the entire operon) and an insertion in the adhesin subunit yielded strains that were outcompeted by wild type when the two were coinoculated in a rat model of ascending cystitis (112). Thus, considerable experimental evidence from animal models supports a role for type 1 fimbriae in the pathogenesis of cystitis. However, a clinical isolate expressing type 1 fimbriae from a plasmid was quickly eliminated from the urine when it was coinoculated with the same strain lacking the plasmid in an experimental human model of cystitis (3). The problems with this experimental approach are discussed above in the section on P fimbriae.

Interesting data have emerged from the study of type 1 fimbriae in other models. In a newborn-rat model of bacteremia, an isogenic mutant lacking type 1 fimbriae could colonize the intestine and cause bacteremia as well as the fimbriated parent when given orally in high doses (15), but when given in extremely low doses, it yielded less colonization of the oral pharynx and intestine and was spread to littermates with lower frequency than the wild-type isolate (16). The investigators suggest that type 1 fimbriae may be important in transmission of *E. coli* because they facilitate colonization of the oral pharynx, where the bacteria are able to replicate in sufficient numbers to breach the gastric barrier and colonize the intestine. In a rat model of peritonitis, a type 1-piliated strain was much less virulent after intraperitoneal injection than an isogenic mutant unable to produce type 1 fimbriae, especially when the piliated strain was grown under conditions favoring piliation (138). Thus, type 1 fimbriae may be detrimental to systemic infections, perhaps because of their phagocytosis-enhancing effect.

In sum, the current state of knowledge, based on studies of the expression of these pili in vitro and in vivo in strains from patients with cystitis and in studies with animal models, suggests that type 1 fimbriae, though ubiquitous, may play an important role in bladder colonization. However, definitive evidence, such as would be supplied by fulfilling the molecular Koch's postulates with isogenic strains in a human model, is lacking. There is currently no evidence that type 1 fimbriae are crucial for the development of pyelonephritis. In fact, they may be detrimental to the bacteria in the upper urinary tract.

## THE *E. COLI* HEMOLYSIN

### Biochemistry and Genetics

Comprehensive reviews of the biochemistry and genetics of the *E. coli* hemolysin have appeared recently (238, 239), so only a brief review of some of the more salient points is given here. Confusion concerning the number of different beta-hemolytic toxins present in *E. coli* continues. H. W. Smith originally designated the erythrolytic activity (beta-hemolytic) present in cell-free filtrates of *E. coli* broth culture supernatants as the $\alpha$-hemolysin and the hemolytic activity that appeared to be cell bound in other strains as the $\beta$-hemolysin (206). As previously bemoaned by Cavalieri et al. (29), this was a poor choice of names because of the ensuing confusion with classic streptococcal hemolytic phenotypes. To make matters worse, the continued use of the term "$\alpha$-hemolysin" by many authors implies that there is a different, $\beta$-hemolysin present among *E. coli* strains. Its been known for more than 15 years that the $\alpha$- and $\beta$-hemolysins are encoded by essentially identical operons (39, 230, 236). The perception of a cell-bound versus a cell-free hemolysin results from differences in expression (39) and secretion of antigenically related hemolysin molecules into the growth medium (237). A 1969 paper reports a beta-hemolytic phenotype among spontaneously occurring nalidixic acid-resistant mutants (231). This activity was named $\gamma$-hemolysin; however, its biochemical or genetic basis has remained uncharacterized.

The *E. coli* hemolysin is a calcium-bound, acylated protein 1,023 amino acids long that is secreted extracellularly without amino-terminal cleavage (21, 55, 56, 88). The estimates of its native molecular size vary from 300 to more than 1,000 kDa (22, 169). There is conflicting evidence that the active hemolysin may be associated with lipopolysaccharide; for details of these studies, see a recent reviewed of this topic in reference 239. It is important that the *E. coli* hemolysin in an active state has not been purified to homogenity as a protein that has been rigorously demonstrated to be free of lipopolysaccharide.

The recombinant introduction of four genes (*hlyCABD*) from a uropathogenic isolate into a nonhemolytic K-12 laboratory strain of *E. coli* is sufficient to produce a beta-hemolytic phenotype for colonies on a blood agar plate and extracellular hemolysin for cells grown in liquid culture (66, 241). The *hlyCABD* genes form an operon (243) that encodes the modification activity, structural protein, and two components of the transport apparatus, respectively (56). In wild-type *E. coli,* these linked genes are loci either on the chromosome of human clinical *E. coli* strains or on plasmids from isolates taken from animal feces (39, 81, 242). Besides the acyl-carrier protein needed for acylation of the toxin (88) and TolC, an outer membrane required for hemolysin secretion (232), the other *E. coli* products needed directly for hemolysin production are unknown. Hemolysin operon (243) expression is positively effected by RfaH (9, 233). This regulator is also a positive effector of lipopolysaccharide core synthesis (186) and the *tra* genes of the F factor (11). The effect on expression is believed to be at the level of transcription antitermination between cistrons of the respective operons. It is intriguing that the possible biochemical interaction between hemolysin and lipopolysaccharide occurs within a background of genetic evidence that the two molecules have a positive regulatory element in common. At present, no modulator of *rfaH* expression is known. However, *hha* is a negative effector of hemolysin expression that putatively acts by changing DNA supercoiling and in turn is responsive to changes in osmolarity. Under low-osmolarity conditions, *E. coli* harboring hemolysin recombinant plasmids shows a more than fivefold increase in hemolysin expression (28, 148). This is a particularly significant discovery, because it suggests that the in vivo expression of hemolysin by uropathogenic *E. coli* could be responsive to changes in the osmolarity of urine and that the differences in urine osmolarity from one individual to another could also have a significant effect on the virulence of diseases such as pyelonephritis and cystitis.

The cytolytic activity of the hemolysin appears to result from the formation of membrane lesions (12, 99, 100, 141). Associated with the lesions in target cells is a rapid influx of calcium ions accompanied by an efflux of potassium ions (101). In erythrocytes, this activity leads to colloid-osmotic lysis. At present, there is no information on possible membrane receptors for the toxin. A large number of studies indicate that cells other than erythrocytes, such as neutrophils and monocytes, are susceptible to the hemolysin. Perhaps more important, concentrations of the hemolysin that do not induce lysis of these cells cause a number of diverse cytotoxic effects (reviewed elsewhere [238–240]). Relevant to the specific topic of this review are studies that indicate that renal tubular cells in primary culture are very sensitive to the cytotoxic effects of the hemolysin (111, 143, 234, 244). This work led Warren and his colleagues to hypothesize that the hemolysin destroys the renal tubular epithelium, leading to invasion of *E. coli* to deeper tissues of the kidney, and that the hemolysin is therefore a critical factor in causing pyelonephritis (217, 234).

### Epidemiology

The initial suggestion that the hemolysin may be a virulence factor for *E. coli* involved in UTI was made in 1917 by Lyon, who observed that isolates of *E. coli* from the urine of patients with cystitis were more frequently hemolytic than those cultured from the feces (133). Studies by Dudgeon et al. of surveys of *E. coli* that caused UTI indicated that nearly 50% of the isolates were hemolytic, in contrast to only 13% of the isolates from feces of healthy individuals (44). Numerous subsequent epidemiological studies infer a similar circumstantial argument: because the hemolysin is seen more frequently in UTI isolates than in normal fecal strains of *E. coli*, it is at least a phenotypic marker of virulent strains and perhaps a virulence factor directly involved in disease.

As mentioned earlier in the analyses of epidemiological studies of the various fimbriae, it is critical to examine in greater depth the host characteristics and types of UTI in order to derive more meaningful information. The first report on the incidence of hemolysin that separated UTI isolates on the basis of pyelonephritis versus cystitis was by Brooks and coworkers (23). They found hemolytic activity in 58% of the pyelonephritis isolates and 27% of the cystitis isolates. The source of their "normal" *E. coli* was the isolates taken from cultures of the periurethral areas of healthy women; only 9% of these strains were hemolytic. The most recent observations concerning a possible difference in the phenotypes of *E. coli* isolates causing pyelonephritis in men and women subjects (222) indicate a problem with the study by Brooks et al., i.e., the pyelonephritis isolates came from both men and women. Still, that study was a historically critical study that suggested that perhaps hemolysin is at least a marker for *E. coli* strains that cause more serious UTIs. Further analysis of the epidemiological studies with data pooled from five different studies (7, 159, 168, 225, 227) indicates that *E. coli* strains from patients with pyelonephritis have hemolysin 54.1% of the time (95% CI, 48.6 to 60.3%) with a relative risk of 3.11 compared to normal fecal strains (Fig. 2). In cystitis, the incidence of hemolysin production is 38.5% (95% CI, 33.5 to 44.2%) with a relative risk of 2.12 compared to the incidence among normal fecal isolates (Fig. 3). These calculations provide clear evidence supporting the observation of Brooks et al. that hemolysin is more common to strains of *E. coli* that cause pyelonephritis than to those that cause cystitis (159, 197). Sandberg et al. differentiated cases of pyelonephritis on the basis of whether or not there were underlying illnesses or anatomical problems but did not detect significant differences between groups (197). One notable survey by Ulleryd et al. (222) involved a phenotypic analysis of *E. coli* strains isolated from male patients alone. The general pattern of a higher incidence of hemolysin-positive strains causing pyelonephritis than cystitis (73 versus 50%) was seen, but for the first time among pyelonephritic isolates, the number of hemolysin-positive strains was higher than that of P-fimbria-producing strains (73 versus 56%). These findings underscore the complexity of the *E. coli* populations that cause extraintestinal diseases and the great pains that are required to perform meaningful surveys of these virulence factors.

## Genetic Evidence for a Role of Hemolysin in UTI

The *E. coli* hemolysin was genetically established as a significant virulence factor for *E. coli* involved in extraintestinal disease with the demonstration that fecal strains of *E. coli* become approximately 500-fold more virulent in a rat model of intra-abdominal sepsis when they are transformed with a recombinant plasmid encoding hemolysin than when they are transformed with the same plasmid with an insertion mutation in the hemolysin structural gene (241). The source of the hemolysin genes used in this study was *E. coli* J96, which is a hemolytic, O6:K6 urine isolate from a woman with pyelonephritis.

In a rat model of ascending UTI, Marre et al. injected rats intravesicularly with $7.5 \times 10^7$ CFU of genetically manipulated derivatives of *E. coli* UTI isolate 536 (136). At 7 days after injection, the rats were sacrificed, histopathology of the kidneys was performed, and the number of CFU per gram of kidney was determined. The number of CFU in a gram of kidney tissue decreased >2,000-fold when the wild-type 536 strain was compared with a double-deletion derivative of 536 (536-21) that was missing both PAIs that encode several P-fimbria-related adhesins, hemolysin, a serum resistance determinant, and an unknown number of other potential virulence factors. Different transformants of 536-21 were constructed, each having high-copy-number recombinant plasmids that encoded S fimbriae, serum resistance, or hemolysin. Successive increases in the number of CFU per gram of kidney were observed in the strains transformed with individual determinants. Strain 536-31/pANN 5311, which had all three virulence factors, achieved an infectivity nearly identical to that of wild-type 536 with just a fourfold reduction in the number of bacteria recovered in the kidney. In retrospect, the deletion of the PAIs means that strain 536-21 has lost approximately 5% of the genomic information present in strain 536. The loss of probably 200 to 250 genes creates a problem in the interpretation and significance of the data in the Marre et al. study.

O'Hanley and colleagues used a murine model of ascending UTI with a different set of *E. coli* recombinant strains and provided perhaps stronger evidence that the hemolysin contributes significantly to the histopathology of pyelonephritis. In these studies, mice were dehydrated for 18 h prior to bladder inoculation with $10^8$ CFU of different strains. At 48 h after infection, the mice were sacrificed, their kidneys were examined histopathologically, and the CFU were semiquantified. A P-fimbriated, nonhemolytic wild-type strain, 3669, successfully colonized the murine kidney without resulting in any deaths. Strain 3669 transformed with the well-studied hemolysin recombinant plasmid pSF4000 caused the death of 63% of the infected mice (157). The mice challenged with 3669 showed some focal inflammation in the kidney, whereas strain 3669/pSF4000 caused segmental inflammation and abscess formation in the kidneys of the surviving mice. When mice were immunized with hemolysin prior to challenge, there was little reduction in the colonization of the kidney, but the hisopathological evidence for pyelonephritis was reduced, with the kidneys appearing nearly normal. Thus, the evidence is strong that the hemolysin of hemolytic uropathogenic *E. coli* contributes to the pathogenesis of upper UTI. Its contribution may involve direct tissue damage and dysfunction of local cellular immune responses such as phagocytosis.

## IRON SIDEROPHORES

Numerous reviews discuss the subject of iron acquisition by *E. coli* (32, 177). Although few studies describe the iron metabolism of bacteria multiplying in urine, epidemiological evidence suggests that a bacterium's ability to acquire iron enhances its growth kinetics. The evidence for this is from studies that show that *E. coli* clinical isolates that produce the iron siderophore aerobactin grow faster in urine than isolates that do not produce aerobactin (145). The second type of evidence comes from multiple surveys that indicate that the genes or the ability to acquire iron via aerobactin production is a trait more common to pyelonephritis isolates than to cystitis isolates and more common to cystitis isolates than to normal fecal isolates. Carbonetti and coworkers used DNA hybridization to examine a set of 516 *E. coli* strains for the genes encoding the aerobactin synthesis and uptake system (27). The expression of aerobactin was also examined by a bioassay system. These strains were from a variety of clinical sources, including blood and urine from patients having one of three different diagnoses (pyelonephritis, symptomatic lower UTI, and asymptomatic bacteruria). For comparison, 67 normal fecal isolates were also examined. Nearly 92% of the strains possessing DNA sequences similar to those of the aerobactin gene probe were positive for aerobactin production in the bioassay. This fact suggests that the presence of aerobactin gene sequences is a very good indication that the aerobactin system is at least expressed in vitro. Detection of the aerobactin system occurred in 69% of the septicemia isolates, 75% of the pylonephritis isolates, 60% of the symptomatic lower UTIs and 63% of the asymptomatic lower UTIs. Because only 34% of the normal fecal isolates harbored the aerobactin system, it was concluded that iron is likely needed for growth in the urinary tract and that the increased incidence of the aerobactin chelator among uropathogenic *E. coli* is an indication that aerobactin is a virulence factor. The age, sex, and possible predisposing conditions of the patients were not noted in this study, nor were the serotypes of the strains known.

In a large study by I. Orskov et al. that involved UTIs of girls 3 months to 15 years of age, the incidence of bioassay aerobactin-positive *E. coli* strains among 467 isolates from patients with pyelonephritis, cystitis, and asymptomatic bacteriuria and from feces of healthy girls were 70, 40, 21, and 34%, respectively (168). The isolates were assayed not only for aerobactin production but also for their O:K:H serotypes. Aerobactin production was associated with particular *E. coli* serotypes (e.g., O1:K1:H7, O2:K1:H4, O4:K12:H5, O7:K1:H-, O16:K1:H-, and O75:K5:H). The majority (>90%) of the UTIs were the first known episode of infection. No attempts were made to establish whether underlying predisposing factors such as anatomical abnormalities were present.

In a second large epidemiological survey published at the same time as the study described above, Jacobson and colleagues found that in children or adult women with primary UTIs, aerobactin production occurred in 72% of the pyelonephritis isolates and 42% of the cystitis isolates (89). The percentage of pyelonephritis aerobactin-positive strains did not differ remarkably in either patient age category. However, 54% of the cystitis isolates from children were aerobactin positive compared to only 30% of the isolates from women. This led Johnson et al. to hypothesize that in children suffering their first infection, the bacterium may need more virulence factors in order to enter and survive in the urinary tract than are needed in women, in whom hormonal changes and sexual activity are predisposing factors for infection.

One of the most comprehensive epidemiological studies of the incidence of aerobactin production among *E. coli* involved in UTIs was reported by Johnson and coworkers. They focused their attention not only on the relative incidence of aerobactin production among *E. coli* from patients with different degrees of urinary tract disease and underlying urological conditions but also on whether these strains caused bacteremia (97). The aerobactin-positive urosepsis isolates constituted 78% of the total 58 strains tested. Moreover, when the bacteremic patients were divided into classes of compromised versus noncompromised states, the patterns of genetic locations of the aerobactin synthesis genes were different. Generally, the genes were found on antibiotic resistance plasmids in strains isolated from patients with underlying anatomical abnormalities or serious medical diseases such as diabetes, but in strains from individuals without predisposing factors, the aerobactin gene loci were chromosomal. The significance of this discovery is that it was already known that genes encoding other known virulence factors common to uropathogenic *E. coli* from noncompromised hosts, such as P fimbriae and hemolysin, are also chromosomal (80, 129, 132, 242). The precise locations of the aerobactin genes on the chromosome are unknown. The strains with plasmid-mediated aerobactin production generally do not have any additional known uropathogenic virulence factors. These data continue to support the hypothesis that *E. coli* strains infecting individuals in general good health possess multiple virulence determinants in order to infect the urinary tract and cause disease. A later study by the Johnson group that included serotyping and identification of aerobactin, P fimbriae, hemolysin, antibiotic resistance, and carboxylesterase B phenotypes and genotypes lent impressive support to this hypothesis (95). In the two epidemiological studies, the patient population was not divided on the basis of sex, although it might be presumed that the majority of isolates were from women. Otto et al. took the sex of the individual into account and found that 83% of the urosepsis isolates from women without underlying complications were aerobactin positive (173). Surprisingly, 100% of the isolates were P fimbriated, but only 33% of these had a hemolytic phenotype. A further indication that there are some curious twists to the epidemiology of *E. coli* virulence factors among UTI isolates arises from the previously mentioned study by Ulleryd et al. (222). They found that, unrelated to underlying complications, the incidence of aerobactin-positive strains was 51% in men with pyelonephritis and the incidences of P fimbriation and hemolysin production in men were 56 and 73%, respectively.

Unfortunately, the aerobactin studies described thus far provide only correlative evidence that iron is a limiting element that is important for the growth of bacteria in urine. This is somewhat enigmatic, considering that iron is present in relatively large amounts in urine (58) and that no definitive experiments show that it is unavailable to bacteria because of being complexed to chelators in urine. A study by Shand et al. demonstrated that the outer membrane profiles of *Klebsiella pneumoniae* and *Proteus mirabilis* strains taken directly from the urine of patients with UTI are similar to the profiles of those two strains grown in vitro under iron stress and dissimilar to the outer membrane protein pattern of the strains grown under iron-replete conditions (202). Although this evidence of iron stress is circumstantial, it does suggest that growth in urine involves a regulatory state different from that used for growth in vitro. Clearly, we need to experimentally establish the importance of iron competition by a comparison of the growth of isogenic aerobactin-positive and -negative strains in urine. Those studies should be followed by a comparison of the colonization abilities and kidney invasiveness of such isogenic strains in the murine model of ascending UTI. Finally, it will be instructive to see whether the aerobactin synthetic genes that are chromosomally located in the common urosepsis clones are linked to other virulence factors on PAIs.

## CNF

CNF1 is a recently discovered protein toxin that has been associated with the *E. coli* serotypes commonly isolated from serious upper UTIs (14, 25, 26). This toxin was originally recognized in isolates of *E. coli* causing enteritis in children (24). A related toxin, CNF2, is produced by *E. coli* causing enteritis in piglets and calves (42, 140). The CNF toxins were originally recognized for their abilities to cause dermonecrotic lesions when injected intradermally in rabbits and multinucleation of CHO, Vero, and HeLa cells in culture (24). The cytopathic effect appears to be due in part to a reorganization of F actin into long, thick filaments called stress fibers (59, 170). The Rho family of GTP-binding proteins appears to be covalently modified by CNF in an unknown way (60, 170). The Rho proteins are thought to modulate the formation of stress fibers in eukaryotic cells (170). The genes encoding CNF1 and CNF2 have been sequenced and shown to encode proteins approximately 114 kDa in size (52, 170). Sequence similarity searches reveal that the amino-terminal halves of the CNFs share high similarity to the dermonecrotic toxin (PMT) produced by *Pasteurella multocida* serotype D. The PMT toxin appears to be important in the pathogenesis of turbinate atrophy in progressive atrophic rhinitis in piglets (179). PMT is a potent mitogen that through coupling in a GTP-binding protein process induces an inositol phosphate secondary-messenger cascade (147). Falzano et al. found that CNF1-treated HEp2 cells are induced to take up latex beads or noninvasive *Listeria innocua*, which suggests that CNF-producing bacteria may be invasive to cells (54). At present, there is no in vivo evidence to indicate that CNF1-producing uropathogenic E. coli invades any cells along the urinary tract. This observation suggests an intriguing new line of study for investigators interested in the pathogenesis of UTI.

The general incidence of CNF1 production among E. coli strains isolated from patients with UTIs follows the general pattern described previously for P fimbriae and hemolysin. For example, although the UTIs in a study by Caprioli and coworkers were not categorized on the basis of upper versus lower tract disease, compromised versus noncompromised states, or sex of the patient, the CNF-positive phenotype occurred in 37% of 91 UTI isolates compared to 3% of 114 normal fecal isolates (25). Caprioli's group also demonstrated the curious epidemiological association between hemolysin and CNF1 among extraintestinal E. coli isolates (26). They found that for strains in the six O serotypes (O2, O4, O6, O22, O75, and O83) that are often associated with serious upper UTI, if a strain is hemolytic, it is almost always CNF1 positive. The exceptions to the apparent rule were O6:K-:H1 and O6:K2:H1 isolates that were hemolysin positive and CNF1 negative; nearly all other O6 strains were positive for both traits. Thus, CNF1 and hemolysin fit within the general clonal pattern of virulence determinants among uropathogenic E. coli. What makes the possibility that these two toxins are significant virulence factors in urinary tract disease even more compelling is their newly discovered side-by-side genetic linkage (51). In screening and subcloning the CNF1 gene from cosmid clones of a genomic library of strain E-B35, an O4:K12:H5 UTI isolate, Falbo et al. (51) found that the hemolysin operon and the CNF1 gene are linked on a continuous 37-kb stretch of the chromosome. They also performed Southern blotting analysis that examined the CNF and hemolysin gene linkage among isolates that are representative of the six uropathogenic E. coli serotypes found in their previous epidemiological studies. In each case, the genes reside on restriction endonuclease fragments of similar size, indicating that their linkage is probably pervasive for this group of uropathogenic E. coli. In subsequent DNA sequence analysis of the CNF gene from E-B35, the Falbo group found that only 945 bp separates the last codon of the last gene of the hly operon from the ATG of the CNF gene (52). Recently, the genes for not only CNF1 and hemolysin but also one of the P-fimbrial variants (Prs fimbriae) were localized to within a PAI present in the well-studied uropathogenic strain J96 (O6:K6) (17). Unpublished DNA sequence data from the Welch laboratory confirm that the CNF gene is present on the smaller of two PAIs in J96 and is linked to the hemolysin operon exactly as described by Falbo et al. for strain E-B35. However, 3' to the hemolysin operon present on the second, larger PAI of J96, the 945-bp intergenic sequence between $hlyD$ and $cnf-1$ is disrupted by insertion of an RHS (recombination hot spot) element (214). Southern blotting of cosmids that cover the second PAI indicates that there are no $cnf-1$-like sequences on that island but there are P-fimbria-like genes. Thus, there is some variability in the hemolysin–P-fimbria–CNF linkages within the E. coli PAIs.

## SEROGROUPS AND SEROTYPES

E. coli strains are serotyped on the basis of a system developed by Kauffmann in the 1940s (110). The three determinants of serotype that are still in use are the O, or somatic, antigen; the K, or capsular, antigen; and the H, or flagellar, antigen (164). The O antigen is composed of the repeating carbohydrate side chains of lipopolysaccharide. The serogroup of a strain is simply its O antigen type, while its serotype refers to all three antigens. The K antigens are acidic polysaccharides distinct from the O antigens that are produced by many strains involved in extraintestinal infections. The

H antigen is determined by the structure of flagellin, the protein that makes up flagella. Not all *E. coli* are motile and produce flagella. Nonmotile mutants may be closely related to, indeed clonally derived from, strains that produce a typeable H antigen (209). Precise serotype determination is a laborious process that involves the use of hundreds of cross-absorbed antisera to determine to which of the 173 O, 80 K, and 56 H types a strain belongs. It has been estimated that as many as 50,000 different *E. coli* serotypes exist, yet, as pointed out decades ago by Kauffmann, a limited number of serotypes account for a large proportion of strains that cause human infection.

Several serogroups and a few defined serotypes are common among *E. coli* strains that cause UTI, especially strains isolated from patients with uncomplicated pyelonephritis (Table 1). Most analyses consist of comparing the proportion of strains belonging to these common serogroups among strains from patients with different categories of illness with the proportion among fecal control strains. Since investigators tested different serogroups, it is not possible to pool the data. However, several serogroups and a handful of serotypes stand out. In addition, nontypeable strains are more common among the fecal flora than among isolates causing UTIs (83, 225). In one study that considered serogroups individually, O8 and O75 each had high odds ratios when isolates of patients with a variety of UTI syndromes were compared to fecal controls (205). In another study, the O6 antigen was more

**TABLE 1** Association of serogroups with UTI[a]

| Authors (reference) | Study group | Control group | Serogroups or serotypes significantly more common in study group |
|---|---|---|---|
| Vaisanen-Rhen et al. (225) | Girls with AP | Fecal isolates | O1 + O2 + O4 + O6 + O16 |
| O'Hanley et al. (159) | Women with AP and cystitis | Fecal isolates | O4 + O6 + O25 + O50 + O75 |
| Stenqvist et al. (209) | Pregnant women with AP | Pregnant women with ABU and cystitis | O1 + O2 + O6 + O16 + O75 |
| Sandberg et al. (197) | Women with uncomplicated AP | Women with complicated AP or cystitis | O1:K1:H7 + O1:K1:H- + O2:K1:H- + O4:K12:H1 + O7:K1:H- + O9:K34:H- + O16:K1:H6 + O16:K1:H- + O75:K5:H- |
| Lomberg et al. (130) | Children without reflux with AP | Children with reflux and AP | O1 + O2 + O4 + O6 + O7 + O8 + O16 + O18 + O25 + O75 |
| Westerlund et al. (247) | Girls with AP | Girls with cystitis | O1 + O2 + O4 + O6 + O16 |
| Siitonen et al. (205) | Adults with various UTIs | Fecal isolates | O2, O6, O8, O18, and O75 (each analyzed separately) |
| Mårild et al. (134) | Infants with febrile UTI | Infants with ABU | O1 + O2 + O4 + O6 + O16 + O18 + O75 |
| Israele et al. (87) | Infants with AP and cystitis | Fecal isolates from infants | O1 + O2 + O4 + O6 + O18 + O25 + O75 |
| Lindberg et al. (128) | Girls with AP or girls with cystitis | Girls with ABU | O1 + O2 + O4 + O6 + O7 + O16 + O18 + O75 |
| Olling et al. (160) | Children with AP | Fecal isolates from children | O1 + O2 + O4 + O6 + O7 + O18 + O75 |

[a] Summary of studies that demonstrate a significant difference in isolation of *E. coli* strains belonging to a collection of serogroups or serotypes in patients with defined syndromes of UTI. AP, acute pyelonephritis; ABU, asymptomatic bacteriuria.

common in cystitis than in pyelonephritis (203), an interesting observation, given the association of O6 with the production of non-P MRHA (205).

The association of particular serogroups with disease is clearly confounded by other potential virulence factors that are found significantly more frequently in the serogroups associated with infection (95, 159, 205, 222, 225). Strains from a particular serogroup may be closely related, especially if they have the same serotype (85, 209, 225). Thus, there is no experimental evidence to support the hypothesis that having a particular O-antigen type per se increases the pathogenic potential of an *E. coli* strain.

## CAPSULE AND SERUM RESISTANCE

The ability to grow in the presence of human serum is a complex phenotype that depends on multigenic factors, including lipopolysaccharide, outer membrane proteins, and the ability to make a carbohydrate capsule (33, 235). The K1, K5, and K54 capsules play a role in serum resistance (33, 184, 195). Capsules also play a role in resistance to phagocytosis in the absence of anticapsular opsonizing antibody (79).

The epidemiological data concerning the occurrence of capsule in strains isolated from patients with UTIs are quite confusing and contradictory. Encapsulated strains are no more common among isolates from the urinary tract than among fecal isolates (87). In fact, a multivariate analysis revealed that the absence of a capsule is significantly more common among cystitis isolates than among fecal isolates (205). However, the production of individual capsular types may be related to urinary tract infectivity. As noted above, at least 80 different capsule antigens may be produced by *E. coli*. Of these, the K1 capsule has received the most attention because of its association with neonatal meningitis (116). Compiled data from multiple studies indicate that the K1 capsule is found in 28.4% (95% CI, 25.0 to 32.3%) of *E. coli* strains that cause pyelonephritis (35, 62, 102, 197, 198, 209, 223, 225). In one study, K1 capsules were found more often in strains associated with pyelonephritis than in those associated with cystitis (197). However, in another analysis, K1 capsule was found no more often in cystitis or other UTI strains than in fecal isolates (205). In yet another report, possession of capsular type K1, K5, or K20 was more common in strains isolated from patients with pyelonephritis than in those from patients with asymptomatic bacteriuria (209), but the presence of K1, K2, K12, or K13 capsule was no more common in isolates from infants with pyelonephritis than in control strains from the fecal flora of infants in another study (87). Pooled results from three independent studies that compared the prevalence of K1 capsules in strains from pyelonephritis patients with the prevalence in fecal isolates do not demonstrate a significantly higher prevalence in the pyelonephritis strains (odds ratio, 1.30; 95% CI, 0.95 to 1.77) (Fig. 2) (35, 102, 225). However, in another analysis of odds ratios, K5 capsules and capsules other than K1 and K5 were significantly more common in UTI strains than in fecal strains (205). Not surprisingly, particular capsular types are associated with certain serogroups and other potential virulence factors. For example, K1 strains are more likely to possess P fimbriae and K5 strains are more likely to have non-P MRHA than are strains with other capsular types (83, 84, 205).

The abilities of *E. coli* isolates from UTI patients and other sources to grow in the presence of serum have been tested in several studies with variable results. Pooled data suggest that serum resistance is found in 63.5% (95% CI, 60.2 to 66.9%) of isolates from patients with pyelonephritis (91,

128, 130, 131, 134, 197, 198, 209). However, the results vary widely between studies, as do the definitions of and methods for measuring serum resistance and the source of the serum. Few individual studies have detected significant differences among isolates from different sources. In one study involving children, serum resistance was significantly more common among isolates from patients with pyelonephritis but no reflux than in isolates from patients with pyelonephritis and vesicoureteral reflux (130). In another study, serum resistance was more common in strains from pregnant women with pyelonephritis than in those from pregnant women with asymptomatic bacteriuria (209). Serum resistance was also more common in strains from patients with pyelonephritis and symptomatic cystitis than in those from patients with asymptomatic bacteriuria (160). However, serum resistance was no more common in strains from girls with pyelonephritis and no renal scarring than in strains from girls with pyelonephritis and scarring (131). Serum resistance was also no more common in patients with pyelonephritis complicated by bacteremia than in those for whom the organism was isolated only from urine (173). Serum resistance was also found no more frequently in isolates from children with pyelonephritis than in those from children with cystitis (197, 203) or in isolates from infants with pyelonephritis than in isolates from infants with asymptomatic bacteriuria (134). Two studies compared strains from patients with pyelonephritis with concurrent fecal control strains. One study found no difference (160). The other study found an unusually high prevalence of serum resistance in the pyelonephritis isolates (87.5%) that was significantly higher than that in the fecal strains (91). Unfortunately, since the former report did not include raw data, it is not possible to calculate pooled odds ratios. Interestingly, in one study, serum resistance was not associated with other putative virulence factors such as P fimbriae, particular O antigens or K capsules, or production of hemolysin, aerobactin, or CNF, but the sample size was probably too small to detect all but the strongest correlations (91). Indeed, other studies have shown a correlation between serogroup and serum resistance (160).

No studies using true isogenic mutants to assess the role of capsules or serum resistance in ascending models of UTIs have been published.

## GROWTH OF *E. COLI* IN URINE

We do not understand the in vivo growth of *E. coli* at a site such as the urinary tract. Experiments that study the growth of *E. coli* in urine provide an approximation of the process and have been reported sporadically for the past three decades (8). Urine does support the growth of *E. coli* quite well, but the variability in pH, osmolality, urea, and organic acids makes its use problematic as a research tool. Traits that enable one strain of *E. coli* to survive and grow better than another strain within that niche would have to be considered virulence factors for uropathogenesis. Gordon and Riley examined that possibility through an epidemiological survey in which the growth kinetics in urine for a set of *E. coli* UTI isolates was compared to that for a set of normal fecal isolates (70). Growth in vitro under moderate aeration and 37°C conditions had a statistically significant shorter lag time and doubling time for the UTI isolates than for the fecal isolates. What genetic factor(s) permits this greater capability is unknown. One specific hypothesis that has been tested is that tolerance to the varying osmolarity of urine would be an advantageous trait for uropathogenic *E. coli*. Kunin and associates tested this hypothesis by examining over 300 *E. coli* isolates for their abilities to grow in minimal medium with its osmolality varied over an NaCl concentration range of 0.1 to 0.7 M (119). The collection of 101 UTI isolates was on average no better at growing at the extremes of osmalitty than 100 bloodstream isolates or 100 normal fecal strains. Patient characteristics for the UTI and bacteremic isolates were not delineated. The ability of *E. coli* to grow in high concentrations of electrolytes and sugars in urine is thought to be mediated by the osmoprotective effect of compatible solutes in urine such as glycine betaine or proline betaine, which *E. coli* cells can actively accumulate intracellularly to protect against loss of water to the environment (36). Therefore, efficient transport of proline/glycine betaine would be an adaptive trait for *E. coli* needing to grow in urine. Culham and colleagues used DNA hybridization and immunoblotting to study the presence and expression of the three known proline/glycine transporters (*putP, proP,* and *proU*) among a collection of *E. coli* isolates (34). Of 63 strains examined, 30 were UTI isolates and 26 were diarrheagenic isolates. Only two isolates from normal feces were studied. All 63 strains possessed sequences similar to that of *putP*, and nearly all had sequences for the other two loci. Therefore, these data support the hypothesis stated above, but since an inadequate number of normal fecal strains was examined, we cannot determine whether these genes are unique determinants of osmoregulation for uropathogenic *E. coli*. It will be interesting to see if the genes present on the PAIs confer selective adaptation to growth in urine.

## NEW APPROACHES FOR IDENTIFYING VIRULENCE GENES FOR UROPATHOGENIC *E. COLI*

The identification of virulence genes among pathogenic bacteria has almost always relied on what may be termed a top-down approach. Assays for pathogenic traits are applied to a pathogen. If the pathogen has a positive virulence-associated phenotype, then the genes or proteins responsible for that phenotype are identified and isolated. The pace of discovery depends on the imagination, technical skills, and materials of the investigators. In the case of *E. coli* involved in extraintestinal disease, it has been known for more than 10 years that the P-fimbrial and hemolysin genes are just small parts of large unique inserts associated with the chromosomes of pathogenic *E. coli* (73, 132). In the last 10 years, except for the putative virulence factor CNF1, no new virulence genes have been identified, and the PAIs remain uncharacterized. Progress toward identifying the virulence genes involved in complex diseases such as pyelonephritis has been unsatisfactory. The time is right to try a bottom-up approach to identifying new virulence gene candidates. The linkage of pili, hemolysin, and CNF genes within PAIs is compelling, and the straightforward DNA sequence analysis of PAIs may reveal many new possible virulence genes. That approach, although laborious, would simply lead to a more comprehensive database for this pathogen. Preliminary data in this regard have been gathered in one of our laboratories, and sequences that are similar to those of several adhesins and another toxin and were not previously known to exist in uropathogenic *E. coli* have been found within two different PAIs (214).

## SUMMARY AND OPINION: WHAT IS A UROPATHOGENIC *E. COLI*?

The concept that certain traits are more common among *E. coli* isolates from patients with UTIs than among other *E. coli* strains is now well accepted. In addition, dramatic outbreaks of nosocomial and community-acquired pyelonephritis and cystitis involving single clones of *E. coli* emphasize the concept that certain strains are uniquely suited to infecting the urinary tract (121, 182, 220). This chapter summarizes what is known about several putative virulence factors that may play a role in the pathogenesis of UTIs. However, as discussed in the Introduction, it is important to remember that none of these factors is present in all cases of pyelonephritis or other UTIs, even when only normal hosts are considered. We do not find this fact surprising. We propose that virtually all *E. coli* strains have the potential to cause pyelonephritis. Different strains of *E. coli* that possess or lack various virulence factors differ not in absolute ability but rather in the probability that they will infect a normal host and cause cystitis or pyelonephritis. The absence of a competing microflora in the urinary tract affords any bacterium that arrives there an undisputed claim to the territory. In this respect, disease of the urinary tract differs greatly from disease of the gastrointestinal tract. Specific virulence attributes undoubtedly contribute in additive and synergistic form to increase the likelihood that a particular strain may cause UTI and to influence the severity of the ensuing response. However, no single method of colonization and no requisite factor for disease accounts for all infections. Alternative strategies that allow urinary tract colonization and damage serve to dilute the epidemiologic association of particular factors with disease. In addition, redundant systems complicate the ability of traditional experimental strategies to provide definitive data on pathogenesis.

When one is considering the role of particular virulence factors in disease, it is often instructive to ponder the selective pressure that maintains the trait in the population. We are not persuaded, however, that infection of the urinary tract per se is part of the survival strategy of particular strains of *E. coli*. While colonization of the urinary tract may allow these strains to avoid competing flora in the colon, this strategy would provide at most only a temporary respite for the bacterium. To succeed, the pathogen must ultimately be transmitted to a new host, which is unlikely to occur through urine. Instead, such infections are likely to be the occasional consequence of strains that possess blocks of genetic material that give them an advantage in a different niche. Unfortunately, the advantage imparted by P fimbriae or other putative virulence determinants of uropathogenic strains and the niche in which they operate are not known.

Given these considerations, what generalizations are possible regarding uropathogenic *E. coli*? First, these strains are a heterogeneous collection that differ greatly in phenotypic properties within the group as well as in comparison to other *E. coli* strains. Second, they often express specific adhesins, most notably P fimbriae for those associated with pyelonephritis and type 1 fimbriae for those associated with cystitis, that may aid in colonization of the urinary tract. Third, they commonly possess toxins (hemolysin and CNF1) that may contribute to inflammation and damage. Fourth, a number of other attributes reported to be common among these strains are actually supported by very little evidence. Last, and perhaps most important, many strains associated with UTI possess vast stretches of genetic information that are absent from many other *E. coli* strains, that have yet to be explored genetically, and that likely contain many other virulence genes that enhance the chances of urinary tract colonization. It is quite obvious that we have much to learn about how *E. coli* can cause these extremely common infections.

## ACKNOWLEDGMENTS

We thank Deborah Bills and Linda Amrhein for clerical assistance and John W. Warren and Harry L. T. Mobley for patience.

This work was supported by Public Health Service grants P01 DK49720 and RO1 AI20323 from the National Institutes of Health.

## REFERENCES

1. **Abraham, J. M., C. S. Freitag, J. R. Clements, and B. I. Eisenstein.** 1985. An invertible element of DNA controls phase

variation of type 1 fimbriae of *Escherichia coli*. *Proc. Natl. Acad. Sci. USA* **82**:5724–5727.
2. **Ahrens, R., M. Ott, A. Ritter, H. Hoschutzky, T. Buhler, F. Lottspeich, G. J. Boulnois, K. Jann, and J. Hacker.** 1993. Genetic analysis of the gene cluster encoding nonfimbrial adhesin I from an *Escherichia coli* uropathogen. *Infect. Immun.* **61**:2505–2512.
3. **Andersson, P., I. Engberg, G. Lidin-Janson, K. Lincoln, R. Hull, S. Hull, and C. Svanborg.** 1991. Persistence of *Escherichia coli* bacteriuria is not determined by bacterial adherence. *Infect. Immun.* **59**:2915–2921.
4. **Archambaud, M., P. Courcoux, and A. Labigne-Roussel.** 1988. Detection by molecular hybridization of *pap, afa,* and *sfa* adherence systems in *Escherichia coli* strains associated with urinary and enteral infections. *Ann. Inst. Pasteur Microbiol.* **139**:575–588.
5. **Archambaud, M., P. Courcoux, V. Ouin, G. Chabanon, and A. Labigne-Roussel.** 1988. Phenotypic and genotypic assays for the detection and identification of adhesins from pyelonephritic *Escherichia coli*. *Ann. Inst. Pasteur Microbiol.* **139**:557–573.
6. **Aronson, M., O. Medalia, L. Schori, D. Mirelman, N. Sharon, and I. Ofek.** 1979. Prevention of colonization of the urinary tract of mice with *Escherichia coli* by blocking of bacterial adherence with methyl alpha-D-mannopyranoside. *J. Infect. Dis.* **139**:329–332.
7. **Arthur, M., C. E. Johnson, R. H. Rubin, R. D. Arbeit, C. Campanelli, C. Kim, S. Steinbach, M. Agarwal, R. Wilkinson, and R. Goldstein.** 1989. Molecular epidemiology of adhesin and hemolysin virulence factors among uropathogenic *Escherichia coli*. *Infect. Immun.* **57**:303–313.
8. **Asscher, A., M. Sussman, W. Waters, R. Davis, and S. Chick.** 1966. Urine as a medium for bacterial growth. *Lancet* **ii**:1037–1041.
9. **Bailey, M. J. A., V. Koronakis, T. Schmoll, and C. Hughes.** 1992. *Escherichia coli* HlyT protein, a transcriptional activator of haemolysin synthesis and secretion, is encoded by the *rfaH(sfrB)* locus required for expression of sex factor and lipopolysaccharide genes. *Mol. Microbiol.* **6**:1003–1012.
10. **Benton, J., J. Chawla, S. Parry, and D. Stickler.** 1992. Virulence factors in *Escherichia coli* from urinary tract infections in patients with spinal injuries. *J. Hosp. Infect.* **22**:117–127.
11. **Beutin, L., P. A. Manning, M. Achtman, and N. Willetts.** 1981. *sfrA* and *sfrB* products of *Escherichia coli* K-12 are transcriptional control factors. *J. Bacteriol.* **145**:840–844.
12. **Bhakdi, S., N. Mackman, J. M. Nicaud, and I. B. Holland.** 1986. *Escherichia coli* hemolysin may damage target cell membranes by generating transmembrane pores. *Infect. Immun.* **52**:63–69.
13. **Bilge, S. S., C. R. Clausen, W. Lau, and S. L. Moseley.** 1989. Molecular characterization of a fimbrial adhesin, F1845, mediating diffuse adherence of diarrhea-associated *Escherichia coli* to HEp-2 cells. *J. Bacteriol.* **171**:4281–4289.
14. **Blanco, J., M. P. Alonso, E. A. Gonzalez, M. Blanco, and J. I. Garabal.** 1990. Virulence factors of bacteraemic *Escherichia coli* with particular reference to production of cytotoxic necrotising factor (CNF) by P-fimbriate strains. *J. Med. Microbiol.* **31**:175–183.
15. **Bloch, C. A., and P. E. Orndorff.** 1990. Impaired colonization by and full invasiveness of *Escherichia coli* K1 bearing a site-directed mutation in the type 1 pilin gene. *Infect. Immun.* **58**:275–278.
16. **Bloch, C. A., B. A. D. Stocker, and P. E. Orndorff.** 1992. A key role for type 1 pili in enterobacterial communicability. *Mol. Microbiol.* **6**:697–701.
17. **Blum, G., V. Falbo, A. Caprioloi, and J. Hacker.** 1995. Gene clusters encoding the cytotoxic necrotizing factor type 1, Prs-fimbriae and alpha-hemolysin form the pathogenicity island II of uropathogenic *Escherichia coli* strain J96. *FEMS Microbiol. Lett.* **126**:189–196.
18. **Blum, G., M. Ott, A. Cross, and J. Hacker.** 1991. Virulence determinants of *Escherichia coli* O6 extraintestinal isolates analysed by Southern hybridizations and DNA long range mapping techniques. *Microb. Pathog.* **10**:127–136.
19. **Blum, G., M. Ott, A. Lischewski, A. Ritter, H. Imrich, H. Taschape, and J. Hacker.** 1994. Excision of large DNA regions termed pathogenicity islands from tRNA-specific loci in the chromosome of an *Escherichia coli* wild-type pathogen. *Infect. Immun.* **62**:606–614.
20. **Bock, K., M. E. Breimer, A. Brignole, G. C. Hannsson, K. A. Karlsson, G. Larson, H. Leffler, B. E. Samuelsson, N. Stromberg, C. Svanborg Eden, and J. Thurin.** 1985. Specificity of binding of a

20. strain of uropathogenic *Escherichia coli* to Galα1-4Gal-containing glycosphingolipids. *J. Biol. Chem.* **8545:**8545–8551.
21. **Boehm, D. F., R. A. Welch, and I. S. Snyder.** 1990. Domains of *Escherichia coli* hemolysin (HlyA) involved in binding of calcium and erythrocyte membranes. *Infect. Immun.* **58:**1959–1964.
22. **Bohach, G. A., and I. S. Snyder.** 1985. Chemical and immunological analysis of the complex structure of *Escherichia coli* α-hemolysin. *J. Bacteriol.* **164:**1071–1080.
23. **Brooks, H. J., F. O'Grady, M. A. McSherry, and W. R. Cattell.** 1980. Uropathogenic properties of *Escherichia coli* in recurrent urinary-tract infection. *J. Med. Microbiol.* **13:**57–68.
24. **Caprioli, A., V. Falbo, L. G. Roda, F. M. Ruggeri, and C. Zona.** 1983. Partial purification and characterization of an *Escherichia coli* toxic factor that induces morphological cell alterations. *Infect. Immun.* **39:**1300–1306.
25. **Caprioli, A., V. Falbo, F. M. Ruggeri, L. Baldassarri, R. Bisicchia, G. Ippolito, E. Romoli, and G. Donelli.** 1987. Cytotoxic necrotizing factor production by hemolytic strains of *Escherichia coli* causing extraintestinal infections. *J. Clin. Microbiol.* **25:**146–149.
26. **Caprioli, A., V. Falbo, F. M. Ruggeri, F. Minelli, I. Ørskov, and G. Donelli.** 1989. Relationship between cytotoxic necrotizing factor production and serotype in hemolytic *Escherichia coli*. *J. Clin. Microbiol.* **27:**758–761.
27. **Carbonetti, N. H., S. Boonchai, S. H. Parry, V. Vaisanen-Rhen, T. K. Korhonen, and P. H. Williams.** 1986. Aerobactin-mediated iron uptake by *Escherichia coli* isolates from human extraintestinal infections. *Infect. Immun.* **51:**966–968.
28. **Carmona, M., C. Balsalobre, F. Munoa, M. Mourino, Y. Jubete, F. D. L. Cruz, and A. Juarez.** 1993. *Escherichia coli* hha mutants, DNA supercoiling and expression of the haemolysin genes from the recombinant plasmid pANN202-312. *Mol. Microbiol.* **9:**1011–1018.
29. **Cavalieri, S., G. Bohach, and I. S. Snyder.** 1984. *Escherichia coli* α-hemolysin: characteristics and probable role in pathogenicity. *Microbiol. Rev.* **48:**326–343.
30. **Conventi, L., G. Errico, S. Mastroprimiano, R. D'Elia, and F. Busolo.** 1989. Characterisation of *Escherichia coli* adhesins in patients with symptomatic urinary tract infections. *Genitourin. Med.* **65:**183–186.
31. **Copenhaver, W. M., R. P. Bunge, and M. B. Bunge.** 1971. The urinary system, p. 518–547. *In Bailey's Textbook of Histology*, vol. 16. The Williams & Wilkins Co., Baltimore.
32. **Crosa, J.** 1989. Genetics and molecular biology of siderophore-mediated iron transport in bacteria. *Microbiol. Rev.* **53:**517–530.
33. **Cross, A. S., K. S. Kim, D. C. Wright, J. C. Sadoff, and P. Gemski.** 1986. Role of lipopolysaccharide and capsule in the serum resistance of bacteremic strains of *Escherichia coli*. *J. Infect. Dis.* **154:**497–503.
34. **Culham, D., K. Emmerson, B. Lasby, D. Mamelak, B. Steer, C. Gyles, M. Villarejo, and J. Wood.** 1994. Genes encoding osmoregulatory proline/glycine betaine transporters and the proline catabolic system are present and expressed in diverse clinical *Escherichia coli* isolates. *Can. J. Microbiol.* **40:**397–402.
35. **Czirok, E., H. Milch, K. Csiszar, and M. Csik.** 1986. Virulence factors of *Escherichia coli*. III. Correlation with *Escherichia coli* pathogenicity of haemolysin production, haemagglutinating capacity, antigens K1, K5, and colicinogenicity. *Acta Microbiol. Hung.* **33:**69–83.
36. **Czonka, L.** 1989. Physiology and genetic responses of bacteria to osmotic stress. *Microbiol. Rev.* **53:**121–147.
37. **Daigle, F., J. Harel, J. M. Fairbrother, and P. Lebel.** 1994. Expression and detection of *pap-*, *sfa-*, and *afa*-encoded fimbrial adhesin systems among uropathogenic *Escherichia coli*. *Can. J. Microbiol.* **40:**286–291.
38. **Dalet, F., T. Segovia, and G. Del Rio.** 1991. Frequency and distribution of uropathogenic *Escherichia coli* adhesins: a clinical correlation over 2,000 cases. *Eur. Urol.* **19:**295–303.
39. **de la Cruz, F., D. Muller, J. M. Ortiz, and W. Goebel.** 1980. Hemolysis determinant common to *Escherichia coli* hemolytic plasmids of different incompatibility groups. *J. Bacteriol.* **143:**825–833.
40. **de Man, P., I. Claeson, I. M. Johanson, U. Jodal, and C. Svanborg Eden.** 1989. Bacterial attachment as a predictor of renal abnormalities in boys with urinary tract infection. *J. Pediatr.* **115:**915–922.
41. **de Ree, J. M., and J. F. van den Bosch.** 1987. Serological response to the P fimbriae of uropathogenic *Escherichia coli* in pyelonephritis. *Infect. Immun.* **55:**2204–2207.
42. **de Rycke, J., J. Guillot, and R. Boivin.** 1987. Cytotoxins in nonenterotoxigenic

strains of *Escherichia coli* isolated from feces of diarrheic calves. *Vet. Microbiol.* **15**:137–150.
43. Dowling, K. J., J. A. Roberts, and M. B. Kaack. 1987. P-fimbriated *Escherichia coli* urinary tract infection: a clinical correlation. *South. Med. J.* **80**:1533–1536.
44. Dudgeon, L. S., E. Wordley, and F. Bawtree. 1921. On *Bacillus coli* infections of the urinary tract, especially in relation to hemolytic organisms. *J. Hyg.* **20**:137–164.
45. Eden, C. S., R. Freter, L. Hagberg, R. Hull, S. Hull, H. Leffler, and G. Schoolnik. 1982. Inhibition of experimental ascending urinary tract infection by an epithelial cell-surface receptor analogue. *Nature* (London) **298**:560–562.
46. Eden, C. S., L. A. Hanson, U. Jodal, U. Lindberg, and A. S. Akerlund. 1976. Variable adherence to normal human urinary-tract epithelial cells of *Escherichia coli* strains associated with various forms of urinary-tract infection. *Lancet* **i**:490–492.
47. Eisenstein, B. I. 1981. Phase variation of type 1 fimbriae in *Escherichia coli* is under transcriptional control. *Science* **214**:337–339.
48. Elo, J., L. G. Tallgren, V. Vaisanen, T. K. Korhonen, S. B. Svenson, and P. H. Makela. 1985. Association of P and other fimbriae with clinical pyelonephritis in children. *Scand. J. Urol. Nephrol.* **19**:281–284.
49. Elsinghorst, E., L. Baron, and D. Kopecko. 1989. Penetration of human intestinal epithelial cells by *Salmonella*: molecular cloning and expression of *Salmonella typhi* invasion determinants in *Escherichia coli*. *Proc. Natl. Acad. Sci. USA* **86**:5173–5177.
50. Enerbäck, S., A.-C. Larsson, H. Leffler, A. Lundell, P. de Man, B. Nilsson, and C. Svanborg-Edén. 1987. Binding to galactose$\alpha$1 → 4galactose$\beta$-containing receptors as potential diagnostic tool in urinary tract infection. *J. Clin. Microbiol.* **25**:407–411.
51. Falbo, V., M. Famiglietti, and A. Caprioli. 1992. Gene block encoding production of cytotoxic necrotizing factor 1 and hemolysin in *Escherichia coli* isolates from extraintestinal infections. *Infect. Immun.* **60**:2182–2187.
52. Falbo, V., T. Pace, L. Picci, E. Pizzi, and A. Caprioli. 1993. Isolation and nucleotide sequence of the gene encoding cytotoxic necrotizing factor 1 of *Escherichia coli*. *Infect. Immun.* **61**:4909–4914.
53. Falkow, S. 1988. Molecular Koch's postulates applied to microbial pathogenicity. *Rev. Infect. Dis.* **10**:S274–S276.
54. Falzano, L., C. Fiorentini, G. Donelli, E. Michel, C. Kocks, P. Cossart, L. Cabanie, E. Oswald, and P. Boquet. 1993. Induction of phagocytic behavior in human epithelial cells by Escherichia coli cytotoxic necrotizing factor type 1. *Mol. Microbiol.* **9**:1247–1254.
55. Felmlee, T., S. Pellett, E. Y. Lee, and R. A. Welch. 1985. The *Escherichia coli* hemolysin is released extracellularly without cleavage of a signal peptide. *J. Bacteriol.* **163**:88–93.
56. Felmlee, T., S. Pellett, and R. A. Welch. 1985. The nucleotide sequence of an *Escherichia coli* chromosomal hemolysin. *J. Bacteriol.* **163**:94–105.
57. Fetherston, J. D., P. Schuetze, and R. D. Perry. 1992. Loss of the pigmentation phenotype in *Yersina pestis* is due to the spontaneous deletion of 102 kb of chromosomal DNA which is flanked by a repetitive element. *Mol. Microbiol.* **6**:2693–2704.
58. Finkelstein, R., C. Sciortino, and M. McIntosh. 1983. Role of iron in microbe-host interactions. *Rev. Infect. Dis.* **5**:759–777.
59. Fiorentini, C., G. Arancia, V. Falbo, F. Ruggeri, and G. Donelli. 1988. Cytoskeletal changes induced in HEp-2 cells by the cytotoxic necrotizing factor of *Escherichia coli*. *Toxicon* **26**:1047–1056.
60. Fiorentini, C., L. Falzano, G. Donelli, E. Oswald, M. Popoff, and P. Boquet. 1993. *E. coli* cytotoxic necrotizing factor 1 (CNF 1) and its effects on cells. *Toxicon* **31**:501.
61. Fujita, K., T. Yamamoto, T. Yokota, and R. Kitagawa. 1989. In vitro adherence of type 1-fimbriated uropathogenic *Escherichia coli* to human ureteral mucosa. *Infect. Immun.* **57**:2574–2579.
62. Funfstuck, R., H. Tschape, G. Stein, H. Kunath, M. Bergner, and G. Wessel. 1986. Virulence properties of *Escherichia coli* strains in patients with chronic pyelonephritis. *Infection* **14**:145–150.
63. Galen, J., and R. Curtiss III. 1989. Cloning and molecular characterization of genes whose products allow Salmonella typhimurium to penetrate tissue culture cells. *Proc. Natl. Acad. Sci. USA* **86**:6383–6387.
64. Gander, R. M., V. L. Thomas, and M. Forland. 1985. Mannose-resistant hemagglutination and P receptor recognition of uropathogenic *Escherichia coli* isolated from adult patients. *J. Infect. Dis.* **151**:508–513.
65. Giron, J. A., T. Jones, F. Millan-Velasco, E. Castro-Munoz, L. Zarate, J. Fry, G.

Frankel, S. L. Moseley, B. Baudry, J. B. Kaper, G. K. Schoolnik, and L. W. Riley. 1991. Diffuse-adhering *Escherichia coli* (DAEC) as a putative cause of diarrhea in Mayan children in Mexico. *J. Infect. Dis.* **163:**507–513.

66. Goebel, W., and J. Hedgpeth. 1982. Cloning and functional characterization of the plasmid-encoded hemolysin determinant of *Escherichia coli*. *J. Bacteriol.* **151:**1290–1298.

67. Goldhar, J., R. Perry, J. R. Golecki, H. Hoschutzky, B. Jann, and K. Jann. 1987. Nonfimbrial, mannose-resistant adhesins from uropathogenic *Escherichia coli* O83:K1:H4 and O14:K?:H11. *Infect. Immun.* **55:**1837–1842.

68. Goldhar, J., R. Perry, and I. Ofek. 1984. Extraction and properties of nonfimbrial mannose-resistant hemagglutinin from a urinary isolate of *Escherichia coli*. *Curr. Microbiol.* **11:**49–54.

69. Goluszko, P., S. Nowicki, A. Kaul, T. Pham, S. Moseley, and B. Nowicki. 1995. Development of experimental chronic pyelonephritis with Dr fimbriae bearing *Escherichia coli* O75:K5:H-, abstr. B-15, p. 168. *Abstr. 95th Gen. Meet. Am. Soc. Microbiol.*

70. Gordon, D., and M. Riley. 1992. A theoretical and experimental analysis of bacterial growth in the bladder. *Mol. Microbiol.* **6:**555–562.

71. Hacker, J., L. Bender, M. Ott, J. Wingender, B. Lund, R. Marre, and W. Goebel. 1990. Deletions of chromosomal regions coding for fimbriae and hemolysins occur *in vitro* and *in vivo* in various extraintestinal *Escherichia coli* isolates. *Microb. Pathog.* **8:**213–225.

72. Hacker, J., H. Kestler, H. Hoschutzky, K. Jann, F. Lottspeich, and T. K. Korhonen. 1993. Cloning and characterization of the S fimbrial adhesin II complex of an *Escherichia coli* causing urinary tract infections. *Infect. Immun.* **61:**544–550.

73. Hacker, J., S. Knapp, and W. Goebel. 1983. Spontaneous deletions and flanking regions of the chromosomally inherited hemolysin determinant of an *Escherichia coli* O6 strain. *J. Bacteriol.* **154:**1145–1152.

74. Hagberg, L., R. Hull, S. Hull, S. Falkow, R. Freter, and C. Svanborg Eden. 1983. Contribution of adhesion to bacterial persistence in the mouse urinary tract. *Infect. Immun.* **40:**265–272.

75. Hagberg, L., U. Jodal, T. K. Korhonen, G. Lidin-Janson, U. Lindberg, and C. Svanborg Eden. 1981. Adhesion, hemagglutination, and virulence of *Escherichia coli* causing urinary tract infections. *Infect. Immun.* **31:**564–570.

76. Haley, R., D. Culver, J. White, W. Morgan, T. Emori, V. Munn, and T. Hooton. 1985. The SENIC 3. The efficacy of infection surveillance and control programs in preventing nosocomial infections in United States hospitals. *Am. J. Epidemiol.* **121:**182–205.

77. High, N. J., B. A. Hales, K. Jann, and G. J. Boulnois. 1988. A block or urovirulence genes encoding multiple fimbriae and hemolysin in *Escherichia coli* O4:K12:H-. *Infect. Immun.* **56:**513–517.

78. Holloway, B. W. 1993. Genetics for all bacteria. *Annu. Rev. Microbiol.* **47:**659–684.

79. Horwitz, M. A., and S. C. Silverstein. 1980. Influence of the *Escherichia coli* capsule on complement fixation and on phagocytosis and killing by human phagocytes. *J. Clin. Invest.* **65:**82–94.

80. Hull, R., S. Bieler, S. Falkow, and S. Hull. 1986. Chromosomal map position of genes encoding P adhesins in uropathogenic *Escherichia coli*. *Infect. Immun.* **51:**693–695.

81. Hull, R. A., S. I. Hull, and S. Falkow. 1982. Genetics of hemolysin of *Escherichia coli*. *J. Bacteriol.* **151:**1006–1012.

82. Hultgren, S. J., T. N. Porter, A. J. Schaeffer, and J. L. Duncan. 1985. Role of type 1 pili and effects of phase variation on lower urinary tract infections produced by *Escherichia coli*. *Infect. Immun.* **50:**370–377.

83. Ikaheimo, R., A. Siitonen, U. Karkkainen, P. Kuosmanen, and P. H. Makela. 1993. Characteristics of *Escherichia coli* in acute community-acquired cystitis of adult women. *Scand. J. Infect. Dis.* **25:**705–712.

84. Ikaheimo, R., A. Siitonen, U. Karkkainen, and P. H. Makela. 1993. Virulence characteristics of *Escherichia coli* in nosocomial urinary tract infection. *Clin. Infect. Dis.* **16:**785–791.

85. Ikaheimo, R., A. Siitonen, U. Karkkainen, J. Mustonen, T. Heiskanen, and P. H. Makela. 1994. Community-acquired pyelonephritis in adults: characteristics of *E. coli* isolates in bacteremic and non-bacteremic patients. *Scand. J. Infect. Dis.* **26:**289–296.

86. Inouye, S., M. G. Sunshine, E. W. Six, and M. Inouye. 1991. Retronphage φR73: an *E. coli* phage that contains a retroelement

and integrates into a tRNA gene. *Science* **252**: 969–971.

87. **Israele, V., A. Darabi, and G. H. McCracken, Jr.** 1987. The role of bacterial virulence factors and Tamm-Horsfall protein in the pathogenesis of *Escherichia coli* urinary tract infection in infants. *Am. J. Dis. Child.* **141**:1230–1234.

88. **Issartel, J.-P., V. Koronakis, and C. Hughes.** 1991. Activation of *Escherichia coli* prohaemolysin to the mature toxin by acyl carrier protein-dependent fatty acylation. *Nature* (London) **351**:759–761.

89. **Jacobson, S., M. Hammarlind, K. Lidefeldt, E. Osterberg, K. Tullis, and A. Brauner.** 1988. Incidence of aerobactin-positive *Escherichia coli* strains in patients with symptomatic urinary tract infection. *Eur. J. Clin. Microbiol. Infect. Dis.* **7**:630–634.

90. **Jacobson, S. H., L.-E. Lins, S. B. Svenson, and G. Kallenius.** 1985. P fimbriated *Escherichia coli* in adults with acute pyelonephritis. *J. Infect. Dis.* **152**:426–427.

91. **Jacobson, S. H., C. G. Ostenson, K. Tullus, and A. Brauner.** 1992. Serum resistance in *Escherichia coli* strains causing acute pyelonephritis and bacteraemia. *APMIS* **100**:147–153.

92. **Johanson, I., R. Lindstedt, and C. Svanborg.** 1992. Roles of the *pap*- and *prs*-encoded adhesins in *Escherichia coli* adherence to human uroepithelial cells. *Infect. Immun.* **60**:3416–3422.

93. **Johnson, J.** 1991. Virulence factors in *Escherichia coli* urinary tract infections. *Clin. Microbiol. Rev.* **4**:80–128.

94. **Johnson, J., P. Goullet, B. Picard, S. Moseley, P. Roberts, and W. Stamm.** 1991. Association of carboxylesterase B electrophoretic pattern with the presence and expression of urovirulence factor determinants and antimicrobial resistance among strains of *Escherichia coli* that cause urosepsis. *Infect. Immun.* **59**:2311–2315.

95. **Johnson, J., I. Orskov, F. Orskov, P. Goulet, B. Picard, S. Moseley, P. Roberts, and W. Stamm.** 1994. O, K, and H antigens predict virulence factors, carboxyesterase B pattern, antimicrobial resistance and host compromise among *Escherichia coli* strains causing urosepsis. *J. Infect. Dis.* **169**:119–126.

96. **Johnson, J., P. Roberts, and W. Stamm.** 1987. P fimbriae and other virulence factors in *Escherichia coli* urosepsis: association with patients' characteristics. *J. Infect. Dis.* **156**:225–229.

97. **Johnson, J. R., S. L. Moseley, P. L. Roberts, and W. E. Stamm.** 1988. Aerobactin and other virulence factor genes among strains of *Escherichia coli* causing urosepsis: association with patient characteristics. *Infect. Immun.* **56**:405–412.

98. **Johnson, J. R., K. M. Skubitz, B. J. Nowicki, K. Jacques-Palaz, and R. M. Rakita.** 1995. Nonlethal adherence to human neutrophils mediated by Dr antigen-specific adhesins of *Escherichia coli*. *Infect. Immun.* **63**:309–316.

99. **Jorgensen, S. E., R. F. Hammer, and G. K. Wu.** 1980. Effects of a single hit from the α-hemolysin produced by *Escherichia coli* on the morphology of sheep erythrocytes. *Infect. Immun.* **27**:988–994.

100. **Jorgensen, S. E., P. F. Mulcahy, and C. F. Louis.** 1986. Effect of Escherichia coli hemolysin on permeability of erythrocyte membranes to calcium. *Toxicon* **24**:559–566.

101. **Jorgensen, S. E., P. F. Mulcahy, G. K. Wu, and C. F. Louis.** 1983. Calcium accumulation in human and sheep erythrocytes that is induced by Escherichia coli hemolysin. *Toxicon* **21**:717–727.

102. **Kaijser, B., L. A. Hanson, U. Jodal, G. Lidin-Janson, and J. B. Robbins.** 1977. Frequency of *E. coli* K antigens in urinary-tract infections in children. *Lancet* **i**:663–666.

103. **Kallenius, G., R. Mollby, S. B. Svenson, I. Helin, H. Hultberg, B. Cedergren, and J. Winberg.** 1981. Occurrence of P-fimbriated *Escherichia coli* in urinary tract infections. *Lancet* **ii**:1369–1372.

104. **Kallenius, G., R. Mollby, S. B. Svenson, J. Winberg, A. Lundblad, S. Svensson, and B. Cedergren.** 1980. The P$^k$ antigen as receptor for the haemagglutinin of pyelonephritic *Escherichia coli*. *FEMS Microbiol. Lett.* **7**:297–302.

105. **Kallenius, G., S. Svenson, R. Mollby, B. Cedergren, H. Hultberg, and J. Winberg.** 1981. Structure of carbohydrate part of receptor on human uroepithelial cells for pyelonephritogenic *Escherichia coli*. *Lancet* **ii**:604–606.

106. **Kallenius, G., S. B. Svenson, R. Mollby, T. Korhonen, J. Winberg, B. Cedergren, I. Helin, and H. Hultberg.** 1982. Carbohydrate receptor structures recognized by uropathogenic *E. coli*. *Scand. J. Infect. Dis. Suppl.* **33**:52–60.

107. **Kao, J., and H. T. Mobley.** Personal communication.

108. **Karkkainen, U., R. Ikaheimo, M. L. Katila, and R. Mantyjarvi.** 1991. P fimbriation of *Escherichia coli* strains from patients

with urosepsis demonstrated by a commercial agglutination test (PF TEST). *J. Clin. Microbiol.* **29:**221–224.
109. **Karr, J. F., B. Nowicki, L. D. Truong, R. A. Hull, and S. I. Hull.** 1989. Purified P fimbriae from two cloned gene clusters of a single pyelonephritogenic strain adhere to unique structures in the human kidney. *Infect. Immun.* **57:**3594–3600.
110. **Kauffmann, F.** 1947. The serology of the coli group. *J. Immunol.* **57:**71–100.
111. **Keane, W. F., R. A. Welch, G. Gekker, and P. K. Peterson.** 1987. Mechanism of *Escherichia coli* α-hemolysin-induced injury to isolated renal tubular cells. *Am. J. Pathol.* **126:**350–357.
112. **Keith, B. R., L. Maurer, P. A. Spears, and P. E. Orndorff.** 1986. Receptor-binding function of type 1 pili effects bladder colonization by a clinical isolate of *Escherichia coli*. *Infect. Immun.* **53:**693–696.
113. **Kisielius, P. V., W. R. Schwan, S. K. Amundsen, J. L. Duncan, and A. J. Schaeffer.** 1989. In vivo expression and variation of *Escherichia coli* type 1 and P pili in the urine of adults with acute urinary tract infections. *Infect. Immun.* **57:**1656–1662.
114. **Knapp, S., J. Hacker, T. Jarchau, and W. Goebel.** 1986. Large, unstable inserts in the chromosome affect virulence properties of uropathogenic *Escherichia coli* O6 strain 536. *J. Bacteriol.* **168:**22–30.
115. **Korhonen, T. K., J. Parkkinen, J. Hacker, J. Finne, A. Pere, M. Rhen, and H. Holthofer.** 1986. Binding of *Escherichia coli* S fimbriae to human kidney epithelium. *Infect. Immun.* **54:**322–327.
116. **Korhonen, T. K., M. V. Valtonen, J. Parkkinen, V. Vaisanen-Rhen, J. Finne, F. Ørskov, I. Ørskov, S. B. Svenson, and P. H. Makela.** 1985. Serotypes, hemolysin production, and receptor recognition of *Escherichia coli* strains associated with neonatal sepsis and meningitis. *Infect. Immun.* **48:**486–491.
117. **Korhonen, T. K., R. Virkola, and H. Holthofer.** 1986. Localization of binding sites for purified *Escherichia coli* P fimbriae in the human kidney. *Infect. Immun.* **54:**328–332.
118. **Korhonen, T. K., R. Virkola, B. Westurlund, H. Holthofer, and J. Parkkinen.** 1990. Tissue tropism of *Escherichia coli* adhesins in human extraintestinal infections. *Curr. Top. Microbiol. Immunol.* **151:**115–127.
119. **Kunin, C., T. Hua, L. White, and M. Villarejo.** 1992. Growth of *Escherichia coli* in human urine: role of salt tolerance and accumulation of glycine betaine. *J. Infect. Dis.* **166:**1311–1315.
120. **Kunin, C. M.** 1994. Urinary tract infections in females. *Clin. Infect. Dis.* **18:**1–12.
121. **Kunin, C. M., T. H. Hua, C. Krishnan, L. Van Arsdale White, and J. Hacker.** 1993. Isolation of a nicotinamide-requiring clone of *Escherichia coli* O18:K1:H7 from women with acute cystitis: resemblance to strains found in neonatal meningitis. *Clin. Infect. Dis.* **16:**412–416.
122. **Labigne-Roussel, A., and S. Falkow.** 1988. Distribution and degree of heterogeneity of the afimbrial-adhesin-encoding operon (*afa*) among uropathogenic *Escherichia coli*. *Infect. Immun.* **56:**640–648.
123. **Labigne-Roussel, A. F., D. Lark, G. Schoolnik, and S. Falkow.** 1984. Cloning and expression of an afimbrial adhesin (AFA-I) responsible for P blood group-independent, mannose-resistant hemagglutination from a pyelonephritis *Escherichia coli* strain. *Infect. Immun.* **46:**251–259.
124. **Latham, R. H., and W. E. Stamm.** 1984. Role of fimbriated *Escherichia coli* in urinary tract infections in adult women: correlation with localization studies. *J. Infect. Dis.* **149:**835–840.
125. **Lee, C., B. Jones, and S. Falkow.** 1992. Identification of a *Salmonella typhimurium* invasion locus by selection for hyperinvasive mutants. *J. Bacteriol.* **89:**1847–1851.
126. **Levin, B. R., and C. S. Eden.** 1990. Selection and evolution of virulence in bacteria: an ecumenical excursion and modest suggestion. *Parasitology* **100:**S103–S115.
127. **Lidefelt, K. J., I. Bollgren, G. Kallenius, and S. B. Svenson.** 1987. P-fimbriated *Escherichia coli* in children with acute cystitis. *Acta Paediatr. Scand.* **76:**775–780.
128. **Lindberg, U., L. A. Hanson, U. Jodal, G. Lidin-Janson, K. Lincoln, and S. Olling.** 1975. Asymptomatic bacteriuria in schoolgirls. II. Differences in *Escherichia coli* causing asymptomatic bacteriuria. *Acta Paediatr. Scand.* **64:**432–436.
129. **Lomberg, H., L. A. Hanson, B. Jacobsson, U. Jodal, H. Leffler, and C. S. Eden.** 1983. Correlation of P blood group, vesicoureteral reflux, and bacterial attachment in patients with recurrent pyelonephritis. *N. Engl. J. Med.* **308:**1189–1192.
130. **Lomberg, H., M. Hellstrom, U. Jodal, H. Leffler, K. Lincoln, and C. Svanborg Eden.** 1984. Virulence-associated traits in *Escherichia coli* causing first and recurrent episodes of urinary tract infection in children

with or without vesicoureteral reflux. *J. Infect. Dis.* **150**:561–569.
131. Lomberg, H., M. Hellstrom, U. Jodal, I. Orskov, and C. Svanborg Eden. 1989. Properties of *Escherichia coli* in patients with renal scarring. *J. Infect. Dis.* **159**:579–582.
132. Low, D., V. David, D. Lark, G. Schoolnik, and S. Falkow. 1984. Gene clusters governing the production of hemolysin and mannose-resistant hemagglutination are closely linked in *Escherichia coli* serotype O4 and O6 isolates from urinary tract infections. *Infect. Immun.* **43**:353–358.
133. Lyon, M. W., Jr. 1917. A case of cystitis caused by *Bacillus coli-hemolyticus*. *JAMA* **69**:353–358.
134. Mårild, S., B. Wettergren, M. Hellstrom, U. Jodal, K. Lincoln, I. Ørskov, F. Ørskov, and C. Svanborg Eden. 1988. Bacterial virulence and inflammatory response in infants with febrile urinary tract infection or screening bacteriuria. *J. Pediatr.* **112**:348–354.
135. Marre, R., and J. Hacker. 1987. Role of S- and common-type I-fimbriae of *Escherichia coli* in experimental upper and lower urinary tract infection. *Microb. Pathog.* **2**:223–226.
136. Marre, R., J. Hacker, W. Henkel, and W. Goebel. 1986. Contribution of cloned virulence factors from uropathogenic *Escherichia coli* strains to nephropathogenicity in an experimental rat pyelonephritis model. *Infect. Immun.* **54**:761–767.
137. Marre, R., B. Kreft, and J. Hacker. 1990. Genetically engineered S and F1C fimbriae differ in their contribution to adherence of *Escherichia coli* to cultured renal tubular cells. *Infect. Immun.* **58**:3434–3437.
138. May, A. K., C. A. Bloch, R. G. Sawyer, M. D. Spengler, and T. L. Pruett. 1993. Enhanced virulence of *Escherichia coli* bearing a site-targeted mutation in the major structural subunit of type 1 fimbriae. *Infect. Immun.* **61**:1667–1673.
139. McDaniel, T. K., K. G. Jarvis, M. S. Donnenberg, and J. B. Kaper. 1995. A genetic locus of enterocyte effacement conserved among diverse enterobacterial pathogens. *Proc. Natl. Acad. Sci. USA* **92**:1664–1668.
140. McLaren, I., and C. Wray. 1986. Another animal *Escherichia coli* cytopathic factor. *Vet. Rec.* **119**:576–577.
141. Moayeri, M., and R. Welch. 1994. Effects of temperature, time and toxin concentration of lesion formation by the *Escherichia coli* hemolysin. *Infect. Immun.* **62**:4124–4134.
142. Mobley, H. L. T., G. R. Chippendale, J. H. Tenney, R. A. Hull, and J. W. Warren. 1987. Expression of type 1 fimbriae may be required for persistence of *Escherichia coli* in the catheterized urinary tract. *J. Clin. Microbiol.* **25**:2253–2257.
143. Mobley, H. L. T., D. M. Green, A. L. Trifillis, D. E. Johnson, G. R. Chippendale, C. V. Lockatell, B. D. Jones, and J. W. Warren. 1990. Pyelonephritogenic *Escherichia coli* and killing of cultured human renal proximal tubular epithelial cells: role of hemolysin in some strains. *Infect. Immun.* **58**:1281–1289.
144. Mobley, H. L. T., K. G. Jarvis, J. P. Elwood, D. I. Whittle, C. V. Lockatell, R. G. Russell, D. E. Johnson, M. S. Donnenberg, and J. W. Warren. 1993. Isogenic P-fimbrial deletion mutants of pyelonephritogenic *Escherichia coli*: the role of $\beta$-Gal(1-4)$\beta$-Gal binding in virulence of a wild-type strain. *Mol. Microbiol.* **10**:143–155.
145. Montgomerie, J. Z., A. Bindereif, J. B. Neilands, G. M. Kalmanson, and L. B. Guze. 1984. Association of hydroxamate siderophore (aerobactin) with *Escherichia coli* isolated from patients with bacteremia. *Infect. Immun.* **46**:835–838.
146. Morschhauser, J., V. Vetter, L. Emody, and J. Hacker. 1994. Adhesin regulatory genes within large, unstable DNA regions of pathogenic *Escherichia coli*: cross-talk between different adhesin gene clusters. *Mol. Microbiol.* **11**:555–566.
147. Murphy, A., and E. Rozengurt. 1992. *Pasteurella multocida* toxin selectively facilitates phosphatidylinositol-4,5-biphosphate hydrolysis by bombesin, vasopressin and endothelin. *J. Biol. Chem.* **267**:25296–25303.
148. Nieto, J. M., M. Carmona, S. Bolland, Y. Jubete, F. de la Cruz, and A. Jaurez. 1991. The *hha* gene modulates haemolysin expression in *Escherichia coli*. *Mol. Microbiol.* **5**:1285–1293.
149. Nowicki, B., J. P. Barrish, T. Korhonen, R. A. Hull, and S. I. Hull. 1987. Molecular cloning of the *Escherichia coli* O75X adhesin. *Infect. Immun.* **55**:3168–3173.
150. Nowicki, B., A. Hart, K. E. Coyne, D. M. Lublin, and S. Nowicki. 1993. Short consensus repeat-3 domain of recombinant decay-accelerating factor is recognized by *Escherichia coli* recombinant Dr adhesin in a model of a cell-cell interaction. *J. Exp. Med.* **178**:2115–2121.
151. Nowicki, B., H. Holthofer, and T. Saraneva. 1986. Location of adhesion sites for P

fimbriated and for O75X-positive *Escherichia coli* in the human kidney. *Microb. Pathog.* **1**:169–180.
152. Nowicki, B., A. Labigne, S. Moseley, R. Hull, S. Hull, and J. Moulds. 1990. The Dr hemagglutinin, afimbrial adhesins AFA-I and AFA-III, and F1845 fimbriae of uropathogenic and diarrhea-associated *Escherichia coli* belong to a family of hemagglutinins with Dr receptor recognition. *Infect. Immun.* **58**:279–281.
153. Nowicki, B., J. Moulds, R. Hull, and S. Hull. 1988. A hemagglutinin of uropathogenic *Escherichia coli* recognizes the Dr blood group antigen. *Infect. Immun.* **56**:1057–1060.
154. Nowicki, B., C. Svanborg-Eden, R. Hull, and S. Hull. 1989. Molecular analysis and epidemiology of the Dr hemagglutinin of uropathogenic *Escherichia coli*. *Infect. Immun.* **57**:446–451.
155. Ofek, I., D. Mirelman, and N. Sharon. 1977. Adherence of *Escherichia coli* to human mucosal cells mediated by mannose receptors. *Nature* (London) **265**:623–625.
156. Ofek, I., and N. Sharon. 1988. Lectinophagocytosis: a molecular mechanism of recognition between cell surface sugars and lectins in the phagocytosis of bacteria. *Infect. Immun.* **56**:539–547.
157. O'Hanley, P., G. Lalonde, and G. Ji. 1991. Alpha-hemolysin contributes to the pathogenicity of piliated digalactoside-binding *Escherichia coli* in the kidney: efficacy of an alpha-hemolysin vaccine in preventing renal injury in the BALB/c mouse model of pyelonephritis. *Infect. Immun.* **59**:1153–1161.
158. O'Hanley, P., D. Lark, S. Falkow, and G. Schoolnik. 1985. Molecular basis of *Escherichia coli* colonization of the upper urinary tract in Balb/c mice. *J. Clin. Invest.* **75**:347–360.
159. O'Hanley, P., D. Low, I. Romero, D. Lark, K. Vosti, S. Falkow, and G. Schoolnik. 1985. Gal-gal binding and hemolysin phenotypes and genotypes associated with uropathogenic *Escherichia coli*. *N. Engl. J. Med.* **313**:414–420.
160. Olling, S., L. A. Hanson, J. Holmgren, U. Jodal, K. Lincoln, and U. Lindberg. 1973. The bactericidal effect of normal human serum on *E. coli* strains from normals and from patients with urinary tract infections. *Infection* **1**:24–28.
161. Opal, S. M., A. S. Cross, P. Gemski, and L. W. Lyhte. 1990. Aerobactin and α-hemolysin as virulence determinants in *Escherichia coli* isolated from human blood, urine, and stool. *J. Infect. Dis.* **161**:794–796.
162. Orndorff, P. E., and C. A. Bloch. 1990. The role of type-1 pili in the pathogenesis of Escherichia-coli infections: a short review and some new ideas. *Microb. Pathog.* **9**:75–79.
163. Orskov, F., and I. Orskov. 1983. Summary of a workshop on the clone concept in the epidemiology, taxonomy, and evolution of the *Enterobacteriaceae* and other bacteria. *J. Infect. Dis.* **148**:346.
164. Orskov, F., and I. Orskov. 1992. *Escherichia coli* serotyping and disease in man and animals. *Can. J. Microbiol.* **38**:699–704.
165. Orskov, I., and F. Orskov. 1983. Serology and *Escherichia coli* fimbriae. *Prog. Allergy* **33**:80–105.
166. Orskov, I., and F. Orskov. 1985. *Escherichia coli* in extraintestinal infections. *J. Hyg.* **95**:551–575.
167. Orskov, I., F. Orskov, A. Birch-Anderson, M. Kanamori, and C. Svanborg-Eden. 1982. O, K, H and fimbrial antigens in *Escherichia coli* serotypes associated with pyelonephritis and cystitis. *Scand. J. Infect. Dis. Suppl.* **33**:18–25.
168. Orskov, I., C. Svanborg Eden, and F. Orskov. 1988. Aerobactin production of serotyped *Escherichia coli* from urinary tract infection. *Med. Microbiol. Immunol.* **177**:9–14.
169. Ostolaza, H., B. Bartoleme, J. Serra, F. de la Cruz, and F. Goni. 1991. α-Hemolysin from *E. coli*: purification and self-aggregation properties. *FEBS Lett.* **280**:195–198.
170. Oswald, E., M. Sugai, A. Labigne, H. C. Wu, C. Fiorentini, P. Boquet, and A. D. O'Brien. 1994. Cytotoxic necrotizing factor type 2 produced by virulent *Escherichia coli* modifies the small GTP-binding proteins Rho involved in assembly of actin stress fibers. *Proc. Natl. Acad. Sci. USA* **91**:3814–3818.
171. Ott, M., J. Hacker, T. Schmoll, T. Jarchau, T. K. Korhonen, and W. Goebel. 1986. Analysis of the genetic determinants coding for the S-fimbrial adhesin (*sfa*) in different *Escherichia coli* strains causing meningitis or urinary tract infections. *Infect. Immun.* **54**:646–653.
172. Ott, M., H. Hoschutzky, K. Jann, I. van Die, and J. Hacker. 1988. Gene clusters for S fimbrial adhesin (*sfa*) and F1C fimbriae (*foc*) of *Escherichia coli*: comparative aspects of structure and function. *J. Bacteriol.* **170**:3983–3990.
173. Otto, G., T. Sandberg, B.-I. Marklund, P. Ulleryd, and C. Svanborg. 1993. Virulence factors and *pap* genotype in *Escherichia*

coli isolates from women with acute pyelonephritis, with or without bacteremia. *Clin. Infect. Dis.* **17**:448–456.

174. Paranchych, W., and L. S. Frost. 1988. The physiology and biochemistry of pili. *Adv. Microb. Physiol.* **29**:53–114.

175. Parkkinen, J., G. N. Rogers, T. Korhonen, W. Dahr, and J. Finne. 1986. Identification of the O-linked sialyloligosaccharides of glycophorin A as the erythrocyte receptors for S-fimbriated *Escherichia coli*. *Infect. Immun.* **54**:37–42.

176. Pawelzik, M., J. Heesemann, J. Hacker, and W. Opferkuch. 1988. Cloning and characterization of a new type of fimbria (S/FIC-related fimbria) expressed by an *Escherichia coli* O75:K1:H7 blood culture isolate. *Infect. Immun.* **56**:2918–2924.

177. Payne, S. 1988. Iron and virulence in the family Enterobacteriaceae. *Crit. Rev. Microbiol.* **16**:81–111.

178. Pecha, B., D. Low, and P. O'Hanley. 1989. Gal-Gal pili vaccines prevent pyelonephritis by piliated *Escherichia coli* in a murine model. *J. Clin. Invest.* **83**:2102–2108.

179. Pedersen, K., and F. Elling. 1984. The pathogenesis of atrophic rhinitis in pigs induced by toxigenic *Pasteurella multocida*. *J. Comp. Pathol.* **94**:203–214.

180. Pere, A., M. Leinonen, V. Vaisanen-Rhen, M. Rhen, and T. K. Korhonen. 1985. Occurrence of type-1C fimbriae on *Escherichia coli* strains isolated from human extraintestinal infections. *J. Gen. Microbiol.* **131**:1705–1711.

181. Pere, A., B. Nowicki, H. Saxen, A. Siitonen, and T. K. Korhonen. 1987. Expression of P, type-1, and type-1C fimbriae of *Escherichia coli* in the urine of patients with acute urinary tract infection. *J. Infect. Dis.* **156**:567–574.

182. Phillips, I., S. Eykyn, A. King, W. R. Gransden, B. Rowe, J. A. Frost, and R. J. Gross. 1988. Epidemic multiresistant *Escherichia coli* infection in West Lambeth health district. *Lancet* **i**:1038–1041.

183. Plos, K., T. Carter, S. Hull, R. Hull, and C. S. Eden. 1990. Frequency and organization of *pap* homologous DNA in relation to clinical origin of uropathogenic *Escherichia coli*. *J. Infect. Dis.* **161**:518–524.

184. Pluschke, G., J. Mayden, M. Achtman, and R. P. Levine. 1983. Role of the capsule and the O antigen in resistance of O18:K1 *Escherichia coli* to complement-mediated killing. *Infect. Immun.* **42**:907–913.

185. Portnoy, D. A., T. Chakraborty, W. Goebel, and P. Cossart. 1992. Molecular determinants of *Listeria monocytogenes* pathogenesis. *Infect. Immun.* **60**:1263–1267.

186. Pradel, E., and C. A. Schnaitman. 1991. Effect of *rfaH* (*sfrB*) and temperature on expression of *rfa* genes of *Escherichia coli* K-12. *J. Bacteriol.* **173**:6428–6431.

187. Reiter, W.-D., P. Palm, and S. Yeats. 1989. Transfer RNA genes frequently serve as integration sites for prokaryotic genetic elements. *Nucleic Acids Res.* **17**:1907–1914.

188. Rhen, M., V. Vaisanen-Rhen, M. Saraste, and T. K. Korhonen. 1986. Organization of genes expressing the blood-group-M-specific hemagglutinin of *Escherichia coli*: identification and nucleotide sequence of the M-agglutinin subunit gene. *Gene* **49**:351–360.

189. Riegman, N., R. Kusters, H. Van Veggel, H. Bergmans, P. Van Bergen en Henegouwen, J. Hacker, and I. Van Die. 1990. F1C fimbriae of a uropathogenic *Escherichia coli* strain: genetic and functional organization of the *foc* gene cluster and identification of minor subunits. *J. Bacteriol.* **172**:1114–1120.

190. Riley, M., and S. Krawiec. 1987. Genome organization, p. 967–981. *In* F. C. Neidhardt, J. L. Ingraham, K. B. Low, B. Magasanik, M. Schaechter, and H. E. Umbarger (ed.), *Escherichia coli and Salmonella typhimurium: Cellular and Molecular Biology*, vol. 2. American Society for Microbiology, Washington, D.C.

191. Roberts, J. A., K. Hardaway, B. Kaack, E. N. Fussell, and G. Baskin. 1984. Prevention of pyelonephritis by immunization with P-fimbriae. *J. Urol.* **131**:602–607.

192. Roberts, J. A., B. Kaack, G. Kallenius, R. Mollby, J. Winberg, and S. B. Svenson. 1984. Receptors for pyelonephritogenic *Escherichia coli* in primates. *J. Urol.* **131**:163–168.

193. Roberts, J. A., M. B. Kaack, G. Baskin, T. K. Korhonen, S. B. Svenson, and J. Winberg. 1989. P-fimbriae vaccines. II. Cross reactive protection against pyelonephritis. *Pediatr. Nephrol.* **3**:391–396.

194. Roberts, J. A., B.-I. Marklund, D. Ilver, D. Haslam, M. B. Kaack, G. Baskin, M. Louis, R. Mollby, J. Winberg, and S. Normark. 1994. The Galα(1-4)Gal-specific tip adhesin of *Escherichia coli* P-fimbriae is needed for pyelonephritis to occur in the normal urinary tract. *Proc. Natl. Acad. Sci. USA* **91**:11889–11893.

195. Russo, T. A., M. C. Moffitt, C. H. Hammer, and M. M. Frank. 1993. Tn*phoA*-mediated disruption of K54 capsular polysaccharide genes in *Escherichia coli* confers serum sensitivity. *Infect. Immun.* **61:**3578–3582.
196. Rydberg, J., and I. Helin. 1991. A simple reliable agglutination test for screening P-fimbriated *Escherichia coli* in children with urinary tract infections gives valuable clinical information. *Scand. J. Infect. Dis.* **23:** 573–575.
197. Sandberg, T., B. Kaijser, G. Lidin-Janson, K. Lincoln, F. Orskov, I. Orskov, E. Stokland, and C. Svanborg-Eden. 1988. Virulence of *Escherichia coli* in relation to host factors in women with symptomatic urinary tract infection. *J. Clin. Microbiol.* **26:** 1471–1476.
198. Sandberg, T., K. Stenqvist, C. Svanborg Eden, and G. Lidin-Janson. 1983. Host-parasite relationship in urinary tract infections during pregnancy. *Prog. Allergy* **33:** 228–235.
199. Schaeffer, A. J., W. R. Schwan, S. J. Hultgren, and J. L. Duncan. 1987. Relationship of type 1 pilus expression in *Escherichia coli* to ascending urinary tract infections in mice. *Infect. Immun.* **55:**373–380.
200. Schmoll, T., J. Morschhauser, M. Ott, I. van Die, and J. Hacker. 1990. Complete genetic organization and functional aspects of the *Escherichia coli* S fimbrial adhesion determinant: nucleotide sequence of the genes *sfa* B, C, D, E, F. *Microb. Pathog.* **9:**331–343.
201. Selander, R. K., T. K. Korhonen, V. Vaisanen-Rhen, P. H. Williams, P. E. Pattison, and D. A. Caugant. 1986. Genetic relationships and clonal structure of strains of *Escherichia coli* causing neonatal septicemia and meningitis. *Infect. Immun.* **52:** 213–222.
202. Shand, G. H., H. Anwar, J. Kadurugamuwa, M. R. W. Brown, S. H. Silverman, and J. Melling. 1985. In vivo evidence that bacteria in urinary tract infection grow under iron-restricted conditions. *Infect. Immun.* **48:**35–39.
203. Siegfried, L., M. Kmetova, H. Puzova, M. Molokacova, and J. Filka. 1994. Virulence-associated factors in *Escherichia coli* strains isolated from children with urinary tract infections. *J. Med. Microbiol.* **41:** 127–132.
204. Siitonen, A. 1992. *Escherichia coli* in fecal flora of healthy adults: serotypes, P and type 1C fimbriae, non-P mannose-resistant adhesins, and hemolytic activity. *J. Infect. Dis.* **166:**1058–1065.
205. Siitonen, A., R. Martikainen, R. Ikaheimo, J. Palmgren, and P. H. Makela. 1993. Virulence-associated characteristics of *Escherichia coli* in urinary tract infections: a statistical analysis with special attention to type 1C fimbriation. *Microb. Pathog.* **15:** 65–75.
206. Smith, H. W. 1963. The hemolysins of *Escherichia coli*. *J. Pathol. Bacteriol.* **85:** 197–211.
207. Stamm, W. E., T. M. Hooton, J. R. Johnson, C. Johnson, A. Stapleton, P. L. Roberts, S. L. Moseley, and S. D. Fihn. 1989. Urinary tract infections: from pathogenesis to treatment. *J. Infect. Dis.* **159:** 400–406.
208. Stapleton, A., S. Moseley, and W. E. Stamm. 1991. Urovirulence determinants in *Escherichia coli* isolates causing first-episode and recurrent cystitis in women. *J. Infect. Dis.* **163:**773–779.
209. Stenqvist, K., T. Sandberg, G. Lidin-Janson, F. Orskov, I. Orskov, and C. Svanborg-Eden. 1987. Virulence factors of *Escherichia coli* in urinary isolates from pregnant women. *J. Infect. Dis.* **156:**870–877.
210. Stromberg, N., B. I. Marklund, B. Lund, D. Ilver, A. Hamers, W. Gaastra, K. A. Karlsson, and S. Normark. 1990. Host-specificity of uropathogenic *Escherichia coli* depends on differences in binding specificity to Gal-alpha(1-4)Gal-containing isoreceptors. *EMBO J.* **9:**2001–2010.
211. Stromberg, N., P. G. Nyholm, I. Pascher, and S. Normark. 1991. Saccharide orientation at the cell surface affects glycolipid receptor function. *Proc. Natl. Acad. Sci. USA* **88:**9340–9344.
212. Sun, J., M. Inouye, and S. Inouye. 1991. Association of a retroelement with a P4-like cryptic prophage (retronphage $\phi$R73) integrated into the selenocystyl tRNA gene of *Escherichia coli*. *J. Bacteriol.* **173:**4171–4181.
213. Swanson, T. N., S. S. Bilge, B. Nowicki, and S. L. Moseley. 1991. Molecular structure of the Dr adhesin: nucleotide sequence and mapping of receptor-binding domain by use of fusion constructs. *Infect. Immun.* **59:** 261–268.
214. Swenson, D., D. Berg, N. Bukanov, and R. Welch. Unpublished observations.
215. Tambic, T., V. Oberiter, J. Delmis, and A. Tambic. 1992. Diagnostic value of a P-fimbriation test in determining duration of therapy in children with urinary tract infections. *Clin. Ther.* **14:**667–671.
216. Tewari, R., T. Ikeda, R. Malaviya, J. I. MacGregor, J. R. Little, S. J. Hultgren,

and S. N. Abraham. 1994. The PapG tip adhesin of P fimbriae protects *Escherichia coli* from neutrophil bactericidal activity. *Infect. Immun.* **62:**5296–5304.
217. **Trifillis, A. L., M. S. Donnenberg, X. Cui, R. G. Russell, S. J. Utsalo, H. L. T. Mobley, and J. W. Warren.** 1994. Binding to and killing of human renal epithelial cells by hemolytic P-fimbriated *E. coli*. *Kidney Int.* **46:**1083–1091.
218. **Trucksis, M., J. E. Galen, J. Michalski, A. Fasano, and J. Kaper.** 1993. Accessory cholera enterotoxin (Ace), the third toxin of a Vibrio cholerae virulence cassette. *Proc. Natl. Acad. Sci. USA* **90:**5267–5271.
219. **Tullus, K., A. Brauner, B. Fryklund, T. Munkhammar, W. Rabsch, R. Reissbrodt, and L. G. Burman.** 1992. Host factors versus virulence-associated bacterial characteristics in neonatal and infantile bacteraemia and meningitis caused by *Escherichia coli*. *J. Med. Microbiol.* **36:**203–208.
220. **Tullus, K., K. Horlin, S. B. Svenson, and G. Kallenius.** 1984. Epidemic outbreaks of acute pyelonephritis caused by nosocomial spread of P fimbriated *Escherichia coli* in children. *J. Infect. Dis.* **150:**728–736.
221. **Tullus, K., S. H. Jacobson, M. Katouli, and A. Brauner.** 1991. Relative importance of eight virulence characteristics of pyelonephritogenic *Escherichia coli* strains assessed by multivariate statistical analysis. *J. Urol.* **146:**1153–1155.
222. **Ulleryd, P., K. Lincoln, J. Scheutz, and T. Sandberg.** 1994. Virulence characteristics of *Escherichia coli* in relation to host response in men with symptomatic urinary tract infection. *Clin. Infect. Dis.* **18:**579–584.
223. **Vaisanen, V., J. Elo, L. G. Tallgren, A. Siitonen, P. H. Makela, C. Svanborg-Eden, G. Kallenius, S. B. Svenson, H. Hultberg, and T. Korhonen.** 1981. Mannose-resistant haemagglutination and P antigen recognition are characteristic of *Escherichia coli* causing primary pyelonephritis. *Lancet* **ii:**1366–1369.
224. **Vaisanen-Rhen, V.** 1989. Fimbria-like hemagglutinin of *Escherichia coli* O75 strains. *Infect. Immun.* **46:**401–407.
225. **Vaisanen-Rhen, V., J. Elo, E. Vaisanen, A. Siitonen, I. Orskov, F. Orskov, S. B. Svenson, P. H. Makela, and T. K. Korhonen.** 1984. P-fimbriated clones among uropathogenic *Escherichia coli* strains. *Infect. Immun.* **43:**149–155.
226. **Valvano, M. A., R. P. Silver, and J. H. Crosa.** 1986. Occurrence of chromosome- or plasmid-mediated aerobactin iron transport systems and hemolysin production among clonal groups of human invasive strains of *Escherichia coli* K1. *Infect. Immun.* **52:**192–199.
227. **van den Bosch, J. F., P. Postma, P. A. R. Koopman, J. De Graaff, and D. M. MacLaren.** 1982. Virulence of urinary and faecal *Escherichia coli* in relation to serotype, haemolysis and haemagglutination. *J. Hyg.* **88:**567–577.
228. **Van der Woude, M. W., B. A. Braaten, and D. A. Low.** 1992. Evidence for global regulatory control of pilus expression in *Escherichia coli* by Lrp and DNA methylation: model building based on analysis of *pap*. *Mol. Microbiol.* **6:**2429–2435.
229. **Virkola, R., J. Parkkinen, J. Hacker, and T. K. Korhonen.** 1993. Sialyloligosaccharide chains of laminin as an extracellular matrix target for S fimbriae of *Escherichia coli*. *Infect. Immun.* **61:**4480–4484.
230. **Wagner, W., M. Vogel, and W. Goebel.** 1983. Transport of hemolysin across outer membrane of *Escherichia coli* requires two functions. *J. Bacteriol.* **154:**200–210.
231. **Walton, J. R., and D. H. Smith.** 1969. New hemolysin ($\gamma$) produced by *Escherichia coli*. *J. Bacteriol.* **98:**304–305.
232. **Wandersman, C., and P. Delepelaire.** 1990. TolC, an *Escherichia coli* outer membrane protein required for hemolysin secretion. *Proc. Natl. Acad. Sci. USA* **87:**4776–4780.
233. **Wandersman, C., and S. Letoffe.** 1993. Involvement of lipopolysaccharide in the secretion of *Escherichia coli* $\alpha$-hemolysin and *Erwinia chrysanthemi* proteases. *Mol. Microbiol.* **7:**141–150.
234. **Warren, J., H. Mobley, J. Hebel, and A. Trifillis.** 1995. Cytolethality of hemolytic *Escherichia coli* to primary human renal proximal tubular cell cultures obtained from different donors. *Urology* **45:**706–710.
235. **Weiser, J. N., and E. C. Gotschlich.** 1991. Outer membrane protein A (OmpA) contributes to serum resistance and pathogenicity of *Escherichia coli* K-1. *Infect. Immun.* **59:**2252–2258.
236. **Welch, R., and S. Falkow.** Unpublished observations.
237. **Welch, R. A.** Unpublished observations.
238. **Welch, R. A.** 1991. Pore-forming cytolysins of Gram-negative bacteria. *Mol. Microbiol.* **5:**521–528.
239. **Welch, R. A.** 1994. Holistic perspective on the *Escherichia coli* hemolysin, p. 351–364. In

V. L. Miller, J. B. Kaper, D. Portnoy, and R. R. Isberg (ed.), *Molecular Genetics of Bacterial Pathogenesis*. ASM Press, Washington, D.C.

240. **Welch, R. A., M. Bauer, A. Kent, J. Leeds, M. Moayeri, L. Regassa, and D. Swenson.** Battling against host phagocytes: the wherefore of the RTX family of toxins? *Infect. Agents Dis.*, in press.

241. **Welch, R. A., E. P. Dellinger, B. Minshew, and S. Falkow.** 1981. Hemolysin contributes to virulence of extra-intestinal *Escherichia coli* infections. *Nature* (London) **294**:665–667.

242. **Welch, R. A., R. Hull, and S. Falkow.** 1983. Molecular cloning and physical characterization of a chromosomal hemolysin from *Escherichia coli*. *Infect. Immun.* **42**:178–186.

243. **Welch, R. A., and S. Pellett.** 1988. Transcriptional organization of the *Escherichia coli* hemolysin. *J. Bacteriol.* **170**:1622–1630.

244. **Welch, R. A., S. Pellett, D. Robbins, W. Keane, G. Gekker, and P. Peterson.** 1989. Epidemiological observations involving the *Escherichia coli* hemolysin, p. 136–143. *In* E. Kass and C. Svanborg-Eden (ed.), *Host-Parasite Interactions in Urinary Tract Infections*. University of Chicago Press, Chicago.

245. **Wenzel, R.** 1991. Epidemiology of hospital-acquired infection, p. 147–150. *In* A. Balows, W. J. Hausler, Jr., K. L. Herrmann, H. D. Isenberg, and H. J. Shadomy (ed.), *Manual of Clinical Microbiology*, 5th ed. American Society for Microbiology, Washington, D.C.

246. **Westerlund, B., P. Kuusela, J. Risteli, L. Risteli, T. Vartio, H. Rauvala, R. Virkola, and T. K. Korhonen.** 1989. The O75X adhesin of uropathogenic *Escherichia coli* is a type IV collagen-binding protein. *Mol. Microbiol.* **3**:329–337.

247. **Westerlund, B., A. Siitonen, J. Elo, P. H. Williams, T. K. Korhonen, and P. H. Makela.** 1988. Properties of *Escherichia coli* isolates from urinary tract infections in boys. *J. Infect. Dis.* **158**:996–1102.

# STRUCTURE, FUNCTION, AND ASSEMBLY OF ADHESIVE P PILI

*C. Hal Jones, Ph.D., Karen Dodson, Ph.D., and Scott J. Hultgren, Ph.D.*

The initiation and persistence of many bacterial infections is thought to require the presentation of adhesins on the surface of the microbe in accessible configurations that promote binding events that dictate whether extracellular colonization, internalization, or other cellular responses will occur (23, 24, 43, 48, 92, 93, 113, 118, 163, 166, 186, 187, 189, 192, 193, 220, 241). Many bacterial adhesins are assembled into hairlike fibers called pili or fimbriae that pro-trude from the bacterial surface (Table 1). Other adhesins are directly associated with the microbial cell surface (nonpilus adhesins). Irrespective of the mode by which adhesins are presented, their recognition of host receptor structures is extremely fine tuned and allows for very selective interactions with the host. Host range, tissue tropism, and target cell specificity demonstrated by a particular microbe are determined at least in part by a stereochemical fit between a bacterial adhesin and specific receptor architectures on host cells (23, 24, 48, 93, 120). The biogenesis of adhesive pili requires a highly conserved secretion apparatus that is composed of periplasmic immunoglobulin-like chaperones and outer membrane ushers (93, 98). This assembly machinery is known to be required for the assembly of at least 26 different types of adhesive organelles in diverse gram-negative bacteria (Table 1). P pili are critical to the ability of uropathogenic strains of *Escherichia coli* to cause disease (111, 139, 152, 237, 238, 245). Type 1 and S pili have also been associated with uropathogenic *E. coli* (2, 99, 116, 125, 136, 186, 249). P, S, and type 1 pili consist of two distinct subassemblies: a thick cylindrical pilus rod joined to a thin, open helical tip fiber called a tip fibrillum (109, 131). The bipartite structure of all three pilus types, the association of the adhesin with a specialized tip fibrillum, and the biogenesis of pilus subassemblies represent common organizational and functional paradigms used by bacteria to present adhesins in configurations that make them accessible for mediating microbial attachment. This chapter reviews in detail the genetics and molecular biology of the expression, synthesis, and assembly of the P pilus. Where possible, the similarities between

---

*C. Hal Jones, Karen Dodson, and Scott J. Hultgren,* Department of Molecular Microbiology, Washington University Medical School, Box 8230, 660 South Euclid Avenue, St. Louis, Missouri 63110-1093.

**TABLE 1** Chaperone-usher strategy for assembly of adhesins and other virulence-associated structures

| Structure | Chaperone/usher[a] | Organism | Associated disease[b] | Adhesin/receptor | Reference(s) |
|---|---|---|---|---|---|
| 7 to 10 nm fiber | | | | | |
| P pilus | PapD/PapC | Escherichia coli | Pyelonephritis/cystitis | PapG/Gal$\alpha$(1-4)Gal moiety in globoseries of glycolipids PapE and fibronectin | 45, 92, 95, 96, 98, 133, 151, 177, 232, 233, 255 |
| Prs pilus | PrsD/PrsC | Escherichia coli | Cystitis? | PrsG/Gal$\alpha$(1-4)Gal moiety in globoseries of glycolipids | 92, 151, 232, 233 |
| Type 1 pilus | FimC/FimD | Escherichia coli, Salmonella species, Klebsiella pneumoniae | Cystitis | FimH/mannose-oligosaccharides laminin, fibronectin | 2, 4, 6, 39, 108, 109, 160, 165, 180, 226, 227 |
| F1C pilus | FocC/FocD | Escherichia coli | Cystitis? | FocH/? | 120, 205, 248 |
| S pilus | SfaE/SfaF | Escherichia coli | UTI, NBM | SfaS/$\alpha$-sialyl-2,3-$\beta$-galactose | 80, 125, 127, 169, 216 |
| Hif pilus | HifB/HifC | Haemophilus influenzae | Otitis media, meningitis | ?/Sialylganglioside-GM1 | 36, 78, 129, 246 |
| Type 2 and type 3 pili | FimB (FhaD)/FimC | Bordetella pertussis | Whooping cough | FimD/not identified | 149, 171, 172, 258 |
| MR/P pilus | MrpD/MrpC | Proteus mirabilis | Nosocomial UTI | ?/Gal$\alpha$(1-4)Gal moiety in globoseries of glycolipids | 17, 260 |
| PMF pilus | PmfC/PmfD | Proteus mirabilis | Nosocomial UTI | ?/? | 16, 158 |
| Pef Pilus | PefD/PefC | Salmonella typhimurium | Gastroenteritis, salmonellosis | ? | 62 |
| 2- to 5-nm fiber | | | | | |
| K99 pilus | FaeE/FaeD | Escherichia coli | Neonatal diarrhea in calves, lambs, and piglets | FanC/N-glycolyl-GM3, N-glycolyl-sialoparagloboside | 18, 185, 225 |
| K88 pilus | FanE/FanD | Escherichia coli | Neonatal diarrhea in piglets | FaeG/glycoprotein or glycolipid of ileal mucous | 18, 57, 162, 170 |
| MR/K (type 3) pilus | MrkB/MrkC | Klebsiella pneumoniae | Pneumonia | MrkD/type V collagen | 8, 65, 183, 184 |
| F17 pilus | F17D/F17PapC | Enterotoxigenic Escherichia coli | Diarrhea | ?/? | 148 |
| CS31A pilus | ClpE/? | Enterotoxigenic Escherichia coli | Diarrhea | ?/? | 69 |

*Continued on following page*

**TABLE 1** *Continued*

| Structure | Chaperone/usher[a] | Organism | Associated disease[b] | Adhesin/receptor | Reference(s) |
|---|---|---|---|---|---|
| CS6 pilus | Css6/CssD | Enterotoxigenic *Escherichia coli* | Diarrhea | ?/? | 124 |
| Nonfimbrial adhesins | | | | | |
| NFA1-6 family of closely related structures | NfaE/NfaC | *Escherichia coli* | UTI, NBM | NfaA/carbohydrate moieties associated with glycophorin A | 72, 77, 90, 104, 105, 190 |
| Afa-1 | AfaB/AfaC | *Escherichia coli* | Pyelonephritis | Afa-1E/determinants of Dr(a) blood group marker, DAF[c] | 137, 178, 179 |
| Dr/Afa-111 | DraE/DraD | *Escherichia coli* | UTI, diarrhea | DraA/determinants of Dr(a) blood group marker | 140 |
| M | BmaB/BmaC | *Escherichia coli* | Pyelonephritis | BmaE/A$^M$ determinant of M blood group marker | 106, 104 |
| Atypical structures | | | | | |
| Sef | SefB/SefC | *Salmonella enteritidis* | Gastroenteritis, salmonellosis | ?/? | 40, 173 |
| Envelope antigen F1 | Caf1M/Caf1A | *Yersinia pestis* | Plague | ?/? | 114 |
| CS3 | Cs3-1/Cs3-104kD | Enterotoxigenic *Escherichia coli* | Traveler's diarrhea | ?/? | 143 |
| PH6 antigen | PsaB/Orf4' | *Yersinia pestis* | Plague | ?/? | 147 |
| Myf | MyfB/MyfC | *Yersinia enterocolitica* | Enterocolitis | ?/? | 100 |
| AAF/1 | AggD/AggC | Enterotoxigenic *Escherichia coli* | Diarrhea | ?/? | 214 |
| ? | EcpD/HtrE | *Escherichia coli* | ? | ?/? | 202 |

[a] Chaperone and usher assignments are based on sequence similarity to PapD and PapC, respectively. All the chaperones share 50% homology, and the ushers share 25% homology. Functional studies have demonstrated chaperone-like activity for FimC (90), SfaE, HifB (unpublished data), and FanE and FaeE (15). Fim D has usherlike activity (unpublished data).
[b] NBM, newborn meningitis.
[c] DAF, decay-accelerating factor.

the related type 1 and S pili will also be discussed.

## HISTORY

Bacterially mediated hemagglutination was first reported in 1908 by Guyot (79), and the visualization of nonflagellar filamentous appendages and their association with hemagglutination by *E. coli* were first reported by Duguid et al. in 1955 (49). Duguid's studies differentiated a collection of 47 *E. coli* strains into four groups based on the pattern of agglutination of erythrocytes from various species. The bacteria that were good agglutinators were covered with filamentous appendages that were wholly different in appearance from flagella as viewed under the electron microscope (49). Such appendages were absent from strains that failed to agglutinate. The "filamentous appendages" identified by Duguid et al. (49) were termed fimbriae, although the designation "pili" has also become associated with these structures (33–35) "Pilus," which was Brinton's (35) designation for the structures associated with conjugative transfer of genetic material (the F pilus), has now become a generic term for all types of nonflagellar filamentous appendages. We will use the term "pilus" in this chapter. In the last 40 years, considerable progress has been made in elucidating the genetics, biochemistry, and structural biology of the development of adhesive organelles and their role in directing adherence to eukaryotic cells. Excellent reviews by Klemm (120) and Miller et al. (164) discuss studies relating to other pilus types and adherence mechanisms.

Pili were originally classified as mannose resistant (MR) or mannose sensitive (MS) depending on the ability of the pilus to direct hemagglutination in the presence of mannosides (46, 182). This functional test differentiates mannose-binding common, or type 1, pili from other pilus types, such as the P pilus, which binds the Gal$\alpha$(1-4)Gal disaccharide (46, 48). The operons responsible for the expression of both P (MR) and type 1 (MS) were cloned from the human urinary tract isolate J96 (91). This clinical isolate also contained a gene cluster for a third pilus type, termed the Prs (P-related sequence) pilus, that was highly related to the P pilus (151). Gene clusters specific for expression of type 1 pili have also been cloned from other clinical sources (38, 94) and laboratory strains (123). Most of the commonly used laboratory strains that are K-12 derivatives contain the type 1 operon and are capable, when grown under appropriate conditions, of producing type 1 pili (53). The related S pilus (MR) gene cluster (formerly X fimbriae) was cloned from a uropathogenic *E. coli* strain and defined by Hacker et al. (80). The cloned pilus operons (P, Prs, type 1, and S) contain all the information necessary to endow on a naive *E. coli* strain the ability to express the given pilus type.

## FUNCTION OF PILUS ADHESINS IN PATHOGENESIS

### P Pilus

The ability of pathogenic bacteria to bind and adhere to host tissue is critical and is potentially the most important step in the initiation of infection (23, 24, 43, 48, 92, 93, 113, 118, 163, 166, 186, 187, 192, 193, 220, 241). The initial inoculum of pathogenic organisms in the uroepithelium must adhere to tissues in a hostile environment that are constantly flushed with urine. In addition, an ascending infection from the bladder to the kidney may also require the expression of a repertoire of adhesins to enable the pathogen to colonize the various tissues in the urinary tract. Studies by several groups have demonstrated the binding of P-piliated *E. coli* to uroepithelial tissue from several sources in situ (128, 231, 253). *E. coli* expressing P pili binds to the globoseries of glycolipids that are distributed throughout the kidney: the glomerulus, Bowman's capsule, proximal and distal tubules, and connecting ducts of the kidney are targets (Fig. 1). In the bladder, only the vessel walls are strongly bound by P-piliated bacteria, although the epithelium and muscular layer are weakly bound (128, 253). The role of P-pilus-mediated binding in the bladder is not clear at present. Most uropathogenic strains of *E. coli* express P pili (111, 139, 152, 237, 238, 245), which are a critical virulence factor in a primate model of pyelonephritis, as discussed below (206, 207, 209). In contrast, P pili were dispensable in a mouse model of pyelonephritis (168). These studies utilized different strains, and it is possible that the strain used in the mouse model expressed other types of adhesins such as the S adhesin, which was able to compensate for the

**FIGURE 1** P-piliated *E. coli* binds to Galα(1-4)Gal-containing isoreceptors on kidney epithelia in situ. Fluorescein isothiocyanate-labeled *E. coli* expressing class II PapG was incubated with kidney sections and examined under fluorescence microscopy (left). Note the extensive binding throughout the section. Preincubation of the bacteria with soluble Galα(1-4)Gal receptor analogs inhibits binding to kidney sections (right). See text and Striker et al. (231) for details.

lack of a P pilus. Nevertheless, these studies point to the complexities of singling out one specific adhesin as being critical in virulence, since many different factors contribute to pathogenesis. The loss of one specific determinant can often be compensated for by the presence of several other factors that can perform the same or similar functions in pathogenesis. For instance, the type 1 pilus is commonly associated with cystitis strains of *E. coli,* and several animal models have implicated type 1 pili as being important in disease (2, 99, 116, 186, 249). S pili have also been linked to urinary tract infection (UTI) isolates of *E. coli* and, more strongly, to neonatal meningitis strains (125, 136). As is discussed later, P, type 1, and S pili dictate binding to specific receptors distributed throughout the body and therefore define the site of colonization and to a large degree the resulting disease.

## Binding Specificity

Specific binding of the P-pilus adhesin to Galα(1-4)Gal moieties present in the globoseries of glycolipids on uroepithelial cells and erythrocytes was first demonstrated in the 1980s (28, 110, 142). Hemagglutination of human erythrocytes and binding of P-piliated bacteria to uroepithelial tissue was inhibitable by pretreatment of bacteria with Galα(1-4)Gal-containing saccharides (28, 142). Lund et al. (150, 151) first demonstrated that the PapG protein in the P-pilus system is the Galα(1-4)Gal adhesin that determines the specificity of binding. The experiment exploited the different binding specificities of the so-called class I and class III PapG adhesins from the Pap and Prs pilus operons, respectively. These two pilus types are of the same F13 serotype and differ only in the specificity of the respective adhesin (discussed in detail below). Complementation of a *papG* mutant P-pilus operon with *prsG* in *trans* changes the binding specificity of the P pilus (class I) to that of the Prs pilus (class III). This experiment demonstrates that the PapG (or PrsG) protein is the sole determinant defining the binding specificity of the pilus and therefore the tropism of the organism expressing the pilus (150, 151, 232–234). Four PapG adhesins representing three different alleles, classes I, II, and III, were examined for their binding specificities to purified glycolipids (233). Two F13 P-pilus isolates expressing PapG (class I) and PrsG (class III) from a human UTI isolate (J96) had been shown to have different binding specificities (150, 151). An additional binding specificity (class II) was identified on the $F7_2$ and F11 serotypes (AD110 and IA2 isolates, respectively) and on a canine UTI isolate (233). All three PapG alleles bound to Galα(1-4)Gal-containing isoreceptors, but they displayed different tissue tropisms (Table 2). In eukaryotic membranes, the Galα(1-4)Gal moiety is linked by a β-glucose residue to a ceramide group that anchors the receptor in the lipid bilayer (82). Different members of the globoseries of glycolipids have additional sugar residues distal to the Galα(1-4)Gal disaccharide (233, 234). The tissue tropism of the G adhesins appears to be determined by the specific member of the globoseries of glycolipids expressed in different cell types and tissues. Differential distribution of the receptor isotypes in different hosts (e.g., dog versus human) also seems to account for host tropisms that are determined by the class of G adhesin expressed.

The molecular basis of these tropisms was explained by the following studies. A series of hemagglutination studies revealed that class I PapG (PapG from J96 isolate) agglutinates only human erythrocytes, class II PapG (PapG from AD110 isolate) agglutinates human erythrocytes well and sheep erythrocytes only poorly, and class III PapG (PrsG from J96 isolate) agglutinates only sheep erythrocytes (Table 2). The three classes of PapG were then tested for binding to uroepithelial cells from humans and dogs. The class III adhesin directed binding to canine (MDCK) uroepithelia, while the class II adhesin bound to

**TABLE 2** Binding specificities of three classes of PapG[a]

| Class | Source/isolate | Species of erythrocyte agglutinated | Tissue bound | Isoreceptor bound in natural membrane |
|---|---|---|---|---|
| I | *pap* F13 (J96) | Human, rabbit | Human bladder | GbO3 |
| II | *pap* $F7_2$, F11 (IA2, AD110) | Human, sheep (weak) | Human kidney,[b] human bladder (weak) | GbO4 |
| III | *prs* F13 (J96) | Sheep | Canine kidney | Forssman antigen (GbO5) |

[a] See Stromberg et al. (233).
[b] See Striker et al. (231).

human uroepithelia (T24 cells, bladder carcinoma) (233). Neither the class I nor the class II adhesin bound to the MDCK cells. Human erythrocytes, kidney, and bladder are rich in globotriaosylceramide (GbO3) and globoside or globotetraosylceramide (GbO4) and lack the so-called Forssman antigen (GbO5), while sheep erythrocytes and canine kidney are rich in Forssman antigen and express only minute amounts of GbO3 and GbO4 (233). A clue to one possible aspect of the observed specificity came when experiments were designed to test binding to purified glycolipids. Thin-layer chromatography was used to separate various glycolipids for incubation with metabolically labeled bacteria expressing different PapG adhesins. In this assay, the three adhesins bound with reduced specificity for the different glycolipids (234). This reduction in specificity was also seen when the glycolipids were immobilized in microtiter wells. In both assays, the class III adhesin maintained specificity for GbO5 and bound much less efficiently to GbO3 and GbO4, but the class I and class II adhesins bound efficiently to all three glycolipids. Moreover, in a competition assay, binding of the class III adhesin to GbO5 could not be inhibited with free Gal$\alpha$(1-4)Gal, which efficiently inhibited binding of the class I adhesin to immobilized GbO3. This result suggests that the target of the class III adhesin is more complex than the Gal$\alpha$(1-4)Gal disaccharide. Binding and inhibitor studies with a panel of glycolipids demonstrated that in addition to the disaccharide, the class III adhesin requires sugar groups distal to the disaccharide. Specifically, in the case of the PrsG adhesin, a distal GalNAc$\beta$ residue is required, although proximal additions in some analogs are also recognized by the class III adhesin (234).

The loss of specificity for globoside that was observed when the glycolipids were immobilized (not contained in native membranes) suggests that the specificity of binding might depend on the accessibility of receptors in native membranes to the adhesin. Therefore, in the case of the Forssman antigen, PapG (class I) may fail to recognize its binding epitope because of the conformation of the glycolipid in the membrane or because of shielding of the epitope by other membrane constituents. However, on a solid surface, the Gal$\alpha$(1-4)Gal epitope is accessible in the Forssman antigen; hence, the class I and class II PapG adhesins bind efficiently. Stromberg et al. (234) showed by molecular modeling that the preferred conformations of GbO3, GbO4, and GbO5 in membranes reveal different epitopes. The orientation of the disaccharide in the receptor rotates from parallel to the membrane to perpendicular to it as sugar groups are added distal to Gal$\alpha$(1-4)Gal. The specificity of class I, II, and III adhesins for glycolipid could be explained in part by the accessibility of the receptor, Gal$\alpha$(1-4)Gal, in the preferred conformation of the glycolipid, as presented in the modeling, to the adhesin.

**Domain Structure of PapG Adhesin**

The two-domain structure of the PapG adhesin molecule was first proposed by Hultgren et al. (96) on the basis of studies in which the PapD-PapG (DG) complex was first identified and purified. The Gal$\alpha$(1-4)Gal disaccharide was linked to Sepharose beads and employed as an affinity matrix to purify a periplasmic complex composed of PapG and the P-pilus chaperone, PapD (a detailed discussion of PapD is presented below). This strategy resulted in the purification of a 1:1 DG complex from the periplasmic space of E. coli (96). A COOH-terminal deletion of PapG (PapG1) that removed the last 13 residues destabilized the protein, resulting in the appearance of several stable PapG truncates. A 24.5-kDa truncate of PapG bound the Gal$\alpha$(1-4)Gal Sepharose column. This truncate contained the amino-terminal 150 residues of PapG, suggesting that the carbohydrate-binding domain is located in the amino-terminal region of the protein. Furthermore, PapD did not copurify with the 24.5-kDa truncate, which suggests that the PapD recognition site(s) is located in the COOH-terminal region of the protein that had been deleted. Two other truncates, of 24 and 26 kDa, also resulted from expression of the PapG1 mutant. These truncates were missing the amino-terminal domain and failed to bind to the Gal$\alpha$(1-4)Gal Sepharose column.

Haslam et al. (86) demonstrated that the amino-terminal domain of PapG is responsible for the fine specificity of binding originally described by Stromberg et al. (233, 234). To get around the expression and purification problems associated with working with PapG, fusions of the amino-terminal 202 amino acid residues of the class I, II, and III adhesins and the maltose-binding protein (MBP) were constructed. The binding activities of the three purified fusion proteins and purified pili bearing each class of adhesin were compared. For the class I and III adhesins, the receptor-binding specificity, as assayed by enzyme-linked immunosorbent assay (ELISA) and thin-layer chromatography binding, was identical to that of pili bearing the homologous adhesins (86). Fusions and pili bearing the class I adhesin bound to GbO3, GbO4, and GbO5, but fusions and pili bearing the class III adhesin bound only to the GbO5 receptor. This result confirms that the PapG protein endows the bacteria with its receptor-binding specificity. However, a difference was seen in the class II fusion. Both the fusion protein and the pili bound well to GbO4 and poorly to GbO5, but the fusion protein also bound well to GbO3, while the pili bound to GbO3 only poorly. This finding suggests that other determinants in the pilus, such as the minor pilins, can affect the fine specificity of binding, at least in the case of the class II adhesin (86).

Lund et al. (150, 151) described a similar dependence of the adhesin on pilus components for receptor binding. These investigators observed that PapG could be surface expressed in pili in the absence of PapF but that the pili were hemagglutination negative. This finding raised the question of the role of PapF in presenting PapG appropriately to allow receptor binding. As discussed below, Jacob-Dubuisson et al. (101) showed that PapF functions as an adaptor to correctly join PapG to the tip fibrillum. Furthermore, it was thought that other components in the tip fibrillum and/or the pilus rod might affect the fine specificity of receptor binding. Haslam's finding with the class II fusion protein supports this contention (86). Such a finding in the type 1 system was presented recently by Madison et al. (153). Using novel mannosides, these investigators uncovered a difference in the specificity of the FimH adhesin depending on whether it is incorporated into type 1 pili from E. coli or Klebsiella pneumoniae. They found that when the E. coli minor pilins (including FimH) are expressed along with the FimA protein from K. pneumoniae, the adhesin specificity shifts toward that of FimH present in the K. pneumoniae pilus. Similarly, expression of K. pneumoniae FimH along with E. coli FimA protein produces pili that bind with the specificity of E. coli FimH. In both cases, the specificity of the adhesin is influenced by the source of the FimA protein (153).

## PapG Adhesin-Binding Paradigm

In order to determine the contribution of functional groups exposed on the receptor to recognition by the P-pilus adhesin, a panel of galabioside analogs in which the functional groups on the disaccharide were replaced with hydrogen, fluorine, or a methoxy group were tested as inhibitors of hemagglutination by E. coli expressing class I P pili (117). The results of this study provided evidence that the interaction between the class I PapG adhesin and the galabiose receptor utilizes a polar ridge on the receptor that is composed of OH groups -6, -2', -3', -4', and -6'. Hultgren et al. (96) showed that a preassembled class I PapG separate from the pilus (in complex with the periplasmic chaperone as discussed in detail below) recognizes the same polar ridge, which argues that PapG folds into its receptor-binding conformation prior to being incorporated into the pilus.

A recent study by Striker et al. (231) demonstrated that class II PapG recognizes a similar polar ridge in interaction with the GbO4 isoreceptor. In addition to this series of contacts, the adhesin requires an interaction with the distal GalNAc group in GbO4, and more important, it participates in specific hydrogen bonds with the glucose residue proximal to the Gal$\alpha$(1-4)Gal disaccharide. Striker et al. suggest that the ability of class II PapG to bind GbO4 but not GbO3 relates to the exposure of the glucose residue in GbO4 and not to a structural difference in the presentation of the Gal$\alpha$(1-4)Gal moiety with respect to the membrane in the two isoreceptors. Thus, in GbO3, the $\beta$-glucose residue is masked by the membrane; therefore, GbO3 is not recognized by class II PapG (231).

## PapG Is a Virulence Determinant

P piliation is the factor best correlated with pyelonephritis in adults (50 to 90%) and children (95%) (111, 245). Early studies demonstrated that immunization of monkeys with heterologous purified pili protected against pyelonephritis after renal inoculation (206, 208). Similar results were reported with a murine pyelonephritis model (181, 197). Additionally, pretreatment of bacteria with soluble Gal$\alpha$(1-4)Gal delays the appearance of pyelonephritis significantly (236). To test the role of the PapG determinant in the pathogenesis of a clinical isolate of *E. coli*, a frameshift mutation was created in the *papG* open reading frame in a clinical isolate, DS17, that was isolated in a Swedish pediatric ward and is capable of expressing a number of virulence determinants (209, 243). The mutant strain, DS17-8, was fully piliated but failed to recognize the globoside receptor (GbO4). Furthermore, DS17-8 was unable to bind to human or monkey kidney in situ. The mutant strain (DS17-8) and the isogenic parent strain (DS17) were tested for the ability to cause cystitis and pyelonephritis in a cynomolgus monkey model system (209). Monkeys inoculated with DS17 had a mean bacteriuria of 21 days compared to 6.8 days for monkeys inoculated with DS17-8. The monkeys receiving the wild-type strain (DS17) had significant kidney pathology, and renal functions were significantly reduced. Kidney function and pathology were unaffected in monkeys receiving the PapG mutant (DS17-8). These studies strongly suggest that the PapG adhesin is required for pyelonephritis to occur in the normal urinary tract (209).

Interestingly, both wild-type and mutant strains colonized the lower urinary tract and caused acute cystitis in the monkey model (209). PapG was also dispensable for colonization of the vagina and persistence in the intestine. Although PapG did not appear to be critical for lower urinary tract colonization, expression of PapG did provide a competitive advantage. Following coinoculation of DS17 and DS17-8 in the bladder, the mutant strain was outcompeted within a few days. Therefore, adhesiveness in the bladder confers a competitive advantage. Similarly, other *E. coli* adhesins, such as the FimH adhesin of type 1 pili and the SfaS adhesin of the S pilus, may confer a survival advantage in the bladder and therefore play a role in the causation of cystitis. A strategy similar to that described above could be used to define additional virulence determinants, including other pilus types (S, type 1, curli), that allow the DS17-8 mutant strain to cause cystitis.

## TYPE 1 PILUS

### Role in Pathogenesis

In 1977, Ofek et al. (180) demonstrated that type 1 pili direct binding to mannosylated structures; in the same year, Salit and Gotschlich (211) observed that type 1-piliated bacteria and purified type 1 pili bind in an MS fashion to monkey kidney cells. This and other observations suggest that type 1-piliated bacteria may play a role in cystitis and pyelonephritis (2, 11, 52, 81, 99, 116). Type 1-fimbriated bacteria bind to a number of sites, including proximal tubular cells of the kidney, epithelial cells in the bladder and intestine, and various inflammatory cells (12, 115, 211, 212, 242). Additional receptors for the type 1 pilus have been reported to include a 65-kDa protein of guinea pig erythrocytes (68), the leukocyte adhesin molecules CD11 and CD18, and the Tamm-Horsfall glycoprotein of human urine (12). With regard to the role of type 1 pili in promoting *E. coli* extraintestinal colonization, a clinical correlation exists between expression of type 1 pilus and the potential for causing cystitis and urethritis. Type 1 pili mediate binding to vaginal mucus, which may influence the initial attachment and subsequent colonization of the vaginal and urinary tract epithelia by *E. coli* (249). A variety of genetic and biochemical tests of colonization in experimental animals have provided support for the role of type 1 pili in pathogenesis (2, 11, 81, 99, 116). Hultgren et al. (99) demonstrated in a murine model system that inoculation of piliated organisms into the bladder results in effective colonization that is blocked by anti-type-1-pilus antibody. In the same study, nonpiliated organisms were poor colonizers of the bladder (99). Similarly, in murine models of colonization, UTI could be blocked by anti-type 1 antibodies or by a mannoside derivative that blocked adherence (2, 11, 81). Type 1-pilus expression on *K. pneumoniae* and *Salmonella typhimurium* has been associated with pathogenesis in rat models (47, 59, 60). Several studies also showed that type 1 pili aid in protecting *E. coli* from phagocytic killing (115, 242), even though the pili promote binding to a variety of phagocytic cells (242). The fact that pili are not associated with septicemic isolates of *E. coli* may suggest that phase variants (nonpiliated) have an advantage in the blood, since they are less well recognized by phagocytic cells. It has been suggested that type 1 binding may disrupt or bypass the normal lytic pathway in the phagocyte, resulting in reduced killing, and that this protection is related specifically to the mannose-binding adhesin FimH (186, 187). Recently, Bloch et al. (25) demonstrated a role for type 1 piliation in oropharyngeal colonization in neonatal rats. They showed that type 1 pili enhance transmission of *E. coli* K1 among littermates, although the role of the pilus in intestinal colonization is minimal. These authors suggest that colonization of the oropharynx is required for the normal fecal-oral cycle of enteric bacteria (25).

Although a strong case can be made for a role for type 1 pili in murine cystitis (2, 11, 81, 99), there are clear differences in the urinary tracts of murine species and humans. Several groups have utilized in vitro adherence of piliated bacteria to tissue sections to support similar roles of type 1 pili in mice and humans. Virkola et al. (251, 253) caution that the presence of receptors and the demonstration of in vitro binding to uroepithelial tissue is not necessarily correlated with pathogenesis in vivo. Mannose-inhibitable binding of type 1-piliated bacteria to human kidney and bladder has been reported (251, 253). In the kidney, binding is evident in the proximal tubule and vessel walls (251), while in the bladder, binding is mostly to the muscular layer and vessel walls (253). Binding in the kidney is not in areas that are correlated with an ascending route of infection (distal tubules, connecting ducts, glomeruli), as was demonstrated for P pili. However, our recent studies using an in situ binding assay showed that type 1 pili mediate the MS attachment of bacteria throughout the kidney. The adherence pattern involves the glomeruli and collecting tubules (unpublished data). Type 1-piliated bacteria also bind avidly to oligosaccharides in urinary slime and to the Tamm-Horsfall protein, which may play a role in preventing adherence to the urinary tract in vivo and may act as a natural defense mechanism (196). Interaction with urinary slime and Tamm-Horsfall protein should not immediately rule out a role for type-1-pilus-mediated adherence in promoting cystitis, because these interactions may represent an initial site of colonization from which to gain access to the urinary epithelium (49a). Pathogenesis is the result of many complicated factors and a constant interplay between host and pathogen; therefore, changes in the host (hormonal fluctuation, etc.) that have an effect on the makeup of the mucosal epithelium may affect the fate of the pathogen, i.e., colonization or displacement from the urinary tract.

## FimH Adhesin

The adhesive determinant of the type 1 pilus cloned from *E. coli* is a minor component of the pilus encoded by the *fimH* gene (130, 160, 165) that is serologically conserved throughout members of the family Enterobacteriaceae (6). The operons required for synthesis of type 1 fimbriae in *K. pneumoniae* and *S. typhimurium* were also cloned and analyzed (39, 201). Although type 1 pili produced by all three organisms direct MS hemagglutination (MSHA), the binding specificities of each pilus (adhesin) are distinguishable by utilization of mannoside analogs in inhibition studies (61, 174, 221). These studies led to the proposal that the adhesin combining site is an extended pocket with an associated hydrophobic binding site and that the preferred oligomannoside receptor is the trisaccharide $\alpha$-D-Manp-(1-3)-$\beta$-D-Manp-(1-4)-D-GlcNAc (61). These studies revealed that the *S. typhimurium* FimH adhesin has a smaller combining site and does not have the associated hydrophobic pocket. Recent studies with novel mannosides demonstrated a subtle difference in the binding specificities of *E. coli* and *K. pneumoniae* FimH adhesins (153). These studies suggest that the FimH adhesin represents a family of mannoside-binding lectins (227).

## FimH Interaction with Inflammatory Mediators

Type 1-piliated bacteria are recognized by neutrophils via the CD11 and CD18 integrins in an MS interaction (64). Further, interaction of type 1-piliated *E. coli* with neutrophils stimulates the cells such that an oxidative bust can be detected (70, 71). The oxidative burst is a cascade of events that ultimately results in the release of the toxic oxygen metabolites $O_2^-$ and $H_2O_2$. Using purified FimH protein, Tewari et al. (242) demonstrated that the binding of FimH protein to neutrophils triggers an oxidative burst. It is noteworthy that although the oxidative burst is triggered, the piliated bacteria seem to be more resistant to killing by neutrophils, perhaps by being held at "arm's length" from the neutrophil by the pili. A recent study demonstrated that although FimH mediates binding to macrophages, type 1-piliated organisms resist phagocytosis (115). These results run counter to those of several past studies, which correlate piliation with enhanced phagocytosis of piliated organisms (27, 222, 235). At this point, there is no real consensus as to the role of type 1 pili in bacterium-phagocyte interactions as they relate to pathogenesis.

## S PILUS

### Role in Pathogenesis

S-piliated strains of *E. coli* can be cultured from individuals with UTIs, although this pilus type is more closely correlated with the causative agent of neonatal sepsis and meningitis (127, 136, 191). S-piliated bacteria bind to the globoseries of glycolipids that are distributed throughout the kidney; i.e., the glomerulus, Bowman's capsule, proximal and distal tubules, and connecting ducts of the kidney are targets (126). In the bladder, S pili bind the epithelium and also bind to connective tissue (253). S pili are less well correlated with UTI, perhaps because of the presence in urine of Tamm-Horsfall glycoprotein, which is bound by S pili and may act as a natural inhibitor of tissue binding in vivo (196). The facts that P and S pili bind similarly to kidney and bladder tissue in vitro and that only P pili are strongly correlated with UTIs lend some support to this model.

### Pilus-Mediated Binding to the Extracellular Matrix

Additional binding determinants associated with P, S, and type 1 pili that allow interaction with extracellular matrix components have been described (134, 226, 252, 254, 255). PapE protein, the major component of the tip fibrillum (see below), binds to the amino and carboxyl termini of immobilized fibronectin (255). This interaction does not require the PapG protein, although both PapE and PapF are required. Westerlund et al. (255) showed that P-piliated bacteria bind to the basolateral aspect of tubuli in rat kidney. This structure is devoid of Gal$\alpha$(1-4)Gal, suggesting that an alternative adherence mechanism is responsible for the binding (255). Both type 1 and S pili adhere to oligosaccharide chains of laminin, although this interaction is via the lectin activity of the respective adhesins (134, 252). On the other hand, FimH appears to be a multifunctional protein binding both to mannose-containing targets and to portions of immobilized fibronectin (226). The binding to fibronectin is not affected by periodate treatment, suggesting a protein-protein interaction. The interaction is, however, sensitive to mannose. Sokurenko et al. (226) suggested that the mannose has an allosteric effect on FimH, altering the conformation of the protein and making it no longer able to bind to fibronectin. Fibronectin-binding FimH protein has been demonstrated only on a subset of the type 1-expressing strains examined, suggesting that the FimH family of type 1 fimbrial adhesins is heterogeneous (227). Amino acid substitutions that distinguish mannose- and fibronectin-binding FimH isolates from isolates expressing FimH that bind only to mannose are clustered in the amino-terminal domain of FimH, but a correlation of the specific amino acid changes to receptor-binding function remain unclear (227).

## PILUS ASSEMBLY

### Genetics and Molecular Architecture

At least 11 genes are involved in the biosynthesis and expression of functional P pili (Fig. 2). Each of the 11 genes has been inactivated in order to assign a function to each gene product (14, 15, 98, 144–146, 150, 177, 239). Regulation of pilus expression is dependent on the *papB* and *papI* genes that are located upstream of the mapped *pap* promoter as well as on three global regulatory proteins: catabolite activator protein, the leucine response protein

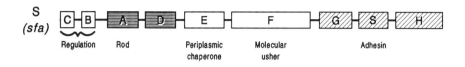

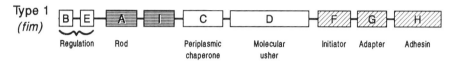

**FIGURE 2** Operons responsible for expression of P, type 1, and S pili share organizational and functional homologies. P-, type 1-, and S-pilus operons are presented, and where known, the roles of each gene product in pilus biogenesis and pilus function are indicated. Tip fibrillar subunits (▨) and rod subunits (☰) are shown.

(Lrp), and H-NS (13, 29–31, 74–76, 176, 247). These elements control expression of the pilus through differential methylation at two sites in the promoter region. Changes in methylation state are correlated with the phase-on and phase-off switches in pilus expression.

The pilus comprises two subassemblies: a rod and a tip fibrillum (131). The rod is a polymer of PapA, and the tip fibrillum is a heteropolymer composed of PapE, PapF, PapK, and PapG (101, 131). The roles of PapA, PapE, PapF, PapG, and PapK are discussed in detail below. Preliminary studies suggest that PapH, a minor pilin, is required to link the pilus rod to the cell membrane and that in doing so, it terminates biogenesis of the rod (14). Mutations in *papJ* have been reported to result in fragile pili. PapJ may function as a cochaperone (240). The assembly of the pilus is dependent on PapD and PapC, the molecular chaperone and usher proteins, respectively, that are essential for pilus assembly (45, 95, 98, 144). These two proteins direct the assembly of the pilus and form a novel protein secretion pathway that is conserved throughout the family *Enterobacteriaceae* (102).

As shown in Fig. 2, the P-, type 1-, and S-pilus operons are organizationally quite similar (80, 123, 188). In many cases, homologous functions have been attributed to similarly located genes in the P-, type 1-, and S-pilus operons (4, 6, 107, 119, 121–123, 130, 160, 161, 165, 169, 188, 210, 216). For example, the major pilus subunit gene is located immediately downstream from the regulatory genes. The gene 3' to the major subunit gene is a minor pilin; however, only PapH has been assigned a function. The next two genes encode the assembly proteins, i.e., the molecular chaperone and usher. The 3'-most cistrons encode gene products that form the tip fibrillum subassemblies as well as the adhesin. The roles of the type 1- and P-pilus gene products in the fibrilla and in pilus biogenesis have been investigated and are discussed below along with S-pilus gene products where information is available.

All three pilus types are subject to multilayered regulatory programs. Phase variation has been demonstrated for P pili (discussed above) and type 1 pili. Phase variation in the type 1 pilus differs from that in the P pilus in that a 314-bp invertible DNA element, which contains the promoter, is controlled in part by two gene products, FimB and FimE (1, 50, 119). The integrative host factor protein is also required for this process (51). Similar to the P-pilus promoter, the S-pilus promoter is subject to catabolite repression and temperature regulation (217). The thermoregulation of P-pilus expression depends on the H-NS protein (75, 76). Regulation of S-pilus production is also affected by osmolarity (217).

### The Tip Fibrillum

High-resolution quick-freeze, deep-etch electron microscopy (87) was used to examine purified P pili; this procedure revealed that the pilus has a heteropolymeric structure in which a thin fibrillar polymer is attached end to end to the right-handed helical rod (131) (Fig. 3A). Immunoelectron microscopy demonstrated that the PapG adhesin is localized to the terminus of the tip fibrillum (131). The tip fibrillum may play a role in the efficient presentation of PapG adhesin so that it has the optimal steric freedom for receptor binding. The same study also demonstrated that the bulk of the fibrillum is composed of the PapE protein. The open helical structure of the fibrillum and its appearance under electron microscopic examination suggest that the fibrillum is a flexible structure (131). This model suggests that placement of the adhesin at the end of the flexible fibrillum optimizes the adhesin's ability to recognize eukaryotic receptors.

### The Roles of PapF and PapK

Jacob-Dubuisson et al. (101) used a biochemical, genetic, and structural approach to dissect the roles of the two minor pilins

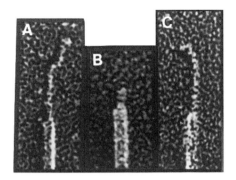

**FIGURE 3** Bipartite structure of P, type 1, and S pili. High-resolution quick-freeze, deep-etch electron microscopy revealed the tip fibrillum present on P (A), type 1 (B), and S (C) pili. In P and type 1 pili, minor pilins, including the adhesin, were localized to the fibrillum. Note the dramatically shorter type 1 fibrillum (16 nm). The fibrilla of the P and S pili range in length from 40 to 80 nm. (Magnification = ×240,000.)

PapF and PapK in the biogenesis of the fibrillum and the pilus rod. It was demonstrated previously that inactivation of papA does not block the ability of bacteria to hemagglutinate human erythrocytes; hence, the PapG adhesin is appropriately exposed on the cell surface in the absence of the pilus rod (145). Since PapG directs binding to galabiose moieties on the uroepithelial cell surface, Galα(1–4)Gal affinity chromatography (96) was used to purify the tip fibrilla from the cell surface and to determine the roles of the minor pilins in the assembly of the pilus structure (101). $F^-$, $E^-$, and $K^-$ tip fibrilla were tested for their abilities to bind to the Galα(1–4)Gal affinity column. In such an assay, binding to the column depends on PapG. In order for subunits to coelute with PapG, they must be joined in the fibrillum. In the absence of PapF, very little PapG bound the Galα(1–4)Gal beads, and few or no PapE or PapK subunits were associated with the PapG that did bind. These findings argue that PapF is required to adapt PapG to the rest of the fibrillum structure. In the papK mutant, PapE and PapF remained joined to PapG and were thus coeluted, similar to what occurred in the wild-type situation. Thus, PapK is probably located at the terminal end of the fibrillum. When *papE* was inactivated, a PapF-PapG moiety that was missing PapK was purified, so PapE subunits are probably located between PapF and PapK. These data allowed us to deduce that the order of the subunits in the tip fibrillum is PapG-PapF-PapE-PapK (101).

PapF is an initiator of pilus formation, since inactivation of *papF* results in a fivefold reduction in pili. The $F^-$ pili are hemagglutination negative because of the absence of PapG from the fibrillum, consistent with the role of PapF in adapting PapG to the fibrillum (101). Wild-type amounts of pili were produced by *papK* mutants, but these mutants were slightly less adhesive than wild-type pili. A *papF papK* double mutant was completely nonpiliated. Thus, PapF by itself is sufficient to initiate pilus formation, and PapK can apparently substitute for this function, albeit poorly, in the absence of PapF. Consistent with the hypothesis that PapK has an initiator function was the finding that only PapK and not PapF, PapE, or PapG was able to initiate the formation of a PapA rod in the absence of all other tip fibrillar genes (101). The incorporation of PapK terminates the growth of the fibrillum subassembly, since in the absence of PapK, the length of the fibrillum is dramatically increased (131), and overexpression of PapK causes a reduction in the average length of the fibrillum (101). Apparently, in the absence of PapK, PapA subunits are able to associate with PapE subunits. However, this association is probably weaker than the PapA-PapK association resulting in an increased number of PapE subunits incorporated into the fibrillum before an incoming PapA is able to terminate fibrillum growth and nucleate the assembly of a pilus rod, a function normally provided by PapK (101).

## Type 1 Minor Pilins—Role in Pilus Biogenesis and Adhesin Presentation

As described above for the P-pilus operon, minor pilins play a role in biogenesis of the pilus and assembly of the adhesin into the fibrillum. In the type 1 pilus, the role of the minor pilins FimF and FimG in pilus biogenesis is somewhat controversial. Investigators in the Orndorff laboratory (161, 210) conducted a detailed mutagenic study of the role of FimF and FimG in type 1-pilus assembly. Specific lesions in *fimF* and *fimG* as well as a double mutant (*fimF fimG*) were constructed on the chromosome, and the effect on piliation was tested (210). None of the mutants affected the assembly of the FimH adhesin into the pilus (210). However, Russell and Orndorff did observe a dramatic effect on pilus biogenesis; FimF appears to initiate piliation, since a *fimF* mutant produces fewer pili, while FimG apparently acts as a terminator of the pilus, since a *fimG* mutant produces pili that are 3.5 times longer than wild-type pili. The double mutant (*fimF fimG*) displayed both phenotypes: production of very few, very long pili (210). It was concluded that FimF is an initiator and FimG is a length regulator or terminator.

Klemm and Christiansen (121) performed a similar analysis but obtained results that differ significantly from those of Russell and Orndorff (210). Klemm and Christiansen found that FimH is not incorporated into $FimF^-$ $FimG^-$ pili. Further, they demonstrated that at least one of the minor pilins (FimF or FimG) is required for the correct incorporation of FimH into the pilus in order for adhesive pili to be formed. These results suggest that FimF and FimG are somewhat interchangeable as adaptors. This system is similar to the P-pilus system, in which PapK and PapF have somewhat overlapping functions in pilus initiation, although only PapF can link PapG to the fibrillum (101). Klemm and Christiansen's (121) studies support the role of the minor type 1 pilins in length regulation and initiation of pilus assembly and a role for FimH in regulating the length of the pilus. Experimental differences between the studies done by Klemm and Christiansen (121) and Russell and Orndorff (210) could account for their different findings. Russell and Orndorff were studying a type 1 operon cloned from a clinical isolate and recombined into the chromosome of a K-12 strain of *E. coli*. Klemm and Christiansen were studying a type 1 operon cloned from a K-12 strain of *E. coli* on a multicopy plasmid.

As discussed above, in the P-pilus system, the adhesin is joined to the fibrillum by a specific adaptor, PapF, that also has a role as an initiator. However, the PapF adapter is not interchangeable with any of the other subunits. In the P pilus, the order of the subunits has been deduced to be PapG-PapF-PapE fibrillum-PapK-PapA rod. The PapA rod is, however, able to join to a K$^-$ fibrillum, although the PapA-PapE association is weaker (101) than a PapA-PapK interaction. In light of the described roles of FimF and FimG in type 1 pilus biogenesis, our knowledge of the bipartite structure of the P pilus raises the question of whether the type 1 pilus also consists of different subassemblies that are joined together.

Following a strategy similar to that of Jacob-Dubuisson et al. (101), we undertook a biochemical and structural approach to this question (109). A type 1 operon lacking the *fimA* structural gene was shown to endow MSHA on a recipient strain, suggesting that the adhesin is appropriately surface exposed (94). A mannose-binding moiety was purified by mannose affinity chromatography and shown to be composed of FimG and FimH (109). The FimG-FimH complex was shown by high-resolution electron microscopy to have a fibrillar structure similar to that of the P fibrillum, although much shorter and stubbier (Fig. 3B). We refer to this structure as the type 1 tip fibrillum. An examination of whole pili from both clinical and recombinant strains revealed that a stubby fibrillar structure is joined to the distal ends of pilus rods and is expressed on every species of the family *Enterobacteriaceae* that was examined (109). This study was consistent with an earlier report by Abraham et al. that demonstrated the conserved nature of FimH in the *Enterobacteriaceae* (6).

The average length of the type 1 fibrillum is 16 nm (the P tip fibrillum is 40 to 60 nm), while the tip fibrillum from a well-characterized *fimH* mutant was 3 nm long. Complementation of the mutant plasmid with *fimH* in *trans* restored both the wild-type adhesive property and the length of the fibrillum (109). This finding strongly suggests that FimH is an oligomer in the tip fibrillum or that in the presence of FimH, FimG and FimH form a short heteropolymer. Abraham et al. (3) reported that a mutation that alters the regulation of FimH results in the formation of FimH oligomers loosely associated with type 1 pili, which those authors referred to as "fimbriosomes." The fimbriosomes are composed only of FimH, suggesting that FimH can oligomerize under some circumstances. We suggest that FimG and FimH minimally form a unique structure at the tip of the type 1 pilus that presents the FimH adhesin in an appropriate conformation for MSHA.

Interestingly, our crude mannose-purified preparation of tip fibrilla contained FimC, the type 1 periplasmic chaperone, and FimF associated with the FimG-FimH tip complex in a putative preassembly chaperone-subunit complex. The role of the chaperone and chaperone-subunit complex formation are discussed in detail below. The FimC-FimF preassembly complex could be displaced from the tip fibrillum by high-pressure liquid chromatography. This finding suggests that FimG has an interactive surface recognized by FimF and that FimF may also be a component of the fibrillum. The localization of FimG and possibly FimF to the fibrillum is consistent with a role for these proteins in pilus biogenesis, although the functions may not be strictly analogous to the roles of PapF and PapK in the biogenesis of the P pilus. An interesting finding (6, 200) suggested that FimH molecules (and possibly the other minor pilins) are intercalated laterally in the pilus shaft. Immunoelectron microscopy revealed FimH at the tips of pili as well as at sites along the shaft (6). Furthermore, the intercalation sites are breakpoints, and Ponniah et al. suggested a model in which pilus fragmentation at these breakpoints would reveal a new FimH adhesin (200). This model was supported by the finding that fragmentation of the pili by repeated freeze-thaw results in an increase in the MSHA titer (200). Type 1 pili lacking FimH are not as susceptible as type 1 pili with FimH to freeze-thaw-induced fragmentation. This finding, interpreted in light of the discovery of the type 1 tip fibrillum (109), reveals new and intriguing complexities in the biogenesis mechanism. We suggest that if FimH is intercalated in the shaft of the pilus, then FimH is in association with FimG and possibly FimF. In the context of the pilus shaft, the type 1 fibrillum is apparently able to package itself into a helical cylinder. This model suggests a mechanism that may enhance the ability of the bacterium to remain associated with the uroepithelium in the face of mechanical shear forces caused by fluid flow. In addition to the ability of the rod to unravel to absorb the shear forces (5) (a model that was also proposed by Bullitt and Makowski [37] for P pili [discussed below]), breakage of the type 1 pilus exposes new adhesins that allow reattachment (200).

## S Pilus Minor Pilins

The third pilus type commonly associated with UTI is the $\alpha$-sialyl-$\beta$-2,3-galactosyl-specific pilus, the S pilus (80, 125–127, 191, 194, 195). An alignment of the P-, type 1-, and S-pilus operons shows a remarkable similarity in genetic organization (Fig. 2). The S pilus has three minor pilin genes (*sfaG, sfaS, sfaH*) in addition to the major pilin gene *sfaA*. Unlike P and type 1 pilins, the larger of the minor pilins (SfaH) is not the adhesin; instead, the 12-kDa protein SfaS seems to contain the sialic acid-binding determinant (169, 216). Moch et al. (169) successfully purified SfaS to homogeneity and demonstrated that the purified protein will hemagglutinate human erythrocytes. The purified adhesin is in a large ($>10^6$-molecular-weight) complex that apparently is multivalent. Interestingly, purified S pili are not multivalent. Those investigators also generated a monoclonal antibody to SfaS and used immunoelectron microscopy to show that SfaS is localized to the tip of the S-pilus rod (169). This monoclonal antibody also blocks hemagglutination by the purified adhesin. Work by Schmoll et al. (216) was aimed at assigning roles to the minor S pilins in S-pilus biogenesis. Mutations were constructed in the three minor pilins, and the mutant derivatives were tested for their abilities to assemble adhesive pili. As expected, a mutation in *sfaS* completely eliminates hemagglutination; however, this mutation also results in a significant reduction in piliation. Mutations in the larger minor pilin, *sfaH*, also affect hemagglutination and the level of fimbriation, while mutations in *sfaG* affect hemagglutination to a lesser degree (216). Therefore, SfaG and SfaH may represent linkers or adaptors for assembly of the SfaS adhesin into the pilus, similar to the role of PapF and FimG in the P-pilus (101) and type 1-pilus (109) systems, respectively. Work in the Hultgren laboratory demonstrated that the S pilus is also a heteropolymeric structure with a tip fibrillum similar to that seen on P pili (Fig. 3C). A reexamination of S-pilin mutations in light of the bipartite S-pilus structure will help to clarify the role of these proteins in pilus and fibrillum biogeneses.

## Structural Diversity of the Tip Fibrillum

Interesting questions arise from the structural and genetic diversity of the P, type 1, and S pili (Fig. 2 and 3). The type 1 and S pili have three fibrillum-associated minor pilins (FimF; FimG and FimH; and SfaG, SfaS, and SfaH), while the P pilus has four fibrillum-associated minor pilins (PapE, PapF, PapK, and PapG). Apparently, the P-pilus operon underwent a gene duplication event to gain the fourth pilin. The PapK subunit may have evolved to better link the PapE fibrillar subassembly to the PapA rod, although this PapK function remains dispensable. Structurally, the S and P fibrilla are very similar in that both are long, open helical conformations that contrast with the type 1 fibrillum, which is a stubby structure, although it is similar in diameter to the other fibrilla. The type 1 fibrillum may be the progenitor to the P pilus, since the type 1 structure is lacking a self-associative pilin similar to PapE, although there is some evidence that FimH may oligomerize (3, 109). In the case of the S pilus, it is clear that one of the minor pilins is self-associative, but the assignment of the polymerizing subunit awaits a high-resolution electron microscopic analysis of mutants. The other clear difference is that the S-pilus adhesin is not the larger minor pilin as in the P and type 1 systems. The larger size of the adhesin in the type 1- and P-pilus systems is due to the two-domain structure of the molecule, which has a sugar-binding domain and a preassembly domain (Fig. 4; discussed in detail below). Such proteins probably arose by fusion of a soluble sugar-binding protein to a pilin; the pilin domain thus allowed assembly of the sugar-binding determinant into the pilus. A detailed study of the role of the large SfaH protein in adhesive function and pilus and fibrillum biogenesis will prove interesting.

## The P-Pilus Rod

Bullitt and Makowski (37) recently reported a three-dimensional reconstruction of the P-pilus rod, which is a polymer composed solely of PapA. The data conform well to previously reported observations using X-ray diffraction (73). The pilus rod appears to be 68 Å (6.8 nm) in diameter and approximately 1 $\mu$m long; there are ~3.3 subunits per turn. The pilus rod also has a 15-Å (1.5-nm) helical cavity winding through the rod and communicating with the outside of the pilus by a set of radial channels. The three-dimensional reconstruction allowed the visualization of a PapA subunit as a pair of globular domains; however, the boundaries between subunits were not clearly defined (E. Bullit, personal communication). Bullitt and Makowski inferred from the structure that PapA subunits interact through four surfaces to form the extremely stable PapA rod. Two of the interactions are best described as head to tail between neighboring subunits: such interactions hold pilin subunits together to form the fibrillar PapA polymer, which is then coiled to form the right-handed helical rod. Two additional interactions are revealed in the Bullitt and Makowski reconstruction: an interaction of a subunit ($n$) with the subunit three residues ahead ($n + 3$) and an interaction with the subunit three residues behind ($n - 3$). Minimally, these interactions result in the transition from the thin fibrillar conformation of the PapA polymer to the right-handed helical rod. Bullitt and Makowski suggest that the $n + 3$ and $n - 3$ interactions could be perturbed by mechanical forces such as fluid flow in the urinary tract. Disruption of the $n + 3$ and $n - 3$ interactions would result in the pilus assuming a more extended and more elastic conformation with increased length. P-piliated bacteria are thought to be resistant to mechanical shear forces in the urinary tract, a property that allows them to remain

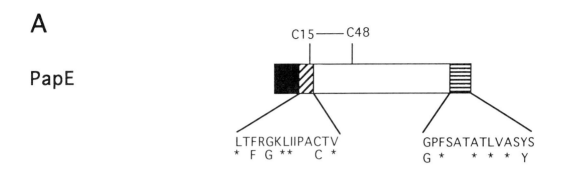

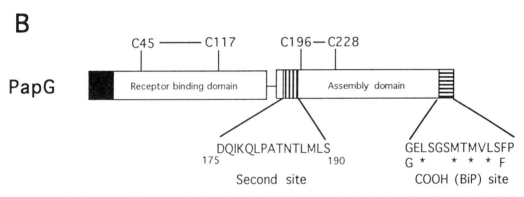

**FIGURE 4** Conserved features of pilus subunits. A diagrammatic depiction of a pilus subunit, PapE (A), and a pilus adhesin, PapG (B), highlighting conserved features. All pilus subunits contain a COOH-terminal motif that in PapG is recognized by the periplasmic chaperone PapD. This motif contains conserved glycine and tyrosine (phenylalanine in PapG) residues separated by a series of alternating hydrophobic residues, the so-called BiP motif. A second conserved sequence (amino-terminal homology region) is located adjacent to the signal cleavage point in subunits (145, 240). This sequence includes an invariant glycine residue and an invariant cysteine residue. The cysteine forms a disulfide bond with another conserved cysteine located approximately 30 residues toward the COOH terminus. Adhesins such as PapG (B) seem to be two-domain proteins. PapG has the conserved COOH-terminal BiP-like motif and a conserved disulfide bridge in which the two cysteines are spaced 32 residues apart in the COOH-terminal domain. Interestingly, a second interaction site has been mapped proximal to cysteine 196, which is positioned similarly to the first cysteine in pilin subunits (A). This so-called second site, however, shares no homology to the conserved amino-terminal site in pilins. Furthermore, the conserved amino terminus of pilins is not found in PapG. Work by Hultgren et al. (96) revealed that PapG truncation, which occurs when PapG is expressed in the absence of PapD, occurs near residues 150 to 160, although the precise clip site is unknown. This truncation event separates the receptor-binding domain, which is active, from the assembly domain. The receptor-binding domain has a second pair of cysteines that form a disulfide bridge. The sugar-binding site in this domain has yet to be mapped.

attached to the uroepithelial surface (190). A "bungee cord" model was presented to account for this resistance to shear force as well as for the breaks, locally unwound segments of the pili, and sharp bends in the pili that were observed by electron microscopy after normal preparation protocols (37). Interestingly, the extended segments of the PapA polymer resembled tip fibrilla; these structures had an open helical structure and dimensions similar to those of tip fibrilla (101, 131). Bullitt and Makowski suggest that the extended conformation of PapA is similar to that of the tip fibrillins PapF and PapE. They also suggest that these pilins have a fibrous and highly extended structure. They propose that the transition from helicoidal to fibrillar conformation of the PapA polymer provides the pilus with a degree of flexibility and allows bacteria expressing the pilus to adhere to and colonize tissues in the urinary tract in the face of fluid flow across the uroepithelium (37).

## Type 1 Pilus Structure

Type 1 pili are approximately 7 nm wide and range from 0.2 to 2.0 $\mu$m in length. The previously described type 1 rod, composed of the FimA major subunit, is arranged in a right-handed helix with 3.125 residues per turn and a helical symmetry identical to that of the recently described P pilus (35, 167). A change in the helical conformation of type 1 pili, resembling that reported by Bullitt and Makowski (37), was reported by Abraham et al. (5), who utilized 50% glycerol to perturb the pilus superstructure and visualized unraveling of the helical conformation of the pilus, which was reversible following dialysis of the glycerol. The unraveled, extended regions of the type 1 pilus, composed of the FimA protein, were 2 to 3 nm in diameter; this width is similar to the diameter of the recently described type 1 tip fibrillum (109).

## Subunit-Subunit Interactions

The ability to dissociate and reassociate the bacterial pilus in vitro is a long-pursued goal of investigators interested in macromolecular assembly and protein-protein interactions. Clues to the assembly of pilus structures may lead to the ability to block steps in the assembly pathway, thereby preventing pilus assembly and blocking bacterial adherence. Eshdat et al. (58) reported that treatment of purified type 1 pili with saturated guanidine hydrochloride completely dissociates the pilus to monomers. Following dialysis of the denaturant, the monomer subunits dimerize. The addition of $MgCl_2$ to the dimeric subunits promotes their polymerization into pilus-like rods. This approach was somewhat efficient (approximately 30% recovery of nativelike structures); however, the biological activity of the reassembled pili was not strictly tested. Attempts to replicate this study with P pili were unsuccessful (229a), and this failure may not be surprising, considering that pili have now been shown to be heteropolymeric structures that require molecular chaperones and ushers for their assembly into adhesive structures in vivo (45, 93, 97, 98, 144).

Another approach to studying the process of pilus assembly was pursued by Striker et al. (230). These investigators demonstrated that a chaperone-subunit complex in the periplasm of piliated bacteria is a true intermediate in the pilus biogenesis pathway (230). Two distinct periplasmic chaperone-subunit complexes were identified: PapD-PapA (DA; 1:1) and PapD-PapA-PapA ($DA_2$; 1:2) in piliated bacteria. These complexes were also detected in the periplasms of strains as a result of coexpression of *papD* and *papA* from compatible plasmids. The two complexes were easily resolved on isoelectric focusing (IEF) gels. A pulse-chase analysis revealed that labeled DA complex could be chased into pili. The role of the $DA_2$ complex in pilus assembly is unclear at this point, although this species does accumulate in pilus-forming bacteria. It is possible that it represents a dead-end or off-pathway product. Alternatively, the DA₂ complex could represent a nucleating species or a sink for unassembled PapA, a possible mechanism in length control whereby PapA subunits are depleted from the periplasm, thus allowing PapH to be incorporated and resulting in the termination of further pilus growth.

Further study of the DA complexes revealed the presence of ordered PapA multimers in the periplasm of strains expressing PapD and PapA (230). Dimers, trimers, and tetramers of PapA uncomplexed to PapD could be visualized by polyacrylamide gel electrophoresis, and these structures were stable in 1.5% sodium dodecyl sulfate (SDS) at 25°C and disrupted by treatment with 1.5% SDS at 95°C (230). Similar multimeric structures were demonstrated with the PapE subunit but not with PapK or PapG. PapE is the subunit that is the bulk of the tip fibrillum and forms an open helical fiber, while PapK and PapG are represented in the pilus in single copy and not as polymers. Therefore, the association of subunits in the periplasm into SDS-stable multimers reflects the fiber-forming and non-fiber-forming properties of the subunit (230). It is unclear whether these assemblies in the periplasm are intermediates in biogenesis or simply form as a result of accumulation in the periplasm in the experimental system. Nevertheless, it has been demonstrated that mutation of amino acid residues essential for piliation also blocks formation of the periplasmic assemblies (106a, 107). In addition, mutations in PapA that abolish its ability to self-associate into a pilus rod abolish the formation of the DA₂ complex but not the DA complex (106a). These findings suggest that the subunit-subunit interactions that occur in periplasmic multimers and in the DA₂ complex reflect the associations that subunits make in the pilus. Therefore, the periplasmic assemblies are a relevant model for studying subunit-subunit interaction (107, 106a).

Purification of the type 1 tip fibrillum (see above) revealed that the heteropolymer forms SDS-stable, heat-sensitive structures. Therefore, homologous or heterologous native assemblies form very stable multimers and provide a start point for a mutagenesis study that will define the residues and interactions required to form the stable subunit-subunit complexes. Initial studies revealed that residues in the carboxyl termini of pilins are important for the formation of subunit-subunit and chaperone-subunit complexes (106a). A detailed study of requirements for the formation of the DG complex has been reported and is discussed below.

## IMMUNOGLOBULIN-LIKE PERIPLASMIC CHAPERONES

### Periplasmic Chaperone Family

Periplasmic chaperones are required for the assembly of the diverse surface fibers produced by many different gram-negative bacteria. To date, the periplasmic chaperone family contains 27 members from many species of the *Enterobacteriaceae* family and from bacterial species outside of this family (99a). Many of the identified PapD homologs are involved in the assembly of piluslike structures, both type 1-like (7- to 10-nm right-handed helical rods) and thin fibrillar structures such as the K88 and K99 pili (2- to 3-nm open helical fibers). Some members of the family are required for the assembly of structures that have not been visualized by electron microscopy (non-fimbrial adhesins). Other members mediate the assembly of very thin fibers whose architectures have not yet been well resolved by microscopic techniques but that seem to coil up in an amorphous mass on the surface of bacteria (Table 1). A few members, such as the EcpD (_E. coli_ PapD) chaperone, which is in a two-gene operon, are not associated with a specific structure; interestingly, the second gene in this operon (*htrE*) is a homolog of the usher family of proteins, of which PapC is the prototype (45, 202). As is indicated by the name, *htrE* is a member of the heat shock regulon (202). The identification of chaperone and usher homologs on the chromosome of *E. coli* suggests a possible role for these proteins in housekeeping functions during bacterial growth. A role in the heat shock response would certainly be appropriate for a chaperone (42, 54–56, 67), although a functional test of this model and attribution of known functions of PapD to EcpD await experimentation.

## Structure

The 2.5-Å (0.25-nm) crystal structure of PapD was solved by Holmgren and Brändén in 1989 (88). The protein is composed of two domains, with each domain conforming to a structural motif referred to as an immunoglobulin fold (Ig fold) (259) (Fig. 5). The Ig fold is a dominant motif among cell surface adhesin molecules, which are organized into two families: the immunoglobulin superfamily and the cytokine receptor superfamily (22, 41, 44, 259). Periplasmic chaperones represent a third family and are the only family of bacteria proteins known to use the Ig fold to display recognition surfaces involved in protein-protein interaction (88). The substructural element of the Ig fold is the $\beta$ barrel (9, 10, 32, 88, 199, 215). The $\beta$ barrel is formed by two sheets of $\beta$ strands that lie across one another (32). The topology, or order, of the $\beta$ strands defines the Ig-fold structure. Domain 1 of PapD is most similar to the variable domain of an immunoglobulin molecule; both are composed of seven strands, of which two are exclusively in the top sheet, three are in the bottom sheet, and two are shared by the sheets (88). The second domain of PapD has a topology identical to the second domain of

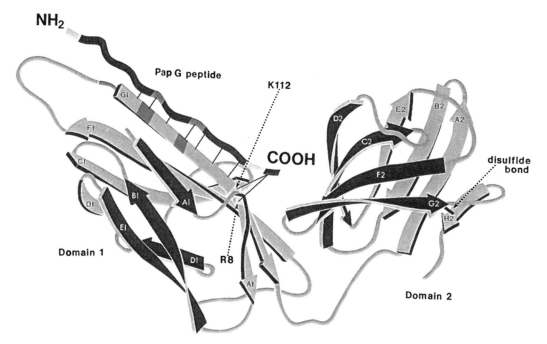

**FIGURE 5** Cocrystal structure of PapD complexed with a PapG COOH-terminal peptide. Both PapD and the PapG 1′-19′ peptide are depicted as ribbon models. The PapG peptide lies along the G1 $\beta$ strand on PapD and extends deep into the cleft between domains 1 and 2 of PapD. See the text and Kuehn et al. (133) for details.

the CD4 molecule, with three strands in the top sheet and four strands in the bottom sheet. Interestingly, PapD has a short fifth β strand at the COOH terminus of the second domain that is disulfide-linked to the β strand that precedes it. Such an intersheet disulfide is not characteristic of immunoglobulins (88). The two domains, linked by a stretch of residues that are referred to as a hinge, are oriented such that the molecule resembles a boomerang (Fig. 5). The amino acid sequences (loops) that link β strands vary in both sequence and number throughout the chaperone family (i.e., some loops are longer than others; see below) and are analogous to the complementarity-determining regions in immunoglobulin molecules. The sheets are organized in the β-barrel motif such that the loops cluster at the ends of the barrel. In immunoglobulins, complementarity-determining region sequences provide the diversity required for the recognition of an untold numbers of antigens to provide an adequate immune response. Whether the loop regions in periplasmic chaperones are part of a specificity-determining structure in chaperone-subunit interactions remains to be determined.

An alignment of the primary sequence from members of the periplasmic family of proteins (89, 99a) revealed the hallmark features of this family of proteins. The alignment, based on the known structure of PapD, takes into account the known limits of the β strands in the domains and reveals that most of the conserved and invariant residues are important in maintenance of the overall fold of the protein and thus are buried in the hydrophobic core of the protein (89). The positioning of four of the loops, which join consecutive β strands, is also a conserved feature of the chaperone family, because four invariant asparagine residues (N24, N39, N145, and N195) that form hydrogen bonds to main-chain atoms are required to orient the loops between β strands B1 and C1, C1 and D1,

B2 and C2, and F2 and G2 (88, 89). Another conserved feature in the chaperone family is an interdomain salt bridge composed of residues R116 (in association with E83) and D196 (88, 89). This interaction is thought to orient the two domains, creating a cleft that participates with subunits in complex formation (see below).

Another group of residues is conserved for no obvious structural reasons. Their side chains protrude into the solvent without interacting with surrounding side chains at all. Three such conserved residues, arginine 8 (R8), threonine 7 (T7), and lysine 112 (K112), are exposed in the cleft (88, 89). Mutations in two of these residues, R8 and K112, abolish or greatly reduce the abilities of the chaperone to form chaperone-subunit complexes and to mediate pilus assembly, arguing that the conserved cleft forms part of the subunit binding site (133, 224). The amino acid substitutions are not expected to have an effect on protein structure, since the R8 and K112 side chains are not involved in interactions with other residues in the protein. The point mutant derivatives of PapD are expressed and stable in the periplasm. These results suggest that the R8 and K112 residues are critical in chaperone function and possibly make direct contacts with subunits.

In addition to the subunit-binding cleft, the variable loops that interconnect adjacent β strands may be important in defining specificity. Jones et al. (108) demonstrated that the *fimC* open reading frame in the type 1-pilus system encodes a periplasmic chaperone required for synthesis of type 1 pili. To further probe the function of the chaperone, a complementation study was used to test the abilities of the PapD and FimC chaperones to assemble heterologous pili. Although FimC failed to assemble P pili, PapD was able to complement a *fimC1* mutation and assemble type 1 pili on the surfaces of bacteria. A high-resolution electron microscopy analysis showed that type 1 pili assembled by PapD are structurally identical to type 1 pili assembled by FimC. A series of PapD mutants were utilized to test whether PapD requires the conserved cleft residue arginine 8 in order to assemble type 1 pili. As predicted, a PapD-R8G mutant failed to complement the *fimC1* mutant, suggesting that type 1-pilin subunits are recognized by the periplasmic chaperone via conserved cleft interactions (108). Recent studies have directly demonstrated that mutations in the invariant cleft residues of FimC block type 1-pilus assembly (107). Interestingly, an E167G (glycine substituted for a glutamic acid at residue 167) mutant of PapD, which has a substitution in the domain 2 C2-D2 loop, was dramatically impaired in its ability to assemble type 1 pili, whereas PapD-E167G assembled P pili almost as well as wild-type PapD did (108). This result suggests that interactions with loop residues do occur, since this substitution should have no effect on the structure of the chaperone. However, the details of these interactions and the reason for the effect on type 1-pilus assembly and not on P-pilus assembly await further study.

## Carboxyl-Terminal Assembly Domain

Hultgren et al. (96) demonstrated that a 24.5-kDa truncate of PapG (N-terminal 150 residues) contains the sugar-binding domain of the adhesin. However, this truncate fails to interact with the PapD chaperone. It was postulated that the COOH-terminal 160 residues function as a preassembly domain, interacting with the periplasmic chaperone and facilitating incorporation of the adhesin into the pilus. The COOH-terminal portion of the adhesin has the hallmarks of a pilin (Fig. 4). An alignment of the immediate COOH-terminal region (30 residues) of 23 pilins (133) revealed several highly conserved and invariant features, including a motif that closely resembles a motif that is recognized by BiP (immunoglobulin binding protein) (26) (BiP-like motif), the sole Hsp70 chaperone in the lumen of the endoplasmic reticulum (67). The BiP-like motif includes a conserved pattern of alternating hydrophobic residues in the COOH-terminal 12 amino acids. In addition, a conserved penultimate tyrosine and a conserved glycine 14 amino acids from the COOH terminus are typical of pilus proteins. Pilin proteins also contain two appropriately spaced (30-residue separation) cysteine residues that form a conserved disulfide bridge (96, 103). The COOH-terminal domain of PapG has all the hallmarks of a pilin (Fig. 4) (96). This PapG variant (PapG1) is highly unstable in wild-type bacteria, which suggests that PapG1 is susceptible to degradation because of an inability to interact with the periplasmic chaperone PapD (96). The protection of subunits from degradation by proteases through chaperone-mediated complex formation in the periplasmic space has since been proven (see below). Genetic and biochemical studies demonstrated that two interactive surfaces are located in the COOH-terminal domain of PapG. Interaction at both regions is essential for the formation of a receptor-binding PapG protein. These studies are described in detail below.

Expression of the type 1-pilus adhesin in wild-type *E. coli* lacking a functional FimC (periplasmic chaperone) results in truncation of the FimH protein to an approximately 16-kDa species (242). This truncate protein has the same amino terminus as full-length FimH and can be purified from the periplasm by mannose-Sepharose affinity chromatography (109). This result suggests that, as in PapG, the carbohydrate-binding region of FimH is located in the amino-terminal domain of the protein. FimH, like all pilins, has conserved features at the C terminus that are hallmarks of a pilin and are thought to be required for interaction with the periplasmic chaperone. These data suggest that the adhesins of P and type 1 pili are two-domain proteins with sugar-binding domains linked to pilinlike preassembly domains.

## Recognition Paradigm

Periplasmic chaperones differ from other classic chaperone proteins (66, 67) such as SecB (135, 141, 203, 257), DnaK (42, 256), and GroEL-ES (63, 85, 154, 250) in that the targets for the chaperone are a defined set of proteins, the pilins (95, 98). As discussed above, several features at the C termini of pilin subunits are highly conserved. These features are hallmarks of a pilin sequence: the conserved penultimate tyrosine and −14 glycine residues and the BiP-like motif, which consists of an alternating pattern of hydrophobic residues (26, 98, 133). Kuehn et al. (133) used an ELISA to test the ability of PapD to bind to peptides corresponding to the COOH terminus of each of the Pap subunits. PapD bound the PapG peptide best, the PapE, PapF, and PapK peptides moderately well, and the PapH peptide not at all. Inhibition of binding with competing peptides showed that the C-terminal seven residues of PapG are sufficient for recognition by the chaperone (133).

The G1′-19′ peptide (the 19-mer peptide is numbered from the COOH terminus such that the COOH-terminal residue is numbered 1′) was used for cocrystallization with purified PapD, and a cocrystal structure was resolved to 3-Å (0.3-nm) resolution (133) (Fig. 5). The invariant R8 and K112 residues of the chaperone form hydrogen bonds with the peptide's COOH terminus, thus anchoring the peptide in the cleft. The BiP-like recognition motif is positioned along the exposed edge of the G1 β strand of PapD, mostly by backbone hydrogen bonds. The alignment of the peptide along the exposed edge of the G1 β strand forms a β-sheet structure between the chaperone and peptide that we call a "beta zipper." The region of contact (peptide residues Met-8 to Phe-2 and PapD residues Glu-104 to Lys-110) involves seven main-chain hydrogen bonds. The alternating pattern of hydrophobic residues in the peptide is mirrored in the G1 strand, allowing hydrophobic interactions between the peptide and the PapD G1 strand. These hydrophobic interactions contribute 20% of the total buried surface area of the complex.

The essential nature of the positioning and spacing of the peptide relative to those of the G1 strand is demonstrated by a PapG peptide lacking the C-terminal proline residue (133). Although an amide terminates the peptide, it is not recognized by PapD. This peptide should be able to form hydrogen bonds with arginine 8 and lysine 112, since a PapG peptide (G1′-19′ amide) in which the C-terminal carboxyl group (of the proline residue) is replaced with an amide group binds efficiently. The C-terminal proline residue also makes a series of van der Waals contacts with residues Thr-7, Thr-152, Ile-154, Thr-170, and Ile-194 (133). Moreover, PapD derivatives containing arginine 8 and lysine 112 substitutions interact poorly with PapG (133, 224). These results suggest that the interactions (along the G1 strand) occur less efficiently when anchor interactions are blocked. Furthermore, spacing between the hydrogen-bonding C terminus (the anchor) and formation of the main-chain hydrogen bonds and hydrophobic interactions seem to be critical.

As mentioned previously, a characteristic of most pilins assembled by PapD-like chaperones is the presence of a conserved penultimate tyrosine. In the PapD peptide crystal structure, the penultimate residue, which in PapG is a phenylalanine, interacts only very weakly with PapD. Phenylalanine 2 interacts in a shallow pocket formed between the two β sheets of domain 1 of PapD (133). Mutations in the penultimate residue of the beta zipper in PapA (Tyr-162) abolish the formation of stable chaperone-subunit complexes, resulting in nonpiliated cells and arguing that this conserved residue is indeed critical in the chaperone-subunit interaction. However, it may be part of a more dynamic process, such as folding of the subunit (106a). The penultimate aromatic residue in the K99 pilin subunit, FanC, is essential for stability of the subunit in the periplasm, a fact that most likely signifies its critical role in interactions (223). Mutation of the penultimate aromatic in PapG (phenylalanine) to a serine also has detrimental effects on the PapD-PapG interaction. This mutation reduces or eliminates the ability to isolate receptor-binding PapG. Thus, it is likely that the penultimate residue plays a critical role in a critical interaction with PapD that may involve folding (107).

### Second-Site Interactions

The cocrystal of PapD with the 19-mer PapG peptide describes one aspect of a series of interactions required for the formation of a stable chaperone-subunit complex. A second DG interaction was recently described by Xu et al. (261). Two separate approaches were used to define amino acid sequence requirements for formation of a DG complex. One approach utilized MBP fusions to various lengths of the COOH terminus of PapG. The MBP-G fusion proteins were coexpressed with PapD, and complex formation was determined by assaying for binding of periplasmic extracts to amylose. If the MBP fusion protein had the sites necessary for interaction with PapD, then PapD would copurify with the fusion protein on the affinity column. Only the fusion that contained the COOH-terminal 140 amino acids of PapG was bound tightly by PapD. Furthermore, coexpression of the largest MBP-G fusion with the *pap* operon inhibited piliation by titrating PapD away from the subunits in vivo. Interestingly, shorter fusions containing the COOH-terminal binding site were dramatically less efficient at binding PapD and inhibiting pilus assembly; therefore, an amino-terminal interaction seemed to be necessary for complex formation to occur. Another approach to dissecting PapD-subunit interactions involved testing the ability of PapD to bind to PapG truncate proteins in vivo (261). This study demonstrated that PapD would form a complex with PapG truncates lacking the COOH-terminal 117 residues but not with a truncate lacking an additional 53 residues (the C-terminal 170 residues). This result correlated nicely with the region identified as important in binding to the MBP fusions. These studies defined an amino-terminal limit to a putative second site recognized by the chaperone, and in combination with the endpoints from the MBP fusion study, the second site was predicted to be within a 20-amino-acid overlap. To define the site, a series of four overlapping peptides conforming to the overlap sequences were synthesized and tested for binding in an ELISA. One of the four peptides bound efficiently to PapD (Fig. 4B), suggesting that the second site acts independently of the COOH-terminal site, although both sites are probably necessary for optimal binding (261). Cocrystallization studies of the site 2 peptide with PapD are under way to define the structural basis of the interaction. These data combined with the detailed knowledge of the COOH-terminal interaction will give a more complete picture of the molecular basis for chaperone-subunit interactions.

### CHAPERONE FUNCTION

Over the years, researchers have suggested many functions as being required for the assembly of the pilus and attributable to the periplasmic chaperone (18, 96–98, 108, 144, 188). These functions include facilitated import of subunits into the periplasmic space, stabilization of subunits in the periplasm, protection of the unfolded state from periplasmic proteases, promotion of folding of subunits, blocking of nonproductive aggregation of subunits, delivery of the subunits to the outer membrane usher, and facilitation of interactions between subunits to form polymers. Several of these suggested functions have been proven to be actual functions of the periplasmic chaperone PapD in P-pilus assembly (45, 132, 133, 224). Limited studies have been carried out with other members of the family (FimC [108, 109] and FaeE [18]).

**Periplasmic Import**
The data that imply a role for chaperones in facilitated or vectorial transport into specialized compartments in eukaryotic cells are considerable. The BiP chaperone functions in the endoplasmic reticulum (83, 175, 213), while the mitochondria (218, 244) and chloroplast (219) each utilize a compartment-specific version of HSP70. These chaperones are responsible for the transport of target proteins into specific organelles. In many experiments, hybrid or fusion protein constructs were used to trap proteins as translocation intermediates (244). These intermediates could be efficiently cross-linked to membrane components that might be parts of a translocation pore. Furthermore, the translocation intermediates interact with a compartment-specific chaperone of the Hsp70 class. In bacteria, a component of the Sec pathway (SecD) involved in the secretion of proteins across the inner membrane is essential for "release" and folding of MBP in the periplasm (159). Following treatment of spheroplasts with a monoclonal antibody against SecD, MBP is localized to the inner membrane and not released in active form into the medium (periplasm). Monoclonal antibodies against other Sec components have no detectable effect on MBP localization. Matsuyama et al. suggested that folding of the protein is dependent on efficient release of the protein from the inner membrane, since trypsin-resistant MBP result only upon release of the protein from the membrane (159).

Utilizing a genetic system, we verified that the DegP protease is responsible for degradation of pilin subunits and subunit aggregates when the subunits are expressed in the absence of the chaperone (18, 107, 228, 229). Furthermore, P-pilin subunits are not efficiently translocated across the inner membrane into the periplasm when they are expressed without a periplasmic chaperone (107). These results suggest that periplasmic chaperones such as PapD are similar to other compartmentalized chaperones in that recognition of nascent translocating intermediates facilitates continued vectorial translocation across a membrane. This interaction may also protect the nascent chain from aggregation and degradation. We suggest that the interactions of a subunit with the chaperone as the subunit emerges from the cytoplasmic membrane are part of a folding pathway that would also contribute to driving the imported subunit into the periplasm.

The driving force of aggregation for unchaperoned subunits may be the exposure of hydrophobic surfaces or premature exposure of the natural polymerization surfaces that are involved in pilus assembly. The former situation suggests that subunit folding assisted by the chaperone is essential for the subunits to achieve a native state, while the latter supports the role of the chaperone in blocking off-pathway interactions, i.e., interactions that occur at the wrong time or location. The answer may be a combination of both situations and may differ for various subunits.

**Complex Formation**
Following periplasmic localization of subunits, chaperone-subunit complexes form. Periplasmic complexes between PapD and PapE (DE; 144), PapD and PapG (96), PapD and PapK (DK; 230), and PapD and PapA (230) were detected and purified to homogeneity. These complexes accumulated in the periplasm during pilus biogenesis and were also detected when the

relevant genes were overexpressed on plasmids. One suggested role of these complexes is the blocking of off-pathway reactions such as premature interaction of subunits that result in aggregation and degradation. A test of this hypothesis was reported by Kuehn et al. (132), who used purified DG complex and IEF gel electrophoresis. PapD has an isoelectric point (pI) of 9.13, PapG has a pI of 5.19, and the DG complex has a pI of 7.3 (132). The DG complex was denatured in urea, and then the denaturant was diluted. After this procedure, the DG complex failed to re-form as assayed on IEF; instead, the proteins aggregated and failed to enter the gel. However, when native PapD was present in the diluent, it was able to bind to PapG and prevent aggregation by re-forming the soluble DG complex, according to IEF. Thus, the native chaperone was able to "cap" interactive surfaces on the unfolded subunits and prevent aggregation. These data support the model that pilin subunits, in this case PapG, during and perhaps after folding expose surfaces that drive aggregation. These surfaces are efficiently covered or capped when the subunit is in a complex with the periplasmic chaperone (132). Presumably, translocating subunits cross the cytoplasmic membrane in a semiunfolded conformation (257) and therefore may tend to aggregate in the periplasm or in association with the inner membrane in the absence of an interaction with the chaperone. Interaction with the chaperone during or immediately following translocation would prevent off-pathway interactions such as aggregation.

The inability to detect or purify native pilin subunits in the absence of the chaperone in wild-type bacteria is well documented. PapA and PapE are completely degraded when they are expressed from high-expression inducible plasmids (144, 230), while in the same situation, PapG and FimH are truncated, as discussed above (96, 108). Coexpression of the chaperone allows purification of all subunits as full-length native subunits in a complex with the chaperone (96, 108, 144, 230). In a strain carrying a *kan* cassette in the *degP* locus, full-length pilin subunits can be expressed without a chaperone, although induction of the subunits results in a profound growth defect (107). The growth defect can be completely suppressed by coexpression of PapD, which suggests that complex formation and possibly import of subunits into the periplasm account for the restoration of growth. This finding also suggests that aggregate formation associated with the membrane localization of the subunits is the cause of toxicity, and it implicates the chaperone in the blocking of aggregate formation (107).

A biochemical analysis of the periplasmic chaperone FaeE, which is required for the assembly of K88 pili, revealed that this member of the chaperone family is a dimer in solution (170). Mol et al. (170) further demonstrated that the dimer interacts with FaeG, the major subunit of the K88 pilus, to form a heterotrimer. The K88 pilus is not structurally related to the type 1, P, and S pili, since the K88 pilus is a thin (2- to 3-nm) fibrillar fiber. The assembly pathway of the fibrillar K88 pilus, as well as of other narrow fibers, may utilize the heterotrimer intermediate, while the assembly pathway of the 7- to 10-nm fibers utilizes the 1:1 stoichiometric complexes demonstrated in the P and type 1 systems (96–98, 108, 132, 133, 144, 230).

## Protein Folding

The fact that unescorted subunits are sensitive to proteolysis in vivo suggests that the subunits are not appropriately folded into a stable tertiary structure (84). A significant amount of data that strengthen the argument that chaperones are involved in catalyzing the folding of target proteins is accumulating (42, 54–56, 63, 67, 85, 138, 155, 156). Protease sensitivity is often a marker of an unfolded structure (84). PapG, when expressed in the absence of PapD, is cleaved into a 24.5-kDa truncate (96). This truncate is stable and possesses receptor-binding activity (see above). Such a result suggests that the COOH-terminal domain, which seems to play a role in assembly of the subunit into the pilus, requires the chaperone template for correct folding; in the absence of the chaperone, it is a target for proteolysis. Full-length PapG could be recovered, however, after expression of PapG in the *degP* strain in the absence of PapD. Interestingly, the fraction of full-length PapG that was localized to the periplasm did not possess receptor-binding activity, which suggests that the adhesin is unable to achieve a receptor-binding conformation (107). These data begin to build a case that PapD provides a template for folding.

## Capping of Associative Surfaces

As discussed above, only fiber-forming subunits (PapA in the rod and PapE in the tip fibrillum) form multimers in vivo in the periplasm (230). Subunits that are present in single or low copy number in the pilus (PapK and PapG) do not form oligomeric aggregates (230). These multimeric structures are characterized by their stability in SDS at 25°C. Purified $DA_2$ and DE complexes were utilized to develop an in vitro assembly system. Striker et al. (106a) demonstrated that repeated freeze-thaw cycles effectively reconstitute pilus subassemblies by dissociating PapD from the purified chaperone-subunit complexes. Dissociation of the chaperone (uncapping) from the rod-forming subunit PapA or the tip fibrillum-forming subunit PapE leads to the formation of pilus rod or tip fibrillum subassemblies, respectively. When these subassemblies are visualized by high-resolution electron microscopy, the PapA rods, approximately 100 subunits long, are indistinguishable from native pili. The PapE subassemblies are open helical in conformation, similar to the tip fibrillum. Uncapping the adapter protein PapK from purified DK does not result in the formation of any oligomeric structures. Moreover, the presence of excess purified PapD blocks the formation of the pilus-like rods, a fact that indicates that PapD caps associative surfaces on the subunit. Mutations in a conserved residue in PapA, the $-14$ glycine, at the leading edge of the beta-zipper motif in PapA greatly reduce subunit-subunit associations both in vivo and in vitro, arguing that this region participates in subunit-subunit interactions after chaperone uncapping. This mutation has no effect on the formation of a DA complex. The complex formed between PapD and mutant PapA was purified, and after uncapping of PapD in vitro, the mutant PapA subunits did not associate into any oligomeric structures. Thus this region probably participates in subunit-subunit interactions after chaperone uncapping (106a). This in vitro assembly system will provide a unique opportunity for further study of the development of a cellular organelle.

## DsbA, an Additional Cellular Factor Required for Piliation

Experiments by Jacob-Dubuisson et al. (103) demonstrated that the *E. coli* periplasmic disulfide isomerase DsbA (19–21) is required for P-pilus assembly. DsbA is required for disulfide bond formation in secretory proteins such as OmpA and $\beta$-lactamase (19, 112). Defects in the assembly of oligomeric structures such as *E. coli* heat-labile enterotoxin, F pili, cholera toxin, and Tcp pili have been reported in strains lacking a functional DsbA (19, 198, 262). The suggested function of DsbA is that of a redox donor (7, 21). DsbA is required for alkaline phosphatase to acquire protease resistance, suggesting that after disulfide bond formation occurs, the protein folds into a native conformation. In the absence of DsbA, alkaline phosphatase is partially degraded in vivo (19, 112).

DsbA acts on both PapD and P-pilus subunits (103). In the case of the subunits, the rapid acquisition of disulfide bonds in PapG, even in the absence of PapD (but in the presence of DsbA), suggests that oxidation precedes chaperone-subunit complex formation. In the absence of PapD, oxidized PapG is subject to a more limited proteolytic degradation than reduced PapG, suggesting that oxidized PapG achieves a more compact conformation or that the interaction with DsbA somewhat protects it. In a *dsbA papD* mutant background, PapG is completely and rapidly degraded. Interestingly, PapD is unable to fold into a native conformation that is able to bind subunits in vivo and mediate pilus assembly in the absence of DsbA. PapD possesses a pair of cysteines spaced only 5 amino acids apart that form an intrasheet disulfide bond between the H2 and the G2 β strands in CD4-like domain 2 as determined by X-ray crystallography. The H2 β strand is not present in most PapD-like chaperones. The conversion of PapD cysteines into serines by site-directed mutagenesis results in misfolded and nonfunctional PapD in vivo, mimicking the effects of the *dsbA* mutation. In contrast, denatured reduced PapD is able to refold and achieve a subunit binding conformation in vitro in the absence of disulfide bond formation. The discrepancy between in vivo and in vitro folding of PapD in the absence of its intramolecular disulfide bond may be due to a more stringent need to control folding (prevent misfolding) of the proteins, in this case PapD, in vivo as they emerge into the periplasmic space from the cytoplasmic membrane. One possibility is that DsbA has both oxidant and chaperone-like functions.

The tertiary structure of DsbA shows an extensive hydrophobic surface close to the active site that may bind partially folded polypeptides in a chaperone-like fashion before the oxidation of cysteine residues (157). In agreement with this proposal, our results suggest that DsbA might bind to nascently translocated PapD, maintaining it in a folding-competent state until the entire protein is exported across the membrane, at which time disulfide bond formation is catalyzed, and correct protein folding ensues. However, it is possible that DsbA acts merely by oxidizing PapD when the cysteines emerge from the cytoplasmic membrane and that the formation of the disulfide bond is a critical event for the in vivo folding of PapD. It is possible that subunit folding in the periplasmic space is a sequential process involving at least two chaperones: DsbA binds the subunit during translocation across the cytoplasmic membrane, and after DsbA has catalyzed the formation of the subunit disulfide bond(s), the subunit is passed onto PapD. Analogs to this type of multicomponent pathway for protein folding have been unveiled in the cytoplasm (63, 138) as well as in eukaryotic organelles, i.e., the endoplasmic reticulum (83).

## OUTER MEMBRANE ASSEMBLY PROTEINS

### Family and Structure

The P-pilus outer membrane protein PapC is required for the transfer of *pap*-encoded subunits from the highly stable chaperone-subunit complexes formed with PapD into the final well-defined architecture of the P pilus (45). PapC and more than 20 homologous proteins from various pathogenic gram-negative bacteria, including *E. coli* and *Klebsiella, Haemophilus, Bordetella,* and *Salmonella* spp., form an ever-increasing family of outer membrane proteins that are required for the formation of extracellular surface structures (Table 1). Each of these proteins is approximately 90 kDa in size and is predicted to have extensive β structure. Pairwise, these proteins share approximately 25% identity and 45% similarity (44a).

### Function of Outer Membrane Proteins

Each outer membrane assembly protein appears to be required in its respective system for the incorporation of subunits into the growing extracellular structure. For instance, in the P-pilus system, if PapC is not present, the subunits are not transferred from the chaperone-subunit complexes into the pilus, and chaperone-subunit complexes thus accumulate in the periplasm (177). This transfer process involves binding of the chaperone-subunit complexes to the outer membrane protein, removal of the chaperone (uncapping), binding of successive subunits to each other, and extrusion of the subunits through the outer membrane (Fig. 6) (45). It may also involve recycling of the chaperone. In addition, in vitro studies suggest that PapC might regulate the ordered targeting of chaperone-subunit complexes into the pilus. For this reason, PapC has been dubbed an "usher." In vitro, DG, DF, and DE complexes are able to bind to PapC, while DK or DA complexes fail to bind to PapC. Furthermore, DG has a greater affinity for PapC than either DF or DE has (45). These differences in binding of the various chaperone-subunit complexes to PapC may describe a mechanism that ensures that every pilus rod has an adhesive tip fibrillum. The current model (Fig. 6) is that after subunit import mediated by PapD and disulfide bond formation mediated by DsbA, DG complexes form and are targeted to empty PapC sites, followed by DF binding which initiates tip assembly. The joining of PapG to PapF is then followed by multiple rounds of DE binding and incorporation to form the bulk of the tip. DK and DA, although apparently unable to bind to an empty PapC site, are hypothesized to be able to bind to PapC with a growing tip fibrillum, thus allowing rod polymerization. Incorporation of PapH terminates rod polymerization (14). As of yet, the generality of the ushering function of PapC to the other pilus systems is not known, since the abilities of the other membrane proteins to differentially bind to their respective chaperone-subunit complexes and thus potentially regulate the ordering of pilus assembly have not been reported.

## VACCINE STRATEGY

It has become increasingly clear, particularly from the recent work of Roberts et al. (209), that adhesive pili are important for pathogenesis. The availability of purified proteins, including adhesins, pili, and tip structures, as well as a monkey model for urinary tract disease now makes it feasible to test whether a vaccine that would prevent or reduce recurrent UTIs can be developed. Roberts et al. (209) showed that a mutant of a pyelonephritogenic clinical isolate that lacks full-length PapG is deficient in its ability to cause pyelonephritis and thus kidney damage in a monkey model. It is therefore logical to target bacteria that are carrying PapG on their surfaces for immune surveillance by vaccinating with either tip complexes that contain PapG or DG complexes that carry PapG in a conformation that is able to bind to its receptor. Vaccination with the tip complex, however, may be advantageous, since this would allow recognition not just of PapG but also of PapE, which binds to fibronectin (255) and thus might also be important in adherence and pathogenesis in vivo.

## PERSPECTIVES

This chapter highlights the extensive groundwork that has been done on the P pilus and other model systems that will allow a detailed understanding of the mechanisms by which gram-negative bacteria are able to elaborate adhesive pilus structures on their extracellular surfaces. Each aspect of the assembly process, including the actions of the chaperone and DsbA at the inner membrane to properly import and fold subunits, the targeting of these complexes to the outer membrane protein, and the subsequent uncapping of the chaperone and incorporation of the subunits into the growing structure, is currently under study. In addition, the subunit surfaces that interact with the chaperone, the outer membrane usher proteins, and each other are being dissected, and the three-dimensional structure of each component is being sought. All of this work will increase our understanding of how pili are made and will allow the rational design

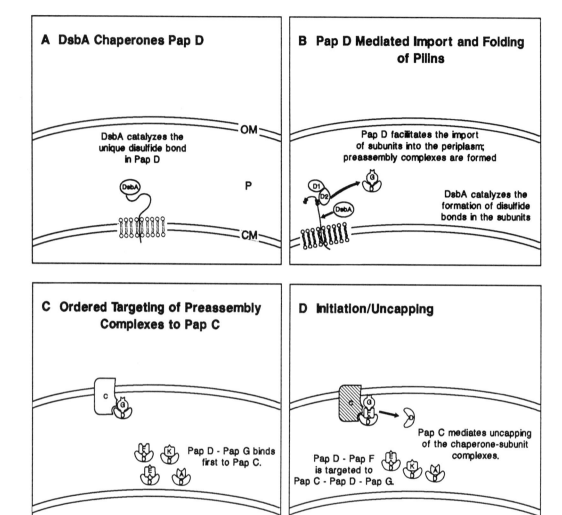

**FIGURE 6** Model of P-pilus biogenesis. The first step (A) in the model involves the import of PapD into the periplasmic space and a requirement for DsbA to catalyze disulfide bond formation in PapD. PapD is required for the import of pilus subunits into the periplasm (B). As indicated, our results suggest that domain 2 interactions mediate subunit import. Complex formation and folding into a nativelike tertiary structure, however, require interactions with both domains. Experimental evidence suggests that disulfide bond formation in the subunits precedes interaction with PapD (103). DsbA catalyzes formation of the subunit disulfide bonds (103). Once chaperone-subunit preassembly complexes are formed, they are targeted to the PapC molecular usher (45) (C). Initiation of the fibrillum requires the formation of a PapC-PapG-PapF complex (101). PapD must be displaced from subunits in order for the subunits to polymerize into the pilus. This process is called uncapping (D). Shading of the usher in panel D indicates that an active complex has formed. PapK regulates the length of the tip fibrillum (E and F) and initiates PapA polymerization into the rod (F and G) (101). The stoichiometry of the DA versus the DH complex regulates the incorporation of PapA into the rod, with polymerization terminated upon incorporation of PapH (14) (H). PapH is also responsible for anchoring the pilus to the outer membrane by an unknown mechanism.

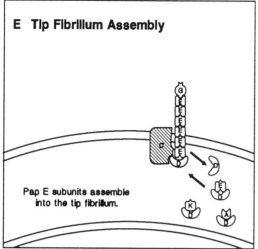
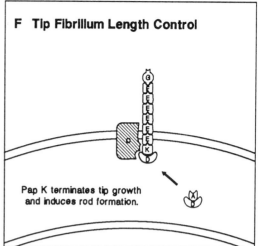
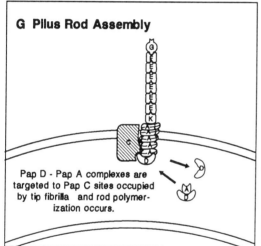
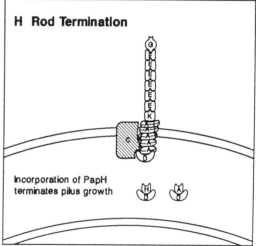

**FIGURE 6** *Continued.*

of compounds to interfere with this process. The detailed understanding of the ultrastructure of the pilus has identified better targets for vaccination against these virulence-associated structures. The studies presented in this review also allow a better appreciation of the host targets recognized by urinary tract pathogens and the complexity of the process that, although it involves more than binding a target, initiates with the pathogen recognizing a specific host component.

### REFERENCES

1. **Abraham, J. M., C. S. Freitag, J. R. Clements, and B. I. Eisenstein.** 1985. An invertible element of DNA controls phase variation of type 1 fimbriae of *Escherichia coli*. *Proc. Natl. Acad. Sci. USA* **82:**5724–5727.
2. **Abraham, S. N., J. P. Babu, C. S. Giampapa, D. L. Hasty, W. A. Simpson, and E. H. Beachey.** 1985. Protection against *Escherichia coli*-induced urinary tract infections with hybridoma antibodies directed against type 1 fimbriae or complementary D-mannose receptors. *Infect. Immun.* **48:**625–628.

3. Abraham, S. N., J. D. Goguen, and E. H. Beachey. 1988. Hyperadhesive mutant of type 1 fimbriated *Escherichia coli* associated with the formation of FimH organelles (fimbriosomes). *Infect. Immun.* **56:**1023–1029.
4. Abraham, S. N., J. D. Goguen, D. Sun, P. Klemm, and E. H. Beachey. 1987. Identification of two ancillary subunits of *Escherichia coli* type 1 fimbriae by using antibodies against synthetic oligopeptides of *fim* gene products. *J. Bacteriol.* **169:**5530–5536.
5. Abraham, S. N., M. Land, S. Ponniah, R. Endres, D. L. Hasty, and J. P. Babu. 1992. Glycerol-induced unraveling of the tight helical conformation of *Escherichia coli* type 1 fimbriae. *J. Bacteriol.* **174:**5145–5148.
6. Abraham, S. N., D. Sun, J. B. Dale, and E. H. Beachey. 1988. Conservation of the D-mannose-adhesion protein among type 1 fimbriated members of the family Enterobacteriaceae. *Nature* (London) **336:**682–684.
7. Akiyama, Y., S. Kamitani, N. Kusukawa, and K. Ito. 1992. *In vitro* catalysis of oxidative folding of disulfide-bonded proteins by the *Escherichia coli dsbA (ppfA)* gene product. *J. Biol. Chem.* **267:**22440–22445.
8. Allen, B. L., G. F. Gerlach, and S. Clegg. 1991. Nucleotide sequence and functions of *mrk* determinants necessary for expression of type 3 fimbriae in *Klebsiella pneumoniae*. *J. Bacteriol.* **173:**916–920.
9. Alzari, P. N., M. B. Lascombe, and R. J. Poljak. 1988. Three dimensional structure of antibodies. *Annu. Rev. Immunol.* **6:**555–580.
10. Amit, A. G., R. A. Marrizzua, S. E. Phillips, and R. J. Poljak. 1986. Three dimensional structure of an antibody-antigen complex at 2.8A resolution. *Science* **233:**747–753.
11. Aronson, M., O. Medalea, L. Schori, D. Mirelman, and I. Ofek. 1979. Prevention of colonization of the urinary tract of mice with Escherichia coli by blocking of bacterial adherence with methyl-α-D-mannopyranoside. *J. Infect. Dis.* **139:**329–332.
12. Baddour, L. M., G. D. Christensen, W. A. Simpson, and E. H. Beachey 1989. Microbial adherence, p. 9–25. *In* G. L. Mandell, R. G. Dangler, and J. E. Bennet (ed.), *Principles and Practice of Infectious Disease,* vol. 2. Churchill Livingstone, New York.
13. Baga, M., M. Goransson, S. Normark, and B. E. Uhlin. 1985. Transcriptional activation of a Pap pilus virulence operon from uropathogenic *Escherichia coli*. *EMBO J.* **4:**3887–3893.
14. Baga, M., M. Norgren, and S. Normark. 1987. Biogenesis of *E. coli* Pap pili: PapH, a minor pilin subunit involved in cell anchoring and length modulation. *Cell* **49:**241–251.
15. Baga, M., S. Normark, J. Hardy, P. O'Hanley, D. Lark, O. Olsson, G. Schoolnik, and S. Falkow. 1984. Nucleotide sequence of the gene encoding the *papA* pilus subunit of human uropathogenic *Escherichia coli*. *J. Bacteriol.* **157:**330–333.
16. Bahrani, F. K., S. Cook, R. Hull, G. Massad, and H. L. T. Mobley. 1993. *Proteus mirabilis* fimbriae: N-terminal amino acid sequence of a major fimbrial subunit and nucleotide sequences of the genes from two strains. *Infect. Immun.* **61:**884–891.
17. Bahrani, F. K., D. E. Johnson, D. Robbins, and H. L. T. Mobley. 1991. *Proteus mirabilis* flagella and MR/P fimbriae: isolation, purification, N-terminal analysis and serum antibody response following experimental urinary tract infection. *Infect. Immun.* **59:**3574.
18. Bakker, D., C. E. Vader, B. Roosendaal, F. R. Mooi, B. Oudega and F. K. de Graaf. 1991. Structure and function of periplasmic chaperone-like proteins involved in the biosynthesis of K88 and K99 fimbriae in enterotoxigenic *Escherichia coli*. *Mol. Microbiol.* **5:**875–886.
19. Bardwell, J. C., K. McGovern, and J. Beckwith. 1991. Identification of a protein required for disulfide bond formation *in vivo*. *Cell* **67:**581–589.
20. Bardwell, J. C. A. 1994. Building bridges: disulphide bond formation in the cell. *Mol. Microbiol.* **14:**199–205.
21. Bardwell, J. C. A., J.-O. Lee, G. Jander, N. Martin, D. Belin, and J. Beckwith. 1993. A pathway for disulfide bond formation *in vivo*. *Proc. Natl. Acad. Sci. USA* **90:**1038–1042.
22. Bazan, J. F. 1990. Structural design and molecular evolution of a cytokine receptor superfamily. *Proc. Natl. Acad. Sci. USA* **87:**6934–6938.
23. Beachey, E. H. (ed.). 1980. *Bacterial Adherence Receptors and Recognition.* Chapman & Hall, London.
24. Beachey, E. H. 1981. Bacterial adherence: adhesion-receptor interactions mediating the attachment of bacteria to mucosal surfaces. *J. Infect. Dis.* **143:**325–345.
25. Bloch, C. A., B. A. Stocker, and P. E. Orndorff. 1992. A key role for type 1 pili in enterobacterial communicability. *Mol. Microbiol.* **6:**697–701.

26. Blond-Elguindi, S., S. E. Cwirla, W. J. Dower, R. J. Lipshutz, S. R. Sprang, J. F. Sambrook, and M.-J. H. Gething. 1993. Affinity panning of a library of peptides displayed of bacteriophages reveals the binding specificty of BiP. *Cell* **75**:717–728.
27. Blumenstock, E., and K. Jann. 1982. Adhesion of piliated *Esherichia coli* strains to phagocytes: differences between bacteria with mannose-sensitive pili and those with mannose-resistant pili. *Infect. Immun.* **35**:264–269.
28. Bock, K., M. E. Breimer, A. Brignole, G. C. Hansson, K.-A. Karlsson, G. Larson, H. Leffler, B. E. Samuelsson, N. Strömberg, C. Svanborg-Edén, and J. Thurin. 1985. Specificity of binding of a strain of uropathogenic *Escherichia coli* to Galα(1-4)Gal-containing glycosphingolipids. *J. Biol. Chem.* **260**:8545–8551.
29. Braaten, B., L. B. Blyn, B. S. Skinner, and D. A. Low. 1991. Evidence for a methylation-blocking factor (*mbf*) locus involved in *pap* pilus expression and phase variation in *Escherichia coli*. *J. Bacteriol.* **173**:1789–1800.
30. Braaten, B. A., X. Nou, L. S. Kaltenbach, and D. A. Low. 1994. Methylation patterns in *pap* regulatory DNA control pyelonephritis-associated pili phase variation in *E. coli*. *Cell* **76**:577–588.
31. Braaten, B. A., J. V. Platko, M. W. Van Der Woude, B. H. Simons, F. K. De Graaf, J. M. Calvo, and D. A. Law. 1992. Leucine-responsive regulatory protein controls the expression of both the *pap* and *fan* pili operons in *Escherichia coli*. *Proc. Natl. Acad. Sci. USA* **89**:4250–4254.
32. Branden, C.-I., and J. Tooze. 1991. *Introduction to Protein Structure*. Garland Publishing, New York.
33. Brinton, C. C. 1959. Non-flagellar appendages of bacteria. *Nature* (London) **183**:782–786.
34. Brinton, C. C., A. Buzzel, and M. Laufer. 1954. Electrophoresis and phage-susceptibility studies on a filament producing variant of E. coli B bacterium. *Biochim. Biophys. Acta* **15**:533.
35. Brinton, C. C., Jr. 1965. The structure, function, synthesis, and genetic control of bacterial pili and a model for DNA and RNA transport in gram negative bacteria. *Trans. N.Y. Acad. Sci.* **27**:1003–1165.
36. Brinton, C. C. J., M. J. Carter, D. B. Derber, S. Kar, J. A. Kramarik, A. C.-C. To, S. C.-M. To, and S. W. Wood. 1989. Design and development of pilus vaccines for *Haemophilus influenzae* diseases. *Pediatr. Infect. Dis.* **8**:554–561.
37. Bullitt, E., and L. Makowski. 1995. Structural polymorphism of bacterial adhesion pili. *Nature* (London) **373**:164–167.
38. Clegg, S. 1982. Cloning of genes determining the production of mannose-resistant fimbriae in a uropathogenic *Escherichia coli* belonging to serogroup O6. *Infect. Immun.* **38**:739–744.
39. Clegg, S., S. Hull, R. Hull, and J. Pruckler. 1985. Construction and comparison of recombinant plasmids encoding type 1 fimbriae of members of the family Enterobacteriacae. *Infect. Immun.* **48**:275–279.
40. Clouthier, S. C., K. H. Muller, J. L. Doran, S. K. Collinson, and W. W. Kay. 1993. Characterization of three fimbrial genes, *sefABC*, of *Salmonella enteriditis*. *J. Bacteriol.* **175**:2523–2533.
41. Cosman, D., S. D. Lyman, R. L. Idzerda, M. P. Beckmann, L. S. Park, R. G. Goodwin, and C. J. March. 1990. A new cytokine receptor superfamily. *Trends Biochem. Sci.* **15**:265–270.
42. Craig, E. A., B. D. Gambill, and R. J. Nelson. 1993. Heat shock proteins: molecular chaperones of protein biognesis. *Microbiol. Rev.* **57**:402–410.
43. de Graaf, F. K., and F. R. Mooi. 1986. The fimbrial adhesins of *Escherichia coli*. *Adv. Microb. Physiol.* **28**:65–143.
44. DeVos, A., M. Ultsch, and A. Kossiakoff. 1992. Human growth hormone and extracellular domain of its receptor: crystal structure of the complex. *Science* **255**:306–312.
44a. Dodson, K., and S. J. Hultgren. Unpublished data.
45. Dodson, K. W., F. Jacob-Dubuisson, R. T. Striker, and S. J. Hultgren. 1993. Outer membrane PapC usher discriminately recognizes periplasmic chaperone-pilus subunit complexes. *Proc. Natl. Acad. Sci. USA* **90**:3670–3674.
46. Duguid, J. P., S. Clegg, and M. I. Wilson. 1979. The fimbrial and non-fimbrial haemagglutinins of *Escherichia coli*. *J. Med. Microbiol.* **12**:213–227.
47. Duguid, J. P., M. R. Dareker, and D. W. F. Wheater. 1976. Fimbriae and infectivity in *Salmonella typhimurium*. *J. Med. Microbiol.* **9**:459–473.
48. Duguid, J. P., and D. C. Old. 1980. Adhesive properties of Enterobacteriacae, p. 186–217. *In* E. H. Beachey (ed.), *Bacterial Adherence Receptors and Recognition*. Chapman & Hall, London.
49. Duguid, J. P., I. W. Smith, G. Dempster, and P. N. Edmunds. 1955. Non-flagellar

filamentous appendages ("fimbriae") and hemagglutinating activity in *bacterium coli*. *J. Pathol. Bacteriol.* **70**:335–348.

49a. Duncan, J. L. 1988. Differential effect of Tamm-Horsfall protein or adherence of *Escherichia coli* to transitional epithelial cells. *J. Infect. Dis.* **158**:1379–1382.

50. Eisenstein, B. I. 1981. Phase variation of type 1 fimbriae in *Escherichia coli* is under transcriptional control. *Science* **214**:337–339.

51. **Eisenstein, B. I., D. S. Sweet, V. Vaughn, and D. I. Friedman.** 1987. Integration host factor is required for the DNA inversion that controls phase variation in *Escherichia coli*. *Proc. Natl. Acad. Sci. USA* **84**:6506–6510.

52. Eisenstein, B. J. 1989. Enterobacteriacae, p. 1658–1673. *In* G. L. Mandell, R. G. Danglers, and J. E. Bennet (ed.), *Principles and Practice of Infectious Disease*, vol. 2. Churchill Livingstone, New York.

53. **Elliott, S. J., N. Nandapalan, and B. J. Chang.** 1991. Production of type 1 fimbriae by *Escherichia coli* HB101. *Microb. Pathog.* **10**:481–486.

54. **Ellis, R. J., and S. M. Hemmingsen.** 1989. Molecular chaperones: proteins essential for the biogenesis of some macromolecular structures. *Trends Biochem. Sci.* **14**:339–342.

55. **Ellis, R. J., and S. van der Vies.** 1991. Molecular chaperones. *Annu. Rev. Biochem.* **60**:321–347.

56. **Ellis, R. J., S. M. van der Vies, and S. M. Hemmingsen.** 1989. The molecular chaperone concept. *Biochem. Soc. Symp.* **55**:145–153.

57. **Erickson, A. K., J. A. Willgohs, S. Y. McFarland, D. A. Benfield, and D. H. Francis.** 1992. Identification of two porcine brush border glycoproteins that bind the K88ac adhesin of *Escherichia coli* and correlation of these glycoproteins with the adhesive phenotype. *Infect. Immun.* **60**:983.

58. **Eshdat, Y., F. J. Silverblatt, and N. Sharon.** 1981. Dissociation and reassembly of *Escherichia coli* type 1 pili. *J. Bacteriol.* **148**:308–314.

59. **Fader, R. C., E. E. Avots-Avotins, and C. P. Davis.** 1979. Evidence for pili-mediated adherence of *Klebsiella pneumoniae* to rat bladder epithelial cells in vitro. *Infect. Immun.* **25**:729–737.

60. **Fader, R. C., and C. P. Davis.** 1982. *Klebsiella pneumoniae* induced experimental pyelitis: the effect of piliation on infectivity. *J. Urol.* **128**:197–201.

61. **Firon, N., I. Ofek, and N. Sharon.** 1983. Carbohydrate specificity of the surface lectins of *Escherichia coli, Klebsiella pneumoniae* and *Salmonella typhimurium*. *Carbohydr. Res.* **120**:235–249.

62. **Friedrich, M. J., N. E. Kinsey, J. Vila, and R. J. Kadner.** 1993. Nucleotide sequence of a 13.9 kb segment of the 90 kb virulence plasmid of *Salmonella typphimurium:* the presence of a fimbrial biosynthetic gene. *Mol. Microbiol.* **8**:543–558.

63. **Frydman, J., E. Nimmesgern, K. Ohtsuka, and F. U. Hartl.** 1994. Folding of nascent polypeptide chains in a high molecular mass assembly with molecular chaperones. *Nature* (London) **370**:111–117.

64. **Gbarah, A., C. G. Gahmberg, I. Ofek, U. Jacobi, and N. Sharon.** 1991. Identification of the leukocyte adhesion molecules CD11/CD18 as receptors for type 1 fimbriated (mannose specific) *Escherichia coli*. *Infect. Immun.* **59**:4524–4530.

65. **Gerlach, G. F., B. L. Allen, and S. Clegg.** 1988. Molecular characterization of the type 3 (MR/K) fimbriae of *Klebsiella pneumoniae*. *J. Bacteriol.* **170**:3547–3553.

66. Gething, M. J. 1991. Molecular chaperones: individualists or groupies? *Curr. Opin. Cell Biol.* **3**:610–614.

67. **Gething, M. J., and J. Sambrook.** 1992. Protein folding in the cell. *Nature* (London) **355**:33–45.

68. **Giampapa, C. S., S. N. Abraham, T. M. Chiang, and E. H. Beachey.** 1988. Isolation and characterization of the receptor for type 1 fimbriae of *Escherichia coli* from guinea pig erythrocytes. *J. Biol. Chem.* **263**:5362–5367.

69. **Girdeau, J. P., M. D. Vartanian, J. L. Ollier, and M. Contrepois.** 1988. CS31A, a new K88-related fimbrial antigen on bovine enteropathogenic and septicemic *Escherichia coli* strains. *Infect. Immun.* **56**:2180–2188.

70. Goetz, M. B. 1989. Priming of polymorphonuclear neutrophilic leukocyte oxidative activity by type 1 pili from Escherichia coli. *J. Infect. Dis.* **159**:533–542.

71. **Goetz, M. B., and F. J. Silverblatt.** 1987. Stimulation of human polymorphonuclear leukocyte oxidative metabolism by type 1 pili from *Escherichia coli*. *Infect. Immun.* **55**:534–540.

72. **Goldhar, J., R. Perry, J. R. Golecki, H. Hoschutzky, B. Jann, and K. Jann.** 1987. Nonfimbrial, mannose-resistant adhesins from uropathogenic *Escherichia coli* O83:K1:H4 and O14:K?:H11. *Infect. Immun.* **55**:1837–1842.

73. Gong, M., and L. Makowski. 1992. Helical structure of Pap adhesion pili from *Escherichia coli*. *J. Mol. Biol.* **228:**735–742.
74. Goransson, M., K. Forsman, P. Nilsson, and B. E. Uhlin. 1989. Upstream activating sequences that are shared by two divergently transcribed operons mediate cAMP-CRP regulation of pilus-adhesin in *Escherichia coli*. *Mol. Microbiol.* **3:**1557–1565.
75. Goransson, M., K. Forsman, and B. E. Uhlin. 1989. Regulatory genes in the thermoregulation of Escherichia coli pili gene transcription. *Genes Dev.* **3:**123–130.
76. Goransson, M., B. Sonden, P. Nilsson, B. Dagberg, K. Forsman, K. Emanuelsson, and B. E. Uhlin. 1990. Transcriptional silencing and thermoregulation of gene expression in *Escherichia coli*. *Nature* (London) **344:**682–685.
77. Grunberg, J., R. Perry, H. Hoschutsky, B. Jann, and K. G. Jann. 1988. Nonfimbrial blood group N-specific adhesin (NFA-3) from *Escherichia coli* O20:KX104:H-, causing systemic infection. *FEMS Microbiol. Lett.* **56:**241.
78. Guerina, N. G., S. Langerman, H. W. Clegg, T. W. Kessler, D. A. Goldmann, and J. R. Gilsdorf. 1982. Adherence of piliated *Hemophilus influenzae* to human oropharyngeal cells. *J. Infect. Dis.* **146:**564.
79. Guyot, G. 1908. Uber die bakterielle Haemagglutination (Bacterio-Haemagglutination). *Zentralbl. Bakteriol. Parasitenkd. Infektionskr. Hyg. Abt. 1 Orig.* **47:**640–653.
80. Hacker, J., G. Schmidt, C. Hughes, S. Knapp, M. Marget, and W. Goebel. 1985. Cloning and characterization of genes involved in production of mannose-resistant neuraminidase-susceptible (X) fimbriae from a uropathogenic O6:K15:H31 *Escherichia coli* strain. *Infect. Immun.* **47:**434–440.
81. Hagberg, L., U. Jodal, T. Korhonen, G. Lidin-Janson, U. Lindberg, and C. Svanborg-Eden. 1981. Adheson, hemagglutination, and virulence of *Escherichia coli* causing urinary tract infections. *Infect. Immun.* **31:**564–570.
82. Hakomori, S.-I. 1990. Bifunctional role of glycosphingolipids: modulators for transmembrane signaling and mediators for cellular interactions. *J. Biol. Chem.* **265:**18713–18716.
83. Hammond, C., and A. Helenius. 1994. Folding of VSV G protein: sequential interaction with BiP and Calnexin. *Science* **266:**456–458.
84. Hardy, S. J., and L. L. Randall. 1991. A kinetic partitioning model of selective binding of nonnative proteins by the bacterial chaperone SecB. *Science* **251:**439–443.
85. Hartl, F. U., J. Martin, and W. Neupert. 1992. Protein folding in the cell: the role of molecular chaperones Hsp70 and Hsp60. *Annu. Rev. Biophys. Biomol. Struct. Adv. Exp. Med. Biol.* **21:**293–322.
86. Haslam, D., T. Boren, P. Falk, D. Ilver, A. Chou, Z. Xu, and S. Normark. 1994. The amino-terminal domain of the P-pilus adhesin determines receptor specificity. *Mol. Microbiol.* **14:**399–409.
87. Heuser, J. 1989. Protocol for 3-D visualization of molecules on mica via the quickfreeze, deep-etch technique. *J. Electron Microsc. Tech.* **13:**244–263.
88. Holmgren, A., and C. Brändén. 1989. Crystal structure of chaperone protein PapD reveals an immunoglobulin fold. *Nature* (London) **342:**248–251.
89. Holmgren, A., M. J. Kuehn, C.-I. Brändén, and S. J. Hultgren. 1992. Conserved imunoglobulin-like features in a family of periplasmic pilus chaperones in bacteria. *EMBO J.* **11:**1617–1622.
90. Hoschutzky, H., W. Nimmich, F. Lottspeich, and K. Jann. 1989. Isolation and characterization of the non-fimbrial adhesin NFA-4 from uropathogenic *Escherichia coli* O7:K98:H6. *Microb. Pathog.* **6:**351–359.
91. Hull, R. A., R. E. Gill, P. Hsu, B. H. Minshaw, and S. Falkow. 1981. Construction and expression of recombinant plasmids encoding type 1 and D-mannose-resistant pili from a urinary tract infection *Escherichia coli* isolate. *Infect. Immun.* **33:**933–938.
92. Hull, R. A., and S. I. Hull. 1994. Adherence mechanisms is urinary tract infections, p. 79–91. In V. L. Miller, J. B. Kaper, D. A. Portnoy, and R. R. Isberg (ed.), *Molecular Genetics of Bacteial Pathogenesis*. ASM Press, Washington, D.C.
93. Hultgren, S. J., S. N. Abraham, M. G. Caparon, P. Falk, J. W. St. Geme III, and S. Normark. 1993. Pilus and non-pilus bacterial adhesins:assembly and function in cell recognition. *Cell* **73:**887–901.
94. Hultgren, S. J., J. L. Duncan, A. J. Schaeffer, and S. K. Amundsen. 1990. Mannose-sensitive hemagglutination in the absence of piliation in *Escherichia coli*. *Mol. Microbiol.* **4:**1311–1318.
95. Hultgren, S. J., F. Jacob-Dubuisson, C. H. Jones, and C.-I. Brändén. 1993. PapD and superfamily of periplasmic immunoglobulin-like pilus chaperones. *Adv. Protein Chem.* **44:**99–123.

96. Hultgren, S. J., F. Lindberg, G. Magnusson, J. Kihlberg, J. M. Tennent, and S. Normark. 1989. The PapG adhesin of uropathogenic *Escherichia coli* contains separate regions for receptor binding and for the incorporation into the pilus. *Proc. Natl. Acad. Sci. USA* **86**:4357–4361.
97. Hultgren, S. J., and S. Normark. 1991. Biogenesis of the bacterial pilus. *Curr. Opin. Genes Dev.* **1**:313–318.
98. Hultgren, S. J., S. Normark, and S. N. Abraham. 1991. Chaperone-assisted assembly and molecular architecture of adhesive pili. *Annu. Rev. Microbiol.* **45**:383–415.
99. Hultgren, S. J., T. N. Porter, A. J. Schaeffer, and J. L. Duncan. 1985. Role of type 1 pili and effects of phase variation on lower urinary tract infections produced by *Escherichia coli*. *Infect. Immun.* **50**:370–377.
99a. Hung, D. Personal communication.
100. Iriarte, M., C. Vanooteghem, I. Delor, R. Diaz, S. Knutton, and G. R. Cornelis. 1993. The Myf fibrillae of *Yersinia enterocolitica*. *Mol. Microbiol.* **9**:507–520.
101. Jacob-Dubuisson, F., J. Heuser, K. Dodson, S. Normark, and S. J. Hultgren. 1993. Initiation of assembly and association of the structural elements of a bacterial pilus depend on two specialized tip proteins. *EMBO J.* **12**:837–847.
102. Jacob-Dubuisson, F., M. Kuehn, and S. Hultgren. 1993. A novel secretion apparatus for the assembly of adhesive bacterial pili. *Trends Microbiol.* **1**:50–55.
103. Jacob-Dubuisson, F., J. Pinkner, Z. Xu, R. Striker, A. Padmanhaban, and S. J. Hultgren. 1994. PapD chaperone function in pilus biogenesis depends on oxidant and chaperone-like activities of DsbA. *Proc. Natl. Acad. Sci. USA* **91**:11552–11556.
104. Jann, K., and H. Hoschutzky. 1990. Nature and organization of adhesins. *Curr. Top. Microbiol. Immunol.* **151**:55.
105. Jann, K., and H. Hoschutzky 1991. Characterization and surface organization of *E. coli* adhesins. *In* E. Z. Ron and S. Rottem (ed.), *Microbial Surface Components and Toxins in Relation to Pathogenesis*. Plenum Press, New York.
106. Jokinen, M., C. Ehnholm, V. Vaisanen-Rhen, T. K. Korhonen, R. Pipkorn, N. Kalkkinen, and C. G. Gahmberg. 1985. Identification of the major human sialylglycoprotein from red cells, glycophorin AM, as the receptor for *Escherichia coli* IH11165 and characterization of the receptor site. *Eur. J. Biochem.* **147**:47.
106a. Jones, C. H., E. Bullitt, G. E. Soto, R. T. Striker, F. Jacob-Dubuisson, M. J. Wick, L. Makowski, and S. J. Hultgren. Development of pilus organelle subassemblies in vitro depends on chaperone uncapping of a beta zipper. Submitted for publication.
107. Jones, C. H., and S. J. Hultgren. Periplasmic chaperones mediate protein import into the periplasmic space in bacteria. Submitted for publication.
108. Jones, C. H., J. S. Pinkner, A. V. Nicholes, L. N. Slonim, S. N. Abraham, and S. J. Hultgren. 1993. FimC is a periplasmic PapD-like chaperone that directs assembly of type 1 pili in bacteria. *Proc. Natl. Acad. Sci. USA* **90**:8397–8401.
109. Jones, C. H., J. S. Pinkner, R. Roth, J. Heuser, A. V. Nicholes, S. N. Abraham, and S. J. Hultgren. 1995. FimH adhesin of type 1 pili is assembled into a fibrillar tip structure in the *Enterobacteriaceae*. *Proc. Natl. Acad. Sci. USA* **92**:2081–2085.
110. Kallenius, G., R. Mollby, S. B. Svenson, J. Windberg, A. Lundblad, S. Svenson, and B. Cedergen. 1980. The $P^k$ antigen as receptor for the haemagglutinin of pyelonephritogenic *Escherichia coli*. *FEMS Microbiol. Lett.* **8**:297–302.
111. Kallenius, G., S. B. Svenson, H. Hultberg, R. Molby, I. Helin, B. Cedergen, and J. Windberg. 1981. Occurrence of P fimbriated *Escherichia coli* in urinary tract infection. *Lancet* **ii**:1369–1372.
112. Kamitani, S., Y. Akiyama, and K. Ito. 1992. Identification and characterization of an *Escherichia coli* gene required for the formation of correctly folded alkaline phosphatase, a periplasmic enzyme. *EMBO J.* **11**:57–62.
113. Kaper, J. B. 1994. Molecular pathogenesis of enteropathogenic *Escherichia coli*, p. 173–197. *In* V. L. Miller, J. B. Kaper, D. A. Portnoy, and R. R. Isberg (ed.), *Molecular Genetics of Bacterial Pathogenesis*. ASM Press, Washington, D.C.
114. Karlyshev, A., E. Galyov, O. Smirnov, A. Guzayev, V. Abramov, and V. Zav'yalov. 1992. A new gene of the *f1* operon of *Y. pestis* involved in the capsule biogenesis. *FEBS Lett.* **297**:77–80.
115. Keith, B. R., S. L. Harris, P. W. Russell, and P. E. Orndorff. 1990. Effect of type 1 piliation on in vitro killing of *Escherichia coli* by mouse peritoneal macrophages. *Infect. Immun.* **58**:3448–3454.

116. Keith, B. R., L. Maurer, P. A. Spears, and P. E. Orndorff. 1986. Receptor-binding function of type 1 pili effects bladder colonization by a clinical isolate of *Escherichia coli*. *Infect. Immun.* **53:**693–696.
117. Kihlberg, J., S. J. Hultgren, S. Normark, and G. Magnusson. 1989. Probing of the combining site of the PapG adhesion of uropathogenic *Escherichia coli* bacteria by synthetic analogues of galabiose. *J. Am. Chem. Soc.* **111:**6364–6368.
118. Klemm, P. 1985. Fimbrial adhesins of *Escherchia coli*. *Rev. Infect. Dis.* **7:**321–329.
119. Klemm, P. 1986. Two regulatory *fim* genes, *fimB* and *fimE*, control the phase variation of type 1 fimbriae in *Escherichia coli*. *EMBO J.* **5:**1389–1393.
120. Klemm, P. (ed.). 1994. *Fimbriae: Adhesion, Genetics, Biogenesis, and Vaccines*. CRC Press, Inc., Ann Arbor, Mich.
121. Klemm, P., and G. Christiansen. 1987. Three *fim* genes required for the regulation of length and mediation of adhesion of *Escherichia coli* type 1 fimbriae. *Mol. Gen. Genet.* **208:**439–445.
122. Klemm, P., and G. Christiansen. 1990. The *fimD* gene required for cell surface localization of *Escherichia coli* type 1 fimbriae. *Mol. Gen. Genet.* **220:**334–338.
123. Klemm, P., B. J. Jorgensen, I. van Die, H. de Ree, and H. Bergman. 1985. The *fim* genes responsible for synthesis of type 1 fimbriae in *Escherichia coli* cloning and genetic organization. *Mol. Gen. Genet.* **199:**410–414.
124. Knutton, S., M. M. Baldini, J. B. Kaper, and A. S. McNeish. 1987. Role of plasmid-encoded adherence factors in adhesion of enteropathogenic *Escherichia coli* to HEp-2 cells. *Infect. Immun.* **55:**78–85.
125. Korhonen, T., V. Vaisanen-Rhen, M. Rhen, A. Pere, J. Parkkinen, and J. Finne. 1984. *Escherichia coli* fimbriae recognizing sialyl galactosides. *J. Bacteriol.* **159:**762–766.
126. Korhonen, T. K., J. Parkkinen, J. Hacker, J. Finne, A. Pere, M. Rhen, and H. Holthofer. 1986. Binding of *Escherichia coli* S fimbriae to human kidney epithelium. *Infect. Immun.* **54:**322–327.
127. Korhonen, T. K., M. V. Valtonen, J. Parkkinen, V. Vaisanen-Rhen, J. Finne, F. Orskov, I. Orskov, S. B. Svenson, and P. H. Makela. 1985. Serotypes, hemolysin production, and receptor recognition of *Escherichia coli* strains associated with neonatal sepsis and meningitis. *Infect. Immun.* **48:**486–491.
128. Korhonen, T. K., R. Virkola, and H. Holthofer. 1986. Localization of binding sites for purified *Escherichia coli* P fimbriae in the human kidney. *Infect. Immun.* **54:**328–332.
129. Krivan, H. C., D. D. Roberts, and V. Ginsburg. 1988. Many pulmonary pathogenic bacteria bind specifically to the carbohydrate sequence GalNac$\beta$1-4Gal found in some glycolipids. *Proc. Natl. Acad. Sci. USA* **85:**6157–6161.
130. Krogfelt, K. A., H. Bergmans, and P. Klemm. 1990. Direct evidence that the FimH protein is the mannose specific adhesin of *Escherichia coli* type 1 fimbriae. *Infect. Immun.* **58:**1995–1999.
131. Kuehn, M. J., J. Heuser, S. Normark, and S. J. Hultgren. 1992. P pili in uropathogenic *E. coli* are composite fibres with distinct fibrillar adhesive tips. *Nature* (London) **356:**252–255.
132. Kuehn, M. J., S. Normark, and S. J. Hultgren. 1991. Immunoglobulin-like PapD chaperone caps and uncaps interactive surfaces of nascently translocated pilus subunits. *Proc. Natl. Acad. Sci. USA* **88:**10586–10590.
133. Kuehn, M. J., D. J. Ogg, J. Kihlberg, L. N. Slonim, K. Flemmer, T. Bergfors, and S. J. Hultgren. 1993. Structural basis of pilus subunit recognition by the PapD chaperone. *Science* **262:**1234–1241.
134. Kukkonen, M., T. Raunio, R. Virkola, K. Lahteenmaki, P. H. Makela, P. Klemm, S. Clegg, and T. K. Korhonen. 1993. Basement membrane carbohydrate as a target for bacterial adhesion: binding of type 1 fimbriae of *Salmonella enterica* and *Escherichia coli* to laminin. *Mol. Microbiol.* **7:**229–237.
135. Kumamoto, C. A. 1991. Molecular chaperones and protein translocation across the Escherichia coli inner membrane. *Mol. Microbiol.* **5:**19–22.
136. Kunin, C. M., H. H. Tong, C. Krishnan, L. Van Arsdale White, and J. Hacker. 1993. Isolation of a nicotinamide-requiring clone of *Escherichia coli* O18:K1:H7 from women with acute cystitis: resemblance to strains found in neonatal meningitis. *Clin. Infect. Dis.* **16:**412–416.
137. Labigne-Roussel, A. F., D. Lark, G. Schoolnik, and S. Falkow. 1984. Cloning and expression of an afimbrial adhesin (AFA-I) responsible for P blood group-independent, mannose-resistant hemagglutination from a pyelonephritic *Escherichia coli* strain. *Infect. Immun.* **46:**251–259.

138. Langer, T., C. Lu, H. Echols, J. Flanagan, M. K. Hayer, and F. U. Hartl. 1992. Successive action of DnaK, DnaJ and GroEL along the pathway of chaperone-mediated protein folding. *Nature* (London) **356**:683–689.
139. Latham, R. H., and W. E. Stamm. 1984. Role of fimbriated *Escherichia coli* in urinary tract infections in adult women: correlation with localization studies. *J. Infect. Dis.* **149**:835–840.
140. Le Bouguenec, C., M. I. Garcia, V. Ouin, J.-M. Desperrier, P. Gounon, and A. Labigne. 1993. Characterization of plasmid-borne *afa-3* gene clusters encoding afimbrial adhesins expressed by *Escherichia coli* strains associated with intestinal or urinary tract infections. *Infect. Immun.* **61**:5106–5114.
141. Lecker, S., R. Lill, T. Ziegelhoffer, C. Georgopoulos, P. J. Bassford, C. A. Kumamoto, and W. Wickner. 1989. Three pure chaperone proteins of Escherichia coli—SecB, trigger factor and GroEL—form soluble complexes with precursor proteins in vitro. *EMBO J.* **8**:2703–2709.
142. Leffler, H., and C. Svanborg-Eden. 1980. Chemical identification of a glycosphingolipid receptor for *Escherichia coli* attaching to human urinary tract epithelial cells and agglutinating human erythrocytes. *FEMS Microbiol. Lett.* **8**:127–134.
143. Levine, M. M., P. Ristaino, G. Marley, C. Smyth, S. Knutton, E. Boedeker, R. Black, C. Young, M. L. Clements, C. Cheney, and R. Patnaik. 1984. Coli surface antigens 1 and 3 of colonization factor antigen II-positive enterotoxigenic *Escherichia coli*: morphology, purification, and immune responses in humans. *Infect. Immun.* **44**:409–429.
144. Lindberg, F., J. M. Tennent, S. J. Hultgren, B. Lund, and S. Normark. 1989. PapD, a periplasmic transport protein in P-pilus biogenesis. *J. Bacteriol.* **171**:6052–6058.
145. Lindberg, F. P., B. Lund, and S. Normark. 1984. Genes of pyelonephritogenic *E. coli* required for digalactoside-specific agglutination of human cells. *EMBO J.* **3**:1167–1173.
146. Lindberg, F. P., B. Lund, and S. Normark. 1986. Gene products specifying adhesion of uropathogenic *Escherichia coli* are minor components of pili. *Proc. Natl. Acad. Sci. USA* **83**:1891–1895.
147. Lindler, L. E., and B. D. Tall. 1993. *Yersinia pestis* pH 6 antigen forms fimbriae and is induced by intracellular association with macrophages. *Mol. Microbiol.* **8**:311–324.
148. Lintermans, P. F., P. Pohl, A. Bertels, G. Charlier, J. Vandekerckhove, J. Van Damme, J. Shoup, C. Schlicker, T. Korhonen, H. De Greve, and M. Van Montagu. 1988. Characterization and purification of the F17 adhesin on the surface of bovine enteropathogenic and septicemic *Escherichia coli*. *Am. J. Vet. Res.* **49**:1794–1799.
149. Locht, C., M.-C. Geoffroy, and G. Renauld. 1992. Common accessory genes for the *Bordetella pertussis* filamentous hemagglutinin and fimbriae share sequence similarities with the *papC* and *papD* gene families. *EMBO J.* **11**:3175–3183.
150. Lund, B., F. Lindberg, B. I. Marklund, and S. Normark. 1987. The PapG protein is the alpha-D-galactopyranosyl-(1-4)-beta-D-galactopyranose-binding adhesin of uropathogenic *Escherichia coli*. *Proc. Natl. Acad. Sci. USA* **84**:5898–5902.
151. Lund, B., B. I. Marklund, N. Stromberg, F. Lindberg, K. A. Karlsson, and S. Normark. 1988. Uropathogenic *Escherichia coli* can express serologically identical pili of different receptor binding specificities. *Mol. Microbiol.* **2**:255–263.
152. Mabeck, C. E., F. Orskov, and I. Orskov. 1971. *Escherichia coli* serotypes and renal involvement in urinary tract infection. *Lancet* **i**:1312–1314.
153. Madison, B., I. Ofek, S. Clegg, and S. N. Abraham. 1994. Type 1 fimbrial shafts of *Escherichia coli* and *Klebsiella pneumoniae* influence sugar-binding specificities of their FimH adhesins. *Infect. Immun.* **62**:843–848.
154. Martin, J., S. Geromanas, P. Tempst, and F. U. Hartl. 1993. Identification of nucleotide-binding regions in the chaperonin proteins GroEL and GroES. *Nature* (London) **366**:279–282.
155. Martin, J., T. Langer, R. Boteva, A. Schramel, A. L. Horwich, and F. U. Hartl. 1991. Chaperonin-mediated protein folding at the surface of groEL through a 'molten globule'-like intermediate. *Nature* (London) **352**:36–42.
156. Martin, J., M. Mayhew, T. Langer, and F. U. Hartl. 1993. The reaction cycle of GroEl and GroES in chaperonin assisted protein folding. *Nature* (London) **366**:228–233.
157. Martin, J. L., J. C. A. Bardwell, and J. Kuriyan. 1993. Crystal structure of the DsbA protein required for disulfide bond

formation in vivo. *Nature* (London) **365**: 464–468.
158. **Massad, G., C. V. Lockatell, D. E. Johnson, and H. L. T. Mobley.** 1994. *Proteus mirabilis* fimbriae: construction of an isogenic *pmfA* mutant and analysis of virulence in a CBA mouse model of ascending urinary tract infection. *Infect. Immun.* **62**:536–542.
159. **Matsuyama, S., Y. Fujita, and S. Mizushima.** 1993. SecD is involved in the release of translocated secretory proteins from the cytoplasmic membrane of *Escherichia coli*. *EMBO J.* **12**:265–270.
160. **Maurer, L., and P. E. Orndorff.** 1985. A new locus, *pilE*, required for the binding of type 1 piliated *Escherichia coli* to erythrocytes. *FEMS Microbiol. Lett.* **30**:59–66.
161. **Maurer, L., and P. E. Orndorff.** 1987. Identification and characterization of genes determining receptor binding and pilus length of *Escherichia coli* type 1 pili. *J. Bacteriol.* **169**:640–645.
162. **Metcalfe, J. W., K. A. Krogfelt, H. C. Krivan, P. S. Cohen, and D. C. Laux.** 1991. Characterization and identification of a porcine small intestine mucus receptor for the K88ab fimbrial adhesin. *Infect. Immun.* **59**:91–96.
163. **Meyer, T. F., C. P. Gibbs, and R. Haas.** 1990. Variation and control of protein expression in *Neisseria*. *Annu. Rev. Microbiol.* **44**:451–477.
164. **Miller, V. L., J. B. Kaper, D. A. Portnoy, and R. R. Isberg (ed.).** 1994. *Molecular Genetics of Bacterial Pathogenesis.* ASM Press, Washington, D.C.
165. **Minion, F. C., S. N. Abraham, E. H. Beachey, and J. D. Goguen.** 1989. The genetic determinant of adhesive function in type 1 fimbriae of *Escherichia coli* is distinct from the gene encoding the fimbrial subunit. *J. Bacteriol.* **165**:1033–1036.
166. **Mirelman, D. (ed.).** 1986. *Microbial Lectins and Agglutinins.* John Wiley & Sons, Inc., New York.
167. **Mitsui, Y., F. P. Dyer, and R. Langridge.** 1973. X-ray diffraction studies on bacterial pili. *J. Mol. Biol.* **79**:57.
168. **Mobley, H., K. Jarvis, J. Elwood, D. Whittle, V. Lockatell, R. Russel, D. Johnson, M. Donnenberg, and J. Warren.** 1993. Isogenic P-fimbriated deletion mutants of pyelonephritogenic *Escherichia coli*: the role of $\alpha$Gal(1-4)$\beta$Gal binding in virulence of a wild-type strain. *Mol. Microbiol.* **10**:143–155.
169. **Moch, T., H. Hoschutzky, J. Hacker, K.-D. Kroncke, and K. Jann.** 1987. Isolation and characterization of the a-sialyl-b-2,3-galactosyl-specific adhesin from fimbriated *Escherichia coli*. *Proc. Natl. Acad. Sci. USA* **84**:3462–3466.
170. **Mol, O., R. W. Vischers, F. K. de Graaf, and B. Oudega.** 1994. *Escherichia coli* periplasmic chaperone FaeE is a homodimer and the chaperone-K88 subunit complex is a heterotrimer. *Mol. Microbiol.* **11**:391–402.
171. **Mooi, F. R., W. H. Jansen, H. Brunings, H. Gielen, H. G. J. van der Heide, H. C. Walvoort, and P. A. M. Guniee.** 1992. Construction and analysis of *Bordetella pertussis* mutants defective in the production of fimbriae. *Microb. Pathog.* **12**:127.
172. **Mooi, F. R., H. G. J. van der Heide, H. C. Walvoort, H. Brunings, W. H. Jansen, and P. A. M. Guinee** 1991. The analysis of *Bordetella pertussis* fimbrial mutants in a rabbit model, p. 69–76. *In* E. Z. Ron and S. Rottem (ed.), *Microbial Surface Components and Toxins in Relation to Pathogenesis.* Plenum Press, New York.
173. **Muller, K. H., S. K. Collinson, T. J. Trust, and W. W. Kay.** 1991. Type 1 fimbriae of *Salmonella enteriditis*. *J. Bacteriol.* **173**: 454–457.
174. **Neeser, J. R., B. Koellreutter, and P. Wuersch.** 1986. Oligomannoside-type glycopeptides inhibiting adhesion of *Escherichia coli* strains mediated by type 1 pili: preparation of potent inhibitors from plant glycoproteins. *Infect. Immun.* **52**:428–436.
175. **Nicchitta, C. V., and G. Blobel.** 1993. Lumenal proteins of the mammalian endoplasmic reticulum are required to complete protein translocation. *Cell* **73**:989–998.
176. **Nilsson, P., and B. E. Uhlin.** 1991. Differential decay of a polycistronic *Escherichia coli* transcript is initiated by RNaseE-dependent endonucleolytic processing. *Mol. Microbiol.* **5**:1791–1799.
177. **Norgren, M., M. Baga, J. M. Tennent, and S. Normark.** 1987. Nucleotide sequence, regulation and functional analysis of the *papC* gene required for cell surface localization of Pap pili of uropathogenic *Escherichia coli*. *Mol. Microbiol.* **1**:169–178.
178. **Nowicki, B., A. Labigne, S. Mosley, R. Hull, S. Hull, and J. Moulds.** 1990. The Dr hemagglutinin, afimbrial adhesins AFA-1 and AFA-III, and F1845 fimbriae of uropathogenic and diarrhea-associated *Escherichia coli* belong to a family of hemagglutinins with Dr receptor recognition. *Infect. Immun.* **58**:279.

179. Nowicki, B., J. Moulds, R. Hull, and S. Hull. 1988. A hemagglutinatinin of uropathogenic *Escherichia coli* reconizes the DR blood group antigen. *Infect. Immun.* **56**:5106.
180. Ofek, I., D. Mirelman, and N. Sharon. 1977. Adherence of *Escherichia coli* to human mucosal cells mediated by mannose receptors. *Nature* (London) **265**:623–625.
181. O'Hanley, P., D. Lark, S. Falkow, and G. Schoolnik. 1985. Molecular basis of *Escherichia coli* colonization of the upper urinary tract in BALB/c mice: Gal-Gal pili immunization prevents *Escherichia coli* pyelonephritis. *J. Clin. Invest.* **83**:2102–2108.
182. Old, D. C. 1972. Inhibition of the interaction between fimbrial hemagglutinatinins and erythrocytes by D-mannose and other carbohydrates. *J. Gen. Microbiol.* **71**:149–157.
183. Old, D. C., and R. A. Adegbola. 1983. A new mannose-resistant haemagglutinatinin in *Klebsiella*. *J. Appl. Bacteriol.* **55**:165.
184. Old, D. C., A. Tavendale, and B. W. Senior. 1985. A comparative study of the type 3 fimbriae of *Klebsiella* species. *J. Med. Microbiol.* **20**:203.
185. Ono, E., K. Abe, M. Nakazawa, and M. Naiki. 1989. Ganglioside epitope recognized by K99 fimbriae from enterotoxigenic *Escherichia coli*. *Infect. Immun.* **57**:907–911.
186. Orndorff, P. E. 1994. *Escherichia coli* type 1 pili, p. 91–111. *In* V. L. Miller, J. B. Kaper, D. A. Portnoy, and R. R. Isberg (ed.), *Molecular Genetics of Bacterial Pathogenesis*. ASM Press, Washington, D.C.
187. Orndorff, P. E., and C. A. Bloch. 1990. The role of type 1 pili in the pathogenesis of *Escherichia coli* infections: a short review and some new ideas. *Microb. Pathog.* **9**:75–79.
188. Orndorff, P. E., and S. Falkow. 1984. Organization and expression of genes responsible for type 1 piliation in *Escherichia coli*. *J. Bacteriol.* **159**:736–744.
189. Orskov, I., A. Birch-Anderson, J. P. Duguid, J. Stenderup, and F. Ørskov. 1985. An adhesive protein capsule of *Escherichia coli*. *Infect. Immun.* **47**:191–200.
190. Orskov, I., F. Orskov, and A. Birch-Andersen. 1980. Comparison of *Escherichia coli* fimbrial antigen F7 with type 1 fimbriae. *Infect. Immun.* **27**:657–666.
191. Ott, M., J. Hacker, T. Schmoll, T. Jarchau, T. K. Korhonen, and W. Goebel. 1986. Analysis of the genetic determinants coding for the S-fimbrial adhesin (*sfa*) in different *Escherichia coli* strains causing meningitis or urinary tract infections. *Infect. Immun.* **54**:646–653.
192. Paranchych, W., and L. S. Frost. 1988. The physiology and biochemistry of pili. *Adv. Microb. Physiol.* **29**:53–114.
193. Paranchych, W., P. A. Sastry, K. Volpel, B. A. Loh, and D. Speert. 1986. Fimbriae (pili): molecular basis of Pseudomonas aeruginosa adherence. *Clin. Invest. Med.* **9**:113–118.
194. Parkkinen, J., J. Finne, M. Achtman, M. Vaisanen, T. K. Korhonen, and W. Goebel. 1983. *Escherichia coli* strains binding neuraminyl a2-3 galactosides. *Biochem. Biophys. Res. Commun.* **111**:456–461.
195. Parkkinen, J., G. N. Rogers, T. K. Korhonen, W. Dahr, and J. Finne. 1986. Identification of the O-linked sialyloligosaccharides of glycophorin A as the erythrocyte receptors for S-fimbriated *Escherichia coli*. *Infect. Immun.* **54**:37–42.
196. Parkkinen, J., R. Virkola, and T. K. Korhonen. 1988. Identification of factors in human urine that inhibit the binding of *Escherichia coli* adhesins. *Infect. Immun.* **56**:2623–2630.
197. Pecha, B., D. Low, and P. O'Hanley. 1989. Gal-Gal pili vaccines prevent pyelonephritis by piliated *Escherichia coli* in a murine model. Single-component Gal-Gal pili vaccines prevent pyelonephritis by homologous and heterologous piliated *E. coli* strains. *J. Clin. Invest.* **83**:2102–2108.
198. Peek, J. A., and R. K. Taylor. 1992. Characterization of a periplasmic thiol:disulfide interchange protein required for the functional maturation of secreted virulence factors of *Vibrio cholerae*. *Proc. Natl. Acad. Sci. USA* **89**:6210–6214.
199. Poljak, R. J., L. M. Amzel, H. P. Avey, B. L. Chen, R. P. Phizackerley, and F. Saul. 1973. Three dimensional structure of the Fab fragment of a human immunoglobulin at 2.8A resolution. *Proc. Natl. Acad. Sci. USA* **70**:3305–3310.
200. Ponniah, S., R. O. Endres, D. L. Hasty, and S. N. Abraham. 1991. Fragmentation of *Escherichia coli* type 1 fimbriae exposes cryptic D-mannose-binding sites. *J. Bacteriol.* **173**:4195–4202.
201. Purcell, B. K., J. Pruckler, and S. Clegg. 1987. Nucleotide sequences of the genes encoding type 1 fimbrial subunits of *Klebsiella pneumoniae* and *Salmonella typhimurium*. *J. Bacteriol.* **169**:5831–5834.
202. Raina, S., D. Missiakas, L. Baird, S. Kumar, and C. Georgopoulos. 1993. Identification and transcriptional analysis of the *Escherichia coli htrE* operon which is homologous to *pap* and related pilin operons. *J. Bacteriol.* **175**:5009–5021.

203. **Randall, L. L.** 1992. Peptide binding by chaperone SecB: implications for recognition of nonnative structure. *Science* **257:** 241–245.
204. **Rhen, M., V. Vaisanen-Rhen, M. Sarasta, and T. K. Korhonen.** 1986. Organization of genes expressing the blood group M-specific hemagglutinin of *Escherichia coli*: identification and nucleotide sequence of the M-agglutinin subunit gene. *Gene* **49:**351.
205. **Riegman, N., R. Kusters, H. Van Veggel, H. Bergmans, P. Van Bergen En Henegouwen, J. Hacker, and I. Van Die.** 1990. F1C fimbriae of a uropathogenic *Escherichia coli* strain: genetic and functional organization of the *foc* gene cluster and identification of minor subunits. *J. Bacteriol.* **172:** 1114–1120.
206. **Roberts, J. A., K. Hardaway, B. Kaack, E. N. Fussell, and G. Baskin.** 1984. Prevention of pyelonephritis by immunization with P-fimbriae. *J. Urol.* **131:**602–607.
207. **Roberts, J. A., B. Kaack, G. Kallenius, R. Mollby, J. Winberg, and S. B. Svenson.** 1984. Receptors for pyelonephritogenic *Escherichia coli* in primates. *J. Urol.* **131:** 163–168.
208. **Roberts, J. A., M. B. Kaack, G. Baskin, T. K. Korhonen, S. B. Svensson, and J. Winberg.** 1989. P-fimbriae vaccines. II. Cross reactive protection against pyelonephritis. *Pediatr. Nephrol.* **3:**391–396.
209. **Roberts, J. A., B.-I. Marklund, D. Ilver, D. Haslam, M. B. Kaack, G. Baskin, M. Louis, R. Mollby, J. Winberg, and S. Normark.** 1994. The Gal α(1-4) Gal-specific tip adhesin of *Escherichia coli* P-fimbriae is needed for pyelonephritis to occur in the normal urinary tract. *Proc. Natl. Acad. Sci. USA* **91:**11889–11893.
210. **Russell, P. W., and P. E. Orndorff.** 1992. Lesions in two *Escherichia coli* type 1 pilus genes alter pilus number and length without affecting receptor binding. *J. Bacteriol.* **174:** 5923–5935.
211. **Salit, I. E., and E. C. Gotschlich.** 1977. Type 1 *Escherichia coli* pili: characterization of binding to monkey kidney cells. *J. Exp. Med.* **146:**1182–1194.
212. **Salit, I. E., and E. C. Gotschlich.** 1977. Hemagglutination by purified type 1 *Escherichia coli* pili. *J. Exp. Med.* **146:**1169–1181.
213. **Sanders, S. L., K. M. Whitfield, J. P. Vogel, M. D. Rose, and R. W. Scheckman.** 1992. Sec61p and BiP directly facilitate polypeptide translocatin into the ER. *Cell* **69:**353–365.
214. **Savarino, S., P. Fox, D. Yikang, and J. P. Nataro.** 1994. Identification and characterization of a gene cluster mediating enteroaggregative *Escherichia coli* aggregative adherence fimbriae I biogenesis. *J. Bacteriol.* **176:**4949–4957.
215. **Schiffer, M., R. L. Girling, K. R. Ely, and A. B. Edmundson.** 1973. Structure of a 1-type Bence Jones protein at 3.5A resolution. *Biochemistry* **12:**4620–4631.
216. **Schmoll, T., H. Hoschutzky, J. Morschhauser, F. Lottspeich, K. Jann, and J. Hacker.** 1989. Analysis of genes coding for the sialic acid-binding adhesin and two other minor fimbrial subunits of the S-fimbrial adhesin determinant of Escherichia coli. *Mol. Microbiol.* **3:**1735–1744.
217. **Schmoll, T., M. Ott, B. Oudega, and J. Hacker.** 1990. Use of a wild-type gene fusion to determine the influence of environmental conditions on expression of the S fimbrial adhesin in an *Escherichia coli* pathogen. *J. Bacteriol.* **172:**5103–5111.
218. **Schneider, H.-C., J. Berthold, M. F. Bauer, K. Dietmeier, B. Guiard, M. Brunner, and W. Neupert.** 1994. Mitochondrial Hsp70/MIM44 complex facilitates protein import. *Nature* (London) **371:** 768–774.
219. **Schnell, D. J., F. Kessler, and G. Blobel.** 1994. Isolation of components of the chloroplast protein import machinery. *Science* **266:** 1007–1012.
220. **Scott, J. R.** 1990. The M protein of group A streptococcus: evolution and regulation, p. 177–199. *In* B. H. Iglewski and V. L. Clark (ed.), *Molecular Basis of Bacterial Pathogenesis*. Academic Press, Inc., New York.
221. **Sharon, N.** 1987. Bacterial lectins, cell-cell recognition and infectious disease. *FEBS Lett.* **217:**145–157.
222. **Silverblatt, F. J., J. S. Dreyer, and S. Schaur.** 1979. Effect of pili on susceptibility of *Escherichia coli* to phagocytosis. *Infect. Immun.* **24:**218–223.
223. **Simons, B., P. Rathman, C. Malij, B. Oudega, and F. K. de Graf.** 1990. The penultimate tyrosine residue of the K99 fibrillar subunit is essential for the stability of the protein and its interaction with the periplasmic carrier protein. *FEMS Microbiol. Lett.* **67:**107–112.
224. **Slonim, L. N., J. S. Pinkner, C. I. Branden, and S. J. Hultgren.** 1992. Interactive surface in the PapD chaperone cleft is conserved in pilus chaperone superfamily and essential in subunit recognition and assembly. *EMBO J.* **11:**4747–4756.

225. Smit, H., W. Gaastra, J. P. Kamerling, J. F. G. Vliegenthart, and F. K. de Graaf. 1984. Isolation and structural characterization of the equine erythrocyte receptor for enterotoxigenic *Escherichia coli* K99 fimbrial adhesin. *Infect. Immun.* **46**:578–584.

226. Sokurenko, E. V., H. S. Courtney, S. N. Abraham, P. Klemm, and D. L. Hasty. 1992. Functional heterogeneity of type 1 fimbriae of *Escherichia coli. Infect. Immun.* **60**: 4709–4719.

227. Sokurenko, E. V., H. S. Courtney, D. E. Ohman, P. Klemm, and D. L. Hasty. 1994. FimH family of type 1 fimbrial adhesins: functional heterogeneity due to minor sequence variations among *fimH* genes. *J. Bacteriol.* **176**:748–755.

228. Strauch, K. L., and J. Beckwith. 1988. An *Escherichia coli* mutation preventing degradation of abnormal periplasmic proteins. *Proc. Natl. Acad. Sci. USA* **85**:1576–1580.

229. Strauch, K. L., K. Johnson, and J. Beckwith. 1989. Characterization of *degP*, a gene required for proteolysis in the cell envelope *Escherichia coli* at high temperature. *J. Bacteriol.* **171**:2689–2696.

229a. Striker, R., and S. J. Hultgren. Unpublished data.

230. Striker, R., F. Jacob-Dubuisson, C. Frieden, and S. J. Hultgren. 1994. Stable fiber forming and non-fiber forming chaperone-subunit complexes in pilus biogenesis. *J. Biol. Chem.* **269**:12233–12239.

231. Striker, R., U. Nilsson, A. Stonecipher, G. Magnusson, and S. J. Hultgren. 1995. Structural requirements for the glycolipid receptor of human uropathogenic E. coli. *Mol. Microbiol.* **16**:1021–1030.

232. Stromberg, N., S. J. Hultgren, D. G. Russell, and S. Normark. 1992. Microbial attachment, molecular mechanisms, p. 1–16. *In* J. Lederberg (ed.), *Encyclopedia of Microbiology*, vol. 3. Academic Press, Inc., New York.

233. Stromberg, N., B. I. Marklund, B. Lund, D. Ilver, A. Hamers, W. Gaastra, K. A. Karlsson, and S. Normark. 1990. Host-specificity of uropathogenic *Escherichia coli* depends on differences in binding specificity to Galα(1-4)Gal-containing isoreceptors. *EMBO J.* **9**:2001–2010.

234. Stromberg, N., P.-G. Nyholm, I. Pascher, and S. Normark. 1991. Saccharide orientation at the cell surface affects glycolipid receptor function. *Proc. Natl. Acad. Sci. USA* **88**:9340–9344.

235. Svanborg, E., L. M. Bjurstsen, R. Hull, S. Hull, K.-E. M. Magnusson, Z. Moldovano, and H. Leffler. 1984. Influence of adhesins on the interactions of *E. coli* with human phagocytes. *Infect. Immun.* **44**: 672–680.

236. Svanborg-Eden, C., B. Andersson, L. Hagberg, L. A. Hanson, H. Leffler, G. Magnusson, G. Noori, J. Dahmen, and T. Soderstrom. 1983. Receptor analogues and anti-pili antibodies as inhibitors of bacterial attachment in vivo and in vitro. *Ann. N.Y. Acad. Sci.* **409**:580–591.

237. Svanborg-Eden, C., B. Eriksson, L. A. Hanson, U. Jodal, B. Kaijser, G. Lidin-Janson, O. Lindberg, and S. Olling. 1978. Adhesion to normal human uroepithelial cells of *Escherichia coli* from children with various forms of urinary tract infection. *J. Pediatr.* **93**:398.

238. Svanborg-Eden, C., L. A. Hanson, U. Jodal, U. Lindberg, and A. Sohl-Akerlund. 1976. Variable adherence to normal urinary tract epithelial cells of *Escherichia coli* strains associated with various forms of urinary tract infection. *Lancet* **ii**:490.

239. Tennent, J. M., S. Hultgren, K. Forsman, M. Goransson, B. I. Marklund, B. E. Uhlin, and S. Normark 1990. Genetics of adhesin expression in *Escherichia coli*, p. 79–110. *In* B. H. Iglewski and V. C. Clark (ed.), *The Bacteria: Molecular Basis of Pathogenesis*. Academic Press, Inc., New York.

240. Tennent, J. M., F. Lindberg, and S. Normark. 1990. Integrity of *Escherichia coli* P pili during biogenesis: properties and role of PapJ. *Mol. Microbiol.* **4**:747–758.

241. Tennent, J. M., and J. S. Mattick 1994. Type 4 pili, p. 127–147. *In* P. Klemm (ed.), *Fimbriae: Adhesion, Genetics, Biogenesis and Vaccines*. CRC Press, London.

242. Tewari, R., J. I. MacGregor, T. Ikeda, J. R. I. Little, S. J. Hultgren, and S. N. Abraham. 1993. Neutrophil activation by nascent FimH subunits of type 1 fimbriae purified from the periplasm of *Escherichia coli. J. Biol. Chem.* **268**:3009–3015.

243. Tullus, K., K. Hortin, S. B. Svenson, and G. Kallenius. 1984. Epidemic outbreaks of acute pyelonephritis caused by nosocomial spread of P fimbriated *Escherichia coli* in children. *J. Infect. Dis.* **150**: 728–776.

244. Ungermann, C., W. Neupert, and D. M. Cyr. 1994. The role of Hsp70 in conferring unidirectionality on protein translocation into mitochondria. *Science* **266**:1250–1253.

245. Vaisanen, V., J. Elo, L. G. Tallgren, A. Siitonen, P. H. Makela, C. Svanborg-Eden, G. Kallenius, S. B. Svenson, H.

Hultberg, and T. Korhonen. 1981. Mannose-resistant hemagglutination and P antigen recognition are characteristics of *Escherichia coli* causing primary pyelonephritis. *Lancet* **ii:**1366–1369.
246. van Alphen, L., L. Geelen-van Den Broek, L. Blaas, M. van Ham, and J. Dankert. 1991. Blocking of fimbria-mediated adherence of *Haemophilus influenzae* by sialyl gangliosides. *Infect. Immun.* **59:**4473–4477.
247. van der Woude, M. W., B. A. Braaten, and D. A. Low. 1992. Evidence of global regulatory control of pilus expression in Escherichia coli by Lrp and DNA methylation: model building based on analysis of pap. *Mol. Microbiol.* **6:**2429–2435.
248. Van Die, I., C. Krammer, J. Hacker, H. Bergmans, W. Jongen, and W. Hoekstra. 1991. Nucleotide sequence of the genes coding for the minor fimbrial subunits of the F1C fimbriae of *Escherichia coli*. *Res. Microbiol.* **142:**653–658.
249. Venegas, M. F., E. N. Navas, R. A. Gaffney, J. L. Duncan, B. E. Anderson, and A. J. Schaeffer. 1995. Binding of type 1-piliated *Escherichia coli* to vaginal mucus. *Infect. Immun.* **63:**416–422.
250. Viitanen, P. V., A. A. Gatenby, and G. H. Lorimer. 1992. Purified chaperonin 60 (groEL) interacts with the nonnative states of a multitude of Escherichia coli proteins. *Protein Sci.* **1:**363–369.
251. Virkola, R. 1987. Binding characteristics of *Escherichia coli* type 1 fimbriae in the human kidney. *FEMS Microbiol. Lett.* **40:**257–262.
252. Virkola, R., J. Parkkinen, J. Hacker, and T. K. Korhonen. 1993. Sialyloligosaccharide chains of laminin as an extracellular matrix target for S fimbriae of *Escherichia coli*. *Infect. Immun.* **61:**4480–4484.
253. Virkola, R., B. Westerlund, H. Holthofer, J. Parkkinen, M. Kekomaki, and T. K. Korhonen. 1988. Binding characteristics of *Escherichia coli* adhesins in human urinary bladder. *Infect. Immun.* **56:**2615–2622.

254. Westerlund, B., and T. Korhonen. 1993. Bacterial proteins binding to the mammalian extracellular matrix. *Mol. Microbiol.* **9:**687–694.
255. Westerlund, B., I. van Die, C. Kramer, P. Kuusela, H. Holthofer, A. M. Tarkkanen, R. Virkola, N. Riegman, H. Bergmans, W. Hoekstra, and T. K. Korhonan. 1991. Multifunctional nature of P fimbriae of uropathogenic *Escherichia coli*: mutations in *fso*E and *fso*F influence fimbrial binding to renal tubuli and immobilized fibronectin. *Mol. Microbiol.* **5:**2965–2975.
256. Wickner, W. 1989. Secretion and membrane assembly. *Trends Biol. Sci.* **14:**280–285.
257. Wickner, W., A. J. M. Driessen, and F.-U. Hartl. 1991. The enzymology of protein translocation across the *Escherichia coli* plasma membrane. *Annu. Rev. Biochem.* **60:**101–124.
258. Willems, R. J. L., H. G. J. van der Heide, and F. R. Mooi. 1992. Characterization of a *Bordetella pertussis* fimbrial gene cluster which is located directly downstream of the filamentous haemagglutinin gene. *Mol. Microbiol.* **6:**2661–2671.
259. Williams, A. F., and A. N. Barclay. 1988. The immunoglobulin superfamily-domains for cell surface recognition. *Annu. Rev. Immunol.* **6:**381–405.
260. Wray, S. K., S. I. Hull, R. G. Cook, J. Barish, and R. A. Hull. 1986. Identification and characterization of a uroepithelial cell adhesin from a uropathogenic isolate of *Proteus mirabilis*. *Infect. Immun.* **54:**43.
261. Xu, Z., C. H. Jones, D. Haslam, J. S. Pinkner, K. Dodson, J. Kihlberg, and S. J. Hultgren. 1995. Molecular dissection of PapD interaction with PapG reveals two chaperone binding sites. *Mol. Microbiol.* **16:**1011–1020.
262. Yu, J., H. Webb, and T. R. Hirst. 1992. A homologue of the *Escherichia coli* DsbA protein involved in disulphide bond formation is required for enterotoxin biogenesis in *Vibrio cholerae*. *Mol. Microbiol.* **6:**1949–1958.

# HOST RESISTANCE TO URINARY TRACT INFECTION

*William Agace, B.Sc. (Hons), Hugh Connell, Ph.D., and Catharina Svanborg, M.D., Ph.D.*

# 8

Urinary tract infections (UTIs) are among the most common bacterial infections in humans. Host factors that determine susceptibility to UTI have been studied at the population level. The frequency of UTI varies with age, gender, and socioeconomic background. Screening detects bacteriuria in about 1% of girls from birth to puberty, in 2% or more of pregnant women, and in 15 to 20% of women at 70 years of age. In addition, symptomatic infections (acute pyelonephritis, acute cystitis) occur frequently in children and sexually active women. Susceptibility is generally higher in females than in males except for young boys and elderly men, in whom the frequency of UTI is comparable to that for females of the same age group. Socioeconomic variables include access to medical care (surgical correction of malformations, antenatal care of expectant mothers, estrogen treatment of women after menopause) and sexual and contraceptive practices (73).

There is additional variation in susceptibility to UTI among individuals of comparable age and socioeconomic status (143).

*William Agace, Hugh Connell, and Catharina Svanborg,* Division of Clinical Immunology, Department of Medical Microbiology, Lund University, Lund, Sweden.

Certain individuals never experience a UTI episode, many others suffer from recurrent infections. Some individuals experience recurrent UTI without sequelae, while others develop scars and impaired renal function or chronic bladder damage (interstitial cystitis). It is embarrassing to admit how little we understand at the molecular level about the mechanisms that control susceptibility to UTI and the tendency to develop chronic sequelae of infection. This chapter summarizes the available information on parameters that have been inferred or proven to influence host resistance to UTI. These parameters are discussed in the context of pathogenesis and in the order in which they are encountered by the bacterial strains that cause UTI.

## STEPS IN THE PATHOGENESIS OF UTI

The *Escherichia coli* clones that cause acute pyelonephritis possess an array of virulence factors that contribute to different stages in pathogenesis; they include adherence factors (P, type 1, S, Dr fimbriae), toxins (lipopolysaccharide [LPS], hemolysin), aerobactin, and capsules (146, 151). The pathogenesis of acute pyelonephritis starts when a pyelonephritogenic *E. coli* clone becomes established in the host at a site outside the urinary tract (often the large intestine). This colonization is partly due to the same adherence mechanisms that make the bacteria virulent for the urinary tract and is influenced by the mucosal receptors expressed by the host. The bacteria spread to the urinary tract and establish bacteriuria; this phase is counteracted by urine flow, secreted receptor analogs that trap type 1- and S-fimbriated bacteria, and bactericidal molecules in the urine and mucosa. Uropathogenic clones overcome these defenses, attach to the mucosa, and ascend to the upper urinary tract, where they elicit an inflammatory response. The bacteria stimulate epithelial and other cells to produce cytokines and other proinflammatory factors. The systemic spread of cytokines such as interleukin 6 (IL-6) leads to fever and the activation of the acute-phase response. Chemotactic cytokines such as IL-8 recruit polymorphonuclear granulocytes (PMNs) to the mucosal surface, and bacteriuria is cleared at the same time. A specific immune response to the infection follows thereafter. In about 30% of patients with acute pyelonephritis, bacteria invade through the mucosa into the bloodstream and cause bacteremia.

Since the arrival of antibiotics, febrile infections have been diagnosed and treated, and they rarely have sequelae. Infections with less typical clinical presentations are often caused by bacteria of reduced virulence. These types of infections often occur in children with vesicoureteral reflux and may cause renal scarring (132, 166).

The pathogenesis of acute cystitis is not as well understood. Spread to the urinary tract and the establishment of bacteriuria presumably occur by the same mechanisms as in pyelonephritis. There are, however, no bacterial parameters that identify "cystitogenic" *E. coli* clones or distinguish them from strains that cause acute pyelonephritis (with the possible exception of hemolysin, type 1 fimbriae, and the $prsG_{J96}$ type of P fimbriae, which occur at higher frequencies in acute cystitis strains than in other *E. coli* strains) (26, 42, 60). We believe that the clinical syndrome of acute cystitis is determined by the host response and that cystitis-prone individuals have developed a specific response pattern that is possibly due to the local accumulation of special inflammatory cells (e.g., mast cells in the bladder mucosa). This possibility needs to be studied further.

Asymptomatic bacteriuria (ABU) may be either the consequence of bacterial attenuation by the host or a primary condition in which bacteria of low virulence stably colonize the urinary tract without activating a host response sufficient to cause symptoms. The bacterial factors that explain this colonization, the host defects that allow it to occur, and the basis for the unresponsiveness of the colonized patients are unknown.

## HOST FACTORS INFLUENCING MUCOSAL COLONIZATION BY UROPATHOGENIC BACTERIA

The large intestine, vaginal introitus, and periurethral areas serve as reservoirs for uropathogenic *E. coli* and other members of the family *Enterobacteriaceae* that cause UTI (12, 41, 80, 117, 154). Early studies defined uropathogenic *E. coli* as the subset of clones that occur more frequently in the urinary tracts of patients with UTI than in the fecal flora of healthy controls (12, 41, 60, 80, 154). This difference suggests that UTI-prone patients have a greater tendency than healthy controls to become colonized by uropathogenic *E. coli*. Stamey and colleagues (38, 137, 138) showed in a series of studies that the introital carriage of *Enterobacteriaceae* is increased in women with recurrent UTI compared to that in controls. Because of these observations, the following question arises: are there differences in the underlying susceptibility to colonization of the intestine between UTI patients and controls, or does UTI occur at random in a fraction of the individuals who encounter a uropathogenic E. coli strain?

In a recent study, we found that children with acute pyelonephritis carry uropathogenic E. coli (defined by the $pap^+$ genotype) in their fecal flora more often than healthy controls (117). This higher carriage rate was evident both at the time of diagnosis and at followup after successful treatment of the UTI episode. This finding suggests that the children with acute pyelonephritis had an increased tendency to carry $pap^+$ strains in their fecal flora at the time of UTI and also during infection-free intervals. The children with ABU had higher intestinal carriage of $pap^+$ strains than the healthy controls at the time of detection of bacteriuria, but the intestinal carriage of $pap^+$ strains decreased during the first year of life, and all the children spontaneously cleared their bacteriuria. The carriage of $pap^+$ strains in the ABU group appeared to be a transient phenomenon coinciding with the time of bacteriuria (117).

These studies with children confirmed and extended earlier observations made in women and children with recurrent UTI. These observations suggest that the tendency to carry uropathogenic bacteria influences susceptibility to UTI. Is this susceptibility a result of predisposing host factors? Can we identify such factors and show that they are more frequent in the UTI prone group?

## The Roles of Adherence and Variation in Receptor Expression

The colonization of mucosal surfaces during the pathogenesis of UTI is influenced by bacterial adherence. Early studies (38, 137, 138) suggested that vaginal epithelial cells from women with recurrent UTI have an increased ability to bind attaching bacteria. Subsequent studies confirmed that uroepithelial cells from women and children with recurrent UTI have a greater receptivity for attaching bacteria than do cells from healthy controls (38, 67, 127, 152). Uropathogenic E. coli expresses an array of adhesins, including P, S, Dr, and type 1 fimbriae (34, 79, 106, 114). The molecular mechanisms of this increased adherence are best characterized for E. coli P fimbriae (127).

P-fimbriated E. coli has enhanced virulence for the urinary tract compared to other E. coli strains (144). P-fimbriated E. coli adheres to human colonic epithelial cells in vitro and persists longer in the large intestines of UTI-prone children than do other E. coli strains (167, 169). P fimbriae mediate adherence to uroepithelial cells, and P-fimbriated E. coli activate an inflammatory response that causes the symptoms and signs of infection (2, 30, 50–53, 145).

P fimbriae recognize as receptors Gal$\alpha$1-4Gal$\beta$- and GalNAc$\beta$-3Gal$\alpha$1-4Gal$\beta$-containing oligosaccharide sequences in the globoseries of glycolipids (66, 78). The fimbriae are encoded by the $pap$ chromosomal gene cluster (57). The $pap$ gene clusters from different E. coli strains show extensive sequence homology except for $papA$, which encodes the antigenically variable fimbrial subunit, and the $papG$ adhesin sequences that determine receptor specificity (8, 81, 92). Several G-adhesin variants (95) share a specificity for the globoseries of glycolipid receptors but differ in isoreceptor specificity, binding to epithelial cells, and disease association (59, 82, 92, 129, 142).

The globoseries glycolipids are present on epithelial and nonepithelial components of the urinary bladder and ureters (18, 78). They are the quantitatively dominating nonacid glycolipids of kidney tissue. The structural prerequisites for fimbria-receptor interactions are therefore present along the urinary tract. P-fimbriated E. coli binds to glycolipid extracts from uroepithelial cells (78). Gal$\alpha$1-4Gal$\beta$-containing glycolipids account for this receptor activity, as shown by thin-layer chromatography (16).

Furthermore, glycolipid extracts from exfoliated uroepithelial cells inhibit the attachment of P-fimbriated *E. coli* to uroepithelial cells from the same donor (78).

The globoseries glycolipids, which are recognized by the P fimbriae, are antigens in the P blood group system. The expression of the globoseries glycolipids on uroepithelial cells varies depending on the P blood group, ABH blood group, and secretor state of the individual (93). According to competitive studies of blood group and glycolipid expression, the P blood group can be used to predict the receptor repertoires of epithelial cells in the urinary tract. The P blood group of an individual can be used in epidemiological studies aimed at clarifying the role of receptor expression for susceptibility to UTI.

## ABSENCE OF RECEPTORS FOR P FIMBRIAE

Individuals of the p blood group phenotype fail to synthesize functional Gal$\alpha$1-4Gal$\beta$-containing glycolipids (93), and therefore uroepithelial cells (78) and erythrocytes (66, 79) from p individuals lack functional receptors for P-fimbriated *E. coli*. By analogy with K88-resistant pigs (40, 124), the absence of functional receptors would be expected to confer resistance to infection with P-fimbriated *E. coli*. The low frequency of p individuals in the population has, however, precluded any evaluation of relative morbidity in infections due to P-fimbriated *E. coli* in individuals of the p and $P_1/P_2$ blood group phenotypes.

## P AND ABH BLOOD GROUP-DEPENDENT RECEPTOR EXPRESSION FOR *prs*G$_{J96}$-POSITIVE STRAINS

P fimbriae of different G-adhesin classes vary in regard to the preferred receptor epitope (59, 79, 82, 83, 92, 129, 142). G adhesins of the *pap*G$_{IA2}$ type recognize most Gal$\alpha$1-4Gal$\beta$-containing glycolipids. They attach to uroepithelial cells from P-positive individuals regardless of the ABH blood group or secretor state of the host (59). G adhesins of the *prs*G$_{J96}$ type prefer a receptor epitope composed of GalNAc$\alpha$ linked to a globoseries core. Their binding to uroepithelial cells requires the Forssman or globo-A glycolipids (59, 79, 82, 83, 92, 129, 142). The Forssman glycolipid is not abundant in the human urinary tract (17). The globo-A glycolipid, however, is expressed on uroepithelial cells from $A_1$ secretor individuals (82, 83). The *prs*G$_{J96}$-encoded P fimbriae attach to uroepithelial cells from A1 secretor individuals but not to cells from non-A or nonsecretor individuals.

This receptor specificity influences the host range of *E. coli* in vivo. Strains with the *prs*G$_{J96}$ type of adhesin cause UTI in blood group $A_1$-positive individuals (83). The frequency of $A_1$ individuals was 100% in the group infected with exclusively *prs*G$_{J96}$-positive strains but only 43% in the population at large.

## $P_1$ BLOOD GROUP AND ACUTE PYELONEPHRITIS

$P_1$ individuals run an 11-fold higher risk of attracting recurrent episodes of acute pyelonephritis with P-fimbriated *E. coli* than $P_2$ individuals (85, 91). This difference was first thought to reflect an increase in receptors for P-fimbriated *E. coli* on uroepithelial cells from $P_1$ children compared to $P_2$ children, but no such difference was found (84). More recent studies have shown that $P_1$ individuals have an increased tendency to carry P-fimbriated *E. coli* strains in the fecal flora compared to individuals of the $P_2$ blood group (117). The mechanism of this increased carriage is not clear. We propose here that $P_1$ individuals express more or better receptors for P-fimbriated *E. coli* in the large intestine and that receptor expression increases the tendency of these individuals to become colonized with P-fimbriated strains.

## SECRETOR STATE

The secretor state influences the derivatization of epithelial glycoconjugates with the A, B, and H blood group determinants. Nonsecretors lack the glycosyltransferase(s) required to elongate the globoseries core structure with the ABH determinants. Nonsecretor individuals run an increased risk of contracting mucosal infections, including infections caused by *Haemophilus influenzae* and *Candida* spp. (14, 15). In addition, nonsecretor individuals are overrepresented among women with a history of recurrent UTI (70a) and among children with UTI who develop renal scarring (90). The mechanism of this association is not known. Attachment to squamous uroepithelial cells has been investigated, because the secretor state influences epithelial-cell glycosylation and receptor expression. The binding of P-fimbriated *E. coli* to squamous uroepithelial cells of nonsecretors is higher than that in secretors (89). Stapleton and coworkers (140) recently demonstrated the presence of two additional sialylated members of the globoseries of glycolipids in nonsecretors; these molecules become fucosylated and elongated with the ABH antigens in secretors. They proposed that these sialylated structures provide additional attachment sites for P-fimbriated *E. coli*.

The mucosae of nonsecretors may be more permeable to toxic bacterial products because of smaller amounts of protective surface polysaccharide. Levels of endotoxin were higher in the circulation of nonsecretors than in that of secretors with UTI (89). This increased level of endotoxin might contribute to the increased tissue damage and renal scarring in these patients.

## Defects in Urine Flow

Susceptibility to UTI is increased in patients with inborn or acquired defects in urine flow. These patients are often infected with a wider spectrum of bacterial species and with bacteria that are avirulent for the healthy urinary tract. Defects in urine flow can arise from malformations, stones, prostatic hyperplasia, indwelling catheters or instrumentation, and neurogenic disorders.

The question of whether urine flow per se is sufficient to maintain the sterility of the urinary tract has been discussed. The efficiency of voiding as a means of eliminating bacteriuria was examined by O'Grady and Pennington with an artificial bladder model (107). They proposed a model for successful bacterial colonization based on variables like bacterial multiplication rates, urine flow rates, bladder volume, and frequency of bladder voiding. They concluded that liquid with a bacterial inoculum of $\sim 10^5$ CFU/ml that wet the bladder surface after voiding was sufficient to reinoculate the next portion of urine and maintain bacteriuria. Cox and Hinman, on the other hand, showed a clear discrepancy between in vitro growth and bacterial colonization in human volunteers (28). A bacterial inoculum of $10^7$ CFU/ml was cleared from the human urinary tract in 72 h and bacteriuria was maintained in an in vitro bladder model. The bladder mucosa was subsequently shown to have bactericidal activity. The urine flow is therefore only one of many factors that contribute to the sterility of the urinary tract.

Vesicoureteral reflux is a major host determinant in the localization, severity, and sequelae of UTI. Reflux can facilitate the ascent of bacteria to the renal pelvis (grade II) or into the kidney tissue (grade III). The contribution of reflux to host susceptibility is difficult to study because of the variable nature of reflux; it may be present during acute infection due to the action of bacteria on the bladder and ureteral mucosa (94, 122) but may be absent during infection-free intervals. Clearly, reflux represents a potential danger to the kidney, and the relative roles of reflux and infection in tissue damage have been discussed elsewhere (55, 119). We found that children with reflux and renal scarring are often infected with bacteria of low virulence, and we proposed that the transport of bacteria into the kidney by refluxing urine reduces the need for fimbria-mediated adherence and other virulence factors (86). This association has not been proven and probably represents an overly simplified view. Patients with reflux but no scarring were subsequently shown to attract fully virulent bacteria, while children with scarring but no reflux are infected with bacteria of low virulence (86). Tissue defense mechanisms in patients with renal scarring may be impaired irrespective of the reflux state, permitting bacteria of reduced virulence to cause acute pyelonephritis.

## Bactericidal Factors of the Urinary Tract Mucosa

Late in the last century, the ability of urine to support growth was recognized (111); however, not all *E. coli* strains are capable of growth in this medium. Kaye showed that isolates from patients with UTI grow well in urine, while most fecal *E. coli* strains are killed (70). This finding prompted a search for antibacterial molecules in urine and the identification of inhibiting factors like urea, organic acids, salts, pH, and osmolarity (7, 70). Asscher et al. showed that urinary isolates of *E. coli* grow optimally at a pH between 6.0 and 7.0 and that growth is inhibited in both alkaline and acidic urines outside this pH range (7). The physiological range of human urine pH is between 4.6 and 7.2. Kass and Zangwill reduced bacterial counts in the urine of patients with chronic UTI by administering DL-methionine, which produces highly acidic urine (69). The inhibition of bacterial growth was due to undissociated organic acids, which exist in high concentrations in acidic urine.

Urine osmolarity also affects the ability of *E. coli* to grow in human urine (7). At high osmolarity (1,200 mosmol/kg), bacterial growth was inhibited by high levels of urea, sodium chloride, sodium sulfate, potassium chloride, and potassium sulfate in the urine. The inhibition of growth is probably due to the hyperosmolarity of the urine rather than to one specific molecule. Urine of low osmolarity ($\leq 200$ mosmol/kg) also inhibits bacterial growth, probably because of the very low nutrient content of urine. This finding supports the idea that high fluid intake assists in the clearance of bacteriuria.

Although urine appears to be inhibitory for bacterial growth, Chambers and Kunin showed that urine confers an osmoprotective effect on *E. coli* (23). Urinary isolates of *E. coli* grown in a defined minimal medium are inhibited by high concentrations of electrolytes and sugars in direct relation to the osmotic strengths of these substances. The addition of human urine and betaine to this medium increases the osmotic resistance of the *E. coli* isolates to these substances. Chambers and Kunin proposed that urine contains low-molecular-weight osmoprotective substances that *E. coli* can use to protect itself against the hypertonic effect of urine (23).

Human urine appears to contain a range of molecules other than electrolytes that are inhibitory for bacterial growth. Norden et al. showed that the bladder mucosae of guinea pigs are capable of killing the mucosa-bound fraction of an *E. coli* inoculum (103). Schulte-Wissermann and coworkers suggested that epithelial cells produce molecules that are bactericidal for *E. coli* and that UTI-prone individuals produce less of this factor than healthy controls (128).

We initially observed marked differences in the abilities of *E. coli* strains to survive in human urine (27). *E. coli* strains from patients with different forms of UTI (acute pyelonephritis, acute cystitis, ABU) and from the intestinal flora of healthy individuals were tested for growth in a pool of male urine. All the UTI isolates attained a cell density of $\geq 10^6$ CFU/ml in 24 h. In contrast, most of the *E. coli* intestinal isolates were killed. This result suggests that the urine contained antibacterial components to which the strains causing UTI were resistant.

To identify the mechanism(s) that explains the observed antibacterial effect, two E. coli strains were selected as a model. E. coli 83972 was the clinical isolate that had successfully established bacteriuria following deliberate colonization of 12 human hosts (6). This strain was able to grow exponentially in pools of male and female urine to a cell density of $10^8$ to $10^9$ CFU/ml of urine by 24 h (27). E. coli HB101 is a K-12 strain of the type that can be found in the fecal flora of healthy carriers. This strain was killed in male urine; at an inoculum of $<10^5$ CFU/ml, no viable bacteria remained at 24 h (27).

Urine was subjected to gel filtration column chromatography to isolate the antibacterial activity (27). Fractions collected from a G-25 Sephadex column were tested for their effects on bacterial growth in a minimal salts and glucose medium with amino acids and vitamins as supplements for the deficiencies caused by auxotrophic mutations in E. coli HB101. A fraction that inhibited the growth of E. coli HB101 but not that of E. coli 83972 was identified. This fraction inhibited the growth of intestinal isolates from healthy individuals, but the UTI strains were able to grow in minimal media supplemented with this fraction.

The inhibitory component was purified further. The active fraction was enriched for the antibacterial component by organic solvent extraction, ion-exchange chromatography, and thin-layer chromatography. The antibacterial component was weakly cationic (one or two positively charged groups), ninhydrin reactive (showing the presence of amine groups), of low molecular weight (between 500 and 1,000), and very hydrophilic (27). This profile is compatible with those of the chemical family of polyamines. Polyamines inhibit DNA replication in bacteria and are taken up through an LPS-dependent transport system (136, 156, 164). Our study suggests that the polyamine-like component we isolated from urine should be added to the list of compounds with neutral antibiotic activity that includes defensins, magainins, cecropins, and cryptdins (35, 77, 112, 170). Variations in the concentrations of this component in the urinary tract may contribute to differences in susceptibility to UTI. Further characterization is being carried out to determine the structure of this compound.

## Secreted Inhibitors of Bacterial Adherence

Like other secretions, urine contains molecules analogous to the cell-bound receptors for bacterial adhesins. These soluble receptor analogs act as competitive inhibitors of attachment. Urine contains a variety of free oligosaccharides and a considerable amount of glycoproteins with receptor activity.

### THP

Tamm-Horsfall glycoprotein (THP; Uromodulin) has a molecular weight of 76,000 and contains 25 to 30% carbohydrate, including mannose and sialic acid residues (36, 37). THP is produced by the luminal cells of the thick ascending loop of Henlé and the early distal tubules and is secreted with urine (130). It is found at the epithelial surface as large aggregates ($\sim 7 \times 10^7$ kDa) and is the most abundant protein in normal human urine (36, 130). THP acts as a receptor matrix for E. coli type 1 and S fimbriae, which recognize mannose and sialic acid residues, respectively (109, 110). THP inhibits the attachment of type 1-fimbriated E. coli to uroepithelial cells by its ability to aggregate type 1-fimbriated E. coli in solution (109). However, these strains bind better to immobilized THP than to soluble protein (110a). This fact may be of consequence in the binding of type 1-fimbriated strains to renal tissue. THP inhibits E. coli S fimbria-mediated agglutination of human erythrocytes, presumably because it contains NeuAc($\alpha$2-3)Gal($\beta$1-4)GlcNAc, the receptor-active epitope for S fimbriae (110a). Soluble THP may therefore prevent attachment of S-fimbriated strains to the urinary tract epithelium. In contrast, THP does not express Gal$\alpha$1-4Gal$\beta$-containing glycolipids and does not interact specifically with P-fimbriated *E. coli*. These lacks have been proposed as reasons why S-fimbriated *E. coli* rarely occurs among pyelonephritogenic strains, despite its ability to bind to the same uroepithelial tissues as P-fimbriated *E. coli* strains in vitro (72, 161). Inter-estingly, THP binds to neutrophils in a calcium-dependent, arginine-glycine-as-partate-mediated mechanism that requires metabolically active cells (157). THP has numerous effects on neutrophils (it increases phagocytosis, complement expression, and arichidonic acid metabolism) and may play a role in modulating neutrophil-bacterium interactions in the kidney.

## LOW-MOLECULAR-WEIGHT COMPOUNDS

Urine contains numerous low-molecular-weight (200 to 2,000) oligosaccharides that strongly inhibit *E. coli* type 1-mediated hemagglutination of guinea pig erythrocytes (110a). $\alpha$-Mannosidase treatment of these oligosaccharides decreases their inhibitory activity, suggesting that they contain mannose residues binding to the adhesin domain of the type 1 fimbriae.

## OLIGOSACCHARIDE OF SECRETORY IgA

Secretory immunoglobulin A (IgA) and IgA myeloma proteins, especially those of the IgA2 subclass, are glycosylated and express terminal mannose residues that act as carbohydrate receptors for the mannose-specific lectin of type 1-fimbriated *E. coli*. Myeloma IgA2 proteins that lack anti-*E. coli* antibody activity inhibit the attachment of type 1-fimbriated *E. coli* to uroepithelial cells in vitro (168). Since IgA2 is secreted into the urine during UTI, such mechanisms may influence type 1 fimbrial interactions with the urinary tract epithelium in vivo.

## INFLAMMATORY RESPONSE TO UTI

Bacteria elicit an inflammatory response in the urinary tract. The magnitude and localization of this inflammatory response may explain many of the clinical features of UTI. Patients with acute pyelonephritis have inflammation of the renal pelvis and kidneys combined with a generalized inflammatory response (fever, C reactive protein, leukocytes) (73). Patients with acute cystitis often have an inflammatory reaction restricted to the lower urinary tract (73). Patients with ABU may show signs of local inflammation in the urinary tract, but the magnitude is not sufficient to make the patients symptomatic (73).

The molecular mechanisms that regulate the inflammatory response have only recently become a focus of study. Information about the bacterial properties involved in this process, the nature of the inflammatory mediators, and the functional consequences of the response is quite limited. This section focuses on the cytokine response to bacteria in the urinary tract.

### Cytokine Responses in UTI

UTI is accompanied by a cytokine response in the infected host. This response was first demonstrated in mice with experimental UTI (31) and in patients who had been colonized with *E. coli* in the urinary tract (2, 48). The discrepancy between cytokine levels in urine and in serum was marked, suggesting local production of cytokines in the urinary tract. Cytokine responses were subsequently shown to occur in children and adults with different forms of UTI (10, 51, 71, 115, 158). IL-6 was found in the urine of children with febrile UTI but not in children with fever of another origin or in children with ABU (10). The highest urine and serum IL-6 levels were detected in children with reflux and renal scarring (10). In adults, IL-6 was detected in the urine of patients with acute pyelonephritis and ABU. The possible use of urine IL-6 levels in the diagnosis of UTI is currently being explored.

UTI also leads to the induction of the chemokine IL-8. Patients deliberately colonized with E. coli in the urinary tract secreted IL-8 into the urine within hours of colonization, but serum IL-8 was not detected (2). In studies of acute pyelonephritis or ABU, IL-8 levels were elevated in the urine of patients with pyuria (71). This study also showed that urinary IL-8 levels are elevated in most patients with UTI, regardless of the bacterial species causing infection. Studies conducted in children with febrile UTI or ABU showed that the frequency of IL-8 responders is higher in children with febrile UTI than in children with ABU (11). The apparent correlation between bacteriuria and pyuria initiated discussion of the usefulness of urine IL-8 measurements in separating "relevant" from "irrelevant" bacteriuria.

## CELLULAR ORIGIN OF URINARY CYTOKINES

The uninfected urinary tract mucosa is dominated by epithelial cells, which, like most cells, secrete cytokines when suitably stimulated. The influx of PMNs, T cells, and other inflammatory cells occurs subsequent to the primary interaction of bacteria with the mucosa. We have demonstrated that epithelial cell lines and nontransformed cells from the human urinary tract produce cytokines when they are exposed to bacteria (1a, 2, 50, 52, 53). Uropathogenic E. coli stimulates de novo synthesis of IL-1$\alpha$, IL-1$\beta$, IL-6, and IL-8 but not of tumor necrosis factor alpha (TNF-$\alpha$) mRNA. Immunofluorescence detected an increase in intracellular IL-1$\alpha$, IL-6, and IL-8. IL-6 and IL-8 are secreted by the cells, but IL-1$\alpha$, IL-1$\beta$, and TNF-$\alpha$ are not (1a, 2, 50, 52). On the basis of these observations, we propose here that epithelial cells are a source of cytokines during the early stages of infection and that the repertoire and magnitude of the epithelial cytokine response influence the subsequent activation of mucosal inflammation and immunity.

The epithelial cytokine response is influenced by the properties of the uropathogenic bacteria that activate the cells. Adherence by type 1 and P fimbriae enhances the response (2, 53). LPS is likely to play a role in cytokine activation, although not in the same manner as for macrophages. LPS alone is a poor stimulant of epithelial-cell cytokine responses (29, 53, 139), perhaps because epithelial cells lack CD-14 or other LPS receptor molecules required for the binding of LPS and the activation of cells (118).

A variety of cells at the mucosa and other cells that migrate to the site in response to infection are activated by bacteria or epithelial cytokines. For example, bacteria stimulate PMNs to secrete IL-8 and immunoregulatory cytokines, which modify the epithelial cell responses to bacteria (see below). These perturbations of the cytokine response need further study.

## Possible Functions of Cytokines in UTI

MUCOSAL CYTOKINE NETWORKS
Nonepithelial cells resident at or recruited to the urinary tract mucosa during the inflammatory process contribute to the mucosal cytokine response to infection. Neutrophils produce large amounts of IL-8 after stimulation with E. coli and are therefore a likely second source of this cytokine during UTI. In addition, neutrophils have been reported to secrete IL-1, TNF, and IL-6 after stimulation with LPS or IL-1 and TNF. Inflammatory cytokines such as IL-1 and TNF induce urinary tract epithelial-cell IL-6 and IL-8 secretion (52), and immunoregulatory cytokines modify bacterially induced cytokine responses (49).

Thus, the production of cytokines by influxing cells may influence epithelial cytokine responses. Epithelial-cell cytokines may in turn affect lymphocyte activities. This type of communication between mucosal cells forms the basis of a mucosal cytokine network.

## NEUTROPHIL INFLUX

Pyuria is one of the classic signs of UTI. The mechanisms of neutrophil recruitment to the urinary tract and the interaction of PMNs with cells at the mucosa are not well understood and have only recently begun to be examined. The influx of neutrophils during UTI involves the generation of a chemotactic gradient from the urinary tract mucosa and neutrophil adherence to the endothelial vessel wall, extravasation into the lamina propria, and movement to the epithelial barrier. Finally, neutrophils cross the urinary tract epithelium into the urine. Epithelial cells were recently shown to participate in neutrophil recruitment in two ways: (i) by secreting neutrophil chemoattractants (2) and (ii) by expressing adhesion molecules involved in neutrophil transmigration (4).

**Neutrophil Chemoattractants.** Urinary tract epithelial cells appear to be an important source of mucosally derived IL-8. The strong correlation between urinary IL-8 levels and neutrophil numbers in the urine of patients with UTI and in patients deliberately colonized with *E. coli* in the urinary tract suggest that IL-8 plays an important role in the influx of neutrophils into the urine. Indeed, Ko and coworkers reported that anti IL-8 antibodies reduce the neutrophil chemotactic ability of infected urine in vitro by an average of 50% (71). In addition, *E. coli*- or IL-1α-induced neutrophil migration across kidney and bladder epithelial-cell layers was completely blocked with Pc anti IL-8 antibodies (1).

Mechanisms of neutrophil recruitment have also been analyzed in a rat model of ascending pyelonephritis (98). Intravenous injection of cobra venom factor (which depletes complement) or addition of phenylbutazone (a competitive antagonist of bacterial chemotactic formyl peptides) significantly reduced the neutrophil influx into kidney tissue 32 h after infection with *E. coli*. This treatment had no effect on neutrophil migration after 72 h of infection. Together, these results suggest that neutrophil migration during UTI is a complex event mediated by an array of chemoattractants originating from both the host and the bacterial pathogen.

**Cell Adhesion Molecules and Transepithelial Neutrophil Migration.** Urinary tract epithelial cells express adhesion molecules involved in transepithelial neutrophil migration. In recent studies in our laboratory, we were able to show that *E. coli* upregulates the expression of ICAM-1 (an adhesion molecule involved in transendothelial neutrophil migration) on the epithelial surface. Antibodies to ICAM-1 blocked from 60 to 80% of *E. coli*-induced neutrophil migration across epithelial layers. The receptor for ICAM-1 on the neutrophil surface was tentatively identified as the $\beta_2$ integrin CD11b/CD18 (MAC-1), since antibodies to CD11b and CD18 but not to CD11a also blocked bacterially induced transepithelial migration (4).

**Cytokines Modify Epithelial-Cell Responses to Bacteria.** T cells and intraepithelial lymphocytes (IELs) are believed to regulate mucosal immune responses; however, the molecular mechanisms of this regulation are not well understood. These cells are localized near epithelial cells, and some of their regulatory effects are achieved, in part, through interactions with nonlymphoid cells in the mucosal layer. T cells and immunoregulatory cytokines produced mainly by T cells influence different cell functions, including the expression of class II molecules and the secretory component (22, 75, 76, 135). Recently, immunoregulatory cytokines were shown to stimulate urinary tract epithelial-cell cytokine production and to modify the epithelial-cell cytokine responses to bacteria (49). In contrast to previous studies showing that the inflammatory cytokines IL-1$\alpha$ and TNF-$\alpha$ stimulate uroepithelial cells to secrete large amounts of IL-6 and IL-8 (46), these cytokines induce only low-level IL-6 and IL-8 secretion (49).

Cells of the $T_H1$ subtype are commonly defined by their abilities to secrete IL-2 and gamma interferon (IFN-$\gamma$). Hedges and coworkers found no effect of IL-2 on epithelial cell IL-6 or IL-8 production, but IFN-$\gamma$ had a stimulatory effect on IL-6 (49). Cells of the $T_H2$ subtype are commonly defined by their ability to secrete IL-4, IL-5, IL-10, and IL-13. These cytokines activate urinary tract epithelial-cell IL-6 (IL-4, IL-5, IL-10, and IL-13) and IL-8 (IL-4 and IL-13) responses. The other immunoregulatory cytokines (transforming growth factor $\beta$ [TGF-$\beta$1] and IL-12) induced IL-6 but not IL-8 production. Whether the lack of IL-8 production and the subsequent lack of PMN chemotaxis are beneficial during some immune processes is not known.

Some of the immunoregulatory cytokines modify the epithelial-cell cytokine responses to bacteria when they are used as costimulants. IFN-$\gamma$ stimulates the bacterially induced IL-6 and inhibits the IL-8 response, while IL-2 has no effect. IL-5, IL-10, IL-13, and TGF-$\beta$1 all enhance the IL-6 response to *E. coli* in an additive manner. IL-4, in contrast, acts in synergy with *E. coli* as an activator of IL-6. Taken together, these results confirm that urinary tract epithelial cells can produce cytokines in response to a variety of stimuli, and they emphasize the selectivity of epithelial-cell responses to different stimuli. In addition, these findings suggest a mechanism whereby T cells or other cells producing immunoregulatory cytokines can control epithelial-cell responses to mucosal microbial challenge.

### Role of Inflammation in Resistance to UTI

Previous studies of host resistance to UTI have focused on specific immunity and the development of UTI vaccines (see below). Inflammation was thought to be detrimental to the integrity of the mucosal barriers. These concepts are contradicted by studies of resistance to experimental UTI in murine models. We found that C3H/HeJ and C57BL/10ScCr mice are more susceptible to experimental UTI than their normal counterparts, C3H/HeN and C57BL/6J mice (3, 148). The susceptible mice are LPS hyporesponders because of an alteration in the *lps* locus on chromosome IV. Spleen cells from these mice do not proliferate when stimulated with LPS, and the mice are generally resistant to many lipid A-induced activities. Mice with this defect were more susceptible to UTI and had significantly lower neutrophil and cytokine responses to experimental UTI than LPS responder mice. The neutrophil influx in the LPS responder mice coincided with the clearance of infection. These observations suggest that the inflammatory response was essential for clearance of bacteria from the urinary tract. Further studies observed that treatment of mice and rats with anti-inflammatory agents severely reduces the clearance of infection. Treatment of rats with antineutrophil serum leads to a 1,000-fold increase of bacteria in the kidneys (100). In contrast, deficient macrophage function does not appear to increase susceptibility to UTI (100, 148). At present, it is not known how bacteria are killed and cleared from the urinary tract. Many cellular components (PMNs, macrophages) and/or secreted components (defensins, NO) of the inflammatory response are likely to contribute to this process.

## SPECIFIC IMMUNITY AND RESISTANCE TO UTI

Infections of the urinary tract activate a mucosal and a systemic antibody response as well as a cellular immune response (44, 149). The role of specific immunity in resistance to UTI remains undefined. We attempt here to summarize the available information and point to areas in need of further study.

### Cell-Mediated Immunity in UTI

The normal urinary tract mucosa contains few T cells. $CD8^+$ T cells are sparsely scattered within the urothelium, while $CD8^+$ and to a lesser extent $CD4^+$ T cells are present in the submucosa and lamina propria (24, 39). $\gamma/\delta$ T cells are not found in bladder, kidney, ureter, and urethra biopsy samples from healthy individuals (24, 163). Early studies by Smith and colleagues demonstrated the presence of T cells in the cellular infiltrate in patients with pyelonephritis (133). In patients with bacterial cystitis, the urothelium and submucosa are infiltrated predominantly by $CD4^+$ T cells, while $\gamma/\delta$ T cells are detected in only occasional sections (24). In a rat model of ascending acute pyelonephritis, Kurnick and coworkers (74) observed a predominant mononuclear cell influx in the kidney interstitium at 4, 8, 15, 21, and 25 days after bacterial inoculation. Most of these cells were $CD4^+$ T cells; a few were $CD8^+$ cells. The cellular infiltrate contained T cells specific to the infecting strain. T-cell expansion in response to E. coli was major histocompatibility complex restricted and was greater in response to non-P-fimbriated strains than P-fimbriated strains (74).

Studies examining the role of cell-mediated immunity in UTI have compared the abilities of athymic animals and their normal counterparts to clear experimental infection. In an acute-UTI model in mice, Swiss (nu/nu) and BALB/c (nu/nu) mice and their normal counterparts showed similar resistance to intravesical infection (148). In addition, cyclosporin A treatment of normal mice did not impair their resistance to experimental UTI (47). Similarly, in chronic-UTI models using T-cell-depleted and athymic rats, the absence of thymus-dependent T cells did not influence the course of infection or the development of pyelonephritic lesions (25, 99). The lack of T-cell involvement in these models was recently brought into question when Bandeira and coworkers showed the majority of murine IELs to be T cells of extrathymic origin (9). However, the numbers of IELs of extrathymic origin is lower in nude mice than in normal mice (80a). It follows that if extrathymic T cells are involved in bacterial clearance, then differences between athymic and normal animals would be observed. The role of T cells of extrathymic origin in the clearance of infection in normal animals needs further study.

### Antibody Response to UTI

Infections of the urinary tract cause a local and sometimes a systemic antibody response to the infecting strain.

#### URINARY ANTIBODY RESPONSE

Uninfected urine contains immunoglobulins and fragments thereof that constitute a large portion of the protein excreted daily into the urine (45). IgA, IgG, and, rarely, IgM are excreted into the urine (20); IgA in its dimeric form is linked to the secretory component (13). These molecules have little specific antibody activity against the bacterial pathogens that cause UTI. A specific urinary antibody response occurs in children with acute pyelonephritis within 7 to 10 days of diagnosis (58, 134). The magnitude of the urinary antibody response is greater in patients with acute pyelonephritis than in those with cystitis or ABU. Antibodies are primarily of the secretory IgA type, suggesting a mucosal origin of antibody production; however, monomeric IgA and IgG are also found (44, 153). A number of these antibodies are specific for the O and K antigens and the fimbriae of the infecting strain.

Antibody production occurs in both the upper and the lower urinary tract (21). Recently, Christmas observed significantly higher numbers of IgA-producing plasma cells in the urothelium and submucosa of patients with bacterial cystitis than in healthy controls, thus confirming the presence of these cells at the mucosa during infection (24). Antibody-secreting cells and B lymphocytes migrate to the kidney during infection; however, the plasma cell infiltrate of the urinary tract has not been well characterized.

## SERUM ANTIBODY RESPONSES TO UTI

Specific antibodies to *E. coli* antigens are found in the circulation of most individuals; however, levels increase during episodes of acute UTI (5, 56, 58, 162). The serum antibody response to UTI is dominated by IgM and IgG antibodies (165). *E. coli*-induced pyelonephritis stimulates a specific serum antibody response to the O and in a few cases the K antigen of the infecting strain (62). Anti-lipid A antibodies of the IgG class are elevated in girls with acute pyelonephritis, acute cystitis and ABU (96). Specific serum antibodies to P fimbriae are produced in patients suffering from pyelonephritis with P-fimbriated *E. coli* (32). In contrast, antifimbrial antibodies are not detected in the sera of healthy controls.

## ROLE OF ANTIBODIES IN PROTECTION AGAINST INFECTION

Despite numerous studies reporting specific antibody responses to UTI, the contribution of antibodies to resistance to infection is not well understood. IgA antibodies isolated from the urine of patients with acute pyelonephritis block the adherence of *E. coli* to urinary tract epithelial cells in vitro (155). Whether IgA antibodies have a similar role during UTI in vivo remains unknown. Circumstantial evidence for a protective role for antibodies has come from vaccination studies in experimental animal models. Vaccine preparations of whole bacteria and isolated bacterial components such as LPS, capsular polysaccharides, and fimbriae induce protection to subsequent challenge with strains carrying the vaccine antigens (19, 65, 97). Although these studies infer a role for specific immunity in protection from subsequent infection, the extent to which specific antibodies are involved in the defense of the human urinary tract remains unclear.

Passive immunization studies in animal models have been used to clarify the role of specific antibodies in resistance to infection. Intraperitoneal injection of pooled ascites fluid containing monoclonal antibodies directed against *E. coli* K13 gave slight protection against intravesical challenge with *E. coli* O6:K13:H1 in rats (63). Monoclonal anti-P-fimbrial antibodies protected mice from experimental infection (131, 147). In contrast, immunization with antisera to lipid A antibody had no effect on outcome of infection in rats (97). Common to these studies was the requirement for threshold serum antibody titers for protection. Passive immunization studies suggest that high-enough serum titers of specific antibodies can influence the course of infection in the urinary tract.

The role of antibodies in protection against UTI remains controversial for a number of reasons. First, levels of specific circulating and local antibodies in individual mice after exposure to antigen show no correlation with outcome of infection (43). Second, in human infections, bacteria often persist despite the presence of high titers of type-specific antibody (162). Third, mice with B-cell immunodeficiencies (CBA/N; *xid;* B lymphocyte deficient) were as able as their normal counterparts to clear experimental *E. coli* UTI (148). Fourth, the frequency of UTI is not increased in patients with hypogammaglobulinemia or other antibody deficiencies.

## PREVENTION OF UTI

### Vaccination

Early observations that vaccination with heat- or formalin-killed *E. coli* induced high levels of antibody in rats and prevented retrograde pyelonephritis (19) led to hopes of developing a vaccine for UTI. Immunization of experimental animals with whole bacteria gave O-type-specific protection (64). The large variation in O antigens coupled with the risk for adverse reactions upon immunization with antigens containing endotoxin led to trials with other *E. coli* antigens. The capsular or K antigens are fewer in number and elicit greater protection in experimental models than O antigens do (61). Unfortunately, K antigens are poor immunogens in humans (44).

The design of a UTI vaccine is complicated by the antigenic variability of uropathogenic *E. coli*. Surveys of patient populations with UTI show that considerable differences exist between the antigenic properties of strains causing first-time and recurrent episodes of acute pyelonephritis and those of strains from patients with and without underlying defects in their host defenses against UTI (85, 120). Strains that cause the first episode of uncomplicated acute pyelonephritis or recurrent episodes in patients without signs of reflux belong to a select group of virulent *E. coli* strains that are ~90% P fimbriated. The high percentage of P-fimbriated strains in these patient populations has led to experimental immunization studies with P fimbriae. Immunization with purified P fimbriae protected mice and monkeys against expermimental pyelonephritis with homologous and heterologous P-fimbriated *E. coli* (108, 113, 123). A vaccine based on the P fimbriae of *E. coli* was therefore proposed to protect children and adults with first or recurrent uncomplicated episodes of UTI due to P-fimbriated *E. coli*.

Strains causing recurrent episodes of acute cystitis or acute pyelonephritis with renal scarring (for which, arguably, vaccination is most needed) express a different range of O and K antigens, and only some 20 to 40% are P fimbriated (85–88). The antigenic diversity of the strains makes it difficult to define a protective antigen or a set of antigens that will induce protective immunity in these patient groups.

### Receptor Analog Treatment

An alternative approach to this problem would be to use receptor analogs as inhibitors of P-fimbrial attachment. Blocking P-fimbrial attachment with globotetraose, a Gal$\alpha$1-4Gal$\beta$-containing receptor analog, reduced the recovery of P-fimbriated *E. coli* from the urinary tracts of mice in an acute-UTI model (150). In this model, globotetraose was mixed with P-fimbriated bacteria before being inoculated into the animals. It remains to be seen whether globotetraose given to animals intravesically or orally affects the outcome of an ongoing infection with P-fimbriated *E. coli*. The use of receptor analogs may have several advantages over vaccination. First, a limited number of structural variants are active against a wide variety of P-fimbriated bacteria, regardless of antigenic variation. Second, the receptor analogs should be less interactive with the host immune system than bacterial antigens are. *E. coli* antigens can trigger an immune response that is cross-reactive with renal tissue and that may participate in tissue damage and renal scarring.

### Alternative Approaches to Prevention

Prevention of recurrent infections is likely to require an approach other than vaccination. Studies examining host defense mechanisms in the urinary tract have highlighted the importance of mucosal inflammation as opposed to specific immunity in the clearance of UTI. While much work remains in understanding the processes involved in the mucosal inflammatory response, identifying the important inflammatory parameters involved in clearance may help us design new ways of improving resistance to infection in these susceptible individuals.

## SPECIFIC GROUPS WITH INCREASED SUSCEPTIBILITY TO UTI

### Pregnancy and Susceptibility to UTI

Bacteriuria in pregnancy is associated with a risk of premature delivery and morbidity in acute pyelonephritis (68). Screening for bacteriuria combined with treatment has successfully prevented those complications in many populations. It is still not well understood to what extent pregnancy is associated with an increased frequency of bacteriuria (reduced resistance to infection) or by what mechanisms this occurs. The acquisition of bacteriuria increases in early pregnancy, suggesting that resistance to infection is reduced before the mechanical effects of the fetus on the urinary tract occur (141). The bacteria found to cause acute pyelonephritis in pregnant women have reduced virulence compared to those in nonpregnant controls, again suggesting that resistance to UTI permits different bacteria to reach and infect the kidneys (126, 141).

Pregnancy is known to be associated with immunosuppression, but immunity to uropathogens has not been studied. We recently compared specific immune responses to *E. coli* strains causing acute pyelonephritis in pregnant and nonpregnant women (115). Acute pyelonephritis in nonpregnant women was accompanied by significant serum and urine antibody responses, but the serum antibody response was significantly lower in the pregnant group. The host cytokine (IL-6) responses to infection in the pregnant and control groups were also compared. The IL-6 levels in serum and urine at diagnosis were significantly higher in the nonpregnant women than in the pregnant women. This fact demonstrates that the immunosuppressive effect of pregnancy includes the mucosal IL-6 and specific antibody responses to acute pyelonephritis caused by *E. coli*.

### Aging and Resistance to UTI

Recurrent UTIs are a problem for many women after menopause. Menopause is accompanied by an atrophy of estrogen-dependent tissues that leads to increased urogenital problems (102). During and following menopause, the vaginal mucosa undergoes atrophy, the pH of the vagina increases, and the indigenous microbiota within the vagina change, with a decrease in lactobacilli and an increase in *Enterobacteriaceae* (101). Symptoms of urogenital atrophy include vaginal dryness, burning, itching, and dyspareunia as well as the urinary symptoms of frequency, urgency, dysuria, incontinence, and recurrent UTI (101). The patients may also suffer a loss of urinary control resulting in urinary incontinence (especially of the urgency type). The urinary mucosa undergoes the same atrophic changes as are observed in the vagina (94). This loss of integrity appears to be a predisposing factor in susceptibility to UTI.

Studies using low-dose estrogen replacement therapy show marked improvements in vaginal and urinary atrophic vasomotor symptoms (54, 125, 159, 160). With the restoration of the atrophic vaginal mucosa and a lowering of the vaginal pH, a corresponding decrease in recurrent UTI has been observed in the same patients.

Raz and Stamm (121) carried out a double-blind, placebo-controlled study of the effects of topically administered estrogen. The incidence of UTI in the group given estradiol was significantly lower than that in the group given placebo. The women given estradiol were also more likely than the placebo group to remain infection free. Analysis of the vaginal flora and vaginal pH prior to the study in all patients showed that lactobacilli were absent from the flora and the pH increased to around 5.5. The patients who recieved estradiol had lactobacilli in their vaginal flora and a corresponding decrease in pH and *Enterobacteriaceae* within 1 month of beginning treatment, whereas the placebo controls did not. It appears from this study that the intravaginal administration of estradiol decrease the rate of recurrent infection in these postmenopausal women. The mode of action by which estrogen prevents recurrent UTI is not known, but it may be related to the decrease in *Enterobacteriaceae* colonizing the introital area, the restoration of the atrophic mucosa to participation in the prevention of infection, and/or an improvement in vasomotor function restoring urinary continence.

Bacteriuria has been discussed as a cause of increased mortality in elderly individuals. Studies of Greek, Finnish, and American patients showed a decreased longevity associated with UTI (33, 104, 116). The patients with UTI were suffering from a variety of diseases other than UTI that might increase their susceptibility to infection as well as their mortality. Nordenstam et al. studied a population of elderly individuals and compared their longevity in relation to bacteriuria (105). There was no increase in mortality in bacteriuric but otherwise healthy individuals. Bacteriuria per se did not appear to be a risk factor. In patients with concomitant disease, bacteriuria was associated with increased mortality. To analyze the contribution of bacteriuria to the mortality of this group, large clinical trials with selective treatment of bacteriuria in these patients would be required.

## SUMMARY

The resistance to UTI is influenced by exposure to uropathogenic bacteria, age, hormonal status, and the conditions that influence urine flow. At the molecular level, susceptibility is influenced by the expression of receptors for attaching bacteria, the production of antibacterial substances in the urine, and the inflammatory response to infection. The role of specific immunity in resistance to infection is unclear, but immunity induced by vaccination protects against UTI in animal models. Elucidation of mechanisms that explain the susceptibility to UTI of certain patient groups can provide novel approaches to diagnosis and treatment of these infections.

## REFERENCES

1. **Agace, W., G. Godaly, S. Hedges, and C. Svanborg.** Unpublished data.
1a. **Agace, W., S. Hedges, U. Andersson, J. Andersson, M. Ceska, and C. Svanborg.** 1993. Selective cytokine production by epithelial cells following exposure to *Escherichia coli*. *Infect. Immun.* **61**:602–609.
2. **Agace, W., S. Hedges, M. Ceska, and C. Svanborg.** 1993. IL-8 and the neutrophil response to mucosal Gram negative infection. *J. Clin. Invest.* **92**:780–785.
3. **Agace, W., S. Hedges, and C. Svanborg.** 1992. Lps genotype in the C57 black mouse background and its influence on the interleukin-6 response to *Escherichia coli* urinary tract infection. *Scand. J. Immunol.* **35**:531–538.
4. **Agace, W. W., M. Patarroyo, M. Svensson, E. Carlemalm, and C. Svanborg.** 1995. *Escherichia coli* induces trans-uroepithelial neutrophil migration by an ICAM-1 dependent mechanism. *Infect. Immun.* **63**:4054–4062.
5. **Andersen, H.** 1966. Studies of urinary tract infections in infancy and childhood. VII. The relation of *Escherichia coli* antibody in pyelonephritis as measured by homologous and common (Kunin) antigens. *J. Pediatr.* **68**:542–550.
6. **Anderson, P., I. Engberg, G. Lidin-Janson, K. Lincoln, R. Hull, S. Hull, and C. Svanborg-Edén.** 1991. Persistence of *Escherichia coli* bacteriuria not determined by bacterial adherence. *Infect. Immun.* **59**:2915–2921.
7. **Asscher, A., M. Sussman, W. Waters, R. Harvard Davis, and S. Chick.** 1966. Urine as a medium for bacterial growth. *Lancet* **ii**:1037–1041.
8. **Båga, M., S. Normark, J. Hardy, P. O'Hanley, D. Lark, O. Olsson, G. Schoolnik, and S. Falkow.** 1984. Nucleotide sequence of the *papA* gene encoding the *pap* pilus subunit of human uropathogenic *Escherichia coli*. *J. Bacteriol.* **157**:330–333.
9. **Bandeira, A., S. Itohara, M. Bonneville, O. Burlen-Derranoux, T. Mota-santos, A. Coutinho, and S. Tonegawa.** 1991.

Extrathymic origin of intestinal intraepithelial lymphocytes bearing T-cell antigen receptor γδ. *Proc. Natl. Acad. Sci. USA* **88**:43.
10. **Benson, M., A. Andreasson, U. Jodal, Å. Karlsson, J. Rydberg, and C. Svanborg.** 1994. Interleukin 6 in childhood urinary tract infection. *Pediatr. Infect. Dis. J.* **13**:612–616.
11. **Benson, M., U. Jodal, W. Agace, A. Andreasson, S. Mårild, E. Stokland, B. Wettergren, and C. Svanborg.** Interleukin-6 and interleukin-8 in children with febrile urinary tract infection and asymptomatic bacteriuria. Submitted for publication.
12. **Bettelheim, K. A., and J. Taylor.** 1969. A study of *Escherichia coli* isolated from chronic urinary tract infection. *J. Med. Microbiol.* **2**:225–236.
13. **Bienenstock, J., and T. Tomasi.** 1968. Secretory IgA in normal urine. *J. Clin. Invest.* **47**:1162–1167.
14. **Blackwell, C., K. Jonsdottir, M. Hanson, W. Todd, A. Chaudhuri, B. Mathew, R. Bettle, and D. Weir.** 1986. Non-secretion of ABO blood group antigens predisposing to infection by *Neisseria meningitidis* and *Streptococcus pneumoniae*. *Lancet* **ii**:284–285.
15. **Blackwell, C., S. Thom, O. Lawrie, D. Weir, D. Wray, and D. Kinane.** 1986. Non-secretion of blood group antigens and susceptibility to oral infections by *Candida albicans*. *J. Dent. Res.* **64**:502.
16. **Bock, K., M. E. Breimer, A. Brignole, G. C. Hansson, K.-A. Karlsson, G. Larson, H. Leffler, B. E. Samuelsson, N. Strömberg, C. Svanborg-Edén, and J. Thurin.** 1985. Specificity of binding of a strain of uropathogenic *Escherichia coli* to Galα1-4Galβ-containing glycosphingolipids. *J. Biol. Chem.* **260**:8545–8551.
17. **Breimer, M. E.** 1985. Chemical and immunological identification of the Forssman pentaglycosylceramide in human kidneys. *Glycoconjugate* **2**:375.
18. **Breimer, M. E., G. C. Hansson, and H. Leffler.** 1985. The specific glycosphingolipid composition of human urethral epithelial cells. *J. Biochem.* **98**:1169–1180.
19. **Brooks, S., J. Lyons, and A. Braude.** 1974. Immunization against retrograde pyelonephritis. *Am. J. Pathol.* **74**:345–354.
20. **Burdon, D.** 1970. Quantitative studies of urinary immunoglobulins in hospital patients, including patients with urinary tract infection. *Clin. Exp. Immunol.* **6**:189–196.
21. **Burdon, D.** 1971. Immunoglobulins of normal human urine and urethral secretions. *Immunology* **21**:363–368.
22. **Cerf-Bensussan, N., A. Quaroni, J. Kurnick, and A. Bhan.** 1984. Intraepithelial lymphocytes modulate Ia expression by intestinal epithelial cells. *J. Immunol.* **132**:2244–2252.
23. **Chambers, S., and C. Kunin.** 1985. The osmoprotective properties of urine for bacteria: the protective effect of betaine and human urine against low pH and high concentrations of electrolytes, sugars and urea. *J. Infect. Dis.* **152**:1308–1316.
24. **Christmas, T.** 1994. Lymphocyte populations in the bladder wall in normal bladder, bacterial cystitis and interstitial cystitis. *Br. J. Urol.* **73**:508–515.
25. **Coles, G., S. Chick, M. Hopkins, R. Ling, and N. Radford.** 1974. The role of the T cell in experimental pyelonephritis. *Clin. Exp. Immunol.* **16**:629–636.
26. **Connell, H., P. de Man, U. Jodal, K. Lincoln, and C. Svanborg.** 1993. Lack of association between hemolysin and acute inflammation in human urinary tract infection. *Microb. Pathol.* **14**:463–472.
27. **Connell, H., I. Wilson, H. Sabharwal, L. Perssson, I. Kockum, M. Zasloff, and C. Svanborg.** Unpublished data.
28. **Cox, C., and F. Hinman.** 1961. Experiments with induced bacteriuria, vesical emptying and bacterial growth on the mechanism of bladder defense to infection. *J. Urol.* **86**:739–748.
29. **Crestani, B., P. Cornillet, M. Dehoux, C. Rolland, M. Guenounou, and M. Aubier.** 1994. Alveolar type II epithelial cells produce interleukin 6 in vitro and in vivo. *J. Clin. Invest.* **94**:731–740.
30. **de Man, P., U. Jodal, K. Lincoln, and C. Svanborg-Edén.** 1988. Bacterial attachment and inflammation in the urinary tract. *J. Infect. Dis.* **158**:29–35.
31. **de Man, P., C. van Kooten, L. Aarden, I. Engberg, H. Linder, and C. Svanborg-Edén.** 1989. Interleukin-6 induced at mucosal surfaces by gram-negative bacterial infection. *Infect. Immun.* **57**:3383–3388.
32. **De Ree, J., and J. van den Bosch.** 1987. Serological response to the P fimbriae of uropathogenic *Escherichia coli* in pyelonephritis. *Infect. Immun.* **55**:2204–2207.
33. **Dontas, A., P. Kasviki-Charvati, P. Papanayiotou, and S. Marketos.** 1981. Bacteriuria and survival in old age. *N. Engl. J. Med.* **304**:939–943.
34. **Duguid, J. P., I. W. Smith, G. Dempster, and P. N. Edmunds.** 1955. Non-flagellar filamentous appendages ("fimbriae") and haemagglutinating activity in *Bacterium coli*. *J. Pathol. Bacteriol.* **70**:335–348.

35. Eisenhauer, P. B., S. S. S. L. Harwig, and R. I. Lehrer. 1992. Cryptdins: antimicrobial defensins of the murine small intestine. *Infect. Immun.* **60**:3556–3565.
36. Fletcher, A., A. Neuberger, and A. Ratcliffe. 1970. Tamm-Horsfall urinary glycoprotein: the chemical composition. *Biochem. J.* **120**:417–424.
37. Fletcher, A., A. Neuberger, and W. Ratcliffe. 1970. Tamm-Horsfall urinary glycoprotein: the subunit structure. *Biochem. J.* **120**:425–432.
38. Fowler, J., and E. Stamey. 1977. Studies of introital colonization in women with recurrent urinary tract infection. VII. The role of bacterial adherence. *J. Urol.* **117**:472–476.
39. Gardiner, R., G. Seymour, M. Lavin, M. G. Strutton, E. Gemmell, and G. Hazan. 1986. Immunohistochemical analysis of the human bladder. *Br. J. Urol.* **58**:19–25.
40. Gibbons, R., R. Sellwood, M. Burrows, and P. Hunter. 1977. Inheritance of resistance to neonatal *Escherichia coli* diarrhoea in the pig: examination of the genetic system. *Theor. Appl. Genet.* **81**:65.
41. Grüneberg, R. 1969. Relationship of infecting urinary organisms to the faecal flora in patients with symptomatic urinary infections. *Lancet* **ii**:766–768.
42. Hagberg, L., U. Jodal, T. K. Korhonen, J. G. Lidin, U. Lindberg, and C. Svanborg-Eden. 1981. Adhesion, hemagglutination, and virulence of *Escherichia coli* causing urinary tract infections. *Infect. Immun.* **31**:564–70.
43. Hagberg, L., H. Leffler, and C. Svanborg-Edén. 1984. Non-antibiotic prevention of urinary tract infection. *Infection* **12**:132–137.
44. Hanson, L., S. Ahlstedt, A. Fasth, U. Jodal, B. Kaijser, P. Larsson, U. Lindberg, S. Olling, A. Sohl-Åkerlund, and C. Svanborg-Edén. 1977. Antigens of *Escherichia coli*, human immune response, and the pathogenesis of urinary tract infections. *J. Infect. Dis.* **135**:144–149.
45. Hanson, L., and E. Tan. 1965. Characterization of antibodies in human urine. *J. Clin. Invest.* **44**:703–715.
46. Hedges, S., W. Agace, M. Svensson, A.-C. Sjögren, M. Ceska, and C. Svanborg. 1994. Uropithelial cells are a part of a mucosal cytokine network. *Infect. Immun.* **62**:2315–2321.
47. Hedges, S., H. Lindner, P. de Man, and C. Svanborg. 1990. Cyclosporin-dependent, *nu* independent mucosal IL-6 response to gram negative infection. *Scand. J. Immunol.* **31**:335–343.
48. Hedges, S., P. Anderson, G. Lidin-Janson, P. de Man, and C. Svanborg. 1991. Interleukin-6 response to deliberate colonization of the human urinary tract with gram-negative bacteria. *Infect. Immun.* **59**:421–427.
49. Hedges, S., M. Bjarnadottir, W. Agace, L. Hang, and C. Svanborg. Immunoregulatory cytokines modify *Escherichia coli* induced epithelial cell IL-6 and IL-8 responses. Submitted for publication.
50. Hedges, S., P. de Man, H. Linder, C. van Kooten, and C. Svanborg-Edén. 1990. Interleukin-6 is secreted by epithelial cells in response to Gram-negative bacterial challenge, p. 144–148. In T. Macdonald (ed.) *Advances in Mucosal Immunology. International Conference of Mucosal Immunity*. Kluwer, London.
51. Hedges, S., K. Stenquist, G. Lidin-Janson, J. Martinell, T. Sandberg, and C. Svanborg. 1992. Comparison of urine and serum concentrations of interleukin-6 in women with acute pyelonephritis or asymptomatic bacteriuria. *J. Infect. Dis.* **166**:653–656.
52. Hedges, S., M. Svensson, W. Agace, and C. Svanborg. 1995. Cytokines induce an epithelial cell cytokine response, p. 189–193. In J. Mestecky, M. Russell, S. Michalek, H. Hognova, and J. Sterzl (ed.), *Recent Advances in Mucosal Immunology*. Plenum Press, New York.
53. Hedges, S., M. Svensson, and C. Svanborg. 1992. Interleukin-6 response of epithelial cell lines to bacterial stimulation in vitro. *Infect. Immun.* **60**:1295–1301.
54. Henriksson, L., M. Stjernquist, L. Boquist, U. Alander, and I. Selinus. 1994. A comparative multicenter study of the effects of continuous low-dose estradiol released from a new vaginal ring versus estriol vaginal pessaries in postmenopausal women with symptoms and signs of urogenital atrophy. *Am. J. Obstet. Gynecol.* **171**:624–632.
55. Hodson, C., T. Maling, P. McManamon, and M. Lewis. 1975. The pathogenesis of reflux nephropathy (chronic atrophic pyelonephritis). *Br. J. Radiol. Suppl.* **13**:1–26.
56. Holmgren, J., and J. Smith. 1975. Immunological aspects of urinary tract infection. *Prog. Allergy* **18**:289–352.
57. Hull, R. A., R. E. Gill, P. Hsu, B. H. Minshew, and S. Falkow. 1981. Construction and expression of recombinant plasmids encoding type 1 or D-mannose resistant pili

from the urinary tract infection *Escherichia coli* isolate. *Infect. Immun.* **33**:933–938.
58. Jodal, U., S. Ahlstedt, B. Carlsson, L. A. Hanson, U. Lindberg, and A. Sohl. 1974. Local antibodies in childhood urinary tract infection: a preliminary study. *Int. Arch. Allergy Appl. Immunol.* **47**:537–546.
59. Johanson, I., R. Lindstedt, and C. Svanborg. 1992. The role of the *pap* and *prs* encoded adhesins in *Escherichia coli* adherence to human epithelial cells. *Infect. Immun.* **60**:3416–3422.
60. Johanson, I.-M., K. Plos, B.-I. Marklund, and C. Svanborg. 1993. *pap, papG* and *prsG* DNA sequences in *Escherichia coli* from the fecal flora and the urinary tract. *Microb. Pathol.* **15**:121–129.
61. Kaijser, B., and S. Ahlstedt. 1977. Protective capacity of antibodies against *Escherichia coli* O and K antigens. *Infect. Immun.* **17**:286–289.
62. Kaijser, B., L. A. Hanson, U. Jodal, J. G. Lidin, and J. B. Robbins. 1977. Frequency of *Escherichia coli* K antigens in urinary-tract infections in children. *Lancet* **i**:663–666.
63. Kaijser, B., P. Larsson, W. Nimmick, and T. Söderström. 1983. Antibodies to *Escherichia coli* K and O antigens in protection against acute pyelonephritis. *Prog. Allergy* **33**:275–288.
64. Kaijser, B., P. Larsson, and S. Olling. 1978. Protection against ascending *Escherichia coli* pyelonephritis in rats and significance of local immunity. *Infect. Immun.* **20**:78–81.
65. Kaijser, B., and S. Olling. 1973. Experimental hematogenous pyelonephritis due to *Escherichia coli* in rabbits. The antibody response and its protective capacity. *J. Infect. Dis.* **128**:41–49.
66. Källenius, G., R. Möllby, S. Svensson, J. Winberg, S. Lundblad, S. Svensson, and B. Cedergren. 1980. The Pk antigen as a receptor for the hemagglutination of pyelonephritogenic *Escherichia coli*. *FEMS Microbiol. Lett.* **7**:297–302.
67. Källenius, G., and J. Winberg. 1978. Bacterial adherence to periurethral epithelial cells in girls prone to urinary tract infection. *Lancet* **ii**:540–542.
68. Kass, E. 1960. Bacteriuria and pyelonephritis of pregnancy. *Arch. Intern. Med.* **105**:194–198.
69. Kass, E., and D. Zangwill. 1960. In E. Kass (ed.), *Biology of Pyelonephritis*, p. 663. Boston.
70. Kaye, D. 1968. Antibacterial activity of human urine. *J. Clin. Invest.* **47**:2374–2390.
70a. Kinane, E., C. Blackwell, R. Brettle, D. Weir, F. Winstanley, and R. Elton. 1982. ABO blood group secretor state and susceptibility to urinary tract infection. *Br. Med. J.* **285**:7–9.
71. Ko, Y. C., N. Mukaida, S. Ishiyama, A. Tokue, T. Kawai, K. Matsushima, and T. Kasahara. 1993. Elevated interleukin-8 levels in the urine of patients with urinary tract infections. *Infect. Immun.* **61**:1307–1314.
72. Korhonen, T., V. Väisänen, H. Saxen, H. Hultberg, and S. Svenson. 1986. Binding of *Escherichia coli* S fimbriae to human kidney epithelium. *Infect. Immun.* **37**:286–291.
73. Kunin, C. 1987. *Detection, Prevention and Management of Urinary Tract Infections.* Lea & Febiger, Philadelphia.
74. Kurnick, J., R. McCluskey, A. Bhan, K. Wright, R. Wilkinson, and H. Rubin. 1988. *Escherichia coli*-specific T lymphocytes in experimental pyelonephritis. *J. Immunol.* **141**:3220–3226.
75. Kvale, D., P. Brandzaeg, and D. Löv-Haug. 1988. Up-regulation of the expression of secretory component and HLA molecules in a human colonic cell line by tumour necrosis factor-α and gamma interferon. *Scand. J. Immunol.* **28**:351–357.
76. Kvale, D., P. Krajci, and P. Brandtzaeg. 1992. Expression and regulation of adhesion molecules ICAM-1 (CD54) and LFA-3 (CD58) in human intestinal epithelial cell lines. *Scand. J. Immunol.* **35**:669–676.
77. Lee, J.-Y., A. Boman, S. Chuanxin, M. Andersson, H. Jörnvall, V. Mutt, and H. Boman. 1989. Antibacterial peptides from pig intestine: isolation of a mammalian cecropin. *Proc. Natl. Acad. Sci. USA* **86**:9159–9162.
78. Leffler, H., and C. Svanborg-Eden. 1980. Chemical identification of a glycosphingolipid receptor for *Escherichia coli* attaching to human urinary tract epithelial cells and agglutinating human erythrocytes. *FEMS Microbiol. Lett.* **8**:127–134.
79. Leffler, H., and C. Svanborg-Edén. 1981. Glycolipid receptors for uropathogenic *Escherichia coli* on human erythrocytes and uroepithelial cells. *Infect. Immun.* **34**:920–929.
80. Lidin-Janson, G., L. Hanson, and B. Kaijser. 1977. Comparison of *Escherichia coli* from bacteriuric patients with those from feces of healthy school children. *J. Infec. Dis.* **136**:346–353.

80a. Lin, T., G. Matsuzaki, T. Nakamura, and K. Nomoto. 1993. Thymus influences the development of extrathymically derived intestinal intraepithelial lymphocytes. *Eur. J. Immunol.* **23**:1968–1974.
81. Lindberg, F., B. Lund, and S. Normark. 1984. Genes of pyelonephrithogenic *Escherichia coli* required for digalactoside specific agglutination of human cells. *EMBO J.* **3**:1167–1173.
82. Lindstedt, R., P. Falk, R. Hull, S. Hull, H. Leffler, E. C. Svanborg, and G. Larson. 1989. Binding specificities of wild-type and cloned *Escherichia coli* strains that recognize globo-A. *Infect. Immun.* **57**:3389–3394.
83. Lindstedt, R., G. Larson, P. Falk, U. Jodal, H. Leffler, and E. C. Svanborg. 1991. The receptor repertoire defines the host range for attaching *Escherichia coli* recognizing globo-A. *Infect. Immun.* **59**:1086–1092.
84. Lomberg, H., B. Cedergren, H. Leffler, B. Nilsson, A.-S. Carlström, and C. Svanborg-Edén. 1986. Influence of blood group on the availability of receptors for attachment of uropathogenic *Escherichia coli*. *Infect. Immun.* **51**:919–926.
85. Lomberg, H., L. Hanson, B. Jacobsson, U. Jodal, H. Leffler, and C. Svanborg-Edén. 1983. Correlation of P blood group phenotype, vesicoureteral reflux and bacterial attachment in patients with recurrent pyelonephritis. *N. Engl. J. Med.* **308**:1189–1192.
86. Lomberg, H., M. Hellström, U. Jodal, H. Leffler, K. Lincoln, and C. Svanborg-Edén. 1984. Virulence-associated traits in Escherichia coli causing first and recurrent episodes of urinary tract infection in children with or without vesicoureteral reflux. *J. Infect. Dis.* **150**:561–569.
87. Lomberg, H., M. Hellström, U. Jodal, I. Ørskov, and C. Svanborg-Edén. 1989. Properties of *Escherichia coli* in patients with renal scarring. *J. Infect. Dis.* **159**:579–582.
88. Lomberg, H., M. Hellström, U. Jodal, and C. Svanborg-Edén. 1986. Renal scarring and non-attaching bacteria. *Lancet* **ii**:1341.
89. Lomberg, H., M. Hellström, U. Jodal, and C. Svanborg-Edén. 1989. Secretor state and renal scarring in girls with recurrent pyelonephritis. *FEMS Microbiol. Immunol.* **47**:371–376.
90. Lomberg, H., U. Jodal, H. Leffler, P. de Man, and C. Svanborg. 1992. Blood group non-secretors have an increased inflammatory response to urinary tract infection. *Scand. J. Infect Dis.* **24**:77–83.
91. Lomberg, H., U. Jodal, C. Svanborg-Edén, H. Leffler, and B. Samuelsson. 1981. P1 blood group and urinary tract infection. *Lancet* **i**:551.
92. Lund, B., B. I. Marklund, N. Strömberg, F. Lindberg, K. A. Karlsson, and S. Normark. 1988. Uropathogenic Escherichia coli can express serologically identical pili of different receptor binding specificities. *Mol. Microbiol.* **2**:255–263.
93. Marcus, D., S. Kundu, and A. Suguki. 1981. The P blood group system: recent progress in immunochemistry and genetics. *Semin. Hematol.* **18**:63–71.
94. Mårild, S., M. Hellström, B. Jacobsson, U. Jodal, and C. Svanborg-Edén. 1989. Influence of bacterial adhesion on ureteral width in children with acute pyelonephritis. *J. Pediatr.* **115**:265–268.
95. Marklund, B. I. 1991. Structural and functional variation among Gal$\alpha$1-4Gal$\beta$ adhesins of *Escherichia coli*. Ph.D. thesis. University of Umeå, Umeå, Sweden.
96. Mattsby-Baltzer, I., I. Claësson, L. Hanson, U. Jodal, B. Kaijser, U. Lindberg, and H. Peterson. 1981. Antibodies to lipid A during urinary tract infection. *J. Infect. Dis.* **144**:319–328.
97. Mattsby-Baltzer, I., L. Hanson, B. Kaijser, and S. Olling. 1982. Experimental *Escherichia coli* ascending pyelonephritis in rats: active peroral immunization with live *Escherichia coli* O6K13H1 and passively transferred anti-lipid A antibodies. *Infect. Immun.* **35**:647–653.
98. Meylan, P., and M. Glauser. 1989. Role of complement derived and bacterial formyl-peptide chemotactic factors in the *in vivo* migration of neutrophils in experimental *Escherichia coli* pyelonephritis in rats. *J. Infect. Dis.* **5**:959–965.
99. Miller, T., G. Findon, and S. Cawley. 1986. Cellular basis of host defence in pyelonephritis. I. Chronic infection. *Br. J. Exp. Pathol.* **67**:12–23.
100. Miller, T., G. Findon, and S. Cawley. 1987. Cellular basis of host defence in pyelonephritis. III. Deletion of individual components. *Br. J. Exp. Pathol.* **68**:377–388.
101. Milsom, I., L. Arvidsson, P. Ekelund, U. Molander, and O. Eriksson. 1993. Factors influencing vaginal cytology, pH and bacterial flora in elderly women. *Acta Obstet. Gynecol. Scand.* **72**:286–291.
102. Molander, U. 1993. Urinary incontinence and related urogenital symptoms in elderly women. *Acta Obstet. Gynecol. Scand. Suppl.* **158**:1–22.
103. Norden, C., G. Green, and E. Kass. 1968. Antibacterial mechanisms of the urinary bladder. *J. Clin. Invest.* **47**:2689–2700.

104. Nordenstam, G., Å. Branberg, A. Odén, C. Svanborg-Edén, and A. Svanborg. 1986. Bacteriuria and mortality in an elderly population. *N. Engl. J. Med.* **314:**1152–1156.
105. Nordenstam, G., V. Sundh, K. Lincoln, A. Svanborg, and C. Svanborg-Edén. 1989. Bacteriuria in representative population samples of persons aged 72–79 years. *Am. J. Epidemiol.* **130:**1176–1186.
106. Nowicki, B., C. Svanborg-Edén, R. Hull, and S. Hull. 1989. Molecular analysis and epidemiology of the Dr hemagglutination of uropathogenic *Escherichia coli*. *Infect. Immun.* **57:**446–451.
107. O'Grady, F., and J. Pennington. 1966. Bacterial growth in an in vitro system simulating conditions in the urinary bladder. *Br. J. Exp. Pathol.* **47:**283–290.
108. O'Hanley, P., P. Lark, S. Falkow, and G. Schoolnik. 1985. Molecular basis of *Escherichia coli* colonization of the upper urinary tract in BALB/c mice. *J. Clin. Invest.* **75:**347–360.
109. Ørskov, F., I. Ørskov, B. Jann, and K. Jann. 1980. Tamm-Horsfall protein or uromucoid is the normal urinary slime that traps type 1 fimbriated *Escherichia coli*. *Lancet* **i:**8173.
110. Parkkinen, J., R. Virkola, and T. K. Korhonen. 1983. *Escherichia coli* strains binding neuraminyl α2-3 galactosides. *Biochem. Biophys. Res. Commun.* **11:**456–461.
110a. Parkkinen, J., R. Virkola, and T. Korhonen. 1988. Identification of factors in urine that inhibit the binding of *Escherichia coli* adhesins. *Infect. Immun.* **56:**2623–2629.
111. Pasteur, L. 1863. Exam du rôle attribué au gaz oxygène atmosphérique dans la destruction des matières animales et végétales après la mort. *C.R. Acad. Sci.* **56:**734–740.
112. Pattersson-Delafield, J., R. Martinez, and R. Lehrer. 1980. Microbicidal cationic proteins in rabbit alveolar macrophages: a potential host defense mechanism. *Infect. Immun.* **30:**180–192.
113. Pecha, B., D. Low, and P. O'Hanley. 1989. Gal-Gal pili vaccines prevent pyelonephritis by piliated *Escherichia coli* in a murine model. Single-component Gal-Gal pili vaccines prevent pyelonephritis by homologous and heterologous piliated *E. coli* strains. *J. Clin. Invest.* **83:**2102–2108.
114. Pere, A., B. Nowicki, H. Saxén, A. Sittonen, and T. Korhonen. 1987. Expression of P, type 1 and type 1C fimbriae of *Escherichia coli* in the urine of patients with acute urinary tract infection. *J. Infect. Dis.* **156:**567–574.
115. Petersson, C., S. Hedges, K. Stenquist, T. Sandberg, H. Connell, and C. Svanborg. 1994. Suppressed antibody and interleukin-6 responses to acute pyelonephritis in pregnancy. *Kidney Int.* **45:**571–577.
116. Platt, R., B. Polk, B. Murdock, and B. Rosner. 1982. Mortality associated with nosocomial urinary tract infection. *N. Engl. J. Med.* **307:**637–642.
117. Plos, K., H. Connell, U. Jodal, B.-I. Marklund, S. Mårild, B. Wettergren, and C. Svanborg. 1995. Intestinal carriage of P fimbriated *Escherichia coli* and the susceptibility to urinary tract infection in young children. *J. Infect. Dis.* **171:**625–631.
118. Pugin, J., M. C. Schürer, D. Leturcq, A. Moriarty, R. J. Ulevitch, and P. S. Tobias. 1993. Lipopolysaccharide activation of human endothelial and epithelial cells is mediated by lipopolysaccharide-binding protein and soluble CD14. *Proc. Natl. Acad. Sci. USA* **90:**2744–2748.
119. Ransley, P., and R. Risdon. 1978. Reflux and renal scarring. *Br. J. Radiol.* **Suppl. 14:**1–38.
120. Ravn Juhl, B. 1985. Semiquantitative immunohistochemical evaluation of H-antigen expression in human ureters of different ABO- and Lewis type. *J. Histochem. Cytochem.* **33:**867–874.
121. Raz, P., and W. Stamm. 1993. A controlled trial of intravaginal estriol in postmenopausal women with recurrent urinary tract infections. *N. Engl. J. Med.* **329:**753–756.
122. Roberts, J. 1975. Experimental pyelonephritis in the monkey. III. Pathophysiology of ureteral malfunction induced by bacteria. *Invest. Urol.* **13:**117–120.
123. Roberts, J., B. Hardaway, E. Kaack, E. Fussell, and G. Baskin. 1984. Prevention of pyelonephritis by immunization with P-fimbriae. *J. Urol.* **131:**602–607.
124. Rutter, J., M. Burrows, R. Sellwood, and R. Gibbons. 1975. A genetic basis for resistance to enteric disease caused by *Escherichia coli*. *Nature* (London) **257:**135.
125. Samsioe, G. 1994. The endometrium: effects of estrogen and estrogen-progestogen replacement therapy. *Int. J. Fertil. Menopausal Stud.* **39**(Suppl. 2):84–92.
126. Sandberg, T., K. Stenquist, C. Svanborg-Edén, and G. Lidin-Janson. 1983. Host-parasite relationship in urinary tract infections during pregnancy. *Prog. Allergy* **33:**228–235.
127. Schaeffer, A., J. Jones, and J. Dunn. 1981. Association of in vitro *Escherichia coli* adherence to vaginal and buccal epithelial cells with susceptibility of women to recurrent urinary tract infection. *N. Engl. J. Med.* **304:**1062–1066.

128. Schulte-Wissermann, H., W. Mannhardt, J. Schwarz, F. Zepp, and D. Bitter-Sauermann. 1985. Comparison of the antibacterial effect of uroepithelial cells from healthy donors and children with asymptomatic bacteriuria. *Eur. J. Pediatr.* **144:** 230–233.
129. Senior, D., N. Baker, B. Cedergren, P. Falk, G. Larson, R. Lindstedt, and C. Svanborg-Edén. 1988. Globo-A—a new receptor specificity for attaching *Escherichia coli. FEBS Lett.* **237:**123–127.
130. Sikri, K., C. Foster, F. Bloomfield, and R. Marshall. 1979. Locolization by immunofluorescence and by light- and electronmicroscopic immunoperoxidase techniques of Tamm-Horsfall glycoprotein in adult hamster kidney. *Biochem. J.* **181:**525–532.
131. Silverblatt, F., and L. Cohen. 1979. Antipili antibody affords protection against experimental ascending pyelonephritis. *J. Clin. Invest.* **64:**333–336.
132. Smellie, J., P. Ransley, I. Normand, N. Prescod, and D. Edwards. 1985. Development of new renal scars: a collaborative study. *Br. Med. J.* **290:**1957–1960.
133. Smith, J., M. Adkins, and D. McGreary. 1975. Local immune response in experimental pyelonephritis in the rabbit. *Immunology* **29:**1067–1076.
134. Sohl-Åkelund, A., S. Ahlstedt, L. Hanson, and U. Jodal. 1979. Antibody responses in urine and serum against *Escherichia coli* O antigen in childhood urinary tract infection. *Acta Pathol. Microbiol. Scand. Sect. C* **87:**29–36.
135. Sollid, L. M., D. Kvale, P. Brantzaeg, G. Markussen, and E. Thorsby. 1987. Inteferon-γ enhances expression of secretory component, the epithelial receptor for polymeric immunoglobulins. *J. Immunol.* **138:** 4303.
136. Srivenugopal, K., and F. Ali-Osman. 1990. Stimulation and inhibition of 1,3-bis(2-chloroethyl)-1-nitrosourea-induced strand breaks and interstrand cross-linking in ColE1 plasmid deoxyribonucleic acid by polyamines and inorganic cations. *Biochem. Pharmacol.* **40:**473–479.
137. Stamey, T., and C. Sexton. 1975. The role of vaginal colonization with enterobacteriacea in recurrent urinary tract infections. *J. Urol.* **113:**214–217.
138. Stamey, T., M. Timothy, M. Miller, and G. Mihara. 1971. Recurrent urinary tract infections in adult women. The role of introital enterobacteria. *Calif. Med.* **115:**1–19.
139. Standiford, T. J., S. L. Kunkel, M. A. Basha, S. W. Chensue, J. Lynch, G. B. Toews, J. Westwick, and R. M. Strieter. 1990. Interleukin-8 gene expression by a pulmonary epithelial cell line. A model for cytokine networks in the lung. *J. Clin. Invest.* **86:**1945–1953.
140. Stapleton, A., E. Nudelman, H. Clausen, S. Hakomori, and W. E. Stamm. 1992. Binding of uropathogenic *Escherichia coli* R45 to glycolipids extracted from vaginal epithelial cells is dependent on histo-blood group secretor status. *J. Clin. Invest.* **90:**965–972.
141. Stenquist, K., I. Dahlén-Nilsson, G. Lidin-Janson, K. Lincoln, A. Odén, S. Rignell, and C. Svanborg Edén. 1989. Bacteriuria in pregnancy: frequency and risk of acquisition. *Am. J. Epidemiol.* **129:** 372–379.
142. Strömberg, N., B.-I. Marklund, B. Lund, D. Ilver, A. Hamers, W. Gaastra, K.-A. Karlsson, and S. Normark. 1990. Host-specificity of uropathogenic *Escherichia coli* depends on differences in binding specificity to Galα-4Galβ-containing isoreceptors. *EMBO J.* **9:**2001–2010.
143. Svanborg, C. 1993. Resistance to urinary tract infection. *N. Engl. J. Med.* **329:**802–803.
144. Svanborg, C., F. Ørskov, and I. Ørskov. 1994. Fimbriae and disease, p. 253–266. *In* P. Klemm (ed.), *Bacterial Fimbriae.* CRC Press, Inc., Boca Raton, Fla.
145. Svanborg, E. C., I. Engberg, S. Hedges, K. Jann, C. van Kooten, P. de Man, H. Linder, and A. Wold. 1989. Consequences of bacterial attachment in the urinary tract. *Biochem. Soc. Trans.* **17:**464–466.
146. Svanborg-Eden, C., and P. de Man. 1987. Bacterial virulence in urinary tract infection. *Infect. Dis. Clin. North Am.* **1:** 731–750.
147. Svanborg-Edén, C., B. Andersson, L. Hagberg, L. A. Hanson, H. Leffler, G. Magnusson, G. Noori, J. Dahmen, and T. Söderström. 1983. Receptor analogues and anti-pili antibodies as inhibitors of bacterial attachment in vivo and in vitro. *Ann. N.Y. Acad. Sci.* **409:**580–592.
148. Svanborg-Edén, C., D. Briles, L. Hagberg, J. McGhee, and S. Michalec. 1984. Genetic factors in host resistance to urinary tract infection. *Infection* **12:**118–123.
149. Svanborg-Edén, C., A. Fasth, and U. Jodal. 1982. Immunology of urinary tract infection, p. 141–162. *In* A. M. Geddes (ed.), *Recent Advances in Infection.* Pittman Press, London.

150. Svanborg-Eden, C., R. Freter, L. Hagberg, R. Hull, S. Hull, H. Leffler, and G. Schoolnik. 1982. Inhibition of experimental ascending urinary tract infection by a receptor analogue. *Nature* (London) 298:560–562.
151. Svanborg-Edén, C., S. Hansson, U. Jodal, G. Lidin-Janson, K. Lincoln, H. Linder, H. Lomberg, P. de Man, S. Mårild, J. Martinell, K. Plos, T. Sandberg, and K. Stenquist. 1988. Host-parasite interaction in the urinary tract. *J. Infect. Dis.* 157:421–426.
152. Svanborg-Edén, C., and U. Jodal. 1979. Attachment of *Escherichia coli* to urinary sediment cells from urinary tract infection prone and healthy children. *Infect. Immun.* 26:837–840.
153. Svanborg-Edén, C., R. Kulhavy, S. Mårild, S. Prince, and J. Mestecky. 1985. Urinary immunoglobulins in healthy individuals and children with acute pyelonephritis. *Scand. J. Immunol.* 21:305–313.
154. Svanborg-Edén, C., G. Lidin-Janson, and U. Lindberg. 1979. Adhesiveness to urinary tract epithelial cells of fecal and urinary *Escherichia coli* isolates from patients with symptomatic urinary tract infections or asymptomatic bacteriuria of varying duration. *J. Urol.* 122:185–188.
155. Svanborg-Edén, C., and A.-M. Svennerholm. 1978. Secretory immunoglobulin A and G antibodies prevent adhesion of *Escherichia coli* to human urinary tract epithelial cells. *Infect. Immun.* 22:790–797.
156. Tjandrawinata, R., L. Hawel III, and C. Byus. 1994. Regulation of putrescine export in lipopolysaccharide or IFN-γ-activated murine monocytic-leukemic RAW 264 cells. *J. Immunol.* 154:3039–3052.
157. Toma, G., J. Bates, and S. Kumar. 1994. Uromodulin (Tamm-Horsfall protein) is a leucocyte adhesion molecule. *Biochem. Biophys. Res. Commun.* 200:275–282.
158. Tullus, K., O. Fituri, L. Burman, B. Wretlind, and A. Brauner. 1994. Interleukin-6 and interleukin-8 in the urine of children with acute pyelonephritis. *Pediatr. Nephrol.* 8:280–284.
159. van der Linden, M., G. Gerretsen, M. Brandhorst, E. Ooms, C. Kremer, and W. Doesburg. 1993. The effect of estriol on the cytology of urethra and vagina in postmenopausal women with genito-urinary symptoms. *Eur. J. Obstet. Gynecol. Reprod. Biol.* 51:29–33.
160. van Leusden, H., G. Albertyn, C. Verlaine, and J. van Ruymbeke. 1993. A comparative multicenter study of two transdermal estradiol replacement therapies in the treatment of postmenopausal symptoms. *Int. J. Fertil. Menopausal Stud.* 38:210–218.
161. Virkola, R., B. Westerlund, H. Holthöfer, J. Parkkinen, M. Kekomäki, and T. K. Korhonen. 1988. Binding characteristics of *Escherichia coli* adhesins in human urinary bladder. *Infect. Immun.* 56:2615–2622.
162. Vosti, K., A. Monto, and L. Rantz. 1965. Host-parasite interaction in patients with infections due to *Escherichia coli*. II. Serologic response of the host. *J. Lab. Clin. Med.* 66:612–626.
163. Vroom, T. M., G. Scholte, F. Ossendorp, and J. Borst. 1991. Tissue distribution of human γδ T cells: no evidence for general epithelial tropism. *J. Clin. Pathol.* 44:1012–1017.
164. Wei, T.-F., W. Bujalowski, and T. Lohman. 1992. Cooperative binding of polyamines induces the *Escherichia coli* single-strand binding protein-DNA binding mode transitions. *Biochemistry* 31:6166–6174.
165. Winberg, J., H. Anderson, L. Hanson, and K. Lincoln. 1963. Studies of urinary tract infection in infancy and childhood. I. Antibody response in different types of urinary tract infections caused by coliform bacteria. *Br. Med. J.* 2:524.
166. Winter, A., B. Hardy, D. Alton, G. Arbus, and B. Churchill. 1983. Acquired renal scars in children. *J. Urol.* 129:1190–1194.
167. Wold, A. E., D. A. Caugant, G. Lidin-Janson, P. de Man, and C. Svanborg. 1992. Resident colonic *Escherichia coli* strains frequently display uropathogenic characteristics. *J. Infect. Dis.* 165:46–52.
168. Wold, A. E., J. Mestecky, and E. C. Svanborg. 1988. Agglutination of *Escherichia coli* by secretory IgA—a result of interaction between bacterial mannose-specific adhesins and immunoglobulin carbohydrate. *Monogr. Allergy* 24:307–309.
169. Wold, A. E., M. Thorssén, S. Hull, and C. Svanborg. 1988. Attachment of *Escherichia coli* via mannose of Galα1-4Galβ containing receptors to human colonic epithelial cells. *Infect. Immun.* 56:2531–2537.
170. Zasloff, M. 1987. Magainins, a class of antimicrobial peptides from Xenopus skin: isolation, characterization of two active forms, and partial cDNA sequence of a precursor. *Proc. Natl. Acad. Sci. USA* 84:5449–5453.

# VIRULENCE OF *PROTEUS MIRABILIS*

Harry L. T. Mobley, Ph.D.

# 9

Urinary tract infections (UTIs) are the most frequently diagnosed kidney and urological disorders. *Escherichia coli* is the most common isolate in healthy individuals, but those with structural abnormalities of the urinary tract are frequently infected with *Proteus mirabilis* (85). Surveys of uncomplicated cystitis or acute pyelonephritis show that *P. mirabilis* is responsible for only a few percent of cases and for only a few percent more than that even in patients with recurrent UTI. Why, then, is it important to understand the molecular mechanisms of the pathogenesis of *P. mirabilis* UTI? The answer lies in the fact that this organism infects much higher proportions of patients with complicated urinary tracts, i.e., those with functional or anatomic abnormalities or with chronic instrumentation (Fig. 1). In these patients, this bacterium causes not only cystitis and acute pyelonephritis (31, 35, 38, 85, 108), but also the production of urinary stones, a hallmark of infection with this organism (39), adds another dimension to the already complicated urinary tract.

*Harry L. T. Mobley*, Division of Infectious Diseases, University of Maryland School of Medicine, Baltimore, Maryland 21201.

*P. mirabilis* is a motile, urease-positive, lactose-negative, indole-negative, gram-negative rod-shaped bacterium that conforms to the general characteristics of the family Enterobacteriaceae (32). The bacterium deaminates phenylalanine and produces abundant hydrogen sulfide. This species, which can differentiate from short vegetative cells into elongated, highly flagellated forms (Fig. 2), is found in soil, water, and the human intestinal tract (40). *P. mirabilis* is probably most familiar to clinical microbiologists, who frequently observe agar plates on which this organism has overtaken the entire surface as a result of swarming differentiation (Fig. 2) (see chapter 10 for a detailed description of this phenomenon). The genus *Proteus* was aptly named by Hauser in 1885 for the character in Homer's *Odyssey* who "has the power of assuming different shapes to escape being questioned" (41, 42, 112).

## PATHOLOGY OF INFECTION

### *Proteus* UTI

*P. mirabilis* is seen in only a few percent of outpatients but in significantly higher numbers of hospitalized patients, who may have received antibiotics or instrumentation (particularly catheterization) of the

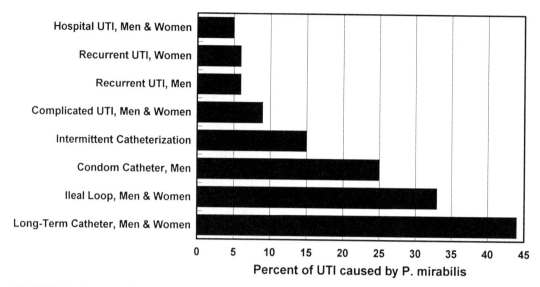

**FIGURE 1** Percent of UTIs caused by *P. mirabilis* in specific studies with selected patient populations. The numbers of specimens for which *P. mirabilis* was cultured per total number of specimens are shown. Actual data and references for each study are as follows: acute cystitis, 4 of 136 patients, 3% (90); hospital-acquired UTI, men and women, $x$ of 25,371 (numerator not provided), 5% (30); recurrent UTI in women, 29 of 518, 6% (102); recurrent UTI in men, 16 of 262, 6% (86); complicated UTI, 12 of 137, 9% (24); intermittent catheterization 7 of 48, 15% (81); condom catheter, 5 of 20, 25% (78); ileal loop, 11 of 34, 32% (29); long-term urethral catheter, 512 of 1,158, 44% (110).

urinary tract (Fig. 1) (85). *Proteus* spp. account for most infections in young uncircumcised boys (89) and has been associated with hyperammonemia with encephalopathy in patients in whom the urinary stream has been diverted into the bowel (25, 87, 100).

An unusual feature of *Proteus* infections, 80 to 90% of which are caused by *P. mirabilis*, is the predilection of the bacterium for the upper urinary tract. In studies in which the bacterium was localized by using bladder washout techniques (33, 49), *P. mirabilis* was localized to the kidney much more often than the most common infecting bacterium, *E. coli*.

*P. mirabilis* is generally susceptible to most commonly used antibiotics, including ampicillin, carbenicillin, cephalothin, chloramphenicol, sulfa, amikacin, and gentamicin (6). Although high-molecular-weight conjugative plasmids can be found in some isolates, multiple antibiotic resistance is uncommon. The bacterium is, however, intrinsically resistant to tetracycline. Despite its susceptibility to most antibiotics, treatment failures are common because of urease-induced stone formation. Organisms become encased in struvite or apatite crystals, which may be impenetrable to antibiotics and thus resistant to clearing.

## Stone Formation

Stone formation, a hallmark of infection with this organism, is caused by the expression of a highly active urease that hydrolyzes urea to ammonia, thus causing a rise in local pH and subsequent precipitation of magnesium ammonium phosphate (struvite) and calcium phosphate (apatite) crystals (Fig. 3) (36, 39, 71, 74). A specific contribution by the *P. mirabilis* capsule has also been implicated (28).

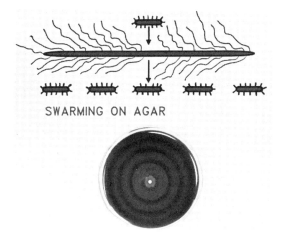

**FIGURE 2** *P. mirabilis* morphology and swarming on agar. Short swimmer cells plated on an agar surface differentiate into elongated, multinuclear, heavily flagellated swarmer cells (up to 80 μm long). Swarmer cells associate with one another and spread away from the point of inoculation. After several hours, swarmer cells consolidate into numerous swimmer cells, thus completing the cycle. Alternating cycles of differentiation and consolidation result in a bull's-eye pattern of swarming on an agar plate.

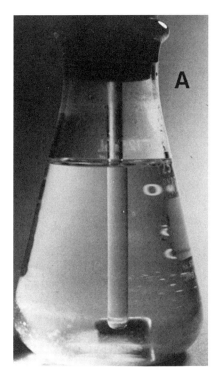
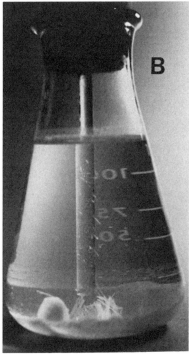

**FIGURE 3** Urease-induced crystal formation in artificial urine. Flasks containing synthetic urine supplemented with 10% Luria broth were inoculated with a *Proteus* strain and incubated statically at 37°C for 48 h. A glass rod served as a nidus for crystal formation. (A) Culture supplemented with acetohydroxamic acid (500 μg/ml), a urease inhibitor that prevented urea hydrolysis and elevation of pH; (B) control culture in which urea was hydrolyzed and pH was elevated. Note crystal formation on the glass rod and at the bottom of flask B.

The stones resulting from aggregation of such crystals complicate infection for three reasons. First, P. mirabilis caught within the interstices of the forming stones is very difficult to clear with only antibiotics. Second, the stone is a nidus for non-P. mirabilis bacteria to establish UTI, which also are difficult to eradicate. Third, the stone can obstruct urine flow; pelvic and renal stones are often associated with pyonephrosis and/or chronic pyelonephritis. For further discussion, see "Role in Virulence" under "Urease" below.

## VIRULENCE DETERMINANTS

A number of virulence determinants that may contribute to pathogenesis of P. mirabilis UTI have been identified (73). These factors have in many instances been systematically examined by identification of each protein, isolation of the corresponding genes, determination of the nucleotide sequences, construction of mutants in the wild-type parental P. mirabilis strains, measurement of an in vitro effect of these mutants on cultured epithelial cells or erythrocytes, and, finally, transurethral challenge of mice with mutant and wild-type strains. Specific proteins that have been analyzed in this fashion include urease, hemolysin, four distinct fimbriae, flagella, amino acid deaminase, and metalloprotease (Fig. 4, Table 1). In addition, the general phenomenon of invasion, most likely a multifactorial phenomenon (65), has been investigated.

## Urease

### ENZYMATIC REACTION

Urease (urea amidohydrolase, EC 3.5.1.5), the most often cited virulence factor of P. mirabilis, catalyzes the hydrolysis of urea to yield ammonia and carbamate. The carbamate spontaneously decomposes to yield carbonic acid and a second molecule of ammonia. Thus, while urease cleaves only one

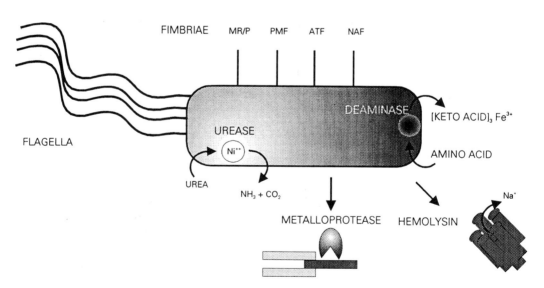

**FIGURE 4** Virulence factors of P. mirabilis. Proteins produced by this species that have either been demonstrated or proposed to contribute to virulence are depicted. Mutants in urease, flagella, hemolysin, MR/P fimbriae, and PMF were constructed by allelic exchange (9, 45, 62, 68, 105). Refer to Table 1 for summary of virulence studies. Modified with permission from *Kidney International*, volume S47, page 5129, 1994 (73).

**TABLE 1** Summary of *P. mirabilis* virulence factor studies

| Virulence factor | Gene(s) cloned | Sequenced | Virulence of mutant in mouse[a] | | | Reference(s) |
|---|---|---|---|---|---|---|
| | | | Urine | Bladder | Kidney | |
| Urease | *ureRDABCEFG* | Yes | 1[b] | 1[b] | 1[b] | 45, 48, 77, 101 |
| Hemolysin | *hpmAB* | Yes | 229 | 58 | 7 | 68, 105, 109 |
| MR/P fimbria | *mrpIABCDEFG* | Yes | 17[b] | 4[b] | 11[b] | 9, 10, 11 |
| PMF | *pmfACDEF* | Yes | 28 | 1[b] | 14 | 7, 62, 63 |
| ATF | *atfA* | No | | | | 60, 61 |
| NAF | | Yes | | | | 107 |
| Flagella | *flaA, flaB, flaD* | Yes | 1[b] | 2[b] | 6[b] | 17 |
| Deaminase | *aad* | Yes | | | | 64 |
| Metalloprotease | *zapA* | Yes | | | | 14 |

[a] Percentage of wild-type CFU per milliliter of urine or per gram of tissue cultured after transurethral challenge of CBA mice.
[b] Mutant values are significantly lower ($P < 0.05$) than values for wild-type control. See text for actual $P$ values.

ammonia group from urea, the net result is liberation of two ammonium ions and a single molecule of carbon dioxide.

## THE ENZYME AND ITS PROPERTIES

The urease of *P. mirabilis* is a cytoplasmic nickel-metalloenzyme of 250 kDa that is composed of three distinct subunits of 11.0, 12.2, and 61.0 kDa in a stoichiometry of (11 kDa-12 kDa-61 kDa)$_3$ (72). Because of its close apparent evolutionary relationship to the urease of *Klebsiella aerogenes*, for which the three-dimensional structure has recently been elucidated (43), the protein is thought to probably be a trimer of trimers. That is, each of three catalytic units present in each urease protein is composed of one copy of each of the 11-, 12-, and 61-kDa subunits. In addition, two nickel ions are coordinated into each of three active sites by residues of the UreC subunit: His-134, His-163, Lys-217, His-246, His-272, and Asp-360 (43).

The *P. mirabilis* urease appears to exhibit simple Michaelis-Menten-type kinetic behavior with no evidence of substrate inhibition or allosteric behavior. The $K_m$s for the ureases of different *P. mirabilis* strains range from 13 to 60 mM (21, 46). Despite the relatively low affinity of urease for its substrate, the $K_m$ is nevertheless appropriate for its niche, in that urea is present at very high concentrations in urine and the enzyme is therefore always saturated and working at the $V_{\max}$.

Urease has been unambiguously localized to the cytoplasm by comparison to control enzymes that partition with the cytoplasm, periplasmic space, and membrane fractions (47). These fractionation data that localize the enzyme to the cytoplasm are consistent with nucleotide sequence data that predict no signal sequences for any of the subunits. Urea is apparently able to diffuse across the bacterial membrane, where it is hydrolyzed. Excess ammonia ($NH_3$) diffuses back out of the bacterial cell, whereas the ammonium ion ($NH_4^+$) is trapped within the cytoplasm and can be directly incorporated into amino acids.

## GENETIC ORGANIZATION

The entire *P. mirabilis* urease gene cluster is encoded on a 6.45-kb DNA sequence (GenBank accession numbers M31834, Z18752, and Z21940) and is one of five urease gene clusters for which the entire nucleotide sequence has been determined (72). Eight contiguous genes make up the

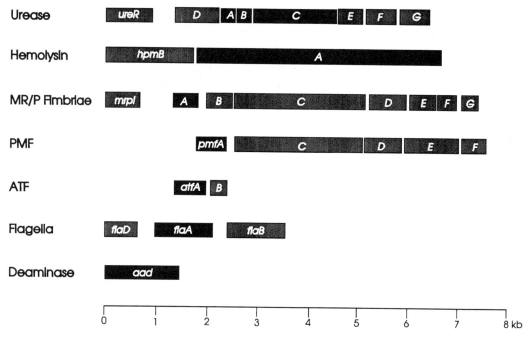

**FIGURE 5** Genetic organization of virulence gene clusters. Genes encoding virulence factors discussed in this chapter for which nucleotide sequences are available are assembled on the same scale. Black boxes indicate genes for the primary structural subunit(s) of each virulence factor. Gray boxes indicate accessory genes necessary for regulation, assembly, or activation of each respective protein. Urease genes localized to 6.5 kb of chromosomal DNA predict eight polypeptides: UreR (33.4 kDa), UreD (31.0 kDa), UreA (11.0 kDa), UreB (12.2 kDa), UreC (61.0 kDa), UreE (17.9 kDa), UreF (23.0 kDa), and UreG (22.4 kDa) (48, 77, 101). Structural subunits of the enzyme are encoded by *ureA, ureB,* and *ureC* and are translated from a single transcript in the order of 11.0, 12.2, and 61.0 kDa, respectively. Transcription is induced by urea and mediated by the positive activator UreR (77). Hpm hemolysin genes are encoded by a 7.2-kb region and predict two polypeptides: HpmB (63.2 kDa) and HpmA (165.9 kDa). The larger polypeptide represents the HpmA hemolysin itself. HpmB is necessary for secretion of an active hemolysin. MR/P fimbriae are encoded by 7.3 kb that predicts eight polypeptides, as discussed in the text. P denotes putative promoters; a stem-loop structure that follows *mrpA* is predicted to attenuate but not terminate transcription. PMF are encoded by the *pmf* gene cluster (5.7 kb), as discussed in the text. PmfF shares 26.9% identity with SfaA, the major structural subunit of S fimbriae. The ATF genes were isolated, and a partial DNA sequence was determined. Polypeptides predicted are AtfA (19.0 kDa) and AtfB (partial sequence available). The region of DNA encoding the flagellin (major flagellar subunit) reveals two flagellin genes (*flaA* and *flaB*) as well as the gene for the flagellar capping protein (*flaD*). Amino acid deaminase is encoded by the single gene *aad*, which predicts Aad (51.2 kDa).

urease gene cluster (Fig. 5) (48, 77, 101). Structural genes *ureABC*, which encode subunits of the enzyme, are flanked immediately upstream by *ureD* and downstream by *ureEFG* genes. The four "accessory genes" appear, on the basis of their homology to the genes of other urease gene clusters (72, 75), to play a role in the insertion of nickel ions into the apoenzyme and the assembly of a catalytically active urease protein.

Urease expression is induced by the presence of urea, and this induction is controlled by *ureR*. The *ureR* gene lies 400 bp upstream of *ureD* and is oriented in the direction opposite to that of the other seven genes. The amino acid sequence predicted by this gene contains a putative helix-turn-helix DNA-binding motif followed 30 residues downstream by an associated AraC family signature (77). This regulatory protein appears to be typical of the AraC DNA-binding regulatory proteins involved in transcriptional activation.

## ROLE IN VIRULENCE

Urea, the principal nitrogenous waste product of humans, is present at 0.4 to 0.5 M in urine (39) and is hydrolyzed by urease ($NH_2$-CO-$NH_2$ + $H_2O$ → $2NH_3$ + $CO_2$). $NH_3$ equilibrates with $H_2O$ to form $NH_4^+OH^-$, which elevates urine pH. At the higher pH, normally soluble ions precipitate to form stones of struvite ($MgNH_4PO_4$) or carbonate-apatite ($Ca_{10}(PO_4)_6 \cdot CO_3$).

A number of investigators (5, 19, 44, 45, 57–59, 76) have used rat or mouse models of infection to study the severity of pyelonephritis caused by P. mirabilis. The effects of urease were studied by injecting acetone-killed organisms that retained urease activity (19); by treating infected animals with oral supplements of acetohydroxamic acid, a specific inhibitor of the enzyme (5, 59, 76); or by inoculation of an ethyl methanesulfonate-generated urease mutant (57). Although all studies supported the supposition that urease played a role in virulence, the use of killed organisms (19) or mutants generated by nonspecific mutagens (57) made interpretation of these data difficult. Additionally, animals in these studies were challenged hematogenously, a procedure that establishes kidney infection by a route that is not now believed to mimic the more natural course of infection that develops by the ascending route.

To specifically evaluate the contribution of urease to virulence, a mutation in the ureC urease structural subunit gene was introduced into a P. mirabilis strain by homologous recombination (45). Virulence was assessed in the CBA mouse model of ascending UTI. Twenty mice were each challenged transurethrally with $1 \times 10^9$ to $2 \times 10^9$ CFU of P. mirabilis HI4320 and its urease-negative derivative. At 48 h, animals were sacrificed, and the mean $log_{10}$ of quantitative cultures of urine (parent, 6.23; mutant, 4.19; $P = 0.0014$), bladder (parent, 6.29; mutant 4.28; $P = 0.0002$), right kidney (parent, 4.11; mutant, 2.43; $P = 0.036$), and left kidney (parent, 4.11; mutant, 1.02; $P = 0.00009$) were all shown to be significantly different (45).

When a longer duration of infection was assessed, mice challenged transurethrally with the parent strain developed significant bacteriuria and struvite renal stones (Table 2) (44). The urease-negative mutant had a 50% infective dose of $>2.7 \times 10^9$ CFU, a value more than 1,000-fold greater than that of the parent strain ($2.2 \times 10^6$ CFU). The urease-positive parent strain reached significantly higher concentrations and persisted significantly longer in the bladder and kidney than did the mutant. Indeed, in the kidney, the parent strain increased in concentration while the numbers of the mutant strain were falling, so that by 1 week, the parent concentration was $10^6$ times that of the mutant. Similarly, the urease-positive parent produced significantly more severe renal pathology than the mutant produced. The initial abnormalities were in and around the pelvis and consisted of acute inflammation and epithelial necrosis. By 1 week, pyelitis was

**TABLE 2** Urolithiasis in CBA mice challenged with P. mirabilis HI4320 and its urease-negative isogenic mutant[a]

| Urease status | No. (%) of mice with visible bladder stones after: | | |
|---|---|---|---|
| | 2 days | 7 days[b] | 14 days[c] |
| Positive | 0/19 | 12/39 (31) | 8/20 (40) |
| Negative | 0/19 | 0/41 | 0/20 |

[a] Data are from reference 44.
[b] $P = 0.0013$.
[c] $P = 0.002$.

more severe, crystals were seen in the pelvis, and acute pyelonephritis with acute interstitial inflammation, tubular epithelial-cell necrosis, and in some cases abscesses had developed. By 2 weeks, more animals had renal abscesses and radial bands of fibrosis. The urease of P. mirabilis is thus a critical virulence determinant for colonization, urolithiasis, and the development of severe acute pyelonephritis.

In patients with long-term urethral catheterization, P. mirabilis urease is also correlated with development of catheter encrustation, including obstruction of the catheterized lumen. This encrustation blocks urine flow and may result in reflux and infection of the upper urinary tract. Among the common urease-positive isolates that infect these patients, including P. mirabilis, Morganella morganii, Providencia stuartii, Klebsiella pneumoniae, Providencia rettgeri, and Proteus vulgaris, the only urease-positive species that is significantly associated with development of obstructions is P. mirabilis (74).

## HpmA Hemolysin

All but a very few strains of P. mirabilis are potently hemolytic when erythrocytes from any number of animal species are incubated with bacterial suspensions (94). Short incubations of 1 h or less can result in complete lysis of the erythrocytes. In bacterial cultures, the activity can first be detected in the early logarithmic phase of growth; it peaks at mid- to late logarithmic phase. No activity is observed in stationary phase (94). The activity does not require the addition of calcium, appears to have a very short (<5-min) half-life, and is associated with the cell surface (94) but has also been found in culture supernatants (104).

### HEMOLYTIC ACTIVITY OF CLINICAL STRAINS

Hemolysin production has been compared for P. mirabilis strains cultured from various clinical sources: 16 patients with acute pyelonephritis, 35 patients with catheter-associated bacteriuria, and 20 fecal isolates (69). The geometric means of reciprocal hemolytic titers were 27.9 for pyelonephritis isolates, 18.0 for urinary catheter isolates, and 55.7 for fecal isolates (none of which were significantly different [$P > 0.1$]). Therefore, strains isolated from patients with serious clinical infections are no more hemolytic than fecal strains, and it must be concluded that in vitro expression of hemolysin is not a reliable index of virulence.

### CYTOTOXICITY OF HpmA HEMOLYSIN

The hemolytic activity is clearly correlated with the expression of a 166-kDa protein that can be identified by using specific antiserum (104). In one study, all of 63 strains exhibited calcium-independent hemolytic activity. A specific mutation of hpmA, constructed in one strain by allelic exchange, resulted in loss of hemolytic activity.

The activity of the hemolysin also extends to that of a more general cytotoxicity (82, 83, 104). As measured by chromium release, cytotoxicity of hemolysin-secreting P. mirabilis was demonstrated for a variety of cell lines, including Daudi, Raji, T24, U937, and Vero. The hpmA mutant was deficient in this cytotoxic activity as well as in the hemolytic activity discussed above.

It can be postulated that Proteus spp. use the HpmA hemolysin to elicit tissue damage that in turn may allow entry of these bacteria into the kidney. In a separate study, strains of P. mirabilis and P. vulgaris and their isogenic hemolysin-negative (hpmA) constructs were overlaid onto primary cell cultures of human renal proximal tubular epithelial cells (70). Cytotoxicity was measured by release of soluble lactate dehydrogenase. Two strains of P. mirabilis inoculated at $10^6$ CFU caused a release of 80% of total lactate dehydrogenase after 6 h (compared to a pyelonephritogenic, hemolytic *E. coli* strain with only 25% release [$P < 0.012$]). Ten selected *P. mirabilis* isolates were all hemolytic and cytotoxic. The HpmA hemolysin is apparently responsible for the majority of cytotoxicity in vitro, since the hemolysin-negative (*hmpA*) mutants of *P. mirabilis* and *P. vulgaris* were significantly less cytotoxic than the wild-type strains.

## GENETICS

The hemolysin genes of *P. mirabilis* were isolated from a cosmid library and found by hybridization studies to be unrelated to the hemolysin genes of *E. coli*, *M. morganii*, and *Citrobacter freundii* (111). The nucleotide sequence demonstrated two open reading frames associated with hemolysin activity; they were designated *hpmB* and *hpmA* (transcribed in that order) (Fig. 5) (109). The determinants, encoded on 7,191 bp, predicted polypeptides of 63,204 and 165,868 Da. The 165,868-Da polypeptide represents the hemolysin itself. The polypeptides have predicted leader peptides of 17 and 19 amino acids, respectively. A Fur-binding site overlaps the $-35$ region, implying regulation by medium iron concentration. These determinants have approximately 50% homology at both the nucleotide and amino acid sequence levels with the *shlA* and *shlB* determinants that encode the hemolysin of *Serratia marcescens*.

The *hpm* genes appear to be the sole hemolysin determinant of *P. mirabilis*; however, a *hlyA* homolog is occasionally found in *P. vulgaris* strains (50, 111).

## ROLE IN VIRULENCE

To assess the role of the HpmA hemolysin in virulence, a hemolysin-negative mutant was constructed as described above (104). In this mutant, a deletion was introduced within *hpmA*, the gene that encodes the hemolysin protein. The parent and mutant strains were tested in the mouse model of ascending UTI, and no difference in virulence was detected between the parent strain and its hemolysin-negative mutant as assessed by quantitative culture and histological examination. The hemolysin-negative strain did, however, have a sixfold-higher 50% lethal dose than the parent strain upon intravenous challenge of C3H mice (105). Using larger numbers of mice, our laboratory also found no significant difference in colonization in urine, bladder, and kidney between the hemolysin-negative mutant and the wild-type strain (68). CBA mice ($n = 40$) were challenged transurethrally with $10^7$ CFU of wild type or mutant. After 1 week, geometric means of $\log_{10}$ CFU per milliliter of urine or per gram of bladder or kidney for wild type and mutant were 5.42 and 5.78, respectively, in urine; 4.19 and 3.95 in bladder; 4.31 and 3.40 in left kidney; and 5.15 and 3.76 in right kidney (no differences were significant; $P > 0.05$). Given the potent in vitro cytotoxicity that has been attributed to the HpmA hemolysin, it is surprising that the relative contribution to colonization and histopathology is not greater.

## Fimbriae and Adhesins

### GENERAL ADHERENCE AND HEMAGGLUTINATION PROPERTIES

Adherence properties of *Proteus* species were first investigated by using suspensions of erythrocytes. A number of investigators noted that suspensions of *P. mirabilis* bacteria agglutinate erythrocytes from various species (23, 27, 97). In addition, electron microscopy revealed fimbriae with different morphologies in this species (23, 27, 41, 97–99). Old and Adegbola (79), however, were the first to correlate the presence of a specific type of fimbria with mannose-resistant hemagglutination properties. The *Proteus* strains investigated hemagglutinated erythrocytes from fowl, guinea pig, horse, human, and sheep and expressed morphologically distinct fimbriae. Because no genetic analyses had been undertaken, no proof could be offered at that point that a specific fimbria was responsible for this specific hemagglutination pattern.

Although the correlation of adherence with virulence is not as strong as that for uropathogenic *E. coli* (1, 37), a few reports have suggested that the adherence of *P. mirabilis* to uroepithelial cells (UEC) contributes to pathogenesis. In an animal model of unobstructed ascending infection, *P. mirabilis* appeared to adhere to renal epithelial cells by fimbriae (98, 99) as well as to human UEC in vitro (36, 54, 99, 103, 114). In animal studies (98, 99), heavily fimbriated organisms initiate infection better than lightly fimbriated organisms. Principally, two hemagglutinins, mannose-resistant *Proteus*-like (MR/P) and mannose-resistant *Klebsiella*-like (MR/K), have been associated with the ability to agglutinate untreated or tannic acid erythrocytes from several animal species. Silverblatt and Ofek (99) found that when rats were inoculated transurethrally with *P. mirabilis* expressing either type IV fimbriae (consistent with our current understanding of MR/P fimbriae) or type III fimbriae (thought at that time to be responsible for MR/K hemagglutination), inocula expressing MR/P fimbriae caused a higher frequency of cortical abscesses at 1 week than inocula expressing predominantly type III fimbriae. This observation suggested that MR/P fimbriae play an important role in the development of pyelonephritis, but this possibility was not proven until some years later (9). Note that the designation type IV is no longer used for MR/P fimbriae; it presently designates a family of fimbriae produced by organisms including enteropathogenic *E. coli* and *Pseudomonas, Moraxella,* and *Neisseria* species.

Thus far, four distinct fimbriae have been identified on *P. mirabilis:* MR/P, *P. mirabilis* fimbriae (PMF), ambient-temperature fimbriae (ATF), and nonagglutinating fimbriae (NAF) (Table 3). Their properties, genetic organizations, and contributions to pathogenesis are summarized below.

## MR/P FIMBRIAE

**Properties.** MR/P fimbriae have been purified from a *P. mirabilis* strain isolated from a patient with acute pyelonephritis (8). Electron microscopy revealed a highly concentrated preparation of fimbriae. Fimbrial structural subunits that require trichloroacetic acid precipitation (or some other harsh denaturant) for denaturation of the intact fimbria were estimated by sodium dodecyl sulfate-polyacrylamide gel electrophoresis (SDS-PAGE) to be 18.5 kDa. N-terminal sequencing revealed that among the first 20 amino acids of the major MR/P subunit, 11 of 20 amino acids matched the predicted amino acid sequence of the *E. coli* P fimbrial structural subunit PapA. MrpA, the major structural subunit, is optimally expressed at 37°C in Luria broth cultured statically for 48 h.

**Genetic Organization.** MR/P fimbrial gene sequences were isolated from a *P. mirabilis* cosmid library by immunoblotting and by hybridization with an oligonucleotide probe based on the N-terminal amino acid sequence of the isolated fimbrial polypeptide ADQGHGTVKFVGSIIDAPCS (10). A clone that reacted strongly both with a monoclonal antibody specific for MR/P fimbriae and with the DNA probe was isolated. *E. coli* transformed with this clone hemagglutinated both tannic acid-treated and untreated chicken erythrocytes in the presence and absence of 50 mM D-mannose (phenotype of MR/P fimbriae) and was shown by transmission electron microscopy to be fimbriated. A 525-bp open reading frame,

**TABLE 3** Fimbriae, hemagglutinins, and adhesins of *P. mirabilis*

| Abbreviation | Full name | Associated with fimbrial structure | Hemagglutination | Adherent to cell culture | Mol wt of major structural subunit | | | Optimal conditions for expression |
|---|---|---|---|---|---|---|---|---|
| | | | | | Apparent | Predicted, unprocessed | Predicted, processed | |
| MR/P | Mannose-resistant *Proteus*-like | Yes | Yes | | 18,500 | 17,900 | 15,700 | Broth, static, 37°C |
| PMF | *P. mirabilis* fimbria | Yes | No | No | 19,500 | 18,900 | 16,700 | Broth, static, 37°C |
| ATF | Ambient-temperature fimbria | Yes | No | | 24,000 | 19,000 | 16,200 | Broth, 23°C |
| NAF | Nonagglutinating fimbria | Yes | No | Yes | 23,000–29,000 | | | Agar, 37°C |
| UCA | Uroepithelial cell adhesin | Yes | | Yes | 17,500 | | | Agar, 37°C |
| MR/K | Mannose-resistant *Klebsiella*-like | No | Yes | | | | | Broth, static, 30°C, 37°C |

designated *mrpA*, predicts a 175-amino-acid polypeptide that includes a 23-amino-acid hydrophobic leader peptide. The unprocessed and processed polypeptides are predicted to be 17,909 and 15,689 Da, respectively. The N-terminal amino acid sequence of the processed fimbrial subunit exactly matched amino acid residues 24 to 43 predicted by the *mrpA* nucleotide sequence. The amino acid sequence of the MrpA polypeptide is 57% identical to that of SmfA, the major fimbrial subunit of *S. marcescens* mannose-resistant fimbriae.

Genes encoding this fimbria were isolated, and the complete nucleotide sequence was determined (Fig. 5) (11). The *mrp* gene cluster encoded by 7,293 bp predicts eight polypeptides: MrpI (22,133 Da), MrpA (17,909 Da), MrpB (19,632 Da), MrpC (96,823 Da), MrpD (27,886 Da), MrpE (19,470 Da), MrpF (17,363 Da), and MrpG (13,169 Da). *mrpI* is upstream of the gene encoding the major structural subunit gene *mrpA* and is transcribed in the direction opposite to that of the rest of the operon. All predicted polypeptides encoded by the *mrp* gene cluster share at least 25% amino acid identity with at least one other enteric fimbrial gene product encoded by the *pap*, *fim*, *smf*, *fan*, or *mrk* gene clusters.

**Role in Virulence in the Mouse Model of UTI.** MR/P fimbriae are expressed in vivo and are recognized by the immune systems of experimentally infected mice (8, 51). An enzyme-linked immunosorbent assay using purified antigens showed a strong reaction between the MR/P fimbriae and the sera of CBA mice challenged transurethrally with *P. mirabilis* (8). This observation suggested a role for MR/P fimbriae in the pathogenesis of UTI that was supported by a previous observation that MR/P fimbriae are expressed preferentially as the sole hemagglutinin type in human pyelonephritis isolates (69).

To investigate the contribution of this fimbrial type to colonization of the urinary tract, an MR/P fimbrial mutant was constructed by allelic exchange (9). A Kan$^r$ cassette was inserted into the *mrpA* open reading frame, and the construct was transferred to the parent *P. mirabilis* strain by conjugation. Following passage on nonselective medium, an allelic exchange double-crossover mutant was isolated and verified by Southern blot. Colony immunoblot, Western blot (immunoblot), and immunogold labeling with a monoclonal antibody to MR/P fimbriae revealed that MrpA was not expressed. Complementation with cloned *mrpA* restored MR/P expression, as shown by hemagglutination, Western blot, and immunogold electron microscopy.

To assess virulence, CBA mice ($n = 40$) were challenged transurethrally with $10^7$ CFU of wild type or MR/P-negative mutant (9). After 1 week, geometric means of $\log_{10}$ CFU per milliliter of urine or per gram of bladder or kidney for wild type and mutant were 7.79 and 7.02 respectively, for urine ($P = 0.035$); 6.22 and 4.78 for bladder ($P = 0.019$); 5.02 and 3.31 for left kidney ($P = 0.009$); and 5.28 and 4.46 for right kidney ($P = 0.039$). Histopathology in the kidney was significantly more severe in wild-type-infected animals than in MP/P fimbriae-deficient mutants. MR/P fimbriae clearly contribute significantly to colonization of the urinary tract and increase the risk of development of acute pyelonephritis. This mutation, however, was not nearly as attenuating as the *ureC* mutation of the urease-negative mutant.

## PMF

**Properties.** In addition to MR/P fimbriae, *P. mirabilis* produces another fimbria, designated PMF. These fimbriae are produced when cultures are passaged statically (i.e., without aeration) for 48 h per passage at 37°C. The predicted N-terminal amino acid sequence of the processed 19.5-kDa-apparent-molecular-size PMF subunit polypeptide, ENETPAPKVSSTK-GEIQLKG (residues 23 to 42 of the predicted polypeptide), is distinct from the MR/P N terminus. The *pmfA* gene encoding the major structural subunit of PMF has been isolated and sequenced for two strains (7). Using an oligonucleotide designed like the *pmfA* open reading frame of strain HU1069, the PMF gene was also isolated and sequenced from a cosmid gene bank clone of strain HI4320. A 552-bp open reading frame predicts a 184-amino-acid polypeptide including a 22-amino-acid hydrophobic leader sequence. The unprocessed polypeptide is predicted to be 18,921 Da; the processed polypeptide is predicted to be 16,749 Da. The nucleotide sequences from the two strains are virtually identical. The predicted amino acid sequence of the polypeptide encoded by *pmfA* displays 36% amino acid sequence identity with the mannose-resistant fimbrial subunit encoded by *smfA* of *S. marcescens* but only 15% exact matches with the predicted sequence encoded by *mrkA* of *K. pneumoniae* (7).

**Genetic Organization.** Genes encoding PMF have been isolated, and the complete nucleotide sequence has been determined (63). The *pmf* gene cluster, encoded by 5,655 bp, predicts five polypeptides: PmfA (18,921 Da), PmfC (93,107 Da), PmfD (28,208 Da), PmfE (38,875 Da), and PmfF (19,661 Da) (Fig. 5). PmfA, PmfC, PmfD, and PmfF have >25% amino acid sequence identity with gene products of the *pap*, *mrp*, and *sfa* fimbrial gene clusters. PmfE shows no similarity to any polypeptide in the SwissProt database. No regulatory genes or regulatory elements are evident in the sequence. The *pmf* cluster shares features with other enteric fimbrial gene clusters but also displays features that are unique.

**Analysis of Virulence in the Mouse Model of UTI.** An isogenic PMF mutant of *P. mirabilis* HI4320 was constructed by marker exchange in a strategy similar to that used for the *mrp* mutant. A Kan$^r$ cassette was cloned into the middle of *pmfA* and used to isolate a double-crossover mutant (62). The isogenic mutant was then used to determine the role of PMF in hemagglutination and virulence in the CBA mouse model of ascending UTI. Hemagglutination patterns of the mutant ruled out involvement of the PMF in both MR/P and MR/K hemagglutination. Similarly, PMF does not appear to be involved in adherence to human exfoliated UEC, since the mutant was as adherent as the wild-type strain (mutant, 14.1 ± 11.7 mean bacteria per UEC, 60% UEC with ≥10 bacteria; wild-type strain, 18.1 ± 16.2 mean bacteria per UEC, 67.5% UEC with ≥10 bacteria; not significantly different). The *pmfA* mutant, which does not express the 19,500-Da major subunit of the PMF, colonized the bladders of transurethrally challenged CBA mice ($n = 20$ per group) in numbers 100-fold less than those of the wild-type strain (mutant, $\log_{10}$ of 4.87 CFU/g; wild-type strain, $\log_{10}$ of 6.79 CFU/g; $P = 0.023$). However, the mutant colonized the kidneys in numbers similar to that of the wild-type strain. These data suggest a role for PMF in colonization of the bladder but not the kidney.

ATF
A third, previously undescribed fimbria of *P. mirabilis*, ATF, has also been identified, purified, and subjected to genetic analysis (60, 64). Electron microscopy of a pure preparation and immunogold-labeled bacterial cells demonstrated that ATF is fimbrial in nature. The major fimbrial subunit of ATF has an apparent molecular weight of 24,000. The N-terminal amino acid sequence, EXTGTPAPTEVTVDGGTIDF, shows no significant similarity to any previously described fimbrial protein. ATF is

expressed by all eight *P. mirabilis* strains that were examined.

Culture conditions affect expression of ATF, with optimal expression observed in static broth cultures at 23°C (60). These fimbriae are not produced by cells grown at 42°C or on solid medium. Expression of ATF assayed by SDS-PAGE and Western blot does not correlate with MR/P or MR/K hemagglutination, and ATF appears to represent a novel fimbria of *P. mirabilis*.

PCR primers based on the N-terminal and an internal amino acid sequence were used to amplify a fragment that was used as a probe to locate a cosmid clone encoding the *atf* major structural subunit (64). Nucleotide sequencing predicts a polypeptide of 19,047 Da with a 28-residue signal peptide; the processed polypeptide is predicted to be 16,219 Da (Fig. 5). This polypeptide, designated AtfA, is characteristic of a typical fimbrial subunit. The *atfA* gene appears to be followed by a gene encoding a chaperonin-like polypeptide, which is typical of the organization of other fimbrial gene clusters of members of the *Enterobacteriaceae*.

### NAF

A fourth fimbrial type, designated NAF, has also been identified and purified (107). The major structural subunit of this fimbria has an apparent molecular weight of 27,000. NAF are expressed by all *P. mirabilis* strains under all growth conditions examined, and the major subunit proteins, which range from 23 to 29 kDa as determined by SDS-PAGE, have highly conserved N-terminal amino acid sequences. The N terminus is identical to the UEC adhesin previously described by Wray and colleagues (114); otherwise, the relationship between these two polypeptides is unclear.

Using purified NAF as an immunogen, NAF-specific monoclonal antibodies were generated (107). Electron microscopy of *P. mirabilis* bacteria, immunogold-labeled by using anti-NAF monoclonal antibodies, localized epitopes to the bacterial cell surface on structures that were consistent with fimbriae. Bacteria expressing NAF as their only fimbrial type adhered strongly to HEp-2 cells in vitro (106). NAF-specific monoclonal antibodies or exogenously added purified NAF markedly reduced *P. mirabilis* attachment. The N terminus of the major structural subunit of NAF is highly conserved among numerous *P. mirabilis* strains. The contribution of NAF to pathogenesis of UTI awaits the construction of isogenic mutants.

## Flagella and Swarming Differentiation

### FLAGELLA

*P. mirabilis* motility is driven by flagella that are typical of enteric bacterial species (general structure reviewed in reference 113). These surface appendages are complex structures composed of numerous and distinct polypeptide subunits. The flagellar filament that extends away from the cell is, however, made up primarily of repeating subunits of a single flagellin monomer (8, 51) of 39 kDa [13, 17]. The filaments range in length from approximately 1 to 4 $\mu$m in swimmer and swarmer cells, respectively (41). The number of flagella per cell can vary from fewer than 10 to more than 1,000 (see below).

### SWARMING MOTILITY

*P. mirabilis* is a dimorphic bacterium that may exist in either of two morphologically and physiologically distinct forms (12, 34, 112). When grown in liquid culture, the bacterium assumes the typical appearance of the *Enterobacteriaceae*: short rods that are fimbriated and have fewer than 10 peritrichous flagella (15, 16). When cultured on solid medium, however, the organism differentiates into elongated, nonseptated, multinuclear swarmer cells that are no longer fimbriated but now express thousands of flagella (one study estimated a range of 500 to 5,000 flagella per cell [41]). This process of differentiation is cyclical; short rods differentiate into swarmer cells and then consolidate into shortened swimmer cells. The typical result on an agar plate inoculated at the center and incubated overnight is a centrifugal spreading with a bull's-eye appearance that represents alternating zones of swarmer cell formation and dedifferentiation into swimmer cells.

The movement of the swarmer cell away from the original inoculum is the result of a coordinated multicellular effort requiring the association of groups of differentiated swarmer cells (18). This differentiation process is initiated by the ability of P. mirabilis to sense cues from the environment, principally an increase in viscosity that prevents the free rotation of the flagellum. This inhibition of flagellar rotation triggers a signal transduction event that results in the production of elongated swarmer cells that produce extraordinarily large amounts of flagellin, resulting in dense flagellum formation. Highly motile swarmer cells associate with one another and migrate across the agar surface until a new signal triggers the division of the elongated form into short swimmer cells. Although reviewed only briefly here, the fascinating phenomenon of swarming differentiation is discussed in detail in chapter 10.

## GENETICS

Numerous genes contribute to the cell's ability to undergo swarming differentiation. Specific genes that have been directly implicated are *flaA*, which encodes flagellin; *flgH*, which encodes the flagellar basal body; *fliG*, which encodes the switch protein; and *fliL*, which encodes a minor flagellar protein (4, 13, 17). In addition, mutations (Tn5 induced) that affect chemotaxis result in abnormal swarming (15).

Thus, the genes required for motility undoubtedly include a very large region of the bacterial chromosome (4, 12, 16). Among these genes are those for flagella, including genes that encode multiple flagellins (*fla*), the major structural subunit. Two *fla* genes plus a portion of the *flaD* gene, which encodes the flagellar capping protein required for filament assembly, have been cloned, and their DNAs have been sequenced (Fig. 5) (GenBank accession number L07270 [17]). All three genes are preceded by putative flagellar gene-specific $\sigma^{28}$ promoters, which suggests that the genes are regulated in a manner similar to those in E. coli. RNA analyses and *lacZ* fusions indicate that the putative $\sigma^{28}$ promoter is active in *flaA* and show that *flaA* transcription is increased eightfold during swarmer cell differentiation. These analyses also show that *flaB* is not ordinarily transcribed. *flaA* mutants are nonmotile, but *flaB* mutants retain wild-type motility, suggesting that FlaA is the expressed form of flagellin in P. mirabilis and *flaB* is a cryptic, unexpressed gene. DNA hybridization and DNA sequence analyses revealed the presence of a third flagellin gene, *flaC*, whose role is not known.

In addition to flagellin, other virulence-associated proteins appear to be coordinately overexpressed by the swarm cell but not by the short swimmer cell (22). Urease, hemolysin, and metalloprotease activities are all dramatically elevated when cells differentiate. The elevation of mRNA levels for urease and hemolysin is commensurate with the rise in activities.

## CONTRIBUTION TO VIRULENCE

To examine the role of flagella in pathogenesis, a nonmotile, nonswarming flagellar mutant of P. mirabilis WPM111 (*hpmA* hemolysin mutant of strain BA6163 [104], chosen because of its lack of in vitro cytotoxicity in the renal epithelial-cell internalization studies described below) was constructed (68). A defined mutation was introduced into the *flaD* gene, which encodes the flagellar cap protein. This mutation does not affect the synthesis of flagellin but instead prevents the assembly of an intact flagellum. To assess virulence, CBA mice ($n = 40$) were challenged transurethrally with $10^7$ CFU of the *hpmA* mutant or the *hpmA flaD* (hemolysin-negative, flagellum-negative) mutant. After 1 week, geometric means of $\log_{10}$ CFU per milliliter of urine or per gram of bladder or kidney for strain WPM111 and the flagellum-negative mutant were 5.78 and 3.52, respectively, for urine; 3.95 and 2.29 for bladder; 3.40 and 2.47 for left kidney; and 3.76 and 2.23 for right kidney. Differences in the kidney were significantly different ($P < 0.01$). Thus, flagella themselves or the swarming differentiation that requires flagellum synthesis contributes significantly to the virulence of *P. mirabilis*.

A similar dependence on swarming differentiation for virulence was inferred by Allison et al. (3), who used transposon mutants deficient in motility and/or swarm cell formation. Mortality rates in mice were lower in the transposon mutants following intravenous injection than in the parent strain. In intravesical challenge studies, mutants were unable to colonize the mouse bladder or kidney.

## FLAGELLAR ANTIGENIC VARIATION

*P. mirabilis* carries at least three flagellin-encoding genes and appears to be capable of antigenically altering the composition of the flagellin protein through rearrangement of the DNA within the *flaA* locus (13). FlaA⁻ mutants are nonmotile because they lack flagellin synthesis. The phenotype of such FlaA⁻ mutants suggests that the *flaA* gene is the principal gene encoding flagella. Interestingly, FlaA⁻ insertional mutants can revert to wild-type motility. Analysis of these motile revertants shows that this phenotypic change in flagellin expression is due to a deletion or rearrangement in the *fla* locus that gives rise to the synthesis of an antigenically distinct flagellin in these revertants. The *flaB* gene is ordinarily silent and has no effect on the motility of *P. mirabilis* but may become active in the reversion process.

### Iron Acquisition

Pathogenic bacteria have developed mechanisms for acquiring iron by synthesizing organic compounds called siderophores, which can outcompete host iron-binding proteins for iron. Unlike many of the *Enterobacteriaceae*, *Proteus* species do not produce the common phenolate-type siderophore enterobactin or the hydroxamate-type siderophore aerobactin. Nor do *Proteus* species form the typical yellow-orange halo when they are grown on the siderophore detection agar of Schwyn and Neilands (91). In addition, the MIC of the iron-chelating agent ethylenediamine dihydroxyphenylacetic acid for *P. mirabilis* is relatively low, further suggesting that this species does not secrete typical siderophores with high affinities for iron.

## IRON AVAILABILITY IN THE URINARY TRACT

Although not much work has examined iron availability in the urinary tract, there is evidence that the urinary tract is an iron-limited environment. Bacteria (*P. mirabilis* and *K. pneumoniae*) isolated directly from the urine of two patients with UTI displayed the outer membrane profile on SDS-PAGE that was similar to the pattern of bands observed for bacteria grown under iron-limiting conditions (96).

## MECHANISMS OF IRON ACQUISITION

*Proteus*, *Providencia*, and *Morganella* species, by the action of amino acid deaminases, produce $\alpha$-keto acids that may act as novel siderophores (26). Amino acids such as phenylalanine and tryptophan are converted to the α-keto acids phenylpyruvic acid and indolylpyruvic acid, respectively, which complex ferric iron. The iron complexes, apparently aided by the hydrophobic side chains, are taken up by bacteria, thus overcoming iron restriction.

## GENETICS

The genes necessary for deaminase activity were cloned from a urinary tract isolate of *P. mirabilis* by screening for a cosmid clone with deaminase activity (64). Deaminase-positive clones were constructed and subjected to nucleotide sequencing. A single open reading frame, designated *aad* (amino acid deaminase), which appears to be both necessary and sufficient for deaminase activity, predicts a 473-amino-acid polypeptide of 51,151 Da (Fig. 5). The predicted amino acid sequence of Aad does not have significant amino acid sequence similarity to any other polypeptide in the PIR and SwissProt databases. Amino acid deaminase activity in both *P. mirabilis* and *E. coli* transformed with *aad*-encoding plasmids is not affected by medium iron concentration or expression of genes in *E. coli* backgrounds with mutations in *fur* (ferric uptake regulation), *cya* (adenylate cyclase), or *crp* (catabolite repression). The gene appears to be present in all *P. mirabilis* strains but not in other species. Deaminase activity is cytosolic in both *P. mirabilis* and *E. coli* containing the *aad* clones. The apparent lack of significant iron regulation of deaminase does not necessarily rule out its role in iron acquisition, since deamination of amino acids may be involved in various metabolic processes.

## Metalloprotease

### THE ENZYME AND ITS PROPERTIES

A high percentage of *P. mirabilis* strains secrete a protease that recognizes and cleaves immunoglobulin A1 (IgA1) and IgA2 as well some other proteins, including casein (55, 66, 93). The EDTA-sensitive 50-kDa protease cleaves the IgA heavy chain outside the hinge region, at sites different from those attacked by other microbial IgA1 proteases, to form two fragments (56).

Experimental evidence demonstrates that IgA protease is produced by the bacterium in the human host (95). In 14 of 21 patients infected with *P. mirabilis,* IgA was detected in the urine by immunoblotting. In 9 of these 14 urine samples, IgA was degraded in a manner identical to that seen in digestion of purified IgA with purified IgA protease, suggesting that the protease is active against endogenously secreted IgA.

## GENETICS

Protease-positive cosmid clones isolated from a genomic library of *P. mirabilis* (14) were identified by plating on skim milk agar. Subclones with recombinant protease activity, detected by a zone of clearing around the colony, were isolated, mapped, and subjected to nucleotide sequencing. The metalloprotease structural gene, designated *zapA*, is 1.4 kb long and predicts a 488-amino-acid polypeptide of 53.7 kDa. The protease gene is part of a gene cluster, and the predicted polypeptide appears to be homologous to the *S. marcescens* zinc-metalloprotease that is secreted via an ATP-dependent transport system (20). These proteases, along with those of *Erwinia* sp. and *Pseudomonas* sp., appear to make up a family of related proteins. The *P. mirabilis* protease requires divalent cations for activity and cleaves serum and secretory IgA1 and IgA2 from both humans and mice (14).

To demonstrate a role in virulence for this enzyme, it will be necessary to use the isolated genes encoding the IgA protease to construct an isogenic mutant lacking this activity and then compare the virulence of the mutant and the wild type in the mouse model of ascending UTI.

## Invasiveness

P. mirabilis localizes in the kidney and damages kidney epithelium. One mechanism whereby P. mirabilis may cross the barrier afforded by the renal tubules is direct invasion of the renal epithelial cells. To test this hypothesis, suspensions of three P. mirabilis strains ($10^8$ CFU) were added to confluent monolayers of primary cultures of human renal proximal tubular epithelial cells, and after 3 h, light and electron microscopy showed that the bacteria had been internalized within membrane-bound vacuoles (22). Internalization of bacteria by renal epithelial cells was corroborated by the gentamicin protection assay. Cytolysis of renal epithelial cells by the HpmA hemolysin, however, was a confounding factor in this assay, so a hemolysin-negative *hpmA* mutant was used in subsequent experiments. The nonhemolytic mutant WPM111 did not disrupt the monolayer and was recovered in numbers that were 10- to 100-fold higher than those of the hemolytic parent BA6163. A previous study (84) presented conflicting results in which the hemolytic titer directly correlated with the level of invasion of Vero cells. Cytochalasin D (20 $\mu$g/ml) does not inhibit this internalization, which suggests that actin polymerization is not necessary for this process (22).

Swarmer cell differentiation and behavior may also be essential for invasion and infection of host cells. Allison and colleagues (2, 3) showed that differentiation is coupled to the ability of P. mirabilis to invade human UEC in vitro. Invasion is reduced but not entirely eliminated in mutants defective in wild-type swarming. On the other hand, in the study that examined the internalization of P. mirabilis by primary cultures of human renal epithelial cells (see above), the swimmer cell of P. mirabilis was internalized within membrane-bound vacuoles and did not undergo any significant replication (22). Indeed, when active swarmer cells were added to cultured renal cells, they rapidly reverted to swimmer cells and were internalized in that form. Thus, whether swarmer or swimmer cells (or both types) are internalized remains an unresolved issue. In vivo studies using mouse models of uropathogenicity have nevertheless demonstrated that mortality rates are lower when mice are infected with mutants defective in swarming than when they are infected with wild-type cells (3, 68).

## MODEL FOR PATHOGENESIS

Infection of the urinary tract by P. mirabilis appears to be governed by the general principles of bacterial pathogenesis. Proteins produced by this species and the swarming differentiation that occurs during infection may contribute to colonization of the host, evasion of host defense, and damage of host tissue.

## Colonization

The source of the bacterium is probably the intestinal tract of the host. Low rates of infection in the healthy host may relate to the rates of intestinal colonization by P. mirabilis, which are lower than those of E. coli. If present, however, Proteus spp. can contaminate the periurethral area of the host. Colonization of the urinary tract then requires movement of P. mirabilis to its niche, attachment to specific receptors, and survival in the urinary tract. At least four distinct fimbrial types that may contribute to this process have been identified in this species (Table 3). MR/P fimbriae and PMF appear to contribute to colonization by P. mirabilis (9, 62). Isogenic mutants deficient in MR/P fimbriae were recovered in lower numbers than the parent strains from the bladder and kidneys of mice 1 week after experimental inoculation of the bladders (Table 1). In similar experiments, the PMF mutant was found at a significantly lower concentration in the bladder only. The contributions of two newly described fimbriae, ATF (60) and NAF (107), have not yet been tested in an animal model.

*P. mirabilis* produces an amino acid deaminase, an enzyme that generates α-keto acids that can bind ferric iron ($Fe^{3+}$) (26) and may allow growth of the bacterium in an otherwise iron-limiting environment (64). Although the affinity of α-keto acids for iron is not predicted to be as high as that of traditional siderophores, production of these compounds may nevertheless confer an advantage on this organism, which lacks siderophores normally produced by members of the *Enterobacteriaceae*.

To move to the site of colonization, *P. mirabilis* may undergo swarmer cell differentiation (i.e., development of an elongated form on solid surfaces) accompanied by production of hundreds of flagella per cell. We postulate that flagellum-mediated motility is required for the cell to ascend the ureters to the kidney. Allison et al. (4) showed that the genes encoding flagellin, urease, and hemolysin are coordinately expressed in these differentiated cells. The expression of each of these virulence genes is very low in the normal vegetative cell but rises dramatically during swarmer cell differentiation. These data suggest that differentiation into swarmer cells is an adaptive response of *P. mirabilis* to the host environment that may facilitate colonization of the kidney.

## Evasion of Host Defense

*P. mirabilis* may avoid host defenses by three possible mechanisms, including production of an IgA-degrading metalloprotease that cleaves secretory IgA produced in response to infection just outside the hinge region of the immunoglobulin protein (55). In addition, expression of MR/P fimbriae may be modulated by a mechanism of phase variation (11), resulting in expression of the fimbriae by some bacteria and no expression by other bacteria within the same population. In addition, the existence of multiple flagellin-encoding genes (13) has been reported and suggests the possibility that *P. mirabilis* elicits an antigenic variation in flagellar epitopes to escape the host immune response. Essential to this hypothesis is the observation that when *flaA*, which encodes the principal flagellin protein of wild-type *P. mirabilis*, is mutated, rendering the bacterium incapable of differentiation and swarming, motile revertants appear over time (13). Analyses of these motile revertants have revealed that the antigenic characteristics of the flagellin have changed, as has the amino acid composition of the protein (13). Genetic analysis of the *flaA* locus of the motile revertants indicates that a deletion or some other genetic rearrangement has occurred, thus producing this antigenically distinct flagellin protein (13). Since the flagellin represents major surface antigens for this species during infection, synthesis of antigenically distinct flagella could represent an effective mechanism for avoiding host defense.

## Damage to Host Tissue

Hemolysin and urease appear to contribute to damage of host tissue. The HpmA hemolysin is a potent cytotoxin in vitro for epithelial cells (105), cytolyzing such primary human renal cell cultures after only brief contact (70). Urease hydrolyzes urea, which is present at a high concentration (0.5 M) in urine; this hydrolysis releases ammonia and raises the local pH, which also damages the epithelium (71).

## Current Model

Our current model of pathogenesis holds *P. mirabilis* to be a highly virulent pathogen that is well adapted for life in the urinary tract (Fig. 4). *P. mirabilis* that contaminates the periurethral area can colonize the bladder epithelium via PMF that may bind to specific (but unknown) receptors on bladder epithelium. We postulate that, once they are established, highly flagellated, differentiated swarmer cells ascend the ureters to the kidney. MR/P fimbriae then are able to bind specifically to renal epithelium (8, 88, 99). As a consequence of binding, a microenvironment that may include biofilm formation can be established (52). During this process, urease hydrolyzes urea in the urine, causing a rise in local pH that initiates precipitation of supersaturated polyvalent cations and anions in the form of struvite or apatite stones (i.e., urolithiasis); epithelial-cell necrosis may follow. Hemolysin, a potent in vitro cytotoxin, may play a subtle role once the organism has reached the kidney parenchyma. In addition, bacteria may invade (or be internalized by) renal tubule epithelial cells, causing further damage that may in turn allow the organism to breach this thin barrier and enter the bloodstream in some cases.

## FEASIBILITY OF A VACCINE

To prevent the serious consequences of infection with *P. mirabilis*, it is clearly possible to develop a vaccine that would protect against infection by this species. Certain criteria make the development of a vaccine both useful and feasible.

First, its usefulness might be judged by a well-defined population who would benefit from immunization. Three categories of patients might constitute this population: (i) those with known anatomically or functionally abnormal urinary tracts, including neurogenic bladders and urinary diversions; (ii) those early in the course of long-term catheterization (urethral, suprapubic, intermittent, and condom); and (iii) women with apparently normal urinary tracts who are experiencing recurrent *E. coli* UTIs (before they develop *P. mirabilis* infection). The last group is included because some patients with struvite stones and recurrent UTI do not have abnormal or instrumented urinary tracts (36). This intimates that *P. mirabilis*, through the process of stone formation, can gradually convert an uncomplicated UTI into a complicated one. Second, infections with *P. mirabilis* are often difficult to clear, since the organism resides within urease-induced crystals, a persistent reservoir for recurrent infection. Third, the combination of stones and infection may result in particularly serious renal damage. Fourth, *P. mirabilis* appears to have a large number of conserved surface antigens that do not differ significantly from strain to strain regardless of whether the bacteria are from feces, urine of asymptomatic individuals, or urine of patients with catheter-associated bacteriuria or acute pyelonephritis. Fifth, *P. mirabilis* is present in the fecal flora of <5% of individuals (92). Thus, a vaccine that clears the organism from the stool would have little effect on the normal fecal flora.

Observations from our laboratory and those of other investigators suggest that *P. mirabilis* vaccination may confer protection against infection with heterologous strains. At least three antigen preparations have been tested. Legagno-Fajardo and colleagues (51) found that parenteral immunization with purified MR/P fimbriae protects mice from transurethral challenge with homologous and heterologous strains. We noted a strong serum immunoglobulin response to MR/P fimbriae when mice were transurethrally inoculated with *P. mirabilis* HI4320 (8), suggesting that this antigen is expressed in vivo and is immunogenic. An outer membrane protein preparation was used by O'Hanley's group (67) to protect BALB/c mice from homologous intravesicular challenge. In addition, some years ago, Pazin and Braude (80) immunized rats parenterally with purified flagella. They demonstrated that antiserum recovered from vaccinated animals immobilized bacteria by binding to flagella. When such vaccinated animals were challenged intrarenally with the homologous *P. mirabilis* strain, they demonstrated that bacteria could not spread from one kidney to the other kidney (i.e., down one ureter, into the bladder, and back up the other ureter), an event that did occur in unvaccinated rats.

## CONCLUSION

Although a model of pathogenesis is emerging, a number of important questions remain unanswered. MR/P fimbriae are critical to the development of acute pyelonephritis, yet the fimbrial adhesin has not been isolated (as it has for *E. coli* P fimbriae [53]), nor has the receptor been identified. In addition, we do not know when, where, or to what degree the proposed virulence factors are expressed in vivo. Are newly described fimbriae, deaminase, and IgA-degrading metalloprotease important in the pathogenesis of UTI? Previous work supports the thesis that *Proteus* pathogenesis is multifactorial, and it is therefore likely that these new factors contribute to the virulence of this organism. Is the swarmer cell truly relevant to infection, and can *P. mirabilis* display numerous antigenically distinct flagellins under the selective pressure of the host immune response? Answers to these questions are necessary to advance our understanding of the pathogenesis caused by *P. mirabilis* in the urinary tract.

## REFERENCES

1. **Adegbola, R. A., D. C. Old, and B. W. Senior.** 1983. The adhesins and fimbriae of *Proteus mirabilis* strains associated with high and low affinity for the urinary tract. *J. Med. Microbiol.* **16:**427–431.
2. **Allison, C., N. Coleman, P. L. Jones, and C. Hughes.** 1992. Ability of *Proteus mirabilis* to invade human urothelial cells is coupled to motility and swarming differentiation. *Infect. Immun.* **60:**4740–4746.
3. **Allison, C., L. Emody, N. Coleman, and C. Hughes.** 1994. The role of swarm cell differentiation and multicellular migration in the uropathogenicity of *Proteus mirabilis*. *J. Infect. Dis.* **169:**1155–1158.
4. **Allison, C., H.-C. Lai, and C. Hughes.** 1992. Co-ordinate expression of virulence genes during swarm-cell differentiation and population migration of *Proteus mirabilis*. *Mol. Microbiol.* **6:**1583–1591.
5. **Aronson, M., O. Medalia, and B. Griffel.** 1974. Prevention of ascending pyelonephritis in mice by urease inhibitors. *Nephron* **12:**94–104.
6. **Atkinson, B. A.** 1986. Species incidence and trends of susceptibility to antibiotics in the United States and other countries: MIC and MBC, p. 995–1162. *In* V. Lorian (ed.), *Antibiotics in Laboratory Medicine,* 2nd ed. The Williams & Wilkins Co., Baltimore.
7. **Bahrani, F. K., S. Cook, R. A. Hull, G. Massad, and H. L. T. Mobley.** 1993. *Proteus mirabilis* fimbriae: N-terminal amino acid sequence of a major fimbrial subunit and nucleotide sequences of the gene from two strains. *Infect. Immun.* **61:**884–891.
8. **Bahrani, F. K., D. E. Johnson, D. Robbins, and H. L. T. Mobley.** 1991. *Proteus mirabilis* flagella and MR/P fimbriae: isolation, purification, N-terminal analysis, and serum antibody response following experimental urinary tract infection. *Infect. Immun.* **59:**3574–3580.
9. **Bahrani, F. K., G. Massad, C. V. Lockatell, D. E. Johnson, J. W. Warren, and H. L. T. Mobley.** 1994. Construction of an MR/P fimbrial mutant of *Proteus mirabilis*: role in virulence in a mouse model of ascending urinary tract infection. *Infect. Immun.* **62:**3363–3371.
10. **Bahrani, F. K., and H. L. T. Mobley.** 1993. *Proteus mirabilis* MR/P fimbriae: molecular cloning, expression, and nucleotide sequence of the major fimbrial subunit gene. *J. Bacteriol.* **175:**457–464.
11. **Bahrani, F. K., and H. L. T. Mobley.** 1994. *Proteus mirabilis* MR/P fimbrial operon: genetic organization, nucleotide sequence, and conditions for expression. *J. Bacteriol.* **176:**3412–3419.
12. **Belas, R.** 1992. The swarming phenomenon of *Proteus mirabilis*. *ASM News* **58:**15–22.
13. **Belas, R.** 1994. Expression of multiple flagellin-encoding genes of *Proteus mirabilis*. *J. Bacteriol.* **176:**7169–7181.
14. **Belas, R.** Unpublished observation.
15. **Belas, R., D. Erskine, and D. Flaherty.** 1991. Transposon mutagenesis in *Proteus mirabilis*. *J. Bacteriol.* **173:**6289–6293.
16. **Belas, R., D. Erskine, and D. Flaherty.** 1991. *Proteus mirabilis* mutants defective in swarmer cell differentiation and multicellular behavior. *J. Bacteriol.* **173:**6279–6288.
17. **Belas, R., and D. Flaherty.** 1994. Sequence and genetic analysis of multiple flagellin-encoding genes from *Proteus mirabilis*. *Gene* **128:**33–41.
18. **Bisset, K. A.** 1973. The motion of the swarm in *Proteus mirabilis*. *J. Med. Microbiol.* **6:**33–35.
19. **Braude, A. L., and J. Siemienski.** 1960. Role of bacterial urease in experimental pyelonephritis. *J. Bacteriol.* **80:**171–179.

20. **Braunagel, S. C., and M. J. Benedik.** 1990. The metalloprotease of *Serratia marcescens* strain SM6. *Mol. Gen. Genet.* **222:** 446–451.
21. **Breitenbach, J. M., and R. P. Hausinger.** 1988. *Proteus mirabilis* urease: partial purification and inhibition by boric acid and boronic acids. *Biochem. J.* **250:**917–920.
22. **Chippendale, G. R., J. W. Warren, A. L. Trifillis, and H. L. T. Mobley.** 1994. Internalization of *Proteus mirabilis* by human renal epithelial cells. *Infect. Immun.* **62:** 3115–3121.
23. **Coetzee, J. N., G. Pernet, and J. J. Theron.** 1962. Fimbriae and haemagglutinating properties in strains of Proteus. *Nature* (London) **196:**497–498.
24. **Cox, C. E.** 1992. A comparison of the safety and efficacy of lomefloxacin and ciprofloxacin in the treatment of complicated or recurrent urinary tract infectins. *Am. J. Med.* **92**(Suppl. 4A):82S–86S.
25. **Drayna, C. J., C. T. Titcomb, R. R. Varma, and K. H. Soergel.** 1981. Hyperammonemic encephalopathy caused by infection in a neurogenic bladder. *N. Engl. J. Med.* **304:**766–768.
26. **Drechsel, H., A. Thieken, R. Reissbrodt, G. Jung, and G. Winkelmann.** 1993. α-Keto acids are novel siderophores in the genera *Proteus, Providencia,* and *Morganella* and are produced by amino acid deaminases. *J. Bacteriol.* **175:**2727–2733.
27. **Duguid, J. P., and R. R. Gillies.** 1958. Fimbriae and haemagglutinating activity in *Salmonella, Klebsiella, Proteus,* and *Chromobacterium. J. Pathol. Bacteriol.* **75:**519–520.
28. **Dumanski, A. J., H. Hedelin, A. Edin-Liljegren, D. Beauchemin, and R. J. C. McLean.** 1994. Unique ability of the *Proteus mirabilis* capsule to enhance mineral growth in infectious urinary calculi. *Infect. Immun.* **62:**2998–3003.
29. **Ehrlich, O., and A. S. Brem.** 1982. A prospective comparison of urinary tract infections in patients treated with either clean intermittent catheterization or urinary diversion. *Pediatrics* **70:**665–669.
30. **Emori, T. G., and R. P. Gaynes.** 1993. An overview of nosocomial infections, including the role of the microbiology laboratory. *Clin. Microbiol. Rev.* **6:**428–442.
31. **Eriksson, S., J. Zbornik, H. Dahnsjo, P. Erlansoon, O. Kahlmeter, H. Fritz, and C. A. Bauer.** 1986. The combination of pivampicillin and pivmecillinam versus pivampicillin alone in the treatment of acute pyelonephritis. *Scand. J. Infect. Dis.* **18:** 431–438.
32. **Ewing, W. H.** 1986. The tribe *Proteeae*, p. 443–459. *In Edwards and Ewing's Identification of the Enterobacteriaceae*, 4th ed. Elsevier Science Publishing Co., Inc., New York.
33. **Fairley, K. F., N. E. Carson, R. C. Gutch, P. Leighton, A. D. Grounds, E. C. Laird, P. H. McCallum, R. L. Sleeman, and C. M. O'Keefe.** 1971. Site of infection in acute urinary-tract infection in general practice. *Lancet* **ii:**615–618.
34. **Falkinham, J. O. I., and P. S. Hoffman.** 1984. Unique developmental characteristics of the swarm and short cells of *Proteus vulgaris* and *Proteus mirabilis. J. Bacteriol.* **158:** 1037–1040.
35. **File, T., J. Tan, S.-J. Salstrom, and J. Johnson.** 1985. Timentin versus piperacillin in the therapy of serious urinary tract infections. *Am. J. Med.* **79:**91–95.
36. **Fowler, J. E.** 1984. Bacteriology of branched renal calculi and accompanying urinary tract infection. *J. Urol.* **131:**213–215.
37. **Fowler, J. E., Jr., and T. A. Stamey.** 1978. Studies of introital colonization in women with recurrent urinary infections. X. Adhesive properties of *Escherichia coli* and *Proteus mirabilis:* lack of correlation with urinary pathogenicity. *J. Urol.* **120:**315–318.
38. **Gentry, L. O. B. A. Wood, M. D. Martin, and J. Smythe.** 1980. Cefamandole alone and combined with gentamicin or tobramycin in the treatment of acute pyelonephritis. *Scand. J. Infect. Dis. Suppl.* **25:** 96–100.
39. **Griffith, D. P., D. M. Musher, and C. Itin.** 1976. Urease: the primary cause of infection-induced urinary stones. *Invest. Urol.* **13:**346–350.
40. **Hoeniger, J. F. M.** 1964. Cellular changes accompanying the swarming of *Proteus mirabilis*. I. Observations on living cultures. *Can. J. Microbiol.* **10:**1–9.
41. **Hoeniger, J. F. M.** 1965. Development of flagella by *Proteus mirabilis. J. Gen. Microbiol.* **40:**29–42.
42. **Hoeniger, J. F. M.** 1966. Cellular changes accompanying the swarming of *Proteus mirabilis*. II. Observations of stained organisms. *Can. J. Microbiol.* **12:**113–122.
43. **Jabri, E., M. B. Carr, R. P. Hausinger, and P. A. Karplus.** 1995. The crystal structure of urease from *Klebsiella aerogenes* at 2 Å resolution. *Science* **268:**998–1004.
44. **Johnson, D. E., R. G. Russell, C. V. Lockatell, J. C. Zulty, J. W. Warren, and**

H. L. T. Mobley. 1993. Contribution of *Proteus mirabilis* urease to persistence, urolithiasis, and renal pathology in a mouse model of ascending urinary tract infection. *Infect. Immun.* **61**:2748–2754.
45. Jones, B. D., C. V. Lockatell, D. E. Johnson, J. W. Warren, and H. L. T. Mobley. 1990. Construction of a urease negative mutant of *Proteus mirabilis*: analysis of virulence in a mouse model of ascending urinary tract infection. *Infect. Immun.* **58**:1120–1123.
46. Jones, B. D., and H. L. T. Mobley. 1987. Genetic and biochemical diversity of ureases of *Proteus, Providencia,* and *Morganella* species isolated from urinary tract infection. *Infect. Immun.* **55**:2198–2203.
47. Jones, B. D., and H. L. T. Mobley. 1988. *Proteus mirabilis* urease: genetic organization, regulation, and expression of structural genes. *J. Bacteriol.* **170**:3342–3349.
48. Jones, B. D., and H. L. T. Mobley. 1989. *Proteus mirabilis* urease: nucleotide sequence determination and comparison with jack bean urease. *J. Bacteriol.* **171**:6414–6422.
49. Kohnle, W., E. Vanek, K. Federlin, and H. E. Franz. 1975. Lokalisation eines Harnwegsinfektes durch Nachweis von antikorperbesetzten Bakterien im Urin. *Dtsch. Med. Wochenschr.* **100**:2598–2602.
50. Koronakis, V., M. Cross, B. Senior, E. Koronakis, and C. Hughes. 1987. The secreted hemolysins of *Proteus mirabilis, Proteus vulgaris,* and *Morganella morganii* are genetically related to each other and to the alphahemolysin of *Escherichia coli. J. Bacteriol.* **169**:1509–1515.
51. Legnani-Fajardo, C., P. Zunino, G. Algorta, and H. F. Laborde. 1991. Antigenic and immunogenic activity of flagella and fimbriae preparations from uropathogenic *Proteus mirabilis. Can. J. Microbiol.* **37**:325–328.
52. Lerner, S. P., M. J. Gleeson, and D. P. Griffith. 1989. Infection stones. *J. Urol.* **141**:753–757.
53. Lindberg, F., B. Lund, L. Hohansson, and S. Normark. 1987. Localization of the receptor-binding protein adhesin at the tip of the bacterial pilus. *Nature* (London) **328**:84–87.
54. Lomborg, H., P. Larsson, R. Leffler, and C. Svanborg-Eden. 1982. Different binding specificities of *P. mirabilis* compared to *E. coli. Scand. J. Infect. Dis. Suppl.* **33**:37–42.
55. Loomes, L. M., B. W. Senior, and M. A. Kerr. 1990. A proteolytic enzyme secreted by *Proteus mirabilis* degrades immunoglobulins of the immunoglobulin A1 (IgA1), IgA2, and IgG isotypes. *Infect Immun.* **58**:1979–1985.
56. Loomes, L. M., B. W. Senior, and M. A. Kerr. 1992. Proteinases of *Proteus* spp.: purification, properties, and detection in urine of infected patients. *Infect. Immun.* **60**:2267–2273.
57. MacLaren, D. M. 1968. The significance of urease in *Proteus* pyelonephritis: a bacteriological study. *J. Pathol. Bacteriol.* **96**:45–56.
58. MacLaren, D. M. 1969. The significance of urease in *Proteus* pyelonephritis: a histological and biochemical study. *J. Pathol.* **97**:43–49.
59. MacLaren, D. M. 1974. The influence of acetohydroxamic acid on experimental *Proteus* pyelonephritis. *Invest. Urol.* **12**:146–149.
60. Massad, G., F. K. Bahrani, and H. L. T. Mobley. 1994. *Proteus mirabilis* fimbriae: identification, isolation, and characterization of a new ambient temperature fimbriae (ATF). *Infect. Immun.* **62**:1989–1994.
61. Massad, G., J. F., Fulkerson, Jr., D. Watson, and H. L. T. Mobley. Submitted for publication.
62. Massad, G., C. V. Lockatell, D. E. Johnson, and H. L. T. Mobley. 1994. *Proteus mirabilis* fimbriae: construction of an isogenic *pmfA* mutant and analyses of virulence in a CBA mouse model of ascending urinary tract infection. *Infect. Immun.* **62**:536–542.
63. Massad, G., and H. L. T. Mobley. 1994. Genetic organization and complete nucleotide sequence of the *Proteus mirabilis* PMF fimbrial operon. *Gene* **150**:101–104.
64. Massad, G., H. Zhao, and H. L. T. Mobley. Submitted for publication.
65. Menard, R., P. Sansonetti, and C. Parsot. 1993. Nonpolar mutagenesis of the *ipa* genes defines IpaB, IpaC, and IpaD and effectors of *Shigella flexneri* entry into epithelial cells. *J. Bacteriol.* **175**:5899–5906.
66. Milazzo, F. H., and G. J. Delisle. 1984. Immunoglobulin a proteases in gram-negative bacteria isolated from human urinary tract infections. *Infect. Immun.* **43**:11–13.
67. Moayeri, N., C. M. Collins, and P. O'Hanley. 1991. Efficacy of a *Proteus mirabilis* outer membrane protein vaccine in preventing experimental *Proteus* pyelonephritis in a BALB/c mouse model. *Infect. Immun.* **59**:3778–3786.
68. Mobley, H. L. T., R. Belas, D. E. Johnson, V. Lockatell, G. Chippendale, and J. W. Warren. Unpublished observation.

69. **Mobley, H. L. T., and G. R. Chippendale.** 1990. Hemagglutinin, urease, and hemolysin production by *Proteus mirabilis* from clinical sources. *J. Infect. Dis.* **161:**525–530.
70. **Mobley, H. L. T., G. R. Chippendale, K. G. Swihart, and R. A. Welch.** 1991. Cytotoxicity of HpmA hemolysin and urease of *Proteus mirabilis* and *Proteus vulgaris* for cultured human renal proximal tubular epithelial cells. *Infect. Immun.* **59:**2036–2042.
71. **Mobley, H. L. T., and R. P. Hausinger.** 1989. Microbial ureases: significance, regulation, and molecular characterization. *Microbiol. Rev.* **53:**85–108.
72. **Mobley, H. L. T., M. D. Island, and R. P. Hausinger.** Molecular biology of microbial ureases. *Microbiol Rev,* in press.
73. **Mobley, H. L. T., M. D. Island, and G. Massad.** 1994. Virulence determinants of uropathogenic *Escherichia coli* and *Proteus mirabilis*. *Kidney Int.* **47**(Suppl. 47)**:**S129–S136.
74. **Mobley, H. L. T., and J. W. Warren.** 1987. Urease-positive bacteriuria and obstruction of long-term urinary catheters. *J. Clin. Microbiol.* **25:**2216–2217.
75. **Mulrooney, S. B., and R. P. Hausinger.** 1990. Sequence of the *Klebsiella aerogenes* urease genes and evidence for accessory proteins facilitating nickel incorporation. *J. Bacteriol.* **172:**5837–5843.
76. **Musher, D. M., D. P. Griffith, D. Yawn, and R. D. Rossen.** 1975. Role of urease in pyelonephritis resulting from urinary tract infection with *Proteus*. *J. Infect. Dis.* **131:**177–181.
77. **Nicholson, E. B., E. A. Concaugh, P. A. Foxall, M. D. Island, and H. L. Mobley.** 1993. *Proteus mirabilis* urease: transcriptional regulation by UreR. *J. Bacteriol.* **175:**465–473.
78. **Nicolle, L. E., G. K. M. Harding, J. Kennedy, M. McIntyre, F. Aoki, and D. Murray.** 1988. Urine specimen collection with external devices for diagnosis of bacteriuria in elderly incontinent men. *J. Clin. Microbiol.* **26:**1115–1119.
79. **Old, D., and R. Adegbola.** 1982. Hemagglutinins and fimbriae of *Morganella, Proteus,* and *Providencia*. *J. Med. Microbiol.* **15:**551–564.
80. **Pazin, G. J., and A. I. Braude.** 1969. Immobilizing antibodies in pyelonephritis. *J. Immunol.* **102:**454–465.
81. **Pearman, J. W., M. Bailey, and L. P. Riley.** 1991. Bladder instillations of trisdine compared with catheter introducer for reduction of bacteriuria during intermittent catheterisation of patients with acute spinal cord trauma. *Br. J. Urol.* **67:**483–490.
82. **Peerbooms, P., A. Verweij, and D. MacLaren.** 1982. Urinary virulence of *Proteus mirabilis* in two experimental mouse models. *Infect. Immun.* **36:**1246–1248.
83. **Peerbooms, P., A. Verweij, and D. MacLaren.** 1983. Investigation of the haemolytic activity of *Proteus mirabilis* strains. *Antonie van Leeuwenhoek* **49:**1–11.
84. **Peerbooms, P., A. Verweij, and D. MacLaren.** 1984. Vero cell invasiveness of *Proteus mirabilis*. *Infect. Immun.* **43:**1068–1071.
85. **Rubin, R. H., N. E. Tolkoff-Rubin, and R. S. Cotran.** 1986. Urinary tract infection, pyelonephritis, and reflux nephropathy, p. 1085–1141. *In* B. M. Brenner and F. C. Rector (ed.), *The Kidney.* The W.B. Saunders Co., Philadelphia.
86. **Sabbaj, J., V. L. Hoagland, and T. Cook.** 1986. Norfloxacin versus co-trimoxazole in the treatment of recurring urinary tract infections in men. *Scand. J. Infect. Dis. Suppl.* **48:**48–53.
87. **Samtoy, B., and M. M. DeBeaukelaer.** 1980. Ammonia encephalopathy secondary to urinary tract infection with *Proteus mirabilis*. *Pediatrics* **65:**294.
88. **Sareneva, T., H. Holthofer, and T. K. Korhonen.** 1990. Tissue-binding affinity of *Proteus mirabilis* fimbriae in the human urinary tract. *Infect. Immun.* **58:**3330–3336.
89. **Saxena, D. R., and D. C. Bassett.** 1975. Sex-related incidence in Proteus infection of the urinary tract in childhood. *Arch. Dis. Child.* **50:**899–901.
90. **Schultz, H. J., L. A. McCaffrey, T. F. Keys, and F. T. Nobrega.** 1984. Acute cystitis: a prospective study of laboratory tests and duration of therapy. *Mayo Clin. Proc.* **59:**391–397.
91. **Schwyn, B., and J. B. Neilands.** 1987. Universal chemical assay for the detection and determination of siderophores. *Anal. Biochem.* **160:**47–56.
92. **Senior, B. W.** 1983. *Proteus morganii* is less frequently associated with urinary tract infections than *Proteus mirabilis*—an explanation. *J. Med. Microbiol.* **16:**317–322.
93. **Senior, B. W., M. Albrechtsen, and M. A. Kerr.** 1987. *Proteus mirabilis* strains of diverse type have IgA protease activity. *J. Med. Microbiol.* **24:**175–180.
94. **Senior, B. W., and C. Hughes.** 1987. Production and properties of haemolysins from clinical isolates of the Proteeae. *J. Med. Microbiol.* **24:**17–25.

95. **Senior, B. W., L. M. Loomes, and M. A. Kerr.** 1991. The production and activity *in vivo* of *Proteus mirabilis* IgA protease in infections of the urinary tract. *J. Med. Microbiol.* **35**:203–207.
96. **Shand, G. H., H. Anwar, J. Kadurugamuwa, M. R. W. Brown, S. H. Silverman, and J. Melling.** 1985. In vivo evidence that bacteria in urinary tract infection grow under iron-restricted conditions. *Infect. Immun.* **48**:35–39.
97. **Shedden, W. I. H.** 1962. Fimbriae and haemagglutinating activity in strains of Proteus hauseri. *J. Gen. Microbiol.* **28**:1–7.
98. **Silverblatt, F.** 1974. Host-parasite interaction in the renal pelvis. A possible role for pili in the pathogenesis of pyelonephritis. *J. Exp. Med.* **140**:1696–1711.
99. **Silverblatt, F. J., and I. Ofek.** 1978. Influence of pili on the virulence of *Proteus mirabilis* in experimental hematogenous pyelonephritis. *J. Infect. Dis.* **138**:664–667.
100. **Sinha, B., and R. Gonzalez.** 1984. Hyperammonemia in a boy with obstructive ureterocele and proteus infection. *J. Urol.* **131**:330–331.
101. **Sriwanthana, B., M. D. Island, and H. L. T. Mobley.** 1993. Sequence of the *Proteus mirabilis* urease accessory gene *ureG*. *Gene* **129**:103–106.
102. **Stamm, W. E., M. McKevitt, P. L. Roberts, and N. J. White.** 1991. Natural history of recurrent urinary tract infections in women. *Rev. Infect. Dis.* **13**:77–84.
103. **Svanborg-Eden, C., P. Larsson, and H. Lomborg.** 1980. Attachment of *Proteus mirabilis* to human urinary sediment epithelial cells in vitro is different from that of *Escherichia coli*. *Infect. Immun.* **27**:804–807.
104. **Swihart, K. G., and R. A. Welch.** 1990. The HpmA hemolysin is more common than HlyA among *Proteus* isolates. *Infect. Immun.* **58**:1853–1860.
105. **Swihart, K. G., and R. A. Welch.** 1990. Cytotoxic activity of the *Proteus* hemolysin, HpmA. *Infect. Immun.* **58**:1861–1865.
106. **Tolson, D.** Personal communication.
107. **Tolson, D. L., D. L. Barrigar, R. J. C. McLean, and E. Altman.** 1995. Expression of a nonagglutinating fimbria by *Proteus mirabilis*. *Infect. Immun.* **63**:1127–1129.
108. **Troilfors, B. M., Jertborn, J. Martineil, G. Norkrans, and G. Lidin-Hanson.** 1982. Mecillinam versus cephaloridine for the treatment of acute pyelonephritis. *Infection* **10**:15–17.
109. **Uphoff, T. S., and R. A. Welch.** 1990. Nucleotide sequencing of the *Proteus mirabilis* calcium-independent hemolysin genes (*hpmA* and *hpmB*) reveals sequence similarity with the *Serratia marcescens* hemolysin genes (*shlA* and *shlB*). *J. Bacteriol.* **172**:1206–1216.
110. **Warren, J. W., H. H. Tenney, J. M. Hoopes, H. L. Muncie, and W. C. Anthony.** 1982. A prospective microbiologic study of bacteriuria in patients with chronic indwelling urethral catheters. *J. Infect. Dis.* **146**:719–723.
111. **Welch, R. A.** 1987. Identification of two different hemolysin determinants in uropathogenic *Proteus* isolates. *Infect. Immun.* **55**:2183–2190.
112. **Williams, F. D., and R. H. Schwarzhoff.** 1978. Nature of the swarming phenomenon in *Proteus*. *Annu. Rev. Microbiol.* **32**:101–122.
113. **Wilson, D. R., and T. J. Beveridge.** 1993. Bacterial flagellar filaments and their component flagellins. *Can. J. Microbiol.* **39**:451–472.
114. **Wray, S., S. Hull, R. Cook, J. Barrish, and R. Hull.** 1986. Identification and characterization of a urinary cell adhesin from a uropathogenic isolate of *Proteus mirabilis*. *Infect. Immun.* **54**:43–49.

# *PROTEUS MIRABILIS* SWARMER CELL DIFFERENTIATION AND URINARY TRACT INFECTION[†]

*Robert Belas, Ph.D.*

## 10

### GENERAL DESCRIPTION OF *PROTEUS MIRABILIS* SWARMING

*Proteus mirabilis* is a motile gram-negative bacterium that is similar in many aspects of its physiology to other members of the family *Enterobacteriaceae* such as *Escherichia coli* and *Salmonella typhimurium*. It was originally described and named by Hauser in 1885 for the character in Homer's *Odyssey* who "has the power of assuming different shapes in order to escape being questioned" (67). *P. mirabilis* is considered an opportunistic pathogen and one of the causes of urinary tract infections (UTIs) in hospital patients with urinary catheters or complicated urinary tracts (28, 29, 44, 48, 50, 97, 102, 113, 119, 121). In these patients, not only does this bacterial species cause cystitis and acute pyelonephritis, but the production of urinary stones can further complicate these infections. It is believed that the ability of *P. mirabilis* to colonize the surfaces of catheters and the urinary tract may be aided by the characteristic first described over a century ago and currently referred to as swarmer cell differentiation.

Unlike swimming behavior, which occurs in liquid environments, swarming is organized movement over a surface and is dependent on a specialized cell that possesses unique characteristics that provide an adaptive advantage for living on such surfaces (66). Swarming motility has been demonstrated in many different bacterial genera, both gram negative and gram positive. Many scientists have seen the end result of *P. mirabilis* swarmer cell differentiation, which is the development of a large, spreading colony made of concentric rings of bacterial growth, as shown in Fig. 1A. Perhaps less known is that this colony is the end product of coordinated gene expression and multicellular behavior (Fig. 1B) that result in a differentiated cell (Fig. 1C) uniquely adapted to life on surfaces, in viscous environments, or on the urinary epithelial mucosa. This chapter focuses on the aspects of *P. mirabilis* swarmer cell differentiation and swarming behavior that generate the differentiated cell and swarming colony and relates this example of bacterial multicellular behavior and prokaryotic differentiation to the

---

[†] Contribution no. 1022 from the Center of Marine Biotechnology.
*Robert Belas,* Center of Marine Biotechnology, University of Maryland Biotechnology Institute, Suite 236, Columbus Center, 701 East Pratt Street, Baltimore, Maryland 21202.

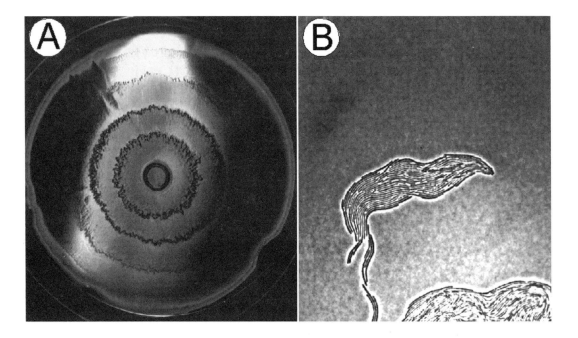
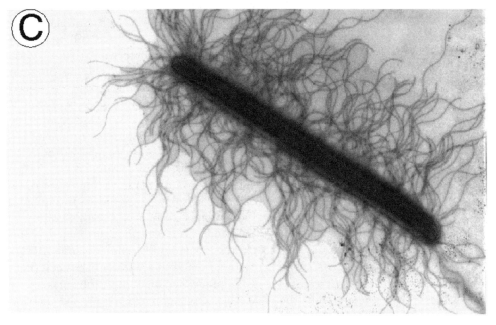

**FIGURE 1** *P. mirabilis* swarming colony formation and swarmer cell morphology. (A) The characteristic bull's-eye colony of latticed zones of bacteria produced by the cyclic events of differentiation, movement, cessation of movement, and dedifferentiation. (B) Movement of a mass of cells from the swarming periphery onto uncolonized agar. The swarming periphery is shown at lower right. (C) Fully differentiated swarmer cell as shown by electron microscopy of a negatively stained specimen taken from the swarming periphery. The cell is approximately 25 $\mu$m long.

pathogenicity of the bacteria in the human urinary tract.

When grown in suitable liquid media, P. mirabilis exists as a 1.5- to 2.0-μm motile cell with 6 to 10 peritrichous flagella. These bacteria, called swimmer cells, display characteristic swimming and chemotactic behavior, moving toward nutrients and away from repellents (1). However, a dramatic change in cell morphology takes place when cells grown in liquid are transferred to a nutrient medium solidified with agar. Shortly after encountering an agar surface, the cells begin to elongate (67–70, 74). This is the first step in the production of a morphologically and biochemically differentiated cell referred to as a swarmer cell. The process of elongation takes place with only a slight increase in cell width and is due to an inhibition in the normal septation mechanism (26). Elongation of the swarmer cell can give rise to cells 60 to >80 μm long. During this process, DNA replication proceeds without any significant change in rate compared to that in the swimmer cell (53). Not surprisingly, the rate of synthesis of certain proteins, i.e., flagellin, is altered markedly in the swarmer cell (10, 14, 15, 49, 71, 79). The result of this process is a very long, nonseptate, polyploid cell with $10^3$ to $10^4$ flagella (Fig. 1C). The number of chromosomes in the swarmer cell is roughly proportional to the increase in length, so that a 40-μm-long swarmer cell has about 20 chromosomes (20). Eventually, septation and division do take place at the ends of the long swarmer cells, producing a microcolony of differentiated cells. Table 1 compares the physical features of swimmer and swarmer cells.

Concurrent with cellular elongation, changes take place in the rate of synthesis of flagella on the swarmer cell (Table 1, Fig. 2). Though swimmer cells have only a few flagella, the elongated swarmer cells are profusely covered by hundreds to thousands of new flagella synthesized specifically as a consequence of growth on the surface (14, 68, 69, 72, 86). The term "flagellin factories" was first used by Hoeniger (68) to describe the tremendous synthesis of new flagella (composed of the protein flagellin) in swarmer cell differentiation. The newly synthesized surface-induced flagella are composed of the same flagellin subunit as the swimmer cell flagella, indicating that the same flagellar species is overproduced upon surface induction. The result of the surface-induced differentiation process is a swarmer cell, which differs from a swimmer cell by having the unique ability to move over solid media in a tranlocation process referred to as swarming (66). However, individual swarmer cells by themselves do not have the ability to swarm (30–32, 34, 45, 46). As shown in Fig. 1B, swarming is the result of the coordinated, multicellular effort of groups of differentiated swarmer cells (30, 31, 42). The process begins when a group of differentiated swarmer cells moves outward as a mass, and it continues until the swarming mass of bacteria is reduced in number by

**TABLE 1** Physical features of swimmer and swarmer cells

| Characteristic | Swimmer cells | Swarmer cells | Reference(s) |
|---|---|---|---|
| Flagella | | | |
|   No./cell | 1–10 | 500–5,000 | 68 |
|   Length (μm) | 1.75 | 5.25 | 68 |
|   No./unit cell length | 3 | 150 | 68 |
| Motility | Tumbling | Smooth | 41, 68 |
| Cell dimensions (μm) | 0.7 by 1–2 | 0.7 by 10–>80 | 68 |
| No. of chromosomes | 1 or 2 | Multiple; correlated with cell length | 69 |

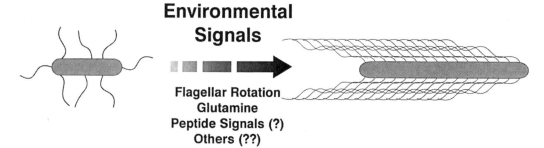

**FIGURE 2** Characteristics of *P. mirabilis* swarmer cell differentiation and swarming motility. Swarmer cell differentiation is controlled through the combined sensing of environmental conditions that reduce wild-type flagellar filament rotation and the sensing of a specific chemical stimulus, the amino acid glutamine. Other signals, e.g., peptide signals and perhaps other compounds, may play a role in this process. The differentiated swarmer cell is characterized by an elongated, polyploid cell that synthesizes numerous flagella in response to these signals.

loss of constituent cells that fall behind on the surface or until the mass reverses direction.

Swarming of *P. mirabilis* is cyclic (Fig. 2 and 3). Once swarmer cells have fully differentiated, the swarming colony moves outward in unison from all points along the periphery for several hours and then stops (30–32, 45, 46). As shown in Fig. 4, this cessation of movement is accompanied by dedifferentiation of the swarmer cell back to swimmer cell morphology, a process referred to as consolidation (30, 31, 67–70, 131). The cycle of swarming and consolidation is then repeated several times until the agar surface is covered by concentric rings formed by the swarming mass of bacteria (46). This cycle of events gives rise to the characteristic "bull's-eye" appearance of *P. mirabilis* colonies (Fig. 1A, 3, and 4). The swarmer cell requires contact with the surface at all times to maintain the differentiated state. When removed from the surface of an agar plate and suspended in liquid medium, cells quickly begin to septate and divide into short cells, and the synthesis of flagella returns to the level observed in swimmer cells (76). Thus, the differentiation process is reversible both as a result of the consolidation process and as

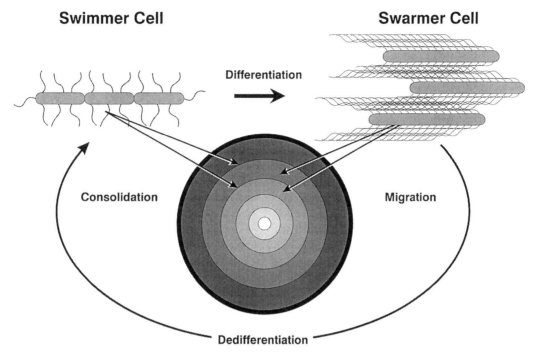

**FIGURE 3** Spatial cycling of *P. mirabilis* swarmer cell differentiation. On agar media, swarmer cell differentiation is observed as a series of ever-expanding concentric rings (see Fig. 1A) that are composed of morphologically and biochemically distinct cell types. During swarming, the leading edge of the swarming zone is composed of completely differentiated swarmer cells. At consolidation, swarming motility stops, and the cells revert to a swimmer cell morphology. This cycle is then repeated, as shown in Fig. 4.

a consequence of the removal of the inducing stimulus from the surface (Fig. 4).

## DIFFERENCES BETWEEN SWIMMER AND SWARMER CELLS

### Cell Wall and Membrane Composition Differences

The suspicion that the cell walls and membranes of swarmer cells may differ significantly from those of swimmer cells arose because of the highly flagellate, elongate, polyploid nature of the swarmer cells and the known involvement of the cell envelope in flagellum function and normal division (13–15). A variety of direct and indirect evidence confirmed this suspicion (Table 2). In comparative studies of swimmer and swarmer cells, the increased permeability demonstrated by leakage of intracellular amino acids and pentose sugars (13), the enhanced sensitivity to deoxycholate (13) and rifampin (hydrophobic molecules normally excluded by the hydrophilic outer membrane of gram-negative organisms) (13), the enhanced sensitivity to physical disruption by sonication (79), the freeze-fracture cleavage and fluidity of the outer membrane (11), the reduction in the number of inner-outer membrane adhesions (Bayer's patches), and phage binding (131) in swarmer cells provided indirect evidence. Changes in the actual composition of the lipopolysaccharide (LPS) (15)

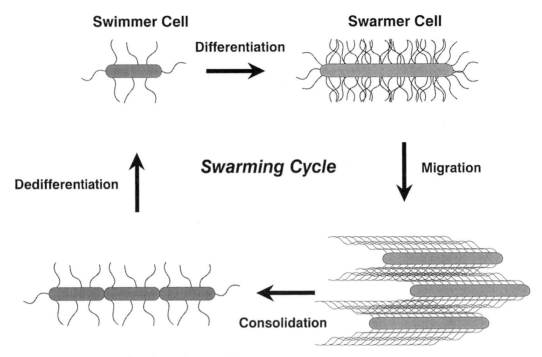

**FIGURE 4** Temporal cycling of *P. mirabilis* swarmer cell differentiation. Swarmer cell differentiation and swarming motility are cyclic. Swimmer cells differentiate into swarmer cells when they sense conditions that induce the expression of swarmer cell-specific genes. Once fully differentiated, the swarmer cells then move en masse away from the initial point of inoculation. Such migration is punctuated by cyclic events of dedifferentiation (referred to as consolidation), whereupon migration stops and the cells revert to a morphology similar to that of the swimmer cell. This process of differentiation and dedifferentiation continues until the agar plate is covered by the bacterial mass.

**TABLE 2** Cell membrane features of swimmer and swarmer cells

| Characteristic | Swimmer cells | Swarmer cells | Reference(s) |
| --- | --- | --- | --- |
| Permeability | Normal | Increased | 13 |
| Sensitivity to chemical and physical disruption | Normal | Increased | 13, 79 |
| Sensitivity to hydrophobic agents | Normal | Increased | 13, 15 |
| Outer membrane | | | |
|   LPS composition | Normal | Higher proportion with long oligosaccharide side chains | 15 |
|   Fluidity | Normal | Increased | 11 |
|   Protein composition | Normal | Proportions change | 49 |
|   Bayer patches | Normal | Reduced | 131 |
| Cytochromes | High in *b*, *a*, and *d* | Low in *b*, deficient in *a* and *d* | 49 |

and outer membrane protein (49) and in the cytochromes of the inner membrane (49) provided direct evidence.

To explain these differences and the apparent contradiction that an increase in hydrophilic long-side-chain LPS in the outer membranes of swarmer cells confers enhanced hydrophobicity, a redistribution of outer membrane LPS associated with the 50-fold increase in flagellar concentration in swarmer cells was proposed. It was suggested that the long-side-chain LPS could aggregate at the bases of the flagella to provide outer membrane stability and prevent membrane damage due to flagellar rotation. As a result, LPS deficiency would occur in other regions of the membrane and create localized exposure of phospholipid on the surface and in lipid bilayer areas in the outer membrane. Both of these features are normally absent in gram-negative bacteria (10–12, 15). The exposed phospholipid would create a surface more hydrophobic, more permeable to hydrophobic antibiotics, and more sensitive to surfactants (11, 13, 15). The lipid bilayer regions would create a cleavable and more flexible outer membrane (11). The LPS aggregation could possibly restrict the LPS available for Bayer patches and LPS-dependent phage-binding sites. Further, because the initial increase in flagellin synthesis is reported to occur before the inhibition of cell division in swarmer cell development, it may be the outer membrane reorganization associated with flagellar development that impairs septation (14). Some of these speculations are supported by recent data demonstrating that genetic lesions directly affecting LPS biosynthesis and, more specifically, chain length result in abnormal cellular elongation during swarming-cell differentiation (26).

## Metabolic Differences

Differences have also been found in some of the metabolic features of swimmer and swarmer cells. Swarmer cells exhibit decreased uptake and incorporation of macromolecular precursors (10, 13) and decreased oxygen consumption (10, 49). The decreased uptake has been attributed to the effect of membrane changes on active transport processes (13). Because of the decreased oxygen consumption, swarmers were initially regarded as nongrowing bacteria (10) of low metabolic activity that expend most of their energy on movement (10).

During the search for other indicators of decreased metabolic activity, the enzyme tryptophanase was found to be repressed and uninducible in swarmer cells (71). Other enzymes, cytochromes, and outer membrane proteins (Table 2) were also examined for differing patterns of expression in the two cell types (49). This work revealed not only differences between swarmer and swimmer cells but also variety in the pattern of protein expression within one cell type. In swarmer cells, for example, tryptophanase is uninducible, but phenylalanine deaminase is inducible, as is urease, and these last two enzymes are both potential virulence factors (80, 81, 100–102). It was this variation in the expression of a number of determinants that resulted in swarming being regarded as an example of prokaryotic differentiation with a common regulatory signal acting at the level of transcription (49). This opinion has subsequently received substantial support (5, 6, 8, 20, 21, 23, 41, 78, 79). In addition, the inducible nature of phenylalanine deaminase and urease indicates that swarmers possess functional transcription and translation. The higher activities of both of these enzymes in swarmer cells indicate that these cells do possess the capacity for metabolic activity. Despite this capacity, transcription and translation do not appear to be necessary for the persistence of migration, for once swarming has been initiated, it continues even in the presence of the transcription and translation inhibitors rifampin and chloramphenicol, respectively (49). Further, no exogenous energy source is necessary for migration once it has been initiated, because swarming cells will continue to swarm if transferred to nonnutrient agar (130). In light of this demonstration of functional transcription and translation and at least the capacity, though not the necessity, for metabolic activity, the decreased respiratory activities and cytochrome contents of swarmer cells were not interpreted, as they were interpreted earlier, as indicating low metabolic activity or a nongrowing status. Rather, it was proposed that the energy required for swarming is derived not from respiration but from fermentation. Other evidence supports this contention, because normal swarming motility occurs aerobically in the presence of cyanide as well as anaerobically (49). Utilization of some kind of fermentable storage material and the catabolism of certain amino acids have been proposed as providing both ATP and the transmembrane proton potential used to drive the flagellar motors (10, 49).

The continuation of swarming when swarmer cells are transferred to nonnutrient agar with low surface tension (agar made with water and detergent) (14) could be related to a stored energy source (122), and the periodicity of swarming could be associated with the depletion and reaccumulation of such a source (131). Consumption of stored energy as the swarm proceeds could account for the differences observed in swarmer cells at different times during a single swarming event. Swarmer cells transferred to fresh solid medium continue to swarm, but the distance traveled after transfer depends on the distance traveled before transfer: early swarmer cells travel further after transfer than do late swarmer cells (130). Early swarmer cells are very motile but become progressively slower as the swarm spreads (45). It has been proposed that the depletion of the energy source could affect the production of slime (131) or cause a drop in membrane potential and thus a decrease in flagellar rotation and cessation of the movement of swarmers (10). Alcian blue- and sudan black B-stainable inclusions could possibly constitute a storage material (131), as could glucuronic acid (49). However, conclusive evidence for the existence of a storage material is lacking.

In contrast to these theories of a stored energy material, it was recently proposed that the temporal and spatial periodicities associated with the formation of the concentric zones are genetically determined and could be due to multicellular interactions within the swarming colony. Such interactions could be mediated by the additive effect of a number of extracellular signal molecules that are repeatedly produced and destroyed in synchronous cycles (20, 23).

## SWARMING MOTILITY

The association between swarming and the development of filamentous cells was recognized in the earliest investigations of the phenomenon (131), but the factors responsible for inducing morphogenesis and the mechanisms involved are still largely a mystery. The investigations of Kvittingen (83, 84) were among the first to specifically address swarmer cell formation, and he concluded that swarmers represented a stage in the normal life cycle of *P. mirabilis*. His conclusion was based partially on the observation of filamentous cells in young broth cultures. On the basis of microscopic observations of living and stained cells, he maintained that only a small fraction of the swarmer cell population remains viable, and he speculated that this fraction is composed of gametes derived from short cells following nuclear reduction or meiosis (84). Subsequent attempts to demonstrate genetic exchange between swarming strains of *P. mirabilis* were not conclusive (85).

Possibly the most influential work on swarming has been that of Lominski and Lendrum (89), which was reported in 1947 (shortly before Kvittingen's first paper). They proposed that swarming of *P. mirabilis* is a negative chemotactic response to toxic metabolites that have accumulated in areas of high population density on a solid medium. Their hypothesis applied specifically to the outward migration of swarmer cells from a central inoculum; this particular aspect is discussed in greater detail below. They implied, however, that the toxic metabolites that act as repellents to the swarmers also influence their development, and this concept has persisted in the literature (39). It was suggested that swarmer cell formation is caused by a volatile metabolite similar in its mechanism to penicillin, but no specific compound has been isolated or identified (75). That certain *Proteus* species produce characteristic volatile amines (110) and specific growth-inhibiting metabolites (58) was reported, and although certain properties of these compounds are similar to those of the swarmer cell-inducing metabolites proposed by Lominski and Lendrum (89), they have not been shown to induce swarmer cell formation.

An extracellular slime postulated to facilitate migration (51, 117) appears to be associated with swarmer cells. The existence of slime was postulated after tracks with a different refractive index were observed on the agar surface behind migrating edge cells (51). Slime has since been visualized in fixed impression smears of the swarm edge by phase-contrast light microscopy and on agar surfaces and converging swarming cells by scanning and transmission electron microscopy. The slime appears to blanket rafts of swarm cells rather than to envelop individual cells, and it appears to persist on the agar surface behind the moving rafts (117, 121). Because of its ruthenium red staining properties, slime is thought to consist of an acidic polysaccharide (117) and a large amount of water (51, 117). Whether slime is absolutely essential for swarming has not been established, but recent evidence from mutants defective in capsular polysaccharide production suggests that it may play an important role in the migration of the swarming colony (73).

## DETERMINANTS OF SWARMING

The advent of the techniques of modern molecular biology has renewed interest in understanding *P. mirabilis* swarmer cell differentiation as it affects the invasiveness and pathogenicity of this organism. Tn5 transposon mutagenesis has been used as a means of constructing mutations in the swarmer cell genes (23, 24, 40). A similar methodology, Tn*phoA* mutagenesis, has been employed in other laboratories (6). We found that Tn5 transposition is random and that once it is integrated into the *P. mirabilis* chromosome, the transposon is stably maintained (24). Characterization of the subsequent swarming-defective mutants (Swr$^-$) revealed several phenotypic classes, including mutants that are defective in (i) swimming motility (Swm$^-$, including defects in flagellin synthesis [Fla$^-$], motor rotation [Mot$^-$], and chemotaxis [Che$^-$]), (ii) swarmer cell elongation (both null mutants [Elo$^-$] and constitutively elongated cells [Elo$^c$]), and (iii) a large group of mutants with an impairment in swarming (Swr$^{cr}$), caused by an unknown defect (23). Although this last group does manifest non-wild-type swarming motility, many of these mutants were altered in their abilities to form discrete consolidation zones. It has been speculated that these mutants arose from transposon insertions in genes coding for production of extracellular signal molecules or the receptors of those signals (20). Localization of the various Tn*phoA* insertions on the chromosomes of swarming mutants by pulse gel electrophoresis revealed that the genes necessary for swarmer cell differentiation and swarming behavior occur on closely linked genetic loci (6).

The genetic lesions that result in the various mutant phenotypes are now being characterized, and the defective genes are being analyzed for regulation and expression during swarmer cell differentiation and multicellular motility and behavior.

The results of these studies are presented in the next section.

## Differentiation to Swarmer Cells

Swarmer cell differentiation and the swarming motility of P. mirabilis are the results of at least four separate phenomena, including (i) the ability to sense cues from the environment, (ii) the production of an elongated swarmer cell, (iii) the synthesis of vastly increased amounts of flagellin (a hallmark of the differentiated swarmer cell), and (iv) the coordinated multicellular interactions that result in cyclic waves of cellular differentiation and dedifferentiation (20). A defect in any of these events results in either abnormal swarming behavior or a complete lack of differentiation and/or motility. The next section deals with the genetic aspects of the first three phenomena. The section "Multicellular Migration" focuses on what is known concerning the fourth aspect of swarming.

## The Surface Signal

### FLAGELLAR ROTATIONAL TETHERING

Studies measuring gene expression in P. mirabilis and other swarming bacteria, e.g., Serratia marcescens and Vibrio parahaemolyticus, convincingly demonstrated that the central environmental stimulus sensed by the cell is physical (2, 7, 26, 27, 95). Swarmer cell genes are induced when swimmer cells are transferred to the surface of solidified medium, suspended in a medium of high viscosity, or agglutinated with antibody to the cell surface. Growth in media amended with polymers such as Ficoll 400 or polyvinylpyrrolidone 360 is as effective at inducing swarmer gene expression as growth on an agar surface (2, 7, 26, 27, 95). These branched polymers increase the microviscosity of the medium, thus creating a matrix that interferes with the normal movement of swimming bacteria. An even more effective inducing condition is the addition of antiflagellar antibody (not preimmune serum) to the growth medium, which results in cell tethering and agglutination (95). McCarter et al. employed an antibody raised against the cell surface of V. parahaemolyticus that recognized primarily the polar flagellum sheath (95). Agglutination with this antibody produced abnormal expression of swarmer cell differentiation in V. parahaemolyticus. Similar results were obtained with P. mirabilis and antisera directed against the flagellar filament (21, 22). What these conditions have in common is that they inhibit the normal rotation of the flagellar filament(s). This observation led to the hypothesis that the flagella function as tactile sensors of external conditions and directly transfer the information they gather into the cell, where the signal is transduced to transcriptionally control the expression of the genes associated with swarmer cell differentiation.

Genetic techniques have strengthened the hypothesis that the rotation of the flagellar filament is the main factor controlling expression of swarmer cell differentiation. Swimmer cells and swarmer cells of P. mirabilis produce the same flagellin protein encoded by the same gene. Belas and Flaherty examined 11 strains and showed that there are three copies of flagellin-encoding genes in P. mirabilis (21, 25). Only one of these flagellin-encoding genes, flaA, is expressed in wild-type cells, either in the swimmer or the swarmer cell phase (25). Mutations that disrupt the function of flaA result in abnormal expression of swarmer cells, thus demonstrating the central role of the flagellar filament in signal transduction (25). In addition, defects in other essential flagellar genes of P. mirabilis result in abnormal swarmer cell differentiation (see below).

### GLUTAMINE

Although chemotaxis is now considered essential for swarmer cell differentiation and motility in all of the swarming bacteria thus far studied, only in P. mirabilis has a very specific interaction linking the amino acid glutamine and swarmer cell differentiation been described (7). By supplementing minimal agar medium insufficient to support swarming migration, Allison et al. identified a single amino acid, glutamine, as sufficient to signal initiation of cell differentiation and migration (7). In contrast, addition of the other 19 common amino acids (excluding glutamine) individually or in combination does not initiate differentiation even after prolonged incubation. In liquid minimal media amended with polyvinylpyrrolidone to increase viscosity and inhibit flagellar rotation (as described above), addition of glutamine also induces swarmer cell differentiation. Furthermore, the induction can be completely inhibited by glutamine analogs, a fact indicating the specificity of the glutamine signal in swarmer cell differentiation. Interestingly, glutamine is chemotactic only for the differentiated swarmer cell and not the swimmer cell (7). These data suggest that glutamine functions in a dual role, both initiating differentiation and directing the migration of swarming cells.

This study indicates that *P. mirabilis* swarmer cells are chemotactic but respond to a more limited range of attractants than swimmer cells do. Moreover, the discovery that amino acid chemoattractants are mutually exclusive for either swimming (e.g., glutamate) or swarming (glutamine) cells may indicate the presence of separate sensory components coupled with the two forms of motility. These results are very tantalizing and suggest that a combination of signals, including inhibition of flagellar rotation and the presence of glutamine, are necessary for the induction of *P. mirabilis* swarmer cell differentiation.

## Genes and Proteins Involved in Differentiation

### FLAGELLAR GENES

***flaA* Locus of *P. mirabilis*.** As described in the first section above, during differentiation from swimmer to swarmer cell, the rates of synthesis of certain proteins undergo dramatic increases. The most evident of these overproduced proteins is flagellin (FlaA, the subunit of the flagellar filament). Although swimmer cells have only a few flagella, the elongated swarmer cells are profusely covered by thousands of newly synthesized flagella (68). In many ways, the increase in flagellin expression is the hallmark of the differentiated swarmer cell, as has been shown not just for *P. mirabilis* but also for *S. marcescens* (2, 107) and *V. parahaemolyticus* (27, 95, 96).

Biochemical studies of flagella isolated from *P. mirabilis* swimmer and swarmer cells (17, 23) along with genetic data from Tn5 mutageneses (23, 24) suggest that *P. mirabilis* synthesizes only a single flagellin species. Recently, Belas and Flaherty reported on the cloning of a region of *P. mirabilis* chromosomal DNA capable of complementing *E. coli* FliC⁻ mutants (25). Nucleotide and deduced amino acid sequence analyses revealed that this region contains three open reading frames (ORFs) that were identified on the basis of their homology to other known flagellar genes. The region includes the 5' end of a putative homolog of *E. coli fliD* (an essential flagellar gene responsible for filament assembly) and two nearly identical flagellin-encoding genes called *flaA* and *flaB*. A third possible flagellin-encoding gene, referred to as *flaC*, was also found in this study by DNA-DNA homology. *flaA* encodes a protein that complements *E. coli* FliC⁻ mutants, but *flaB* fails to complement any *E. coli* defects (25). Moreover, *flaB* encodes a protein that is larger than was predicted from its deduced amino acid sequence when the gene was used in *E. coli* minicell protein-labeling experiments. These data suggest that although *flaA* is functional in *E. coli*, *flaB* is not.

The discovery of multiple flagellin genes in *P. mirabilis* (25) raises provocative questions concerning their regulation and function in association with swarmer cell differentiation. These issues gain further significance because the overproduction of flagella during swarmer cell differentiation is considered an important prerequisite for colonization and invasion by and the ultimate pathogenicity of this organism (3, 8). Many bacterial species possess multiple copies of flagellin genes. For example, *Salmonella typhimurium fliC* and *fliB* (111, 120, 132) and *Campylobacter coli flaA* and *flaB* (9, 59, 60) each encode two separate flagellin species that play a role in antigenic variation of the flagellum. Since flagella and specifically flagellin (H antigen) are extremely antigenic, changes in flagellin antigenicity may provide the bacteria with an effective means of sidestepping the immune response of the host (35).

The functions of the gene products of *flaD*, *flaA*, and *flaB* were established by constructing mutations in *P. mirabilis*. Mutations in *flaA* completely abolish all motility as well as swarmer cell differentiation, while *flaB* mutations cause no demonstrable change in the wild-type phenotype. These observations emphasize the central role of FlaA flagellin in swarmer cell differentiation and behavior. Presumably, the cell responds to environmental conditions that prevent the normal rotation of the FlaA flagella (5, 20, 23). Loss of FlaA filaments results inappropriately in an undifferentiated swimmer cell under conditions that should elicit swarmer cell differentiation. This suggests that *flaA* is required for the induction of swarmer cell differentiation, because mutants defective in FlaA do not differentiate.

As indicated above, FlaA$^-$ mutants do not synthesize flagellin. This observation indicates that the third *P. mirabilis* flagellin-encoding gene, *flaC*, is not actively transcribed. Although the nucleotide sequence of *flaC* has not been determined and the transcription of this gene has not been assessed, the evidence obtained from FlaA$^-$ mutants argues that *flaC* is not transcribed in a *flaA* mutation or a wild-type cell or

that, if it is transcribed, the protein is not a functional flagellin. So, both *flaB* and *flaC* are ordinarily silent copies of flagellin-encoding genes.

Interestingly, at a low frequency, Mot$^+$ revertants were found emanating as flares from *flaA* colonies on semisolid Mot agar plates. Moreover, *flaA* Mot$^+$ revertants are capable of movement through media to which anti-FlaA polyvalent antiserum has been added (Fig. 5). This observation in and of itself suggests that the flagella synthesized by the revertants are antigenically distinct from those produced by wild-type cells. Since the antiserum used is polyvalent and is produced in response to

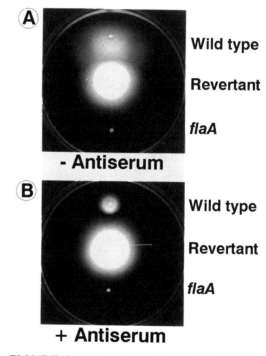

**FIGURE 5** Antigenic variation of *P. mirabilis* flagellin. Swimming motility of the wild type, a *flaA* Mot$^+$ revertant, and the parent *flaA* strain is shown after 24 h of incubation at 37°C in semisolid Mot agar (A) or in Mot agar amended with a 1:500 dilution of anti-FlaA antiserum (B). The swimming zone of the wild type is severely affected by the addition of the anti-FlaA antiserum, but the motility of the *flaA* Mot$^+$ revertant is unaffected.

whole flagella rather than denatured flagellin (23), it may be expected to contain antibodies capable of binding to many different flagellin epitopes. During such binding, bacteria may be tethered together flagellum to flagellum and thus be prevented from achieving wild-type swimming or swarming motility. This is exactly what happens when anti-FlaA is added to cultures of wild-type *P. mirabilis* (Fig. 5A): the bacteria become tethered by flagellum-to-flagellum binding (22). In contrast, *flaA* Mot$^+$ revertants are only loosely bound when the same antiserum is applied to cell suspensions, which indicates that *flaA* Mot$^+$ revertants synthesize flagella containing only a subset of possible FlaA epitopes (Fig. 5B).

Analyses of Southern blots of *flaA* Mot$^+$ revertants reveal that a large deletion of variable size within the *flaAB* locus apparently causes the reversion from Mot$^-$ to Mot$^+$. For example, for one such Mot$^+$ revertant, the deletion removes over 50% of *flaA* and all of *flaB*. This observation suggests that the reversion process is a one-way event in which a deletion permanently removes a portion of DNA downstream from *flaA* and reaching into *flaB* and even further, into genes downstream from *flaB*. Thus, the mutation may result in a hybrid gene fusion in which the 5' end of *flaA* is fused to the 3' end of *flaC* to yield a functional flagellin.

The evidence gathered from sodium dodecyl sulfate-polyacrylamide gel electrophoresis immunoblotting of V8 protease-digested flagellin, N-terminal amino acid sequencing, and amino acid composition analyses strongly suggests that FlaA and the revertant flagellin have identical N-terminal ends but different C termini. The hypothetical model used to explain the events producing the revertant flagellin predicts that any splice between the 5' end of *flaA* and either *flaB* or *flaC* that produces a functional flagellum will result in a motile revertant phenotype. According to this model, the splice site joining FlaA with FlaC is probably located at or near *flaA*.

Spontaneous mutations giving rise to an antigenically distinct flagellin would be equally as likely to occur in vitro as in vivo and may very well occur in FlaA$^+$ cells, as they occur in Mot$^-$ cells. Such antigenic changes would increase the survivability of a urinary pathogen. For example, urinary pathogens are confronted by secretory immunoglobulin A (IgA) as the bacteria attempt to colonize the bladder. Since flagellin is strongly antigenic, a major binding epitope for the immunoglobulins could be the flagellum. Tethering of the bacteria via their flagella would effectively prevent their motility and impose the same selective pressures in this case as occur in vitro. A spontaneous deletion that gave rise to an antigenically distinct flagellum would thus provide the bacterium with an avenue of escape from immobilization by the immunoglobulins. This would be a successful survival strategy prolonging the chances of colonization by the bacteria.

**Other Flagellar Genes.** As indicated in an earlier section of this chapter, inhibition of flagellar rotation is known to cause induction of swarmer cell differentiation (27, 95). It is therefore not surprising to find that mutations in flagellar genes (other than *flaA*) result in abnormal swarmer cell differentiation. For example, Belas et al. characterized the Tn5 insertion sites in *P. mirabilis* mutants defective in swarmer cell elongation (26). Most of the mutations characterized in their study were in genes associated with flagellar biosynthesis. As shown in Table 3, Tn5 insertions were identified in (i) *fliL* (the homolog of which in *Caulobacter crescentus* is required for flagellar gene expression and normal cell division [118]), (ii) *fliG* (a component of the flagellar switch), and (iii) *flgH* (encoding

**TABLE 3** Genetic loci associated with P. mirabilis swarming differentiation, motility, and behavior

| Genetic locus or gene | Type of mutation | Mutant phenotype | Reference(s) |
|---|---|---|---|
| flaA | Allelic exchange | Swm$^-$ Swr$^-$ Elo$^-$ | 21, 25 |
| flaB | Allelic exchange | Wild type | 21, 25 |
| flaD | Allelic exchange | Swm$^-$ Swr$^-$ Elo$^-$ | 21, 25 |
| flhA | Tn5 insertion | Swm$^-$ Swr$^-$ Elo$^-$ | 61 |
| fliG | Tn5 insertion | Swm$^+$ Swr$^{cr}$ Elo$^-$ | 26 |
| fliL | Tn5 insertion | Swm$^+$ Swr$^{cr}$ Elo$^c$ | 26 |
| flgH | Tn5 insertion | Swm$^+$ Swr$^{cr}$ Elo$^c$ | 26 |
| gidA | Tn5 insertion | Swm$^+$ Swr$^{cr}$ Elo$^-$ | 26 |
| cld locus | Tn5 insertion | Swm$^+$ Swr$^{cr}$ Elo$^-$ | 26 |
| rfaCD | Tn5 insertion | Swm$^+$ Swr$^{cr}$ Elo$^-$ | 26 |
| galU | Tn5 insertion | Swm$^+$ Swr$^{cr}$ Elo$^-$ | 26 |
| dapE | Tn5 insertion | Swm$^+$ Swr$^{cr}$ Elo$^-$ | 26 |
| cpsF | Tn5 insertion | Swm$^+$ Swr$^{cr}$ | 73 |
| pepQ | Tn5 insertion | Swm$^+$ Swr$^{cr}$ Elo$^-$ | 26 |
| Urease locus | Northern (RNA) blot | NA$^a$ | 8 |
| Hemolysin locus | Northern (RNA) blot | NA | 8 |

$^a$ NA, not applicable.

the basal-body L ring) and were shown to play a significant role in swarmer cell elongation (26). This suggests that subtle effects on the flagellar motor may cause major perturbations in swarming behavior.

Similarly, Gygi et al. analyzed P. mirabilis mutants defective in flhA (61). FlhA is necessary for flagellar biosynthesis (93) and is a member of a newly identified family of putative signal-transducing receptors that have been implicated in diverse cellular processes (36). Other members of this family include LcrD of Yersinia pestis and Yersinia enterocolitica, FlbF of Caulobacter crescentus, FlhA of Bacillus subtilis and E. coli, MxiA and VirH of Shigella flexneri, InvA of S. typhimurium, HrpC2 of Xanthomonas campestris, and Hrp of phytopathogenic bacteria (36, 47, 52, 67, 87, 98, 124, 129).

Like flaA, flaB, and flaD, P. mirabilis flhA possesses a flagellar-gene-specific $\sigma^{28}$ promoter (61). Mutations affecting the function of FlhA result in a lack of flagellar synthesis and an abnormal expression of swarmer cell differentiation (61). Thus, in general, mutations that prevent the normal function or regulation of flagellar expression in P. mirabilis result in the abnormal expression of swarmer cells and point to the central role of flagellar function and filament rotation in maintaining proper sensing of environmental stimuli during swarmer cell differentiation and motile behavior.

## LPS AND CAPSULAR POLYSACCHARIDE GENES

Another class of genes important in swarmer cell diffentiation and swarming behavior is involved in the synthesis of LPS (O antigen) and capsular polysaccharide. Belas et al. found that the transposon insertion point of some Tn5-generated mutants defective in wild-type swarmer cell elongation is located in an ORF homologous to the hypothetical 43.3-kDa protein in the E. coli locus that is responsible for the LPS chain length determinant (26). As described above, LPS chain length is though to be important in swarmer cell function (11, 13, 15). The cld locus confers a modal distribution of chain length on the O-antigen component of LPS (19). This protein is thought to have a dehydrogenase activity, as indicated by its homology to UDP-glucose dehydrogenase from Streptococcus pyogenes and Streptococcus pneumoniae, which was confirmed in the *P. mirabilis* homolog by amino acid sequence comparison of the deduced amino acid sequence (26). Since *cld* is composed of several ORFs, it is possible that such Tn5 insertion mutants of *P. mirabilis* are defective in maintaining the preferred O-antigen chain length. Alternatively, the mutation may be in the *rfb* gene cluster (O antigen), which is closely linked to *cld* in *E. coli* and *S. typhimurium* (19).

In a second *P. mirabilis* mutant, also phenotypically Elo$^-$, a mutation had occurred in *rfaD*, which encodes ADP-L-glycero-D-mannoheptose-6-epimerase (26). In *E. coli* and *S. typhimurium*, this mutation results in altered heptose (L-glycero-D-mannoheptose) and LPS biosynthesis and increased outer membrane permeability (108). The nucleotide sequence at the distal end of the cloned insert was determined to be highly homologous to *rfaC*, which encodes heptosyltransferase I (116). In *S. typhimurium*, this mutation leads to heptoseless LPS and rough-colony phenotype (37, 116). In other bacteria, such rough mutants have been associated with defects in motility, which may explain the Mot$^-$ phenotype of this particular mutant. *rfaC* is genetically linked to *rfaD*, a fact that supports the finding that the mutation is in *rfaD* and suggests that the defect affects LPS structure and outer membrane permeability.

Interestingly, all of these mutations appear to affect swarmer cell elongation by preventing normal synthesis and rotation of the flagella. However, while swarming motility is affected by these mutations, swimming is not. Moreover, impairment of the flagella should result in the induction of transcription of the swarmer cell regulon, although each of these mutants in Elo$^-$. Thus, there may be a close connection between LPS synthesis and regulation, signal transduction, and swarmer cell regulation in *P. mirabilis*, as has been shown by others (11, 13, 15).

Bacteria often produce extracellular polysaccharides (capsules and slime) that aid cells in their adhesion to substrates. Many swarming colonies produce a clear extracellular fluid and often have a glistening, mucoid appearance. In *P. mirabilis*, this material consists of a polysaccharide matrix (5), but its composition in other bacteria has not been determined, nor have defects in swarming been correlated with specific defects in slime production. For example, *Serratia marcescens* excretes a surfactant (94) that is not essential for swarming (63, 64).

Recently, Gygi et al. cloned and determined the nucleotide and deduced amino acid sequences for a genetic locus of *P. mirabilis* responsible for production of a capsular polysaccharide that is thought to be important in swarming motility (62). This region has strong homology to the *Streptococcus pneumoniae* type 19F capsular polysaccharide biosynthesis genes, particularly *cpsF*. The relevance and relationship of capsular polysaccharide biosynthesis swarming migration may now be assessed, because *cpsF* mutations have been constructed in *P. mirabilis* and the swarming characteristics of the mutants have been assessed. (Some preliminary results are described below in "Multicellular Migration.")

## PEPTIDOGLYCAN AND CELL DIVISION GENES

As part of an analysis of the defects responsible for abnormal swarmer cell elongation, Belas et al. identified several mutations in genes required for cell wall peptidoglycan biosynthesis, cell division, and chromosome replication (26). Two of the mutations identified were in *galU*, which affects glucose-1-phosphate uridylyltransferase and cell wall synthesis (77, 88, 103, 123), and in a gene homologous to *dapE* (33). The *dapE*-homologous gene encodes N-succinyl-L-diaminopimelic acid desuccinylase, an enzyme that catalyzes the synthesis of LL-diaminopimelic acid, one of the last steps in the diaminopimelic acid-lysine pathway that leads to the development of peptidoglycan (33). That mutations in cell wall biosynthesis genes produce abnormal swarmer cell elongation is not unusual, because defects in such genes can have overall effects on the ability of the cell to function.

One of the more interesting mutations that produces the Elo$^-$ Mot$^-$ Swr$^{cr}$ phenotype is in *gidA* (glucose-inhibited division), a nonessential gene in *E. coli* that is very near *E. coli oriC* (26, 106, 127). The homology between *P. mirabilis* GidA and its *E. coli* homolog is one of the strongest observed (26). In *E. coli, gidA* mutations are silent on complex media; however, when grown on glucose-containing media, *E. coli gidA* strains produce long filamentous cells (125–127). Furthermore, there is evidence that *gidA* transcription is regulated by ppGpp and is involved in initiation of chromosomal replication (16, 106). Thus, *gidA* may function to connect glucose metabolism, ribosome function, chromosome replication, and cell division (115). The function of *gidA* in swarmer cell differentiation and elongation is obscure but evidently essential for swarmer cell elongation and wild-type swarming behavior.

## SIGMA FACTORS AND OTHER UPSTREAM REGULATORY SEQUENCES

Nucleotide sequence analysis of cloned swarmer cell differentiation genes from *P. mirabilis* (and other swarming bacteria) has been ongoing for several years. As part of these analyses, regulatory regions of each gene have been scrutinized for evidence of unique regulatory mechanisms that control swarmer cell differentiation and behavior. Although it is too early to draw conclusions from these analyses, two aspects of the upstream regulatory regions of swarmer cell differentiation genes associated with flagellar synthesis can be discussed.

The upstream regulatory regions of many flagellar genes from *B. subtilis* (99), *E. coli* (18), and *S. typhimurium* (65) have a unique promoter region for a flagellar-gene-specific RNA polymerase. An alternate $\sigma$ subunit of RNA polymerase, referred to as $\sigma^{28}$ ($\sigma^F$) in *E. coli* and $\sigma^D$ in *B. subtilis*, is responsible for this specificity (65). Thus, it is perhaps not unexpected that the upstream region in front of the start codon to the *P. mirabilis flaA, flaB,* and *flaD* genes (25) and the *flhA* gene (61) also contains a nucleotide sequence that is very similar (if not identical) to the consensus $\sigma^{28}$ promoter, 5'-TAAA-N$_{15}$-GCCGATAA-3', of *E. coli*. The homology between the *P. mirabilis* sequences and the consensus sequence is very good, with the $\sigma^{28}$ promoter for *flaA* a direct match to the *E. coli* consensus sequence. The $\sigma^{28}$ promoter of *flaD* has a single mismatch with the consensus sequence, and the *flaB* promoter has two mismatches. This suggests that these genes (and probably most of the flagellar genes of *P. mirabilis*) are regulated in a manner similar to that demonstrated in *E. coli*.

What, then, is different about *P. mirabilis* flagellar-gene regulation that might help explain surface-inducible flagellin synthesis in the swarmer cell? The single most notable difference between the *E. coli fliC* regulatory region and those of *flaA* and *flaB* is the presence of a dual, direct tandem repeat (DTR) sequence 5' to the *P. mirabilis* $\sigma^{28}$ promoters (21, 25). This sequence, ATAAAAA repeated twice, is ca. 90 bp upstream from the midpoint of the −35 region of each $\sigma^{28}$ promoter. The *flaA* DTR sequence is 5'-ATAAAAATAATA-TAAAAAAATAA-3' and has two overlapping direct repeats, ATAAAAA and ATAAAAATAA. The *flaB* DTR sequence is on the strand opposite to the *flaA* DTR and has the nucleotide sequence 3'-AT-AAAAAAAGAGAGGTAGATAAAAA-

CAAAAAAGA-5'. The *flaB* DTR has two direct repeats as well. The first of these repeats is identical to that of *flaA*, ATAAAAA, while the second, AAAA-AAGA, does not share sequence identity with the *flaA* DTR. Searches of GenBank bacterial nucleotide sequences failed to find similar sequences in front of any other flagellar gene, but a homologous sequence is found in the upstream regulatory region of *ureR*, the regulatory gene for urease expression (105). Urease and flagellin are coordinately regulated as part of swarmer cell differentiation (8). Although the function of the DTR sequences is currently unknown, it is tempting to speculate, because of sequence conservation and placement, that these sequence have a function in swarmer cell-specific gene expression, perhaps as surface-induced enhancers of transcription (43, 54–56, 82).

## Multicellular Migration

### CONTROL OF SWARMER CELL BEHAVIOR: MIGRATION CYCLE AS A MODEL OF EXTRACELLULAR SIGNALS

In contrast to recent advances at the genetic level in characterizing the genes required for swarmer cell differentiation, little is known or understood about the molecular mechanisms that control swarmer cell motile behavior and, more important, the cyclic events of differentiation, migration, dedifferentiation, and consolidation. Mutant phenotypes produced by transposon-insertion mutagenesis implicate a series of multicellular signaling events that presumably regulate the cyclic nature of consolidation in these bacteria, although characterization of these loci has thus far been limited. Although the role of signals (if they exist at all) is yet to be proven, in the following section I provide a brief synopsis of the data and a possible model to explain the observations. I stress that such a model is merely speculative but hope it will point toward experiments designed to answer questions regarding multicellular swarming migration.

One of the most astonishing observations to emerge from efforts to understand the regulation of swarmer cell differentiation and multicellular swarming behavior in *P. mirabilis* is that many of the mutants defective in wild-type swarming are not null mutants; i.e., they are not mutants completely lacking the ability to swarm on an agar surface (Fig. 6A). Rather, many of the mutants are wild type for the ability to differentiate into swarmer cells and rotate the flagellar filaments in a normal manner (5, 6, 23). What makes these strains interesting appears to be defects in one or more of the genes that regulate the multicellular interactions associated with the formation of the characteristic bull's-eye colony (Fig. 6B to D). Such mutants, which have been referred to in my laboratory as swarming crippled mutants (Swr$^{cr}$), have also been constructed in other laboratories (5, 6). Swr$^{cr}$ mutants do indeed possess the ability to differentiate and swarm on the appropriate surfaces, yet they are defective in orchestrating the proper series of steps required to form distinct, periodic consolidation zones (Fig. 6). The category of crippled mutants is, by its nature, broadly defined and somewhat pleiotropic. Individual strains within the Swr$^{cr}$ group possess a wide variety of mutant phenotypes, with the central theme being a defect in the ability to form evenly spaced or well-defined consolidation zones. As shown in Fig. 6, when compared to a swarming null mutant (Fig. 6A), Swr$^{cr}$ strains fall into phenotypic classes that produce either (i) nonuniform consolidation zones (Fig. 6B), (ii) spatially narrow or broad zones (Fig. 6C), or (iii) indeterminate consolidation zones (Fig. 6D). The first two phenotypic classes (nonuniform and narrow- or broad-spacing strains) appear to have defects in the spatial or temporal control of the multicellular signaling presumed to control the

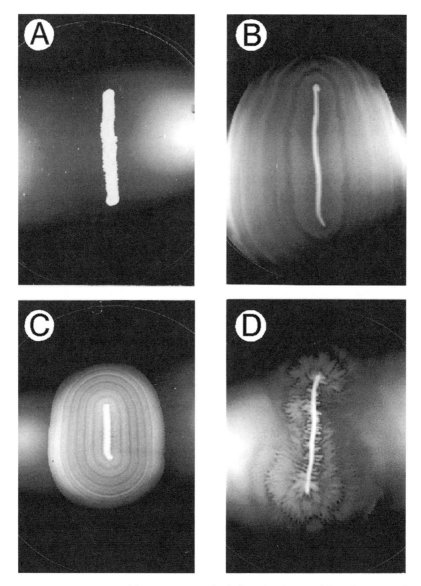

**FIGURE 6** *P. mirabilis* mutants with defects in the spatial and temporal control of swarming behavior. Bacteria were inoculated as a 3-cm line at the center of fresh L-agar medium and incubated for 48 h at 30°C. (A) Swarming null mutant (Swr$^-$ Swm$^-$ Elo$^-$); (B) swarming mutant with infrequent and variable consolidation (Swr$^{cr}$ Swm$^+$ Elo$^+$); (C) swarming mutant with increased consolidation frequency (Swr$^{cr}$ Swm$^+$ Elo$^+$); (D) swarming mutant lacking clearly defined consolidation, referred to as an indeterminate swarming mutant (Swr$^{cr}$ Swm$^+$ Elo$^+$).

sequence of events of dedifferentiation that give rise to the consolidation phase of swarming. It may be that in such mutants, the putative signals either are generated more rapidly than in wild type, giving rise to faster consolidation and narrower zones, or are synthesized slowly, resulting in broad zones that are due to a slower consolidation process. The last class of Swr$^{cr}$ mutants appears to be completely lacking in the signals or, more likely, in the receptors for the signals that control consolidation.

Armed with these observations, I described (20) a hypothetical scenario that may help us understand the unusual Swr$^{cr}$ mutants that produce uneven spacing in consolidation zones and from which we may extrapolate to the nature of the genetic defects in indeterminate mutant strains. Such a model assumes the presence of a set of extracellular signals (in this particular case, three signals, though the number was arbitrarily set). Each signal is assumed to be generated by the swarming colony, increases to a peak level, and then diminishes, perhaps because it is broken down by enzymes or other catalytic processes. As developed, the model requires that each of the three signals be produced, crest, and then diminish simultaneously with the other signals; hence, they are synchronous. Further, according to the model, the cells, which can sense the amplitudes of the signals, would regulate the differentiation cycle as a response to the sum of all of the incoming signals. These cycles of differentiation and dedifferentiation would therefore be regulated in reference to some maximum and minimum value of the sum of the signals, with differentiation commencing at high signal intensity and dedifferentiation occurring at a low signal intensity. Theoretically, such changes could be produced by regulatory mutations that affect the rate of production or destruction of one or more of the signal molecules. The threshold signal level for consolidation would thus become arhythmic. The net outcome would produce a combination of narrow and broad zones, as seen in Fig. 6B. The predictions of this model then make it feasible to consider the indeterminate consolidation class of mutants (Fig. 6A and 6B) as lacking all signals or as possessing a central defect, such as a mutations in the receptor for these signal molecules.

It is evident that the models do simulate some of the swarming patterns observed in *P. mirabilis*. It goes without saying that the use of such models is very limited and that interpretation of such depictions of signal intensity may not mirror the real world. Many different possible explanations can fit the data presented. Nonetheless, modeling does serve as a way of focusing ideas for developing experimental approaches and understandings on the nature of defective Swr$^{cr}$ mutants.

## GENES AND MUTANT PHENOTYPES

Several of the genes described in the first section of this chapter are also needed for wild-type multicellular migration; i.e., defects that affect flagellar biosynthesis and result in the failure of the cell to synthesize flagella are nonmotile and cannot participate in migration events. However, some of the genes associated with cellular differentiation play slightly different roles in migration. Those differences, along with descriptions of some genes thought to be solely involved in multicellular migration, are examined in the next section.

**Capsular Polysaccharide and Surface Migration.** *P. mirabilis* swarmer cells secrete substantial amounts of a viscous biofilm that defines the leading edge of the migrating population. This substance consists of a thus far uncharacterized carbohydrate that is assumed to assist migration, possibly by acting as a surfactant (117). Recently, a mutation that causes frequent consolidation was characterized, and the defect was located in a gene, *cpsF*, involved in the synthesis of a major new capsular polysaccharide, referred to as CPS I (73). The mutant fails to polymerize CPS I, and precursors accumulate intracellularly. However, a second, minor capsular polysaccharide (CPS II) still gets produced and forms a thin capsule on the cell surface. Detailed analysis of the swarming cycle shows that CPS I$^-$ cells differentiate faster than wild type. CPS I$^-$ mutants do not have changes in the temporal control of consolidation pattern formation but instead are affected by a reduction in the motility of the cells; i.e., the spatial placement of the rings is shortened. These data suggest that CPS I is important in reducing friction and acts as a surfactant, perhaps performing a function similar to that of serrawettin, a surfactant of *Serratia marcescens* (94).

## The Glutamine Signal: Possible Roles for a Metalloprotease and a Proline Peptidase?

*P. mirabilis* strains of diverse types produce an extracellular, EDTA-sensitive metalloprotease that is able to cleave serum and secretory IgA1 and IgA2, IgG, and a number of nonimmunological proteins such as gelatin and casein (90–92, 112, 114). The protease activity on IgA is such that the heavy chain of the immunoglobulin is cleaved, a result different from that of classic microbial IgA protease activity (109). An enzyme with the ability to cleave immunoglobulin molecules has the potential to be a virulence factor and, indeed, is frequently found in the urine of patients with *P. mirabilis* urinary infections (112).

Researchers in my laboratory recently cloned into *E. coli* a *P. mirabilis* genetic locus that confers on the recombinant bacterium all of the properties associated with the metalloprotease in wild-type *Proteus* cells (128). Genetic analysis using Tn5 mutagenesis of *P. mirabilis* DNA indicates that a region of approximately 4.5 kb is required for expression of the metalloprotease in *E. coli*. Nucleotide primers to IS50L and IS50R regions of the transposon are being used in analyses of nucleotide and deduced amino acid sequences. Thus far, these analyses have revealed the presence of an operon with three ORFs within the 4.5-kb region. The genes associated with the ORFs correspond to a zinc metalloprotease and two ATP-dependent membrane transport proteins required for the secretion of the metalloprotease to the external milieu.

It is quite likely that this enzyme functions as a virulence factor during UTI. Allison et al. demonstrated that the activity of the metalloprotease is coordinately expressed with cycles of swarmer cell differentiation (3, 4, 8). But does this metalloprotease have any other function? One role it may play is to actually generate the glutamine signal shown to be required for swarmer cell differentiation and migation (7). If it does so, then understanding it represents a significant advance in our understanding of multicellular migration and swarming behavior. Experiments to measure the transcriptional control of this gene and to assess its role in migration are in progress.

One of the Elo$^-$ strains that my laboratory recently examined (26) is the result of a mutation in the *P. mirabilis* homolog to *pepQ*. This gene encodes X-proline dipeptidase (104) and shows strong identity to other proline dipeptidases. What makes this PepQ$^-$ mutant interesting is that in addition to being defective in swarmer cell elongation (Elo$^-$), the mutant produces abnormal consolidation patterns similar to that shown in Fig. 6B. One possible interpretation of these data is that the mutation in *pepQ* functions to generate the signal by cleaving larger polypeptides into transportable peptides. PepQ$^-$ defects may prevent normal uptake of these important signal molecules used by *P. mirabilis* to control swarming behavior and consolidation (20). The interaction (if any) between the metalloprotease and PepQ may be significant in the multicellular signaling that occurs during the cyclic events of consolidation in *P. mirabilis* swarming colonies.

## *P. MIRABILIS* SWARMER CELL DIFFERENTIATION AND UROPATHOGENICITY

*P. mirabilis* expresses virulence factors (see chapter 9 in this book) that are distinct from those described for *E. coli*, the most common uropathogen. Swarmer cell differentiation and behavior may be essential for invasion and infection of host cells. Allison et al. showed that differentiation is coupled to the ability of *P. mirabilis* to invade uroepithelial cells in vitro (4). Invasion is reduced but not entirely eliminated in mutants defective in wild-type swarming. On the other hand, in a study that examined the internalization of *P. mirabilis* by primary cultures of human renal epithelial cells, the swimmer cell of *P. mirabilis* was internalized within membrane-bound vacuoles and did not undergo significant replication (38). Indeed, when active swarmer cells were added to cultured renal cells, the swarmer cells rapidly reverted to swimmer cells and were internalized in that form. Thus, whether swarmer or swimmer cells (or both types) are internalized remains an unresolved issue. In vivo studies using mouse models of uropathogenicity nevertheless demonstrated that mortality rates are reduced when mice are infected with mutants defective in swarming rather than wild-type cells (4).

Virulence factors of *P. mirabilis* that have been shown or implied to be important in virulence are the membrane-damaging hemolysin toxin, a urease that generates ammonia from urea and thus precipitates kidney stones, a metalloprotease that degrades IgA, multiple fimbrial and flagellar adhesins, and a capsular polysaccharide. Allison et al. demonstrated that the hemolysin urease, and protease activities are induced in swarmer cells to levels about 30- to 80-fold higher than those in swimmer cells (3, 8). This increase in enzyme expression occurs in parallel with the increased expression of flagellin (as shown in Fig. 7). Substantial reductions in virulence factor activities in mutants defective in swarming confirmed the correlation between swarmer cell differentiation and virulence (3, 8). For example, Allison et al. showed that swarming-specific induction of virulence and motility is affected by coordinated differential gene expression (Fig. 7) and also that this induction is preferential and specific, not part of a general or "housekeeping" phenomenon (3, 8).

## CONCLUSIONS AND FUTURE DIRECTIONS

For most of the time during which swarming motility has been observed and studied, this form of multicellular prokaryotic behavior has been considered a curious oddity, usually more of a nuisance than a wonder, and certainly not a phenomenon with any connection to uropathogenicity. What is now becoming apparent is that swarmer cell differentiation and behavior are aspects of a complex signal transduction and genetic regulatory pathway, the mechanisms of which almost certainly have implications for the pathogenesis of *P. mirabilis* UTI. Although a model to explain swarmer cell differentiation and its function in uropathogenicity can be constructed, a number of important questions remain unanswered (Fig. 8). We know that inhibition of flagellar rotation is essential for sensing the environment and inducing the expression of swarmer cell-specific genes, but what role do the flagella play in sensing the environment in the urinary tract? Is flagellar function important in establishing infections of *P. mirabilis*? Does *P. mirabilis* display numerous antigenically

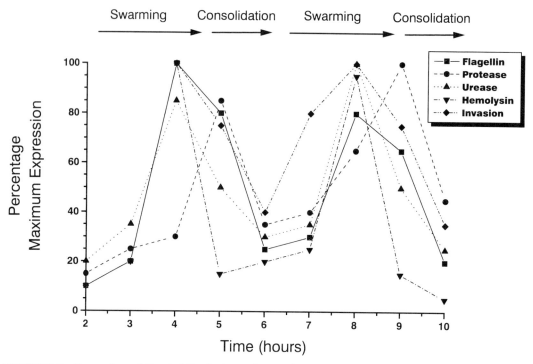

**FIGURE 7** Expression of *P. mirabilis* virulence factors during cyclic swarmer cell differentiation. The expression of flagellin, metalloprotease, urease, and hemolysin and the ability to invade tissue culture cells are shown over two cycles of differentiation and consolidation. All virulence components were regulated coordinately with swarmer cell differentiation. Adapted from reference 8.

distinct flagellins under the selective pressure of the host immune response? In addition, although we have some limited information regarding the expression and transcriptional control of swarmer cell-specific genes, e.g., *flaA* (21), most of these genes remain uncharacterized and with their means of regulation unknown. How are these genes regulated in situ during pathogenesis? Is differential expression dependent on host cell type? When and where during the infection are swarmer cell-specific genes expressed? It is intuitive that a complex series of events must occur for the periodic cycles of differentiation and dedifferentiation. Such processes must somehow link all of the cells into one global network of communication, so that each cell starts and stops the differentiation cycle at the same time. Is extracellular communication via signal molecules important during colonization and invasion, and if so, what is the mechanism? Is the IgA specificity of the metalloprotease important to *P. mirabilis* virulence, and how does the metalloprotease function in differentiation during pathogenesis? We do not have clear answers to any of these questions at present. The answers will extend our understanding of the role of the swarmer cell in pathogenesis in the urinary tract.

Several research groups are actively pursuing such answers by using detailed molecular analyses of the genes and mutants that affect multicellular swarming behavior. It is safe to say that many of the answers to the questions raised in this chapter will be found in the next several years.

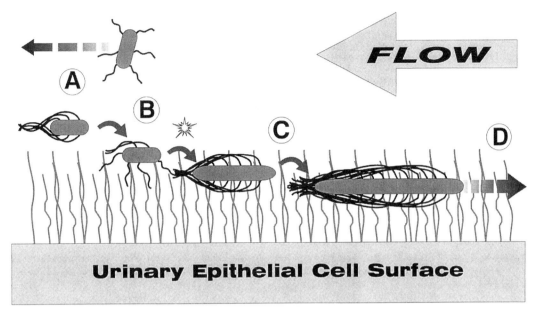

**FIGURE 8** Hypothetical model of *P. mirabilis* adaptation to life as a uropathogen. The human urinary tract imposes severe constraints on the abilities of bacterial pathogens to colonize and invade urinary tissues. Swarmer cell differentiation may be a means of overcoming some of the barriers of this hostile environment. Urine flow through the ureter and a mucous layer overlying the urinary epithelial cells prevent many motile bacteria from colonizing urinary epithelial cells (A). The highly viscous mucous layer traps many motile bacteria. If *P. mirabilis* swimmer cells are trapped in this mucus (B), their flagellar rotation is impaired, thus inducing swarmer cell differentiation (C). The swarmer cell can move through the mucus, thus overcoming a physical barrier (D). Additionally, induction of swarmer cell differentiation results in the expression of several virulence factors (urease, metalloprotease, hemolysin, etc.) that aid the bacteria in thwarting the defenses of the host and in establishing and maintaining an active infection.

What new questions those data will bring forth and what new mechanisms of signal transduction and genetic regulation will be unveiled can only be surmised. Whatever answers are found, however, are very likely to have major and profound implications on the field of bacterial pathogenicity and genetic regulation.

### ACKNOWLEDGMENTS

This work was supported by grants from the National Science Foundation (MCB-9206127) and the National Institutes of Health (AI27107).

### REFERENCES

1. **Adler, J.** 1983. Bacterial chemotaxis and molecular neurobiology. *Cold Spring Harbor Symp. Quant. Biol.* **2**:803–804.
2. **Alberti, L., and R. M. Harshey.** 1990. Differentiation of *Serratia marcescens* 274 into swimmer and swarmer cells. *J. Bacteriol.* **172**:4322–4328.
3. **Allison, C., N. Coleman, P. L. Jones, and C. Hughes.** 1992. Ability of *Proteus mirabilis* to invade human urothelial cells is coupled to motility and swarming differentiation. *Infect. Immun.* **60**:4740–4746.
4. **Allison, C., L. Emody, N. Coleman, and C. Hughes.** 1994. The role of swarm cell differentiation and multicellular migration in the uropathogenicity of *Proteus mirabilis*. *J. Infect. Dis.* **169**:1155–1158.
5. **Allison, C., and C. Hughes.** 1991. Bacterial swarming: an example of prokaryotic differentiation and multicellular behavior. *Sci. Prog.* **75**:403–422.
6. **Allison, C., and C. Hughes.** 1991. Closely linked genetic loci required for swarm cell differentiation and multicellular migration

by *Proteus mirabilis*. *Mol. Microbiol.* **5:** 1975–1982.
7. **Allison, C., H. C. Lai, D. Gygi, and C. Hughes.** 1993. Cell differentiation of *Proteus mirabilis* is initiated by glutamine, a specific chemoattractant for swarming cells. *Mol. Microbiol.* **8:**53–60.
8. **Allison, C., H. C. Lai, and C. Hughes.** 1992. Co-ordinate expression of virulence genes during swarm-cell differentiation and population migration of *Proteus mirabilis*. *Mol. Microbiol.* **6:**1583–1591.
9. **Alm, R. A., P. Guerry, M. E. Power, and T. J. Trust.** 1992. Variation in antigenicity and molecular weight of *Campylobacter coli* VC167 flagellin in different genetic backgrounds. *J. Bacteriol.* **174:**4230–4238.
10. **Armitage, J. P.** 1981. Changes in metabolic activity of *Proteus mirabilis* during swarming. *J. Gen. Microbiol.* **125:**445–450.
11. **Armitage, J. P.** 1982. Changes in the organization of the outer membrane of *Proteus mirabilis* during swarming: freeze-fracture structure and membrane fluidity analysis. *J. Bacteriol.* **150:**900–904.
12. **Armitage, J. P., R. J. Rowbury, and D. G. Smith.** 1974. The effects of chloramphenicol, nalidixic acid and penicillin on the growth and division of swarming cells of *Proteus mirabilis*. *J. Med. Microbiol.* **7:**459–464.
13. **Armitage, J. P., R. J. Rowbury, and D. G. Smith.** 1975. Indirect evidence for cell wall and membrane differences between filamentous swarming cells and short non-swarming cells of *Proteus mirabilis*. *J. Gen. Microbiol.* **89:**199–202.
14. **Armitage, J. P., and D. G. Smith.** 1978. Flagella development during swarmer differentiation in *Proteus mirabilis*. *FEMS Microbiol. Lett.* **4:**163–165.
15. **Armitage, J. P., D. G. Smith, and R. J. Rowbury.** 1979. Alterations in the cell envelope composition of *Proteus mirabilis* during the development of swarmer cells. *Biochim. Biophys. Acta.* **584:**389–397.
16. **Asai, T., M. Takanmi, and M. Imai.** 1990. The AT richness and *gid* transcription determine the left border of the replication origin of the *E. coli* chromosome. *EMBO J.* **9:**4065–4072.
17. **Bahrani, F. K., D. E. Johnson, D. Robbins, and H. L. Mobley.** 1991. *Proteus mirabilis* flagella and MR/P fimbriae: isolation, purification, N-terminal analysis, and serum antibody response following experimental urinary tract infection. *Infect. Immun.* **59:**3574–3580.
18. **Bartlett, D. H., B. B. Frantz, and P. Matsumura.** 1988. Flagellar transcriptional activators FlbB and FlaI: gene sequences and 5′ consensus sequences of operons under FlbB and FlaI control. *J. Bacteriol.* **170:**1575–1581.
19. **Bastin, D., G. Stevenson, P. Brown, A. Haase, and P. Reeves.** 1993. Repeat unit polysaccharides of bacteria: a model for polymerization resembling that of ribosomes and fatty acid synthetase, with a novel mechanism for determining chain length. *Mol. Microbiol.* **7:**725–734.
20. **Belas, R.** 1992. The swarming phenomenon of *Proteus mirabilis*. *ASM News* **58:**15–22.
21. **Belas, R.** 1994. Expression of multiple flagellin-encoding genes of *Proteus mirabilis*. *J. Bacteriol.* **176:**7169–7181.
22. **Belas, R.** 1995. Unpublished data.
23. **Belas, R., D. Erskine, and D. Flaherty.** 1991. *Proteus mirabilis* mutants defective in swarmer cell differentiation and multicellular behavior. *J. Bacteriol.* **173:**6279–6288.
24. **Belas, R., D. Erskine, and D. Flaherty.** 1991. Transposon mutagenesis in *Proteus mirabilis*. *J. Bacteriol.* **173:**6289–6293.
25. **Belas, R., and D. Flaherty.** 1994. Sequence and genetic analysis of multiple flagellin-encoding genes from *Proteus mirabilis*. *Gene* **148:**33–41.
26. **Belas, R., M. Goldman, and K. Ashliman.** 1995. Genetic analysis of *Proteus mirabilis* mutants defective in swarmer cell elongation. *J. Bacteriol.* **177:**823–828.
27. **Belas, R., M. Simon, and M. Silverman.** 1986. Regulation of lateral flagella gene transcription in *Vibrio parahaemolyticus*. *J. Bacteriol.* **167:**210–218.
28. **Bidnenko, S. I., E. P. Bernasovskaia, I. Anisimova, I. Barshtein, and E. V. Mel'nitskaia.** 1985. Enteropathogenicity of *Proteus mirabilis* bacteria and pathogenesis of experimental intestinal infections caused by them. *Mikrobiol. Zh.* **47:**81–88.
29. **Bidnenko, S. I., E. V. Mel'nitskaia, A. V. Rudenko, and L. V. Nazarchuk.** 1985. Serological diagnosis and immunological aspects of *Proteus* infection. V. Design and trial of polyvalent antigenic preparations. *Zh. Mikrobiol. Epidemiol. Immunobiol.* **2:**49–53.
30. **Bisset, K. A.** 1973. The motion of the swarm in *Proteus mirabilis*. *J. Med. Microbiol.* **6:**33–35.
31. **Bisset, K. A.** 1973. The zonation phenomenon and structure of the swarm colony in *Proteus mirabilis*. *J. Med. Microbiol.* **6:**429–433.

32. **Bisset, K. A., and C. W. Douglas.** 1976. A continuous study of morphological phase in the swarm of *Proteus. J. Med. Microbiol.* **9:**229–231.

33. **Bouvier, J., C. Richaud, W. Higgins, O. Bogler, and P. Stragier.** 1992. Cloning, characterization, and expression of the *dapE* gene of *Escherichia coli. J. Bacteriol.* **174:**5265–5271.

34. **Brogan, T. D., J. Nettleton, and C. Reid.** 1971. The swarming of *Proteus* on semisynthetic media. *J. Med. Microbiol.* **4:**1–11.

35. **Brunham, R. C., F. A. Plummer, and R. S. Stephens.** 1993. Bacterial antigenic variation, host immune response, and pathogen-host coevolution. *Infect. Immun.* **61:**2273–2276.

36. **Carpenter, P. B., and G. W. Ordal.** 1993. *Bacillus subtilis* FlhA: a flagellar protein related to a new family of signal-transducing receptors. *Mol. Microbiol.* **7:**735–743.

37. **Chen, L., and W. Coleman.** 1993. Cloning and characterization of the *Escherichia coli* K-12 *rfa-2* (*rfaC*) gene, a gene required for lipopolysaccharide inner core synthesis. *J. Bacteriol.* **175:**2534–2540.

38. **Chippendale, G. R., J. W. Warren, A. L. Trifillis, and H. L. Mobley.** 1994. Internalization of *Proteus mirabilis* by human renal epithelial cells. *Infect. Immun.* **62:**3115–3121.

39. **Coetzee, J. N.** 1972. Genetics of the *Proteus* group. *Annu. Rev. Microbiol.* **26:**23–54.

40. **De Lorenzo, M., M. Herrero, U. Jakubzik, and K. N. Timmis.** 1990. Mini-Tn5 transposon derivatives for insertion mutagenesis, promoter probing, and chromosomal insertion of cloned DNA in gram-negative eubacteria. *J. Bacteriol.* **172:**6568–6572.

41. **Dick, H., R. G. Murray, and S. Walmsley.** 1985. Swarmer cell differentiation of *Proteus mirabilis* in fluid media. *Can. J. Microbiol.* **31:**1041–1050.

42. **Dienes, L.** 1946. Reproductive processes in *Proteus* cultures. *Proc. Soc. Exp. Biol. Med.* **63:**265–270.

43. **Dingwall, A., J. W. Gober, and L. Shapiro.** 1990. Identification of a *Caulobacter* basal body structural gene and a *cis*-acting site required for activation of transcription. *J. Bacteriol.* **172:**6066–6076.

44. **Dlugovitzky, D. G., O. G. Scharovsky, O. A. Molteni, J. C. Morini, and M. V. Londner.** 1988. Effect of *Proteus mirabilis* on liver and spleen weight and the hemagglutinin response to SRBC in rats. *Rev. Latinoam. Microbiol.* **30:**31–35.

45. **Douglas, C. W.** 1979. Measurement of *Proteus* cell motility during swarming. *J. Med. Microbiol.* **12:**195–199.

46. **Douglas, C. W., and K. A. Bisset.** 1976. Development of concentric zones in the *Proteus* swarm colony. *J. Med. Microbiol.* **9:**497–500.

47. **Dreyfus, G., A. W. Williams, I. Kawagishi, and R. M. Macnab.** 1993. Genetic and biochemical analysis of *Salmonella typhimurium* FliI, a flagellar protein related to the catalytic subunit of the F0F1 ATPase and to virulence proteins of mammalian and plant pathogens. *J. Bacteriol.* **175:**3131–3138.

48. **Ebringer, A., S. Khalafpour, and C. Wilson.** 1989. Rheumatoid arthritis and *Proteus*: a possible aetiological association. *Rheumatol. Int.* **9:**223–228.

49. **Falkinham, J. O. I., and P. S. Hoffman.** 1984. Unique developmental characteristics of the swarm and short cells of *Proteus vulgaris* and *Proteus mirabilis*. *J. Bacteriol.* **158:**1037–1040.

50. **Frolov, A. F., L. V. Parkhomenko, and I. G. Lukach.** 1986. Sensitivity of *Proteus mirabilis* strains to the bactericidal action of human serum. *Mikrobiol. Zh.* **48:**23–26.

51. **Fuscoe, F. J.** 1973. The role of extracellular slime secretion in the swarming of *Proteus*. *Med. Lab. Technol.* **30:**373–380.

52. **Galan, J. E., C. Ginocchio, and P. Costeas.** 1992. Molecular and functional characterization of the *Salmonella* invasion gene *invA*: homology of InvA to members of a new protein family. *J. Bacteriol.* **174:**4338–4349.

53. **Gmeiner, J., E. Sarnow, and K. Milde.** 1985. Cell cycle parameters of *Proteus mirabilis*: interdependence of the biosynthetic cell cycle and the interdivision cycle. *J. Bacteriol.* **164:**741–748.

54. **Gober, J. W., R. Champer, S. Reuter, and L. Shapiro.** 1991. Expression of positional information during cell differentiation of *Caulobacter*. *Cell* **64:**381–391.

55. **Gober, J. W., and L. Shapiro.** 1990. Integration host factor is required for the activation of developmentally regulated genes in *Caulobacter*. *Genes Dev.* **4:**1494–1504.

56. **Gober, J. W., and L. Shapiro.** 1992. A developmentally regulated *Caulobacter* flagellar promoter is activated by 3' enhancer and IHF binding elements. *Mol. Biol. Cell.* **3:**913–926.

57. **Gough, C. L., S. Genin, V. Lopes, and C. A. Boucher.** 1993. Homology between the HrpO protein of *Pseudomonas solanacearum* and bacterial proteins implicated in a

signal peptide-independent secretion mechanism. *Mol. Gen. Genet.* **239**:378–392.
58. **Grabow, W. O. K.** 1972. Growth-inhibiting metabolites of *Proteus mirabilis*. *J. Med. Microbiol.* **5**:191–204.
59. **Guerry, P., R. A. Alm, M. E. Power, S. M. Logan, and T. J. Trust.** 1991. Role of two flagellin genes in *Campylobacter* motility. *J. Bacteriol.* **173**:4757–4764.
60. **Guerry, P., S. M. Logan, and T. J. Trust.** 1988. Genomic rearrangement associated with antigenic variation in *Campylobacter coli*. *J. Bacteriol.* **170**:316–319.
61. **Gygi, D., M. Bailey, C. Allison, and C. Hughes.** 1995. Requirement for FlhA in flagella assembly and swarm-cell differentiation by *Proteus mirabilis*. *Mol. Microbiol.* **15**:761–769.
62. **Gygi, D., H. Lai, and C. Hughes.** 1995. *Proteus mirabilis* (*cpsF*) gene, complete sequence. GenBank submission L36873.
63. **Harshey, R.** 1994. Bees aren't the only ones: swarming in gram-negative bacteria. *Mol. Microbiol.* **13**:389–394.
64. **Harshey, R., and T. Matsuyama.** 1994. Dimorphic transition in *E. coli* and *S. typhimurium*: surface-induced differentiation into hyperflagellate swarmer cells. *Proc. Natl. Acad. Sci. USA* **91**:8631–8635.
65. **Helmann, J. D.** 1991. Alternative sigma factors and the regulation of flagellar gene expression. *Mol. Microbiol.* **5**:2875–2882.
66. **Henrichsen, J.** 1972. Bacterial surface translocation: a survey and a classification. *Bacteriol. Rev.* **36**:478–503.
67. **Hoeniger, J. F. M.** 1964. Cellular changes accompanying the swarming of *Proteus mirabilis*. I. Observations on living cultures. *Can. J. Microbiol.* **10**:1–9.
68. **Hoeniger, J. F. M.** 1965. Development of flagella by *Proteus mirabilis*. *J. Gen. Microbiol.* **40**:29–42.
69. **Hoeniger, J. F. M.** 1966. Cellular changes accompanying the swarming of *Proteus mirabilis*. II. Observations of stained organisms. *Can. J. Microbiol.* **12**:113–122.
70. **Hoeniger, J. F. M., and E. A. Cinits.** 1969. Cell wall growth during differentiation of *Proteus* swarmers. *J. Bacteriol.* **148**:736–738.
71. **Hoffman, P., and J. I. Falkinham.** 1981. Induction of tryptophanase in short cells and swarm cells of *Proteus vulgaris*. *J. Bacteriol.* **148**:736–738.
72. **Houwink, A. L., and W. van Iterson.** 1950. Electron microscopical observations on bacterial cytology. II. A study of flagellation. *Biochim. Biophys. Acta* **5**:10–16.
73. **Hughes, C.** 1994. Personal communication.
74. **Hughes, W. H.** 1956. The structure and development of the induced long forms of bacteria. *Symp. Soc. Gen. Microbiol.* **6**:341–360.
75. **Hughes, W. H.** 1957. A reconsideration of the swarming of *Proteus vulgaris*. *J. Gen. Microbiol.* **17**:49–58.
76. **Jeffries, C. D., and H. E. Rogers.** 1968. Enhancing effect of agar on swarming by *Proteus*. *J. Bacteriol.* **95**:732–733.
77. **Jiang, X., B. Neal, F. Santiago, S. Lee, L. Romana, and P. Reeves.** 1991. Structure and sequence of the *rfb* (O antigen) gene cluster of *Salmonella typhimurium* (strain LT2). *Mol. Microbiol.* **5**:695–713.
78. **Jin, T., and R. G. Murray.** 1987. Urease activity related to the growth and differentiation of swarmer cells of *Proteus mirabilis*. *Can. J. Microbiol.* **33**:300–303.
79. **Jin, T., and R. G. E. Murray.** 1988. Further studies of swarmer cell differentiation of *Proteus mirabilis* PM23: a requirement for iron and zinc. *Can. J. Microbiol.* **34**:588–593.
80. **Johnson, D. E., R. G. Russell, C. V. Lockatell, J. C. Zulty, J. W. Warren, and H. L. Mobley.** 1993. Contribution of *Proteus mirabilis* urease to persistence, urolithiasis, and acute pyelonephritis in a mouse model of ascending urinary tract infection. *Infect. Immun.* **61**:2748–2754.
81. **Jones, B. D., C. V. Lockatell, D. E. Johnson, J. W. Warren, and H. L. Mobley.** 1990. Construction of a urease-negative mutant of *Proteus mirabilis*: analysis of virulence in a mouse model of ascending urinary tract infection. *Infect. Immun.* **58**:1120–1123.
82. **Kustu, S., A. K. North, and D. S. Weiss.** 1991. Prokaryotic transcriptional enhancers and enhancer-binding proteins. *Trends Biochem. Sci.* **16**:397–402.
83. **Kvittingen, J.** 1949. Studies of the life-cycle of *Proteus* Hauser. *Acta Pathol. Microbiol. Scand.* **26**:24–40.
84. **Kvittingen, J.** 1949. Studies of the life-cycle of *Proteus* Hauser. Part 2. *Acta Pathol. Microbiol. Scand.* **26**:855–878.
85. **Kvittingen, J.** 1953. Studies of the life-cycle of *Proteus* Hauser. Part 3. *Acta Pathol. Microbiol. Scand.* **32**:170–186.
86. **Leifson, E., S. R. Carhart, and M. Fulton.** 1955. Morphological characteristics of flagella of *Proteus* and related bacteria. *J. Bacteriol.* **69**:73–80.
87. **Lidell, M. C., and S. W. Hutcheson.** 1994. Characterization of the *hrpJ* and *hrpU* operons of *Pseudomonas syringae* pv. *syringae*

Pss61: similarity with components of enteric bacteria involved in flagellar biogenesis and demonstration of their role in Harpin Pss secretion. *Mol. Plant-Microbe Interact.* **7**:488–497.

88. **Liu, D., A. Haase, L. Lindqvist, A. Lindberg, and P. Reeves.** 1993. Glycosyl transferases of O-antigen biosynthesis in *Salmonella enterica*: identification and characterization of transferase genes of groups B, C2, and E1. *J. Bacteriol.* **175**:3408–3413.

89. **Lominski, I., and A. C. Lendrum.** 1947. The mechanism of swarming of *Proteus. J. Pathol. Bacteriol.* **59**:688–691.

90. **Loomes, L. M., M. A. Kerr, and B. W. Senior.** 1993. The cleavage of immunoglobulin G in vitro and in vivo by a proteinase secreted by the urinary tract pathogen *Proteus mirabilis. J. Med. Microbiol.* **39**:225–232.

91. **Loomes, L. M., B. W. Senior, and M. A. Kerr.** 1990. A proteolytic enzyme secreted by *Proteus mirabilis* degrades immunoglobulins of the immunoglobulin A1 (IgA1), IgA2, and IgG isotypes. *Infect. Immun.* **58**:1979–1985.

92. **Loomes, L. M., B. W. Senior, and M. A. Kerr.** 1992. Proteinases of *Proteus* spp.: purification, properties, and detection in urine of infected patients. *Infect. Immun.* **60**:2267–2273.

93. **Macnab, R. M.** 1992. Genetics and biogenesis of bacterial flagella. *Annu. Rev. Genet.* **26**:131–158.

94. **Matsuyama, T., K. Kaneda, Y. Nakagawa, K. Isa, H. Hara-Hotta, and Y. Isuya.** 1992. A novel extracellular cyclic lipopeptide which promotes flagellum-dependent and -independent spreading growth of *Serratia marcescens. J. Bacteriol.* **174**:1769–1776.

95. **McCarter, L., M. Hilmen, and M. Silverman.** 1988. Flagellar dynamometer controls swarmer cell differentiation of *V. parahaemolyticus. Cell* **54**:345–351.

96. **McCarter, L., and M. Silverman.** 1990. Surface-induced swarmer cell differentiation of *Vibrio parahaemolyticus. Mol. Microbiol.* **4**:1057–1062.

97. **McLean, R. J., J. C. Nickel, V. C. Noakes, and J. W. Costerton.** 1985. An in vitro ultrastructural study of infectious kidney stone genesis. *Infect. Immun.* **49**:805–811.

98. **Miller, S., E. C. Pesci, and C. L. Pickett.** 1994. Genetic organization of the region upstream from the *Campylobacter jejuni* flagellar gene *flhA. Gene* **146**:31–38.

99. **Mirel, D. B., and M. J. Chamberlin.** 1989. The *Bacillus subtilis* flagellin gene (*hag*) is transcribed by the $\sigma^{28}$ form of RNA polymerase. *J. Bacteriol.* **171**:3095–3101.

100. **Mobley, H. L., G. R. Chippendale, K. G. Swihart, and R. A. Welch.** 1991. Cytotoxicity of the HpmA hemolysin and urease of *Proteus mirabilis* and *Proteus vulgaris* against cultured human renal proximal tubular epithelial cells. *Infect. Immun.* **59**:2036–2042.

101. **Mobley, H. L. T., and G. R. Chippendale.** 1990. Hemagglutinin, urease, and hemolysin production by *Proteus mirabilis* from clinical sources. *J. Infect. Dis.* **161**:525–530.

102. **Mobley, H. L. T., and J. W. Warren.** 1987. Urease-positive bacteriuria and obstruction of long-term urinary catheters. *J. Clin. Microbiol.* **25**:2216–2217.

103. **Morona, R., M. Mavris, A. Fallarino, and P. Manning.** 1994. Characterization of the *rfc* region of *Shigella flexneri. J. Bacteriol.* **176**:733–747.

104. **Nakahigashi, K., and H. Inokuchi.** 1990. Nucleotide sequence between *fadB* and *rrnA* from *Escherichia coli. Nucleic Acids Res.* **18**:6439.

105. **Nicholson, E. B., E. A. Concaugh, P. A. Foxall, M. D. Island, and H. L. Mobley.** 1993. *Proteus mirabilis* urease: transcriptional regulation by UreR. *J. Bacteriol.* **175**:465–473.

106. **Ogawa, T., and T. Okazaki.** 1991. Concurrent transcription from the *gid* and *mioC* promoters activates replition of an *Escherichia coli* minichromosome. *Mol. Gen. Genet.* **230**:193–200.

107. **O'Rear, J., L. Alberti, and R. M. Harshey.** 1992. Mutations that impair swarming motility in *Serratia marcescens* 274 include but are not limited to those affecting chemotaxis or flagellar function. *J. Bacteriol.* **174**:6125–6137.

108. **Pegues, J., L. Chen, A. Gordon, L. Ding, and W. Coleman, Jr.** 1990. Cloning, expression, and characterization of the *Escherichia coli* K-12 *rfaD* gene. *J. Bacteriol.* **172**:4652–4660.

109. **Plaut, A.** 1983. The IgA1 proteases of pathogenic bacteria. *Annu. Rev. Microbiol.* **37**:603–622.

110. **Proom, H., and A. Woiwod.** 1951. Amine production in the genus *Proteus. J. Gen. Microbiol.* **5**:930–938.

111. **Scott, T. N., and M. I. Simon.** 1982. Genetic analysis of the mechanism of the *Salmonella* phase variation site specific recombination system. *Mol. Gen. Genet.* **188**:313–321.

112. **Senior, B., L. Loomes, and M. Kerr.** 1991. The production and activity *in vivo* of *Proteus mirabilis* IgA protease in infections of the urinary tract. *J. Med. Microbiol.* **35:**203–207.
113. **Senior, B. W.** 1983. *Proteus morgani* is less frequently associated with urinary tract infections than *Proteus mirabilis*—an explanation. *J. Med. Microbiol.* **16:**317–322.
114. **Senior, B. W., M. Albrechtsen, and M. A. Kerr.** 1987. *Proteus mirabilis* strains of diverse type have IgA protease activity. *J. Med. Microbiol.* **24:**175–80.
115. **Shapiro, J.** 1994. Personal communication.
116. **Sirisena, D., K. Brozek, P. MacLachlan, K. Sanderson, and C. Raetz.** 1992. The *rfaC* gene of *Salmonella typhimurium*: cloning, sequencing, and enzymatic function in heptose transfer to lipopolysaccharide. *J. Biol. Chem.* **267:**18874–18884.
117. **Stahl, S. J., K. R. Stewart, and F. D. Williams.** 1983. Extracellular slime associated with *Proteus mirabilis* during swarming. *J. Bacteriol.* **154:**930–937.
118. **Stephens, C., and L. Shapiro.** 1993. An unusual promoter controls cell-cycle regulation and dependence on DNA replication of the *Caulobacter fliLM* early flagellar operon. *Mol. Microbiol.* **9:**1169–1179.
119. **Story, P.** 1954. *Proteus* infections in hospitals. *J. Pathol. Bacteriol.* **68:**55–62.
120. **Szekely, E., and M. Simon.** 1983. DNA sequence adjacent to flagellar genes and evolution of flagellar-phase variation. *J. Bacteriol.* **155:**74–81.
121. **Toshkov, A., A. Kuiumdzhiev, S. Zakharieva, D. Georgiev, and I. Gumpert.** 1977. Experimental pyelonephritis from *Proteus mirabilis* L forms in rats. *Acta Microbiol. Virol. Immunol.* **6:**42–48.
122. **VanderMolen, G., and F. Williams.** 1977. Observation of the swarming of *Proteus mirabilis* with scanning electron microscopy. *Can. J. Microbiol.* **23:**107–112.
123. **Varon, D., S. Boylan, K. Okamoto, and C. Price.** 1993. *Bacillus subtilis gtaB* encodes UDP-glucose pyrophosphorylase and is controlled by stationary phase transcription factor sigma-B. *J. Bacteriol.* **175:**3964–3971.
124. **Vogler, A. P., M. Homma, V. M. Irikura, and R. M. Macnab.** 1991. *Salmonella typhimurium* mutants defective in flagellar filament regrowth and sequence similarity of FliI to $F_0F_1$, vacuolar, and archaebacterial ATPase subunits. *J. Bacteriol.* **173:**3564–3572.
125. **von Meyenburg, K., and F. Hansen.** 1980. The origin of replication, *oriC*, of the *Escherichia coli* chromosome: genes near *oriC* and construction of *oriC* deletion mutants. *ICN-UCLA Symp.* **19:**137–159.
126. **von Meyenburg, K., and F. Hansen.** 1987. Regulation of chromosome replication, p. 1555–1577. *In* F. C. Neidhardt, J. L. Ingraham, K. B. Low, B. Magasanik, M. Schaechter, and H. E. Umbarger (ed.), *Escherichia coli and Salmonella typhimurium: Cellular and Molecular Biology*. American Society for Microbiology, Washington, D.C.
127. **von Meyenburg, K., B. Jorgensen, J. Neilsen, and F. Hansen.** 1982. Promoters of the *atp* operon coding for the membrane-bound ATP synthase of *Escherichia coli* mapped by Tn*10* insertion mutations. *Mol. Gen. Genet.* **188:**240–248.
128. **Wassif, C., D. Cheek, and R. Belas.** Molecular cloning and genetic analysis of a metalloprotease from *Proteus mirabilis*. Submitted for publication.
129. **Wei, Z. M., and S. V. Beer.** 1993. HrpI of *Erwinia amylovora* functions in secretion of harpin and is a member of a new protein family. *J. Bacteriol.* **175:**7958–7967.
130. **Williams, F. D., D. M. Anderson, P. S. Hoffman, R. H. Schwarzhoff, and S. Leonard.** 1976. Evidence against the involvement of chemotaxis in swarming of *Proteus mirabilis*. *J. Bacteriol.* **127:**237–248.
131. **Williams, F. D., and R. H. Schwarzhoff.** 1978. Nature of the swarming phenomenon in *Proteus*. *Annu. Rev. Microbiol.* **32:**101–122.
132. **Zieg, J., M. Silverman, M. Hilmen, and M. Simon.** 1977. The metabolism of phase variation, p. 25–35. *In* G. Wilcox (ed.), *Molecular Approaches to Eucaryotic Genetic Systems*. Academic Press, Inc., New York.

# VIRULENCE DETERMINANTS OF UROPATHOGENIC *KLEBSIELLA PNEUMONIAE*

*Carleen M. Collins, Ph.D., and
Sarah E. F. D'Orazio, Ph.D.*

# 11

*Klebsiella pneumoniae* is a gram-negative, nonmotile rod that can colonize the human gastrointestinal tract (57, 74); the urogenital areas of spinal cord-injured patients (58); and the noses and pharynges of neonates, the aged, and acutely ill hospital patients (57). Colonization of these sites predisposes individuals to infection with this organism (57, 74), with the urinary tract being the most common site of infection. In the community setting, *K. pneumoniae* is reported to cause from 2 to 15% of cystitis cases (5, 34, 49), and the incidence of *K. pneumoniae* urinary tract infection (UTI) increases in the hospital setting. With specific groups of patients, such as those with diabetes mellitus or neuropathic bladders resulting from spinal cord injuries, *K. pneumoniae* can be found in 20 to 40% of all UTIs (8, 21, 47). The increased occurrence of infection in these last groups results either from the immunosuppressive effects of diabetes mellitus or from repeated instrumentation of the urinary tract.

*K. pneumoniae* is second only to *Escherichia coli* as the cause of gram-negative bacteremias. The portal of entry for most of cases of *K. pneumoniae* bacteremia is the urinary tract (28). Urosepsis can lead to infections at secondary sites (79) and is associated with mortality rates of 10 to 12% (28). These secondary infections are most common in diabetics, the aged, and other immunocompromised patients. *K. pneumoniae* is also associated with both lobar and bronchopneumonias, usually in patients with impaired respiratory host defenses (24). *K. pneumoniae* infections are most severe in newborns (57), and outbreaks of *K. pneumoniae* on neonatal and intensive care wards and in chronic care facilities have been reported. In conclusion, this bacterium is predominantly an opportunistic or nosocomial pathogen associated with a high incidence of infection and severe disease in specific patient populations.

## *KLEBSIELLA* VIRULENCE FACTORS

Natural host defenses such as urine flow and mucous secretions eliminate most of the bacteria that enter the urinary system. In order to colonize the urinary tract, bacteria must possess virulence determinants to overcome these defensive strategies. The infecting bacterium must adhere to the

---

*Carleen M. Collins and Sarah E. F. D'Orazio,* Department of Microbiology and Immunology, University of Miami School of Medicine, Miami, Florida 33101.

uroepithelium and avoid the immune response of the host. Klebsiellae produce fimbriae that mediate attachment to host mucosal surfaces; a capsule that protects against phagocytosis and other immune responses; and, similar to all gram-negative organisms, immunosuppressive lipopolysaccharide (LPS). *K. pneumoniae* is able to scavenge iron and to enhance its own survival in the acidic environment of the urinary tract by producing urease. In addition, the incidence of antibiotic-resistant *K. pneumoniae* isolates has increased in recent years, thus complicating treatment of these infections. The contribution of each of these factors to the virulence of *K. pneumoniae* is discussed below.

## Adhesins

The observation that bacteria freshly isolated from patients with symptomatic UTI frequently express surface structures known as fimbriae or pili led to the hypothesis that these adhesin molecules are responsible for mediating bacterial attachment to uroepithelial cells. Using rat models of cystitis and pyelitis, Fader and Davis demonstrated that piliated *K. pneumoniae* strains adhere to the surface of both bladder and kidney to a greater extent than nonpiliated strains do (25, 26). Two types of fimbriae, characterized by their interactions with mannose, have been detected on *Klebsiella* species. Type 1 fimbriae are sometimes referred to as mannose-sensitive hemagglutinins because of their abilities to bind to mannose and to agglutinate erythrocytes in the absence of mannosides. Type 3 fimbriae, or mannose-resistant hemagglutinins, react only with tannin-treated erythrocytes and are not inhibited by mannosides.

Most members of the family *Enterobacteriaceae*, including *Klebsiella* species, can produce type 1 fimbriae. The results of several studies show that at least 75% of *Klebsiella* urinary isolates express these fimbriae on their surfaces (69, 71, 83). Two distinct type 1 fimbrial gene clusters, originally found in uropathogenic *K. pneumoniae* IA565 and IA551, have been described (30). These two gene clusters encode fimbrial subunits with 84% amino acid identity; however, some regions with significant variability appear to be correlated with different immunogenic epitopes. Tarkkanen et al. found that the IA565-like type 1 fimbrial gene cluster predominates among urinary isolates of *K. pneumoniae* (83). About 20% of the strains hybridize with DNA probes from both fimbrial gene clusters. The significance of the multiple fimbrial gene clusters is not clear at this time.

Synthesis of mannose-sensitive hemagglutinin adhesins is dependent on environmental conditions and subject to phase variation. In *E. coli*, an invertible DNA element controls phase variation of type 1 fimbriae (1). The presence of identical inverted repeats upstream of the gene encoding the *K. pneumoniae* major fimbrial subunit is suggestive of a similar function for *Klebsiella* strains (30). Maayan et al. used a mouse model of ascending UTI to show that *K. pneumoniae* with a mannose-sensitive adherence phenotype has a selective growth advantage in the bladder but not in the kidney (48). This result agrees with the data for *E. coli* UTI, which suggest that type 1 fimbriae are virulence factors for infections of the lower but not the upper urinary tract (37, 38).

Type 3 fimbriae are also known as mannose-resistant *Klebsiella*-like hemagglutinins (MR/K HA). These fimbriae are found on a wide variety of gram-negative bacteria, but they are not produced by *E. coli*. Six genes are required for functional expression of type 3 fimbriae. *mrkA* encodes the major fimbrial subunit, and *mrkD* encodes the adhesin subunit (2). The other four genes (*mrkBCEF*) code for accessory proteins that facilitate transport and assembly of the fimbrial subunits. Antisera raised against MR/K HA from a single *K. pneumoniae* isolate reacts with most fimbriated klebsiellae (63); thus, the major type 3 fimbrial subunit appears to be highly conserved.

The majority of *K. pneumoniae* urinary isolates express MR/K HA on their surfaces (69, 83). These fimbriae can mediate attachment to the basement membranes and basolateral surfaces of both renal and pulmonary epithelial cells. In the kidney, purified type 3 fimbriae bind effectively to tubular basement membranes, Bowman's capsule, and interstitial connective tissue (82). Type 3 fimbriae are also associated with adherence to urinary catheters. *Providencia stuartii* strains expressing MR/K HA persist longer in the urine of chronically catheterized patients and adhere to catheter material in vitro to a greater extent than *Providencia stuartii* strains that do not express MR/K HA (55). Isolates bearing only type 1 fimbriae do not adhere well to urinary catheters.

It was recently shown that the target for the *mrkD* gene product is type V collagen, a component of the epithelial basement membrane (82). Recombinant *E. coli* strains expressing either *K. pneumoniae* type 3 fimbriae or *mrkD* in association with the *E. coli* P-fimbrial (*pap*-encoded) filament specifically adhere to immobilized type V collagen and not to other collagens, fibronectin, or laminin. Since tannin-treated erythrocytes probably do not have type V collagen on their surfaces, the actual target for MR/K HA may include several proteins with a common domain. This domain is likely to be rich in positively charged amino acids, since the polyamines spermine and spermidine can inhibit the attachment of type 3 fimbriae to human buccal and tracheal cells (35).

The clinical isolate *K. pneumoniae* IA565 carries a plasmid-borne *mrk* gene cluster and has an *mrkA* gene on the bacterial chromosome (36). The chromosomal *mrkA* may be part of an additional *mrk* gene cluster, since loss of the plasmid-encoded *mrkD* gene product does not reduce fimbrial expression but does change the adherence phenotype. This *mrkD* gene product, though frequently found in *Klebsiella oxytoca* strains, is only rarely associated with *K. pneumoniae* fimbriae (73). MrkD may belong to a larger family of MR/K HA adhesins. If this is the case, it will be interesting to determine whether *Klebsiella* strains can incorporate heterologous adhesins into their fimbrial appendages.

Early observations suggested that MR/K HA-expressing *Klebsiella* spp. could adhere to many different substrates, including yeasts, fungi, cellulose fibers, and glass (22, 44). Although type 3 fimbriae may mediate attachment to a wide variety of surfaces, one common feature of this adherence seems to be that the target component is often not exposed on the intact cell surface. For example, erythrocytes must be treated with tannin for type 3 fimbriae to mediate mannose-resistant hemagglutination, and human buccal cells must be trypsinized in order to demonstrate binding by type 3 fimbriae (35). Therefore, it is possible that in vivo, epithelial linings must be damaged or altered in some way before *Klebsiella* species can adhere. Extracellular-matrix components that are exposed after the epithelium is compromised could provide the target(s) for type 3 fimbrial adhesins. Uroepithelial cells may be injured during the placement of a urinary catheter or by the accumulation of ammonium ions that are released by the action of urease (see below).

## Capsule

The presence of capsular polysaccharides (CPS) is widely believed to be an important virulence factor for *Klebsiella* species. The majority of clinically isolated *K. pneumoniae* strains have a well-defined capsule composed of two distinct layers. Electron microscopy studies indicate that the inner layer is formed by densely packed bundles of thick fibers extending at right angles from the surface of the outer membrane

(3). The outer layer contains a loose network of thinner filaments. Laasko et al. demonstrated that the outer membrane to which CPS are attached plays little part in determining the fine structure of the capsule (45). *E. coli* transconjugants that contain either the *E. coli* O9:K(A30) or the *K. pneumoniae* O1:K20 genetic determinants express CPS that are chemically and serologically indistinguishable. Electron microscopy revealed structural differences within the capsules, however, suggesting that the morphology of the CPS layer may be influenced by the CPS genes alone.

Three virulence functions have been proposed for the capsule: (i) CPS may act as a barrier to the deposition of serum killing factors such as antibodies or complement components, (ii) CPS may prevent phagocytosis by neutrophils and macrophages, and (iii) CPS may have suppressive effects on the immune system. Serum resistance is probably a multifactorial phenomenon in vivo, since a number of peripheral components have been implicated, including CPS, LPS, and various bacterial outer membrane proteins. Most evidence, however, suggests that *K. pneumoniae* capsular antigens are not involved in determining susceptibility to the bactericidal effects of serum. Meno and Amako showed that anti-O antibody penetrates through the capsular layer to the surfaces of the outer membranes in strains with various degrees of capsule thickness (52). Some complement components can also diffuse through CPS. Thus, the capsule probably does not function as a barrier to the deposition of serum bactericidal factors.

The physical and chemical properties of CPS are important for antiphagocytic activity. If a bacterial surface is more hydrophilic than the surface of the engulfing neutrophil or macrophage, the bacterium can resist phagocytosis (85). The binding of specific antibodies or complement components renders encapsulated bacteria more hydrophobic, which allows them to be more readily phagocytosed. The surface hydrophobicity of *K. pneumoniae* strains correlates well with virulence (53). Capsule thickness and fimbriation were ruled out as causes for the various degrees of hydrophobicity noted among *Klebsiella* isolates. Chemical modifications, such as O acetylation of the CPS layer, are probably responsible for the differences in phagocytic uptake that have been observed for *Klebsiella* strains.

At least 77 different capsular (K-antigen) serotypes have been described (64). Some of the K serotypes are isolated at significantly higher frequencies than others. There apparently is no strict correlation, however, between K serotype and the site of isolation or any particular disease state. In addition, capsular serotypes and antibiotic resistance patterns do not appear to be associated. Many investigators have attempted to classify the K serotypes of *Klebsiella* bacteremic, urinary, respiratory, fecal, and environmental isolates (69, 72, 77, 83). Together, these studies examined 307 *Klebsiella* strains isolated from patients with UTIs. The most common capsular types were K2 (11%); K24 (5%); K9, K18, and K27 (4% each); and K55 (3%). Nearly all of the K serotypes were isolated at least once, however, suggesting that K-antigen type alone does not greatly enhance virulence in the urinary tract.

Encapsulated *E. coli* persists in the kidneys longer than unencapsulated mutants (80). The role of capsule in the pathogenicity of *Klebsiella* UTI, however, is not clearly understood. Camprubi et al. found that both K2 and K66 strains and their isogenic K-antigen mutant strains are present in equally high numbers in rat bladders and kidneys 5 days after inoculation (10). They concluded that the capsule is not essential for infection of the urinary tract. Capsules may contribute to the establishment of UTIs, however, by mediating nonspecific adherence to the uroepithelium. Bruce et al. demonstrated that although many fimbriated bacteria can adhere to uroepithelial cells, only encapsulated uropathogens can also attach to urinary mucopolysaccharides (9). Unlike fimbria-mediated attachment, this adherence required no specific cellular receptors.

The rapid clearance of certain *K. pneumoniae* serotypes from serum-poor environments such as the urinary tract and the respiratory tract may be due in part to lectinophagocytosis. In the absence of specific opsonins, lectinophagocytosis can occur after an interaction between lectins on the surface of the phagocytic cell and certain components of the CPS layer of an encapsulated bacterium. Athamna et al. showed that *Klebsiella* strains that produce CPS with certain repeating mannose or rhamnose sequences (Man2/3Man or L-Rha2/3-L-Rha) readily bind to a mannose-specific lectin commonly found on tissue macrophages and are internalized and then killed (6). In contrast, *K. pneumoniae* serotypes (including K1, K2, K7, K12, K24, K32, and K55) that do not contain these forms of either mannose or rhamnose show only negligible binding in serum-free media. Further studies confirmed that this nonopsonic recognition by macrophage is determined by the capsule type, since recombinant strains that express heterologous CPS genes display the macrophage-binding phenotype of the donor (42). Thus, *Klebsiella* serotypes that are recognized by the macrophage lectin would be expected to be rapidly cleared, while those that are not recognized by the lectin could exhibit high or low virulence depending on their genetic backgrounds. In fact, three of the K serotypes that do not bind effectively to macrophage (K2, K24, and K55) are among those commonly isolated from patients with UTI.

The amount of CPS produced by a *Klebsiella* strain may affect that strain's virulence. Capsule size greatly influences the virulence of K1 and K2 strains used in rodent models of lobar pneumonia, burn wound sepsis, and peritonitis; highly encapsulated strains are more virulent (15, 18, 23). Treatment with bismuth or salicylate reduces *K. pneumoniae* capsule expression and results in greater phagocytic uptake by human peripheral blood cells or rat alveolar macrophage (20). Domenico et al. proposed that such compounds might be used in vivo as a means of enhancing phagocytosis of encapsulated bacteria (20). Other studies, however, indicated that capsule size may not be important for virulence. Meno and Amako demonstrated that while some strains with high 50% lethal doses for the mouse are only slightly encapsulated, many other strains with thin capsules are considered virulent in the mouse peritonitis model, and thus capsule thickness alone cannot account for virulence potential (53).

Encapsulated *K. pneumoniae* can also produce large quantities of cell-free CPS. The release of CPS may enhance virulence by causing K-specific antibodies to be complexed away from the bacteria. In one study, circulating capsular antigen was found in about 50% of patients with *Klebsiella* infections (70). The presence of circulating CPS seemed to correlate with an extravascular (i.e., UTI, wounds, and pneumonia) focus of infection. Since the shedding of capsule is influenced by pH and cation concentration (19), local environmental conditions may cause greater production of extracellular CPS for infections localized to these sites.

Two *K. pneumoniae* regulatory genes, *rmpA* and *rmpB*, appear to control expression of the mucoid phenotype (61, 86). When these genes were introduced into either nonmucoid *E. coli* or slightly mucoviscous strains of *K. pneumoniae*, the resultant bacterial colonies were highly mucoid. Further examination revealed that the recombinant strains do not have a well-defined capsule, but they do produce large amounts of exopolysaccharide. *rmpA* encodes a transcriptional regulator of CPS synthesis that displays some homology to NtrC (86). *rmpB* may encode a positive regulator of *rmpA* expression (61). Nassif et al. showed that these two genes are encoded on a 180-kb plasmid that also encodes aerobactin production (60). The *rmpA* coding sequence has a much lower GC content than most *Klebsiella* genes, and the nucleotide sequence upstream of *rmpA* is homologous to an IS3 insertion sequence. These observations suggest that *rmpA* may have been introduced into *Klebsiella* by a transposon-like element from another organism. *Klebsiella* strains that carry these genes would be expected to have a selective growth advantage in the host, since RmpA allows the overproduction of CPS, which enhances antiphagocytic activity.

## LPS

The serum resistance of *Klebsiella* strains is mediated primarily by the core polysaccharide (O antigen) of LPS. In general, O antigens are more immunogenic than K antigens; thus, it is not surprising that O antigen serves as one of the principal targets for complement components. C3b attaches to LPS and activates the alternative complement pathway; C5b binds to O antigens that serve as a nucleation site for the membrane attack complex. The side chains of the core polysaccharide are critical for resistance to the bactericidal effect of nonimmune serum. Attachment of sialic acid residues to O antigens prevents the formation of C3 convertase, similar to the effect observed for capsules with a high sialic acid content. Changes in the length of LPS O-antigen side chains can prevent effective formation of the membrane attack complex. Side chain length may also affect earlier stages of the alternative complement pathway, since C3b preferentially attaches to the longest O-antigen side chains in *E. coli* and *Salmonella* species (12).

LPS is also important for virulence in extravascular compartments. Camprubi et al. showed that spontaneous O-antigen mutants of *K. pneumoniae* have a 50%-lower infection rate in a rat model of ascending UTI than the isogenic wild-type strains have (10). At least 2-log-fewer organisms were recovered from the bladders and kidneys of rats infected with O-antigen mutant strains. Thus, LPS appears to function as a virulence factor for *Klebsiella* UTIs.

## Iron-Scavenging Systems

Iron is required for the growth of most pathogenic bacteria. In response to iron deprivation, many *Enterobacteriaceae* produce siderophores and their specific outer membrane receptors in order to solubilize and transport iron into the cell. Two types of siderophores have been described: enterochelin, which is a phenolate compound, and aerobactin, which is a hydroxamate compound. In *E. coli,* a plasmid-encoded, aerobactin-mediated iron uptake system has an epidemiologic association with pyelonephritogenic isolates (65). However, the selective advantage that aerobactin production confers on strains that already produce enterochelin is not well understood. Aerobactin may be more efficient in sequestering transferrin-bound iron in body fluids (43, 88).

Most clinically isolated *Klebsiella* strains produce enterochelin, but only a few isolates produce aerobactin. Tarkkanen et al. examined 32 *K. pneumoniae* urinary isolates and found that all of the strains secrete enterochelin (83). No evidence of aerobactin production was found either by siderophore bioassay or by DNA hybridization with an *E. coli* aerobactin gene probe. A larger-scale study of urinary isolates showed that only 5 (3%) of 133 *K. pneumoniae* strains secrete aerobactin (69). Podschun et al. screened 481 *Klebsiella* strains from various sources and found that only 6% of the *K. pneumoniae* isolates produce aerobactin (68). The aerobactin-producing strains included clinical, fecal, and environmental isolates, suggesting that the aerobactin system is not used as a primary mechanism for iron supply in *Klebsiella* spp.

Nassif and Sansonetti were able to show a correlation between aerobactin production and virulence in the mouse peritonitis model for *K. pneumoniae* K1 and K2 strains (62). Each of the virulent strains carried a 180-kb plasmid with homology to pColV-K30. pColV-K30 is an *E. coli* plasmid that contains the aerobactin biosynthesis genes (*iucABCD*) and *iutA,* which codes for a 74-kDa outer membrane protein that functions as a ferric-aerobactin receptor (11). Another study also demonstrated the existence of aerobactin genes on large R plasmids in *K. pneumoniae*. However, when 86 different nosocomial strains were examined, only 3 hybridized with the aerobactin gene probe (16). Although each of the three strains was multiply drug resistant, the restriction endonuclease cleavage patterns of their plasmid DNAs differed, suggesting that they carried different R plasmids.

*K. pneumoniae* may be able to scavenge ferric aerobactin without actually synthesizing the chelator itself. Williams et al. showed that some *K. pneumoniae* strains that produce enterochelin and not aerobactin are nevertheless sensitive to the bacteriocin cloacin DF13 (87). The aerobactin receptor also functions as a receptor for cloacin DF13, and thus, bacteria that bear the receptor may be susceptible to cloacin-mediated killing (84). Although these strains do not hybridize with a *iutA* gene probe, they do express a 76-kDa outer membrane protein that cross-reacts with sera raised against the 74-kDa pColV-K30-encoded aerobactin receptor. In addition, mutant derivatives of these strains that are unable to synthesize enterochelin are able to grow in iron-deficient media supplemented with aerobactin (87). The authors concluded that these *K. pneumoniae* strains produce a novel aerobactin receptor that might confer a selective advantage at infection sites at which aerobactin produced by other bacteria could be utilized. Further work will be required to determine whether this receptor is present in all aerobactin-negative strains or if a correlation can be made between the presence of the 76-kDa protein and the sources of various *Klebsiella* isolates.

## Urease

Urease is a virulence factor for many bacterial pathogens, and the role of this enzyme in UTI can be inferred both from clinical observations on human patients and from animal studies with ureolytic uropathogens. Close to 100% of *K. pneumoniae* UTI isolates are urease producers (69), and as cited below, there is ample evidence that urease is a virulence determinant for uropathogenic *K. pneumoniae*. However, no studies that evaluated the role of urease in *K. pneumoniae* infection by using isogenic urease-positive and urease-negative strains in an animal model system have been reported.

When urease, which catalyzes the hydrolysis of urea to ammonia and carbamate, is produced by uropathogens in an infected urinary tract, the breakdown of urea increases the ammonium concentration in the urine and results in the elevation of urine pH. The elevated urine pH can lead to a number of pathogenic effects, the most damaging of which is the production of a urinary stone or calculus formed by the precipitation of magnesium ammonium phosphate salts (struvite) (33). Stone formation can cause urinary obstruction and interfere with voiding, thereby making it more difficult to clear the infecting organism from the urinary tract (46, 56). Stones can also harbor the infecting bacteria in a protected site, which in many instances reduces the effectiveness of antibiotic treatment (27). Struvite precipitates can be found in the renal pelvis and bladder and encrusted on urinary catheters. Undiagnosed asymptomatic renal calculi can serve as a reservoir for urosepsis (79).

Prolonged survival of ureolytic bacteria in the urinary tract is seen even in the absence of stone formation. Recent studies examined the virulence of isogenic pairs of urease-positive and urease-negative strains of *Proteus mirabilis* and *Staphylococcus saprophyticus* in rodent model systems (29, 40, 41). These studies indicate that UTIs with urease-producing organisms are increased in duration; have greater numbers of bacteria colonizing the bladder, urine, and kidney; and result in more damage to kidney tissue. In addition to investigations with urease-negative mutants, rodents have been treated with urease inhibitors such as acetohydroxamic acid (AHA) or flurofamide in an effort to define the role of urease in UTI. Treatment of UTI with urease inhibitors decreases bacterial colonization of the kidneys, severity of kidney lesions, and incidence of bacteremia resulting from infection (32, 54, 59, 81). Unfortunately, urease inhibitors have many adverse side effects and are not useful for treating infections in humans.

The exact mechanism responsible for the increased survival and damage associated with urease can only be inferred. Increased bacterial colonization of the urinary tract might result from the generation of an easily assimilated nitrogen source and/or from alkalinization of the urine to a pH more favorable for growth (51). Ammonia can inactivate the fourth component of complement and thus might prevent the immune system from functioning efficiently (7). Tissue damage associated with the infection can result either from direct damage of the renal cells by ammonia (49) or from an unidentified indirect mechanism.

Struvite stone formation has been reported in patients with *K. pneumoniae* as the sole infecting organism. In one study of risk factors for stone formation in spinal cord injury patients, DeVivo and Fine stated that patients with *K. pneumoniae* as the infecting agent are 7.2 times more likely to develop urinary stones than patients without *K. pneumoniae* infection (17). In that study, urease-negative *E. coli* did not increase the risk of renal calculi. Both Stamey (two cases) and Fowler (one case) documented patients with struvite stone formation who had *K. pneumoniae* as the single infecting organism, and Griffith et al. and McCartney et al. also showed an association between *K. pneumoniae* infection and stone formation (27, 32, 50, 78).

The urease genes from *K. pneumoniae* have been isolated (14). Seven tandem urease genes (*ureDABCEFG*) are necessary for urease synthesis. This gene organization is similar to that of the urease gene clusters found in other enteric uropathogens such as *P. mirabilis* and *Providencia stuartii* (13). *ureABC* encode the structural polypeptides UreA, UreB, and UreC, respectively. X-ray crystallographic studies indicate that the subunits come together in a (UreA-UreB-UreC)$_3$ stoichiometry to form the native cytoplasmic enzyme with a molecular weight of 249,100 (39). Urease is nickel metalloenzyme, and UreD, UreE, UreF, and UreG are believed to be involved in the proper assembly of the metallocenter (66).

*K. pneumoniae* urease genes are regulated by the global nitrogen regulation system (*ntr*) (14). This system is a complex cascade that senses the nitrogen status of the cell. In nitrogen-limiting conditions, the *ntr* system activates the transcription of genes encoding enzymes that can generate either ammonia or glutamine, the preferred nitrogen sources; this system also represses transcription of genes encoding enzymes that facilitate the assimilation of ammonium, such as glutamine dehydrogenase. *K. pneumoniae* urease genes are positively regulated by a member of this cascade termed Nac (nitrogen assimilation control) (31). Transcription of the *nac* gene, in turn, is controlled by two integral members of the *ntr* cascade: the transcriptional activator NtrC and the alternative sigma factor NtrA (RpoN).

The dependence of *K. pneumoniae* urease gene expression on the exogenous nitrogen concentration suggests that *K. pneumoniae*

**TABLE 1** Expression of *K. pneumoniae* urease in urine

| *K. pneumoniae* strain[a] | Exponential phase cells | | Stationary phase cells | |
|---|---|---|---|---|
| | Urease activity $(10^5)$[b] | pH | Urease activity $(10^5)$ | pH |
| PG, urease positive | 1.9 | 7.0 | 5.2 | 9.0 |
| SA, urease negative | 0.1 | 6.5 | 0.2 | 7.0 |
| PG, urease positive + 5 mM AHA | 0.3 | 6.5 | 1.0 | 7.0 |
| Urine + 5 mM AHA | | 6.5 | | |
| Urine alone[c] | | 6.5 | | |
| Urine + [NH$_4$] (4 mM) | | 6.5 | | 6.5 |

[a] Immediately after collection, urine was centrifuged at 2,000 rpm for 5 min to remove any particulate matter and then filter sterilized through a 0.45-$\mu$m-pore-size nitrocellulose filter. *K. pneumoniae* strains were grown in the urine to the indicated growth phase at 37°C with aeration, and then samples were removed and the pH and cell concentration were determined. Each sample was washed three times with a phosphate buffer and then assayed for urease activity. The urease assay measures the production of ammonia, a product of urea hydrolysis, and is based on the chromogenic reaction between ammonia and phenol in the presence of hypochlorite, as described in reference 14. *K. pneumoniae* PG is an isolate from an intermittently catheterized spinal cord-injured patient. *K. pneumoniae* SA is a naturally occurring urease-negative isolate.

[b] Urease activity is expressed in millimoles of ammonia produced per minute per measure of bacterial cell concentration (optical density at 550 nm).

[c] The ammonia concentration of urine used in the experiment was 4 mM.

urease may not be synthesized in an infected urinary tract. Although it is difficult to predict the nitrogen concentration of urine in the kidneys, the fact that *K. pneumoniae*-associated struvite stones are found suggests that low nitrogen conditions can exist in the tubules and renal pelvis. In addition, we have evidence that *K. pneumoniae* urease is produced in normal human urine. As shown in Table 1, *K. pneumoniae* produces urease activity with growth in urine. This activity is not seen with a naturally occurring urease-negative isolate or when the urease inhibitor AHA is present in the medium. It is significant that the pH of the urine increases, since the local pH is primarily responsible for struvite stone formation. Clearly, since the nitrogen status of urine changes depending on the consumption of the individual, urease activity and pH values in Table 1 will vary from experiment to experiment. However, it appears that, similar to other uropathogens, *K. pneumoniae* can produce urease in the urinary tract and thus increase its own virulence.

## Antibiotic Resistance

In recent years, the incidence of drug-resistant *K. pneumoniae* isolates has increased. Most *Klebsiella* strains are inherently resistant to ampicillin and amoxicillin; however, in some settings, 25% or more of the isolates are resistant to expanded-spectrum cephalosporins (47). This resistance is believed to be due to the production of broad-spectrum $\beta$-lactamases that in many strains are encoded on self-transmissible plasmids (4, 67, 76). *K. pneumoniae* can be resistant to antibiotics other than beta-lactams, and isolates that are resistant to tetracycline, chloramphenicol, gentamicin, kanamycin, and trimethoprim-sulfamethoxazole have been reported (5, 16, 28, 34). In one hospital, only 33% of *K. pneumoniae* isolates were susceptible to trimethoprim-sulfamethoxazole, a drug often used to treat UTI (5). An outbreak of *K. pneumoniae* UTI with a strain susceptible only to amikacin and colistimethate was reported (75). In general, nosocomial isolates are more resistant to commonly used antibiotics than are isolates from community-acquired infections (5). The increased incidence of multidrug-resistant strains raises the obvious concern that effective, appropriate antibiotics for treatment of these infections will no longer be available. In addition, hospital patients taking antibiotics can be colonized, usually in the gastrointestinal tract, with drug-resistant *K. pneumoniae*.

This gastrointestinal colonization predisposes these patients to infections with drug-resistant *K. pneumoniae* and provides a reservoir for recurrent infection (74).

## CONCLUSIONS

*K. pneumoniae* is a common pathogen of the urinary tract in both community and hospital settings. Infections with this organism occur most often in hospitalized, chronically catheterized, or diabetic patients, and these infections can be severe and possibly life-threatening because of the potential for urosepsis. *K. pneumoniae* has a number of virulence determinants, including fimbriae, capsule, iron-scavenging systems, and urease. Type 3 fimbriae, urease activity, and enterochelin are repeatedly found in isolates from human UTIs. However, these factors are also found in respiratory, bacteremic, and environmental *Klebsiella* isolates. This finding suggests that *K. pneumoniae* strains cannot be separated into clonal pathogenic groups. The common occurrence of these features, as well as the heterogeneity of capsular antigen types among the varied isolates, may simply reflect the opportunistic nature of these infections.

## ACKNOWLEDGMENTS

The laboratory of C.M.C. is supported by Public Health Service grant DK 59495 from the National Institutes of Health.

## REFERENCES

1. **Abraham, J. M., C. C. Freitag, J. R. Clements, and B. I. Eisenstein.** 1985. An invertible element of DNA controls phase variation of type-1 fimbriae of *Escherichia coli*. *Proc. Natl. Acad. Sci. USA* **82:**5724–5727.
2. **Allen, B. L., G.-F. Gerlach, and S. Clegg.** 1991. The nucleotide sequence and functions of *mrk* determinants necessary for expression of type 3 fimbriae in *Klebsiella pneumoniae*. *J. Bacteriol.* **173:**916–920.
3. **Amako, K., Y. Meno, and A. Takade.** 1988. Fine structures of the capsules of *Klebsiella pneumoniae* and *Escherichia coli* K1. *J. Bacteriol.* **170:**4960–4962.
4. **Arlet, G., M. Rouveau, I. Casin, P. J. M. Bouvet, P. H. Lagrange, and A. Philippon.** 1994. Molecular epidemiology of *Klebsiella pneumoniae* strains that produce SHV-4 β-lactamase and which were isolated in 14 French hospitals. *J. Clin. Microbiol.* **32:**2553–2558.
5. **Ashkenazi, S., S. Even-Tov, Z. Samra, and G. Dinari.** 1991. Uropathogens of various childhood populations and their antibiotic susceptibility. *Pediatr. Infect. Dis. J.* **10:**742–746.
6. **Athamna, A., I. Ofek, Y. Keisari, S. Markowitz, G. G. S. Dutton, and N. Sharon.** 1991. Lectinophagocytosis of encapsulated *Klebsiella pneumoniae* mediated by surface lectins of guinea pig alveolar macrophages and human monocyte-derived macrophages. *Infect. Immun.* **59:**1673–1682.
7. **Beeson, P. B., and D. Rowley.** 1959. The anticomplementary effect of kidney tissue. Its association with ammonia production. *J. Exp. Med.* **110:**695–698.
8. **Bennett, C. J., M. N. Young, and H. Darrington.** 1995. Differences in urinary tract infection in male and female spinal cord injury patients on intermittent catheterization. *Paraplegia* **33:**69–72.
9. **Bruce, A. W., R. C. Y. Chan, D. Pinkerton, A. Morales, and P. Chadwick.** 1983. Adherence of gram-negative uropathogens to human uroepithelial cells. *J. Urol.* **130:**293–298.
10. **Camprubi, S., S. Merino, V.-J. Benedi, and J. M. Tomas.** 1993. The role of the O-antigen lipopolysaccharide and capsule on an experimental *Klebsiella pneumoniae* infection of the rat urinary tract. *FEMS Microbiol. Lett.* **111:**9–14.
11. **Carbonetti, N. H., and P. H. Williams.** 1984. A cluster of five genes specifying the aerobactin iron uptake system of plasmid ColV-K30. *Infect. Immun.* **46:**7–12.
12. **Ciurana, B., and J. M. Tomas.** 1987. Role of lipopolysaccharide and complement in susceptibility of *Klebsiella pneumoniae* to nonimmune serum. *Infect. Immun.* **55:**2741–2746.
13. **Collins, C. M., and S. E. F. D'Orazio.** 1993. Bacterial ureases: structure, regulation of expression and role in pathogenesis. *Mol. Microbiol.* **9:**907–913.
14. **Collins, C. M., D. M. Gutman, and H. Laman.** 1993. Identification of a nitrogen-regulated promoter controlling expression of *Klebsiella pneumoniae* urease genes. *Mol. Microbiol.* **8:**187–198.

15. **Cryz, S. J., Jr., E. Furer, and R. Germanier.** 1984. Experimental *Klebsiella pneumoniae* burn wound sepsis: role of capsular polysaccharide. *Infect. Immun.* **43:**440–441.
16. **Darfeuille-Michaud, A., C. Jallat, D. Aubel, D. Sirot, C. Rich, J. Sirot, and B. Joly.** 1992. R-plasmid-encoded adhesive factor in *Klebsiella pneumoniae* strains responsible for human nosocomial infections. *Infect. Immun.* **60:**44–55.
17. **DeVivo, M. J., and P. R. Fine.** 1986. Predicting renal calculus occurrence in spinal cord injury patients. *Arch. Phys. Med. Rehabil.* **67:**722–725.
18. **Domenico, P., W. G. Johanson, Jr., and D. C. Straus.** 1982. Lobar pneumonia in rats produced by clinical isolates of *Klebsiella pneumoniae*. *Infect. Immun.* **37:**327–335.
19. **Domenico, P., R. J. Salo, A. S. Cross, and B. A. Cunha.** 1994. Polysaccharide capsule-mediated resistance to opsonophagocytosis in *Klebsiella pneumoniae*. *Infect. Immun.* **62:**4495–4499.
20. **Domenico, P., R. J. Salo, D. C. Straus, J. C. Hutson, and B. A. Cunha.** 1992. Salicylate or bismuth salts enhance opsonophagocytosis of *Klebsiella pneumoniae*. *Infection* **20:**66–72.
21. **Donovan, W. H., R. Hull, D. X. Cifu, H. D. Brown, and N. J. Smith.** 1990. Use of plasmid analysis to determine the source of bacterial invasion of the urinary tract. *Paraplegia* **28:**573–582.
22. **Duguid, J. P.** 1959. Fimbriae and adhesive properties of *Klebsiella* strains. *J. Gen. Microbiol.* **21:**271–286.
23. **Ehrenwort, L., and H. Baer.** 1956. The pathogenicity of *Klebsiella pneumoniae* for mice: the relationship to the quantity and rate of production of type-specific capsular polysaccharide. *J. Bacteriol.* **72:**713–717.
24. **Eisenstein, B. I.** 1990. *Enterobacteriaceae*, p. 1658–1673. *In* G. L. Mandell, R. G. Douglas, and J. E. Bennett (ed.), *Principles and Practice of Infectious Disease*. Churchill Livingstone, New York.
25. **Fader, R. C., and C. P. Davis.** 1980. Effect of piliation on *Klebsiella pneumoniae* infection in rat bladders. *Infect. Immun.* **30:**554–561.
26. **Fader, R. C., and C. P. Davis.** 1981. *Klebsiella pneumoniae*-induced experimental pyelitis: the effect of piliation on infectivity. *J. Urol.* **128:**197–201.
27. **Fowler, J. E., Jr.** 1984. Bacteriology of branched renal calculi and accompanying urinary tract infection. *J. Urol.* **131:**213–215.
28. **Garcia de la Torre, M., J. Romero-Vivas, J. Martinez-Beltran, A. Guerrero, M. Meseguer, and E. Bouza.** 1985. *Klebsiella* bacteremia: an analysis of 100 episodes. *Rev. Infect. Dis.* **7:**143–150.
29. **Gatermann, S., J. John, and R. Marre.** 1988. *Staphylococcus saprophyticus* urease: characterization and contribution to uropathogenicity in unobstructed urinary tract infection of rats. *Infect. Immun.* **57:**110–116.
30. **Gerlach, G.-F., and S. Clegg.** 1988. Characterization of two genes encoding antigenically distinct type-1 fimbriae of *Klebsiella pneumoniae*. *Gene* **64:**231–240.
31. **Goss, T. J., and R. A. Bender.** 1995. The nitrogen assimilation control protein, NAC, is a DNA-binding transcription activator in *Klebsiella aerogenes*. *J. Bacteriol.* **177:**3546–3555.
32. **Griffith, D. P., F. Khonsari, J. H. Skurnick, K. E. James, and V. A. C. S. Group.** 1988. A randomized trial of acetohydroxamic acid for the treatment and prevention of infection-induced urinary stones in spinal cord injury patients. *J. Urol.* **140:**318–324.
33. **Griffith, D. P., D. M. Musher, and C. Itin.** 1976. Urease: the primary cause of infection-induced urinary stones. *Invest. Urol.* **13:**346–350.
34. **Gruneberg, R. N.** 1990. Changes in the antibiotic sensitivities of urinary pathogens, 1971–1989. *J. Antimicrob. Chemother.* **26:**3–11.
35. **Hornick, D. B., B. L. Allen, M. A. Horn, and S. Clegg.** 1992. Adherence to respiratory epithelia by recombinant *Escherichia coli* expressing *Klebsiella pneumoniae* type 3 fimbrial gene products. *Infect. Immun.* **60:**1577–1588.
36. **Hornick, D. B., J. Thommandru, W. Smits, and S. Clegg.** 1995. Adherence properties of an *mrkD*-negative mutant of *Klebsiella pneumoniae*. *Infect. Immun.* **63:**2026–2032.
37. **Hultgren, S. J., T. N. Porter, A. J. Schaeffer, and J. L. Duncan.** 1985. Role of type 1 pili and effects of phase variation on lower urinary tract infections produced by *Escherichia coli*. *Infect. Immun.* **50:**370–377.
38. **Iwahi, T., Y. Abe, M. Nakao, A. Imada, and K. Tsuchiya.** 1983. Role of type 1 fimbriae in the pathogenesis of ascending urinary tract infection induced by *Escherichia coli* in mice. *Infect. Immun.* **39:**1307–1315.

39. Jabri, E., M. B. Carr, R. P. Hausinger, and P. A. Karplus. 1995. The crystal structure of urease from *Klebsiella aerogenes*. *Science* **268**:998–1004.
40. Johnson, D. E., G. Russell, C. V. Lockatell, J. C. Zulty, J. W. Warren, and H. L. T. Mobley. 1993. Contribution of *Proteus mirabilis* urease to persistence, urolithiasis, and acute pyelonephritis in a mouse model of ascending urinary tract infection. *Infect. Immun.* **61**:2748–2754.
41. Jones, B. D., C. V. Lockateil, D. E. Johnson, J. W. Warren, and H. L. T. Mobley. 1990. Construction of a urease-negative mutant of *Proteus mirabilis*: analysis of virulence in a mouse model of ascending urinary tract infection. *Infect. Immun.* **58**:1120–1123.
42. Kabha, K., L. Nissimov, A. Athamna, Y. Keisari, H. Parolis, L. A. S. Parolis, R. M. Grue, J. Schlepper-Schafer, A. R. B. Ezekowitz, D. E. Ohman, and I. Ofek. 1995. Relationships among capsular structure, phagocytosis, and mouse virulence in *Klebsiella pneumoniae*. *Infect. Immun.* **63**:847–852.
43. Konopka, K., A. Bindereif, and J. B. Nielands. 1982. Aerobactin-mediated utilization of transferrin iron. *Biochemistry* **21**:6503–6508.
44. Korhonen, T. K., E. Tarkka, H. Ranta, and K. Haahtela. 1983. Type 3 fimbriae of *Klebsiella* sp.: molecular characterization and role in bacterial adhesion to plant roots. *J. Bacteriol.* **155**:860–865.
45. Laasko, D. H., M. K. Homonylo, S. J. Wilmot, and C. Whitfield. 1988. Transfer and expression of the genetic determinants for O and K antigen synthesis in *Escherichia coli* O9:K(A)30 and *Klebsiella* sp. O1:K20, in *Escherichia coli* K12. *Can. J. Microbiol.* **34**:987–992.
46. Lerner, S. P., M. J. Gleeson, and D. P. Griffith. 1989. Infection stones. *J. Urol.* **141**:753–759.
47. Lye, W. C., R. K. T. Chan, E. J. C. Lee, and G. Kumarasinghe. 1992. Urinary tract infections in patients with diabetes mellitus. *J. Infect.* **24**:169–174.
48. Maayan, M. C., I. Ofek, O. Medalia, and M. Aronson. 1985. Population shift in mannose-specific fimbriated phase of *Klebsiella pneumoniae* during experimental urinary tract infection in mice. *Infect. Immun.* **49**:785–789.
49. MacLaren, D. M., and P. G. H. Peerbooms. 1986. Urinary infections by urea-splitting micro-organisms, p. 183–195. *In* A. W. Asscher and W. Brumfitt (ed.), *Microbial Diseases in Nephrology*. John Wiley & Sons, Inc., New York.
50. McCartney, A. C., J. Clark, and H. J. E. Lewi. 1985. Bacteriological study of renal calculi. *Eur. J. Clin. Microbiol.* **4**:553–555.
51. McLean, R. J. C., J. C. Nickel, K.-J. Cheng, and J. W. Costerton. 1988. The ecology and pathogenicity of urease-producing bacteria in the urinary tract. *Crit. Rev. Microbiol.* **16**:37–79.
52. Meno, Y., and K. Amako. 1990. Morphological evidence for penetration of anti-O antibody through the capsule of *Klebsiella pneumoniae*. *Infect. Immun.* **58**:1421–1428.
53. Meno, Y., and K. Amako. 1991. The surface hydrophobicity and avirulent charcter of an encapsulated strain of *Klebsiella pneumoniae*. *Microbiol. Immun.* **35**:841–848.
54. Millner, O. E. J., J. A. Andersen, M. E. Appler, C. E. Benjamin, J. G. Edwards, D. T. Humphrey, and E. M. Shearer. 1982. Flurofamide: a potential inhibitor of bacterial urease with a potential clinical utility in the treatment of infection induced urinary stones. *J. Urol.* **127**:346–350.
55. Mobley, H. L. T., G. R. Chippendale, J. H. Tenney, A. R. Mayrer, L. J. Crisp, J. L. Penner, and J. W. Warren. 1988. MR/K hemagglutination of *Providencia stuartii* correlates with adherence to catheters and with persistence in catheter-associated bacteriuria. *J. Infect. Dis.* **157**:264–271.
56. Mobley, H. L. T., and J. W. Warren. 1987. Urease-positive bacteriuria and obstruction of long-term urinary catheters. *J. Clin. Microbiol.* **25**:2216–2217.
57. Montgomerie, J. Z. 1979. Epidemiology of *Klebsiella* and hospital-associated infections. *Rev. Infect. Dis.* **1**:736–753.
58. Montgomerie, J. Z., D. S. Gilmore, M. A. Ashley, D. G. Schick, and E. M. Jimenez. 1989. Long-term colonization of spinal cord injury patients with *Klebsiella pneumoniae*. *J. Clin. Microbiol.* **27**:1613–1616.
59. Musher, D. M., C. Saenz, and D. Griffith. 1974. Interaction between acetohydroxamic acid and 12 antibiotics against 14 gram-negative pathogenic bacteria. *Antimicrob. Agents Chemother.* **5**:106–110.
60. Nassif, X., J. M. Fournier, J. Arondel, and P. J. Sansonetti. 1989. Mucoid phenotype of *Klebsiella pneumoniae* is a plasmid-encoded virulence factor. *Infect. Immun.* **57**:546–552.
61. Nassif, X., N. Honore, T. Vasselon, S. T. Cole, and P. J. Sansonetti. 1989. Positive

control of colanic acid synthesis in *Escherichia coli* by *rmpA* and *rmpB*, two virulence-plasmid genes of *Klebsiella pneumoniae*. *Mol. Microbiol.* **3:**1349–1359.

62. **Nassif, X., and P. J. Sansonetti.** 1986. Correlation of the virulence of *Klebsiella pneumoniae* K1 and K2 with the presence of a plasmid encoding aerobactin. *Infect. Immun.* **54:**603–608.

63. **Old, D. C., A. Tavendale, and B. W. Senior.** 1985. A comparative study of the type 3 fimbriae of *Klebsiella* species. *J. Med. Microbiol.* **20:**203–214.

64. **Orskov, I., and M. A. Fife-Asbury.** 1977. New *Klebsiella* capsular antigen, K82, and the deletion of five of those previously assigned. *Int. J. Syst. Bacteriol.* **27:**386–387.

65. **Orskov, I., C. Svanborg-Eden, and F. Orskov.** 1988. Aerobactin production of serotyped *Escherichia coli* from urinary tract infections. *Med. Microbiol.* **177:**9–14.

66. **Park, I.-S., and R. P. Hausinger.** 1995. Evidence for the presence of urease apoprotein complexes containing UreD, UreF, and UreG in cells that are competent for in vivo enzyme activation. *J. Bacteriol.* **177:**1947–1951.

67. **Petit, A., D. Sirot, C. Chanal, J. Sirot, R. Labia, G. Gerbaud, and R. Cluzel.** 1988. Novel plasmid-mediated β-lactamase in clinical isolates of *Klebsiella pneumoniae* more resistant to ceftazidime than to other broad-spectrum cephalosporins. *Antimicrob. Agents Chemother.* **32:**626–630.

68. **Podschun, R., A. Fischer, and U. Ullmann.** 1992. Siderophore production of *Klebsiella* species isolated from different sources. *Int. J. Med. Microbiol. Virol. Parasitol. Infect. Dis.* **276:**481–486.

69. **Podschun, R., D. Sievers, A. Fischer, and U. Ullmann.** 1993. Serotypes, hemagglutinins, siderophore synthesis, and serum resistance of *Klebsiella* isolates causing human urinary tract infections. *J. Infect. Dis.* **168:**1415–1421.

70. **Pollack, M.** 1976. Significance of circulating capsular antigen in *Klebsiella* infections. *Infect. Immun.* **13:**1543–1548.

71. **Przondo-Hessek, A., and G. Pulverer.** 1983. Hemagglutinins of *Klebsiella pneumoniae* and *Klebsiella oxytoca*. *Zentralbl. Bakteriol. Mikrobiol. Hyg. Abt 1 Orig. A Med. Mikrobiol. Infektionskr. Parasitol.* **255:**472–478.

72. **Riser, E., and P. Noone.** 1981. *Klebsiella* capsular type versus site of isolation. *J. Clin. Pathol.* **34:**552–555.

73. **Schurtz, T. A., D. B. Hornick, T. K. Korhonen, and S. Clegg.** 1994. The type 3 fimbrial adhesin gene (*mrkD*) of *Klebsiella* species is not conserved among all fimbriate strains. *Infect. Immun.* **62:**4186–4191.

74. **Selden, R., S. Lee, W. L. L. Wang, J. V. Bennett, and T. C. Eickhoff.** 1971. Nosocomial Klebsiella infections: intestinal colonization as a reservoir. *Ann. Intern. Med.* **74:**657–664.

75. **Sewell, C. M., M. A. Koza, R. J. Luchi, and E. J. Young.** 1988. Risk factors associated with a cluster of urinary tract infections in a geriatric unit caused by *Klebsiella pneumoniae* resistant to multiple antibiotics. *Am. J. Infect. Control* **16:**66–71.

76. **Sirot, D., J. Sirot, R. Labia, A. Morand, P. Courvalin, A. Darfeuille-Michaud, R. Perroux, and R. Cluzel.** 1987. Transferable resistance to third-generation cephalosporins in clinical isolates of *Klebsiella pneumoniae*: identification of CTX-1, a novel β-lactamase. *J. Antimicrob. Chemother.* **20:**323–334.

77. **Smith, S. M., J. T. Digori, and R. H. K. Eng.** 1982. Epidemiology of *Klebsiella* antibiotic resistance and serotypes. *J. Clin. Microbiol.* **16:**868–873.

78. **Stamey, T. A.** 1980. Infection stones, p. 430–474. In T. A. Stamey (ed.), *Pathogenesis and Treatment of Urinary Tract Infections*. The Williams & Wilkins Co., Baltimore.

79. **Stotka, J. L., and M. E. Rupp.** 1991. *Klebsiella pneumoniae* urinary tract infection complicated by endophthalmitis, perinephric abscess, and ecthyma gangrenosum. *South. Med. J.* **84:**790–793.

80. **Svanborg-Eden, C., and P. de Man.** 1987. Bacterial virulence factors in urinary tract infections. *Infect. Dis. Clin. North Am.* **1:**731–750.

81. **Takeuchi, H., K. Kobashi, and O. Yoshida.** 1980. Prevention of infected urinary stones in rats by urease inhibitor. *Invest. Urol.* **18:**102–105.

82. **Tarkkanen, A.-M., B. L. Allen, B. Westerlund, H. Holthofer, P. Kuusela, L. Ristell, S. Clegg, and T. K. Korhonen.** 1990. Type V collagen as the target for type 3 fimbriae, enterobacterial adherence organelles. *Mol. Microbiol.* **4:**1353–1361.

83. **Tarkkanen, A.-M., B. L. Allen, P. H. Williams, M. Kauppi, K. Haahtela, A. Siitonen, I. Orskov, F. Orskov, S. Clegg, and T. K. Korhonen.** 1992. Fimbriation, capsulation, and iron-scavenging systems of

*Klebsiella* strains associated with human urinary tract infection. *Infect. Immun.* **60:** 1187–1192.

84. **Tiel-Menkveld, C. J. V., J. K. Mentjox-Vervuust, B. Oudega, and F. K. de Graaf.** 1982. Siderophore production by *Enterobacter cloacae* and a common receptor protein for the uptake of aerobactin and cloacin DF13. *J. Bacteriol.* **150:**490–497.

85. **van Oss, C. J.** 1978. Phagocytosis as a surface phenomenon. *Annu. Rev. Microbiol.* **32:** 19–39.

86. **Wacharotayankun, R., Y. Arakawa, M. Ohta, K. Tanaka, T. Akashi, M. Mori, and N. Kato.** 1993. Enhancement of extracapsular polysaccharide synthesis in *Klebsiella pneumoniae* by RmpA2, which shows homology to NtrC and FixJ. *Infect. Immun.* **61:** 3164–3174.

87. **Williams, P., M. A. Smith, P. Stevenson, E. Griffiths, and J. M. T. Tomas.** 1989. Novel aerobactin receptor in *Klebsiella pneumoniae*. *J. Gen. Microbiol.* **135:**317–3181.

88. **Williams, P. H., and N. H. Carbonetti.** 1986. Iron, siderophores and the pursuit of virulence: independence of the aerobactin and enterochelin iron uptake systems in *Escherichia coli*. *Infect. Immun.* **51:**942–947.

# VIRULENCE FACTORS OF *STAPHYLOCOCCUS SAPROPHYTICUS*, *STAPHYLOCOCCUS EPIDERMIDIS*, AND ENTEROCOCCI

Sören G. Gatermann, M.D., Ph.D.

## 12

## ENTEROCOCCI

The genus *Enterococcus* currently comprises more than 15 species, two of which (*Enterococcus faecalis* and *Enterococcus faecium*) cause the majority of human infections. Most species are very hardy organisms that withstand extreme environmental conditions such as sodium azide, 6.5% sodium chloride, heat (45°C), and drying. Enterococci, especially *E. faecalis* and *E. faecium*, are members of the indigenous flora of the human bowel. They are only rarely associated with primary infections in the noncompromised host. In hospitalized or otherwise compromised patients, they cause increasingly problematic nosocomial infections (88, 101); the problem is augmented by the development of resistance to almost any antibiotic, including vancomycin and ampicillin (2, 52). Enterococci account for 7.3% of nosocomially acquired bacteremias, and the incidence of enterococcal bacteremia is about 1.2/1,000 admissions (88). Many of these infections are thought to originate from previous colonization or infection of the urinary tract (40, 43, 88, 133). The frequency of isolation of enterococci from the urinary tracts of hospitalized patients has risen from 6% in 1975 to 16% in 1984 in one study (101) or from 11.1% in 1980 to 20.8% in 1985 in another (43). Long-term urinary catheterization (80) is a well-known factor predisposing to enterococcal infection or colonization of the urinary tract.

## Virulence Factors of Enterococci

### ADHESINS AND SURFACE FACTORS

*E. faecalis* can exchange plasmids that may code for resistance determinants or a hemolysin-bacteriocin system by conjugal exchange. This species possesses a unique sex pheromone system whereby a strain that does not possess a certain plasmid produces and excretes a short hydrophobic peptide that is sensed by a donor strain carrying the corresponding plasmid (13, 148). In response to the sex pheromone, the donor strain produces a surface protein called aggregation substance that causes clumping of donor with recipient cells, thereby facilitating conjugative plasmid transfer. After the plasmid has been transferred, synthesis and excretion of the sex

*Sören G. Gatermann, Institut für Medizinische Mikrobiologie, Hochhaus am Augustusplatz, 55101 Mainz, Germany.*

pheromone and, consequently, of the aggregation substance cease, making both cells possible future donors. The major function of this system is probably to collect and distribute plasmids between strains of *E. faecalis*; recent data, however, indicate that the aggregation substance may also mediate adhesion to eukaryotic cells. Electron micrographs of bacteria expressing the aggregation substance are shown in Fig. 1.

The gene for one aggregation substance (*asa1*) codes for a protein of 1,296 amino acids. The deduced amino acid sequence (24) possesses the typical LPXTG membrane anchor sequence of gram-positive cell surface proteins and also has the glycine-rich region in its C-terminal part (Fig.

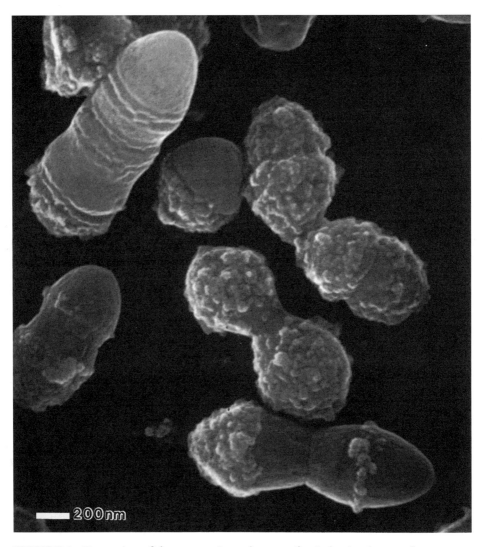

**FIGURE 1** Expression of the aggregation substance after induction by sex pheromones. Expression was induced by the addition of chemically synthesized sex pheromone to growing cells. The aggregation substance was detected with antibody to it and gold-labeled protein A.

2). No further similarities to surface proteins of gram-positive bacteria are found. Within the amino acid sequence are one RGDS and one RGDV motif. These motifs are typically found in the matrix proteins (e.g., fibronectin, fibrinogen) of higher organisms. The matrix proteins bind to their receptors, the integrins, on the eukaryotic cell via these sequences. Therefore, the aggregation substance may also function as an adhesin to eukaryotic cells expressing integrins.

Enterococci expressing the aggregation substance bind to a pig renal tubular cell line more efficiently than those not expressing the surface protein (77; Fig. 3). In addition, adhesion could be inhibited by the RGDS peptide, which causes a 34% reduction in adherence. Because expression of the surface protein requires induction by the corresponding pheromone, one would expect the presence of such peptides to be necessary. However, as-yet-unidentified substances present in serum and serum-free cell culture media can induce production of the aggregation substance. These observations make it conceivable that conditions that allow expression of the adhesin within the human host do exist. Functional analyses of the aggregation substance have shown that sequences needed for the clumping reaction are located in the N-terminal domain of the protein, whereas the recognition sequence for integrins is located in the C-terminal half (Fig. 2).

Guzman et al. (45) reported that strains of enterococci isolated from endocarditis adhere more efficiently to Girardi heart cells than do enterococci isolated from patients with urinary tract infections (UTIs). In contrast, UTI strains show better adherence to human embryonic kidney cells. When the bacteria are grown in the presence of serum instead of brain heart infusion, adhesion to all cell types increases, with the most dramatic increase (eightfold) being observed with urinary tract isolates and adherence to Girardi heart cells. A subsequent report showed that adherence of *E. faecalis* is mediated by carbohydrates present on the surface of the bacterial cell. Those authors found that D-galactose and L-fucose are present only on strains isolated from endocarditis patients and that these carbohydrates mediate adherence to Girardi heart cells. In contrast, urinary tract isolates express on their surfaces D-mannose- and D-glucose-containing adhesins that allow efficient adhesion to cells from the urinary tract. When these strains are grown in serum, expression of the surface molecules is modulated, and the

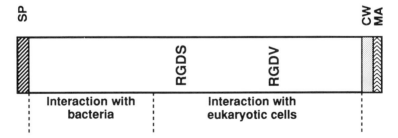

**FIGURE 2** Structure of the aggregation substance Asa1. Domains of the aggregation substance as determined from the deduced amino acid sequence or by functional studies are outlined. MA, membrane anchor region at the C terminus; CW, cell wall-spanning region; SP, signal peptide; RGDS and RGDV, approximate positions of these motifs. The regions responsible for interactions with bacteria or eukaryotic cells are also delineated. Reproduced from reference 148 with permission.

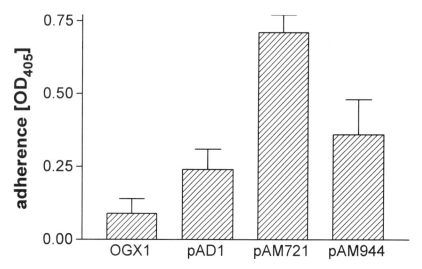

**FIGURE 3** The aggregation substance contributes to adhesion. A plasmid-free *E. faecalis* strain (OGX1) does not express the aggregation substance; strain OGX1 containing plasmid pAD1 inducibly expresses the aggregation substance; with plasmid pAM721, this strain produces the aggregation substance constitutively; and with plasmid pAM944, a truncated adhesin is produced, of which the majority is released into the medium and only a small amount is retained. Adherence to a renal tubular cell line (LLC-PK$_1$) was determined with an ELISA. OD$_{405}$, optical density at 405 nm. Modified from reference 77 with permission.

bacteria began to express D-galactose- and L-fucose-containing adhesins, thus facilitating attachment to Girardi heart cells.

In addition to the aggregation substance and the carbohydrates, both of which may serve as adhesins that directly interact with the target cells, *E. faecalis* is able to bind fibronectin and albumin (134). The bacterial receptor for fibronectin apparently contains protein and carbohydrates, but it has not been characterized in detail or purified. The same holds true for the albumin-binding structure. Binding of fibronectin or albumin has been reported for many gram-positive bacteria and is thought to be a virulence factor in endocarditis (122), wound infections, or catheter-associated infections. It has not yet been established for *E. faecalis* whether fibronectin binding facilitates adhesion to host tissues. It was, however, suggested that binding of albumin, which decreases the surface hydrophobicity of *E. faecalis,* may conceal bacterial surface antigens from the immune system (134).

## TOXINS

Many clinical isolates of *E. faecalis,* isolated from patients with a wide variety of infections, produce a cytolysin that lyses human, rabbit, and horse erythrocytes (68, 78). This cytolysin can also lyse a wide variety of gram-positive bacteria. The system consists of two components that have been called A and L substances. Component A (CylA), which has homologies to serine proteinases, is believed to play a role in activation of the precursor of cytolytic component L (CylL) (66, 131). Recent molecular analysis showed that a third component, CylB, is required for externalization of the cytolysin precursor (37), CylL. Activation of the cytolysin occurs after externalization by CylA (66). The activator apparently also confers immunity to the cytolysin on the producing cell. The cytolysin-bacteriocin system is encoded by the plasmid pAD1 and similar plasmids that also carry determinants needed for conjugative transfer of the plasmid. Hemolysins or cytolysins of a wide variety of bacteria contribute to virulence of the organisms (5). Besides destroying cellular layers, thereby allowing access to the underlying tissue, the toxins may also liberate iron from erythrocytes or may cause dysfunction of other host systems. In a mouse model, *E. faecalis* rendered nonhemolytic by transposon insertions into pAD1 exhibited much higher 50% lethal doses than strains that showed normal hemolytic activity. Virulence of a hyperhemolytic plasmid copy mutant was increased (67). Since those authors did not find any evidence for systemic hemolysis, they suggested that death of the animals was not due to depletion of erythrocytes.

In an endophthalmitis model with cytolytic and noncytolytic strains of *E. faecalis,* the presence of the hemolysin increased the retinal inflammatory response, leading to destruction of tissue (71).

Although both studies showed that expression of the hemolysin significantly contributes to virulence of *E. faecalis,* they did not establish the mechanism by which the toxin causes this damage. In clinical surveys, the hemolytic phenotype of *E. faecalis* was detected more often in isolates causing infection (68) and in strains with high levels of aminoglycoside resistance (65) than in susceptible strains or in enterococci isolated from feces.

The sex pheromones, which normally function in the plasmid collection system, may also contribute to pathogenesis by triggering an inflammatory response. Some of these hydrophobic peptides are able to induce a chemotactic response in neutrophils, induce polarization of the cells, and trigger superoxide production (19, 118). The sex pheromones act through the *N*-formylmethionyl receptor on the leukocyte membrane (118). Peptide cPD1 is a much better inducer than the less hydrophobic pheromone cAD1 (19). These results not only show that the sex pheromones have ancillary functions during an enterococcal infection but also indicate that N formylation of prokaryotic peptides is not an absolute prerequisite for induction of chemotaxis.

## Pathogenesis of Infections with Enterococci

Knowledge of the virulence factors of enterococci and the pathogenesis of enterococcal infections is comparatively scarce. Only a few reports used animal models to assess the virulence of enterococci or to study the relevance of putative virulence factors. Studies focusing on endocarditis suggested that the combination of hemolysin and aggregation substance is associated with increased mortality, whereas the weight of the vegetations formed on cardiac valves correlates with production of the aggregation substance (10). These conclusions, obtained by experimental infection of rabbits, were challenged recently by experiments with rats that did not find any influence by expression of the aggregation substance or the hemolysin on vegetation weight or mortality (149). However, many facts still have to be reconciled, such as the influence of the animal model and of the different strains used for infection. Production of the hemolysin is evidently associated with tissue destruction in endophthalmitis and with mortality after intraperitoneal challenge. In addition, there are indications that hemolytic enterococci have a greater propensity than other enterococcal strains to cause kidney infections (100).

Although it is clear from clinical data that enterococci can cause UTIs, very large inocula are needed to induce infection in animals (53). Lower numbers of enterococci may contribute to the pathogenesis of UTIs by enhancing the virulence of gram-negative rods in mixed infections (143).

Because enterococci bind to exfoliated uroepithelial cells, human embryonic kidney cells, and porcine renal tubular cells, this species obviously possesses adhesive properties, which are regarded as a prerequisite for UTI. Adhesion may be mediated by the RGDS motif of the aggregation substance or by carbohydrate-containing adhesins. It is of special interest that growth in serum modulates expression of the surface adhesins, giving rise to cells that are able to adhere to heart cells. It is thus conceivable that after colonizing the urinary tract, *E. faecalis* gains access to the vascular system, where a change in the expression of surface factors allows the bacterium to colonize endothelia and cause endocarditis. This sequence of events, however, is still speculative, and much more work is needed to define possible virulence factors of enterococci and assess the function of these factors during the infectious process. Because of the advent of multiresistant, almost untreatable microorganisms, such knowledge may be crucial in the development of new antimicrobial strategies.

## STAPHYLOCOCCUS SAPROPHYTICUS

In 1962, Torres Pereira reported the isolation of coagulase-negative staphylococci from the urine of female patients suffering from acute UTI (142). The isolates appeared to be homogeneous, since they all possessed a common antigen (arbitrarily named antigen 51), which was determined by conventional serologic techniques, and were novobiocin resistant. In subsequent years, several reports of staphylococci as urinary tract pathogens were published. The organism was found to belong to *Micrococcus* subgroup 3 (later called *Staphylococcus saprophyticus* subgroup 3) (92, 95, 98) of the Baird-Par-ker scheme. The species was later reclassified as *Staphylococcus saprophyticus* (123).

### Infections with *S. saprophyticus*

*S. saprophyticus* mainly causes UTIs, especially in young female outpatients. Notably, these infections are very uncommon in hospitalized patients or in males (95, 98). Torres Pereira already had reported that the isolates were mainly from females (142), and later surveys confirmed this finding. Maskell found 82 infections in women but only 1 in a male patient (92); Digranes and Oeding (17) reported 59 of 60 isolates as being from women. They also pointed out that most (55 of 59) strains came from outpatients, a fact that was corroborated by Wallmark et al. (145) and Marrie et al. (91), who showed that *S. saprophyticus* accounts for less than 1% of bacteriurias in hospitalized patients although it is frequently isolated from female outpatients. *S. saprophyticus* was found in 42.3% of all cases of bacteriuria in women aged 16 to 25 years (145). The infections tend to occur more often during late summer and fall (92, 145), an incidence that parallels the incidence of sexually transmitted diseases (150). Rather severe symptoms, including hematuria, pyuria, and flank pain, are commonly observed in infections with *S. saprophyticus* (48, 59, 75, 92, 145). Signs of renal involvement are not uncommon, and reduced renal concentration capacity that returns to normal after appropriate treatment has been reported (61, 81). That the kidneys may be infected is also suggested by the isolation of *S. saprophyticus* from renal calculi (22). Pyelonephritis with septicemia (38, 79) or endocarditis (135) may occur but apparently is uncommon.

Although the great majority of infections with *S. saprophyticus* occur in women, isolation from men with UTI has been described. Hovelius et al. (57) reported that, as with UTIs caused by other organisms, *S. saprophyticus* infections are more often found in patients with predisposing conditions such as indwelling urinary catheters or obstructions. Their patients also tended to be older, and many of them (21 [41%] of 51) were hospitalized, which is in stark contrast to the situation seen in women. In men without predisposing conditions, the symptoms were very similar to those observed in women. It was also suggested that *S. saprophyticus* may cause urethritis in men (62). Hovelius et al. isolated the organism more often from patients presenting with symptoms of urethritis than from patients without symptoms or from healthy controls (20.8, 14.9, and 7.1%, respectively).

## Epidemiology of *S. saprophyticus*

As pointed out above, UTIs with *S. saprophyticus* are more frequent during late summer and fall. During those parts of the year, urethral and rectal cultures contain the organism more often (111, 116). In cases of acute UTI, *S. saprophyticus* can be found on the mucous membranes of the urogenital tract or in rectal cultures (50, 73, 90, 116). Plasmid profiles of isolates grown from the rectums of infected patients resembled those isolated from the urinary tract (50). These data suggest that infection with *S. saprophyticus* proceeds by the same route as infection with other urinary pathogens. However, in a prospective study including 19 female subjects colonized by *S. saprophyticus,* Rupp et al. (116) failed to identify any progression to symptomatic UTI. Several authors have noted that many women suffering from UTI with *S. saprophyticus* report recent sexual intercourse (36, 116). Hormonal influences are suggested by the finding that infected women tend to have had their menstrual periods more recently and to have a concurrent diagnosis of vaginal candidosis (116). Hedman and Ringertz (48) found that infection is associated with prior outdoor swimming and with an occupation in meat processing or meat production. This finding is in concord with the observation that *S. saprophyticus* can be isolated from the carcasses of slaughtered animals (50), from the gloves of meat handlers (50), and from rectal cultures, udders, and fodder of pigs, cattle, and goat (49, 51, 90). It was therefore suggested that ingestion of contaminated meat precedes colonization and infection with *S. saprophyticus;* however, infections in vegetarians are not exceptionally rare (48).

## Virulence Factors of *S. saprophyticus*

Soon after *S. saprophyticus* became an established cause of UTIs, suggestions concerning possible virulence factors appeared. Hovelius et al. (61) described the typical microscopic appearance of urine infected with *S. saprophyticus:* clusters of staphylococci adhering to exfoliated epithelial cells and to hyaline or cellular casts. Studies of the adherence of *S. saprophyticus* to various eukaryotic cells and to extracellular material ensued. The organism was found to bind to sheep erythrocytes, causing hemagglutination (58), and to attach to various epithelial cells (1, 14, 89). When *S. saprophyticus* was isolated from the renal pelvis of a patient with urinary calculi (61), it was noted that the organism produces the enzyme urease, which is implicated in the pathogenesis of UTI by *Proteus mirabilis* (104).

## Surface Properties

### ADHESION TO EUKARYOTIC CELLS

*S. saprophyticus* adheres to exfoliated cells from the urinary tract in higher numbers than *Escherichia coli, Enterobacter aerogenes,* or *Staphylococcus epidermidis,* and only a very small proportion of cells do not carry bacteria (30, 89). No differences have been found between the mean numbers of bacteria adhering to exfoliated uroepithelial cells from male and female donors (14). However, a higher proportion of female cells carry bacteria. In the same study, exfoliated buccal cells and cells scraped off the skin were used for comparison. *S. saprophyticus* adhered in higher numbers to uroepithelial cells than to those from other sources. A later survey (74) studied the adherence of *S. saprophyticus* isolated from urine, skin, and the respiratory tract to epithelial cells exfoliated from these organs. No significant differences in adhesion capabilities were found, although *S. saprophyticus* isolated from the respiratory tract tends to adhere more strongly to respiratory epithelia. *S. saprophyticus* also attaches to organ cultures of human male urethra (15). Interestingly, lowering the pH from 7.5 to 5.5 during the attachment phase increases the numbers of bacteria bound to exfoliated cells or to organ cultures. This finding is interpreted as an indication of reduced surface charges at acidic pH, which allows closer contact between prokaryotic and eukaryotic cells.

Various transformed eukaryotic cell lines such as HEp-2, HeLa, Vero, MDCK, and LLC-PK$_1$ have also been used (1, 28, 30, 97). The highest numbers of bacteria per cell are usually achieved with HEp-2 cells. Several investigators noted a marked variation in adherence capabilities among clinical isolates of *S. saprophyticus* (30, 97). Strains that were almost nonadherent and others that adhered in very high numbers were found. Adhesion to HeLa, Vero, and MDCK cells was stronger at 37°C than at 25 or 4°C (1). When compared, the adherence of *S. saprophyticus* was usually much stronger than that of *S. epidermidis*.

These phenomenological studies suggest that *S. saprophyticus* possesses the ability to adhere to eukaryotic cells and that it may have a preference for certain cell types. They do not give any indication of the nature of the adhesin. Teti et al. (139) showed that lipoteichoic acids (LTA) isolated from *S. saprophyticus* inhibit binding of two strains to exfoliated uroepithelial cells; deacylated LTA is not effective. Although this suggests that, similar to group A streptococci (3) or *S. aureus* (8), LTA mediates adhesion, other groups reported that adherence of *S. saprophyticus* to serum proteins deposited on polyetherurethane disks (146) or to renal tubular cells (LLC-PK$_1$, derived from pig [28]) could be inhibited by *N*-acetyl-D-galactosamine. A surface receptor specific for structures possessing *N*-acetylgalactosamine-containing moieties was therefore proposed. In this context, it is of interest that urothelia express surface structures containing *N*-acetylgalactosamine (146).

## HEMAGGLUTINATION

In 1979, Hovelius and Mårdh (58) reported hemagglutination of sheep erythrocytes by 28 of 30 strains of *S. saprophyticus*. In contrast, *S. epidermidis* and *Staphylococcus aureus* hemagglutinate only rarely. This property is heat labile (86°C, 10 min) and sensitive to trypsin. Hemagglutination titers are reduced by treatment with trichloroacetic acid (10%) but not with EDTA (0.1 M). These properties indicate that the hemagglutinin is probably a surface-exposed protein of *S. saprophyticus*.

Human erythrocytes or those from cattle or guinea pigs are usually not agglutinated (58). One group (4), however, described two subsets of strains: one that agglutinated horse erythrocytes as well and one that interacted with rabbit erythrocytes. This finding implies that at least two different hemagglutinins exist in *S. saprophyticus*. That hemagglutination titers differ substantially between clinical isolates (30, 97) points to a similar conclusion: either one hemagglutinin is differentially expressed, or more than one hemagglutinin is involved in binding.

Interestingly, the hemagglutinin is expressed only when the bacteria are grown in liquid media; agar-grown bacteria will not hemagglutinate (58). It is not unusual that efficient expression of surface proteins requires carefully defined culture conditions. Culture on solid or in liquid media induces different surface proteins in *S.*

*aureus* (9), and the type 1 pili of *Escherichia coli* are expressed on solid media only (119).

Many surface appendages of gram-negative organisms bind to structures on the eukaryotic cell that contain carbohydrates. Binding can therefore be inhibited by these sugars. By analogy, a carbohydrate specificity of the *S. saprophyticus* hemagglutinin was sought. Gunnarsson et al. (44) reported that structures containing terminal $\beta$-D-galactose-$p$-(1-4)-$\beta$-D-2-acetamido-2-deoxyglucose-$p$-(1- are good inhibitors of hemagglutination (at concentrations of 200 to 300 $\mu$g/ml). However, other authors (4), using different strains, were not able to show inhibition by $N$-acetyllactosamine even at much higher concentrations (0.1 M); they reported activity of a combination of $N$-acetylgalactosamine and $N$-acetylglucosamine or of $N$-acetylneuraminic acid (sialic acid) and $N$-acetylglucosamine. Inhibition of hemagglutination by mannose, lactose, and, for some strains, $N$-acetyllactosamine was also reported (97) (all sugars were employed at 5 mg/ml and 0.1 M). In our group, we were not able to show any inhibition by these sugars or by combinations thereof.

The structures mediating adhesion and hemagglutination appear to be different. Teti et al. (139) reported inhibition of adherence but not of hemagglutination by LTA. Strains can be found that do not cause hemagglutination but that do adhere to epithelial cells (30, 97). Moreover, growth on agar abolishes hemagglutination but increases adherence to HEp-2 cells (30). Accordingly, we did not see a correlation between hemagglutination titers and adherence capacities in this study. In contrast, Fujita et al. found good correlation between adherence to human uretheral epithelium, as quantitated by electron microscopic enumeration, and hemagglutination (23).

## SURFACE HYDROPHOBICITY

Expression of hydrophobic surfaces may facilitate attachment of bacteria to artificial devices (e.g., catheters) and host tissues. Accordingly, hydrophobic properties are more prevalent in *S. aureus* strains isolated from patients with infections than in those from cultures of the anterior nares of healthy laboratory personnel (82). In studies using the BATH (bacterial adhesion to hydrocarbons) test, many (79 of 100) strains of *S. saprophyticus* isolated from patients with UTIs exhibited a hydrophobic surface (127); only 2 of 100 were not hydrophobic. Hydrophobicity is associated with expression of hemagglutination and is probably mediated by a protein (96). In nonhemagglutinating strains, the expression of this property can be effected by culture in liquid media. Thus, many strains of *S. saprophyticus* possess the propensity to exhibit a hydrophobic surface that may, in part, explain the adhesive properties of the organism.

## BINDING OF EXTRACELLULAR MATRIX PROTEINS

Many bacteria bind to human extracellular matrix proteins such as fibronectin or laminin. Fibronectin binding has been found in a variety of gram-positive and gram-negative bacteria and has been implicated in the pathogenesis of infections caused by these organisms (147). Binding to *S. aureus* has been studied most extensively, and two fibronectin-binding proteins have been found and characterized (72). In coagulase-negative staphylococci, binding of fibronectin has been described for several species, including *S. saprophyticus* (138), but no structures associated with this property have been identified. Switalski et al. (138) used fibronectin purified from plasma and labeled with $^{125}$I to demonstrate binding in 11 of 21 strains. Later experiments that employed fibronectin bound to latex particles found agglutination in only a low percentage of strains (107); those authors reported agglutination by laminin-coated latex spheres instead. These conflicting data prompted us to reassess binding of *S.*

*saprophyticus* to fibronectin. In our experiments, hemagglutinating strains bound to fibronectin immobilized on microtiter plates, but no binding was seen with nonhemagglutinating strains (31). Binding was found to be saturable by increasing the number of bacterial cells added. Our hypothesis that the hemagglutinin is responsible for fibronectin binding is supported by the observation that antibody to the hemagglutinin inhibits the interaction, while an antiserum to the surface-associated protein of *S. saprophyticus* does not. In addition, the purified hemagglutinin binds soluble labeled fibronectin. Interestingly, hemagglutination of *S. saprophyticus* is not inhibited by the addition of soluble fibronectin. This indicates that the domains on the hemagglutinin responsible for hemagglutination and those necessary for fibronectin binding are different. Heparin, the D3 peptide (an analog of the fibronectin-binding sequence of the *S. aureus* fibronectin receptor), or RGDS-containing peptides (analogs of the cell attachment site of fibronectin) do not inhibit binding of fibronectin; neither does deglycosylation of fibronectin. The binding site on the fibronectin molecule therefore remains unknown. The data also indicate that the hemagglutinin of *S. saprophyticus* is an at-least-bifunctional molecule that mediates binding to erythrocytes and fibronectin.

Multiple specificities are not uncommon in the surface proteins of gram-positive and gram-negative bacteria. The M protein of group A streptococci binds several serum proteins (20, 126), the YadA protein of *Yersinia enterocolitica* interacts with cellular fibronectin (128) and collagen (129), and a surface protein of *S. aureus* binds various matrix proteins (93). Multispecific receptors may be advantageous to microorganisms that exist in several environments, obviating the need for a quickly responding regulation system. Notably, *S. saprophyticus* has been isolated from various environments, including live and slaughtered animals, their fodder, and humans.

## Surface Structures

### *S. SAPROPHYTICUS* SURFACE-ASSOCIATED PROTEIN (Ssp)

Interactions with eukaryotic cells such as hemagglutination or adhesion are mediated by distinct surface structures in many bacteria. Especially in gram-negative organisms, a plethora of surface organelles such as fimbriae and fibrilla as well as nonfimbrial adhesins have been identified and characterized. The structure often consists of small subunits that have distinct functions such as structural integrity or adherence. Some gram-positive bacteria also possess proteinaceous surface appendages. These proteins are usually larger and possess several domains with different functions. The group A streptococci express the fibrillar M protein that mediates adhesion to eukaryotic cells and matrix proteins and plays a role in the pathogenesis of sequelae associated with infections caused by this bacterial species (20). In *Streptococcus sanguis*, fimbriae and fibrilla were demonstrated by electron microscopy (46), and the aggregation substance of enterococci has a distinctive appearance when it is visualized by scanning electron microscopy (25). Although many surface proteins have been identified and characterized in *S. aureus*, knowledge of the surface structures of coagulase-negative staphylococci is comparatively scarce. *S. epidermidis* produces extracellular, surface-associated structures whose chemical composition, regulation, and genetics remain a conundrum.

It is therefore not surprising that most studies of the surface properties of *S. saprophyticus* have been purely phenomenological. Only a few results indicate that surface appendages on the cells might exist (12, 125). Christiansen and Mårdh (12) described fuzzy surface protrusions that were associated with a hemagglutinating strain but lacking in a nonhemagglutinating one. In none of these studies, however, was the isolation or characterization of the molecules associated with the observed structures attempted.

In 1989, we serendipitously discovered that S. saprophyticus produces vast amounts of a previously undescribed protein when it is grown under appropriate conditions, i.e., when it is cultured on dialysis membranes placed on top of brain heart infusion agar (27). Only vortexing was necessary to shear the protein from the wall. This protein has an apparent molecular weight of 95,000 when it is run under reducing conditions and exhibits a native molecular weight of about 500,000 under nonreducing conditions in the presence of 8 M urea. Most clinical isolates of S. saprophyticus produce this protein; in fact, we only found 2 of more than 100 strains that did not. One was isolated from a woman with a typical UTI; the other is the type strain of S. saprophyticus (CCM 883, ATCC 15305). When one of these strains (CCM 883) and other strains producing the protein were compared by electron microscopy, unequivocal differences became apparent. Bacteria capable of producing the protein exhibit copious amounts of surface-associated material, whereas the nonproducer shows a smooth surface. The appendages are similar in length (50 to 75 nm) but have no determinable width and thus match the definition of fibrils. They are most prominent between adjacent cells, and they tend to clump. Scanning electron micrographs are even more impressive (Fig. 4). They reveal that the septation areas of dividing cells are not covered with this material (27, 32), a situation similar to that seen with the aggregation substance of E. faecalis. Using an enzyme-linked immunosorbent assay (ELISA) system, we found that the protein bound to tubular epithelial cells (LLC-PK$_1$) in a concentration-dependent manner (32). This protein, designated Ssp (for S. saprophyticus surface-associated protein), may therefore function as an adhesin of S. saprophyticus.

## THE HEMAGGLUTININ AND THE FIBRONECTIN-BINDING PROTEIN

Purified Ssp does not inhibit hemagglutination and will not cause direct hemagglutination. In addition, hemagglutination is preferentially seen in broth-grown bacteria, whereas production of Ssp requires growth on dialysis membranes. With some strains, and particularly with some media, hemagglutination is poorly reproducible. This problem can be overcome by growing the bacteria on dialysis membranes or in broth in medium containing micromolar amounts of EDTA; the optimal concentration of EDTA is dependent on the medium and the strain. The zinc content of media most likely exerts a major influence on the protein yield (32). It is not yet known whether this ion regulates expression of the hemagglutinin or is required by an unidentified protease that degrades the protein. When strain CCM 883, which hemagglutinates but does not produce Ssp, is grown in the presence of EDTA, surface structures become apparent (33). From these cells, a protein with an approximate molecular weight of 160,000 was purified. Antibody to the protein reacted with the surface structures, as shown by immunogold staining (Fig. 5), whereas antiserum to the Ssp did not. In addition, only antibody to the 160-kDa polypeptide inhibited hemagglutination. From these data, it was concluded that the 160-kDa surface polypeptide is the hemagglutinin of S. saprophyticus. Later, it was shown that this protein also binds fibronectin (31).

## Secreted Factors and Toxic Products

### HEMOLYSIN

S. saprophyticus has been generally described as a nonhemolytic species. No hemolysis is observed after growth on agar containing sheep, rabbit, ox, or human erythrocytes. One group, however, reported hemolytic activity toward human and guinea pig erythrocytes in cell-free culture supernatants of 9 of 14 strains

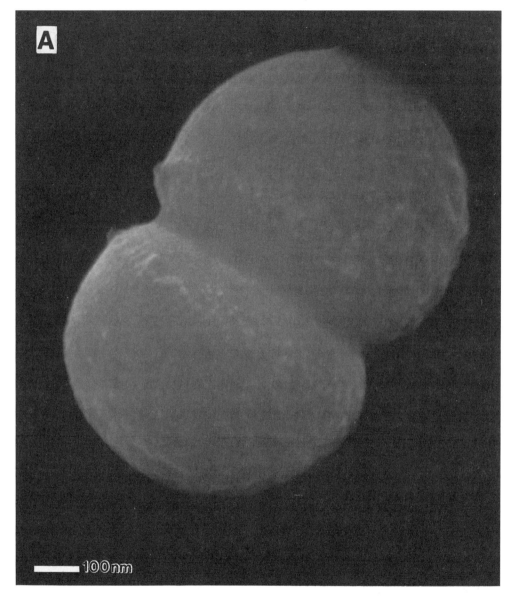

**FIGURE 4** *S. saprophyticus* surface-associated protein (Ssp). A strain (CCM 883) not producing the Ssp (A) and a strain producing this protein (7108) (B) were grown on dialysis membranes, fixed, and subjected to scanning electron microscopy. The protein covers the entire surface of strain 7108, but no surface structures can be seen in strain CCM 883.

(34, 35). The toxin was relatively heat stable and could be neutralized by the presence of lecithin, thus resembling the δ toxin of *S. aureus*. The same strains also caused damage to mouse fibroblasts (35).

## UREASE

Ureases are widely distributed among microorganisms (for a review, see reference 99). The enzymes hydrolyze urea to yield ammonia and carbon dioxide. Ammonia

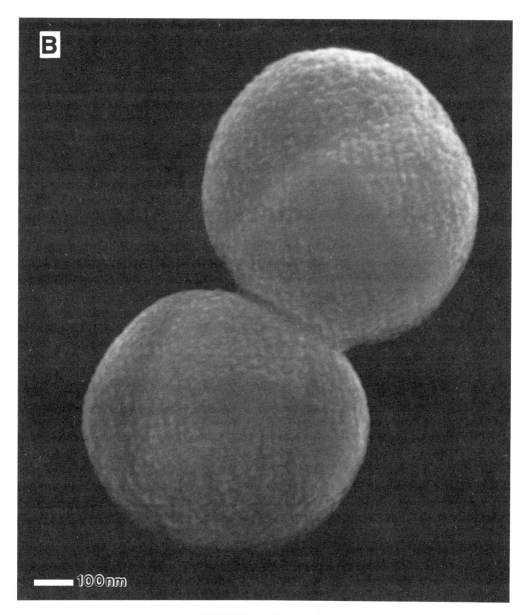

**FIGURE 4** *Continued.*

can be used as a nitrogen source by the urease-producing organism as well as by other microorganisms. In aqueous environments, such as the urinary tract, ammonium ions are formed. This leads to alkalinization, which may cause precipitation of salts like struvite ($MgNH_4PO_4$) or carbonate apatite [$Ca_{10}(PO_4CO_3OH)_6$-$(OH)_2$], i.e., may cause formation of concretions (41). In addition, the alkaline pH and ammonia as well as the ammonium ions can exert direct toxic effects toward the eukaryotic cell and may modulate the immune responses of polymorphonuclear

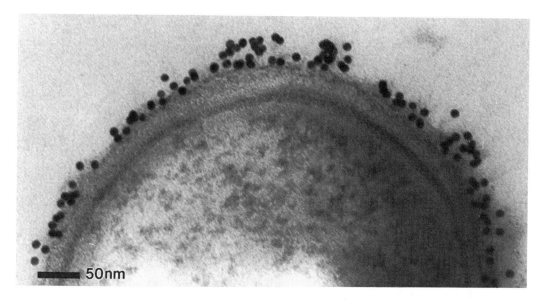

**FIGURE 5** The 160-kDa polypeptide of *S. saprophyticus* is a surface protein. Cells were incubated with antibody to the purified 160-kDa protein, and binding was detected with gold-conjugated protein A.

neutrophils (7, 39). It has therefore been proposed that ureases act as virulence factors in urinary pathogens. *S. saprophyticus* also elaborates this enzyme, and the bacterium has been isolated from urinary stones and from the pelvic urine of a patient with a ureteral concretion. This prompted us to study this enzyme in detail.

The urease of *S. saprophyticus* is a 420,000-Da molecule that consists of three different subunits of 72.4, 20.4, and 13.9 kDa (120). Its $K_m$ is 6.64 mM urea, and its $V_{max}$ is 4.59 μmol of $NH_3$ per min/mg (26). About 5.3 kbp of DNA that code for the structural subunits and several auxiliary peptides are required for expression of enzyme activity. This is in agreement with findings for many other microbial ureases. The additional polypeptides are necessary for nickel incorporation or regulation.

To assess the contribution of the enzyme to the virulence of *S. saprophyticus,* we generated a urease-negative mutant by nitrosoguanidine mutagenesis (26). Virulence of the parent and the mutant strain was evaluated in a rat model of ascending, unobstructed UTI. In this model, bacterial suspensions are instilled into the bladder via the urethra, which leads to a vesicoureteral reflux that permits colonization of the kidneys. On days 3 and 7, bacteriuria and leukocyturia are determined, and then the rats are sacrificed. The numbers of bacteria present in bladder and kidney tissue, spleens, and blood are then determined. Organs of animals infected with the parent strain yield higher bacterial counts and are larger than those challenged with the mutant. Also, bladders of animals that received the parent strain show more severe lesions on histological sections than those from rats infected with the mutant (Fig. 6). Moreover, urinary calculi consisting of struvite are seen in animals infected with the parent strain only. Since the differences of kidney bacterial counts and kidney weights are not statistically significant but the differences between bladder bacterial

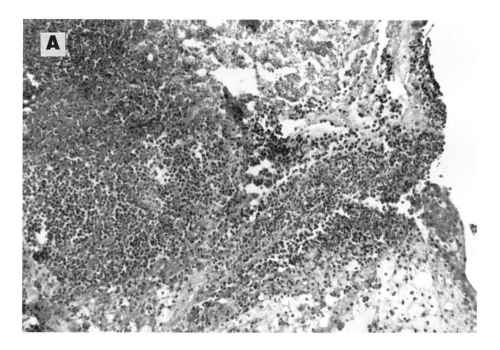

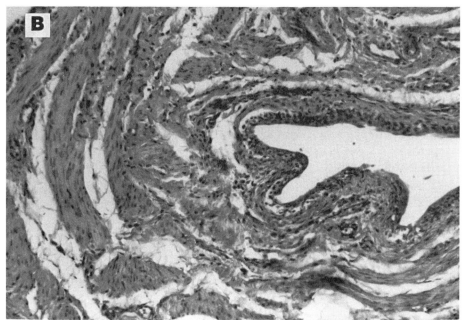

**FIGURE 6** The urease contributes to cystopathogenicity. Histological sections of bladders of rats infected with the urease-positive parent strain (A) or the urease-negative mutant (B) were stained with periodic acid-Schiff stain. Large, destructive abscesses were found with the parent strain; in addition, the bladder wall was thickened, and its normal structures were hardly discernible. With the mutant, there were only scanty subepithelial infiltrations of leukocytes, but otherwise the bladders appeared normal.

counts and weights are, it was concluded that the urease of *S. saprophyticus* contributes mainly to cystopathogenicity, i.e., damage to the bladder. In subsequent experiments, these findings were confirmed by introduction of the cloned urease genes into the urease-negative mutant followed by experimental infections (29). The urease-positive parent strain and the mutant containing the urease plasmid exhibited similar bacterial counts in bladder tissue; bacterial counts for these urease-positive strains differed significantly from that observed with the urease-negative mutant. These experiments therefore established that the urease functions as the major virulence factor during UTI with *S. saprophyticus*.

## Miscellaneous Virulence Factors

Production of an extracellular slime substance has been reported for many coagulase-negative staphylococci, including *S. saprophyticus*. Slime production is observed in artificial or natural urine only and requires the presence of urea (55). Other constituents of the medium such as iron or sex hormones exert no apparent influence. The expression of slime is, however, inhibited by alkaline pH. Since the urease of *S. saprophyticus* probably causes alkalinization of the urine during infection, the significance of slime production remains unclear. Other authors (110), using Congo red agar to detect slime production, found slime production in only 11% of their strains.

The presence of a capsule has been reported over and over for *S. saprophyticus*. Knowledge about the expression of this capsule, let alone its composition, is scant. However, it is worth mentioning that protease digestion of bacteria expressing Ssp unravels an amorphous, protease-resistant surface layer that might represent capsular material (27). Studies concerning the nature and relevance of this material are still wanting.

Hjelm and Lundell-Etherden (54) showed that extracellular, probably proteinaceous products of *S. saprophyticus* exert T-cell mitogenic activity after prolonged (5-day) incubation. The clinical relevance of this phenomenon, however, is obscure.

Another potentially important but still unsubstantiated finding is that *S. saprophyticus* may enter HEp-2 cells (124). The mechanisms that cause internalization are unknown, as is the clinical relevance of the data, because there are no reports on intracellular appearance of *S. saprophyticus* in uroepithelial cells.

The binding of *S. saprophyticus* to mucus was analyzed by using ferret nasal mucin and bovine submaxillary gland mucin. Attachment was inhibited by pretreatment of the bacteria with trypsin or with sodium *meta*-periodate, indicating involvement of proteins and carbohydrates (or glycoproteins) in staphylococcal binding to mucus (117). During UTI with *S. saprophyticus*, bacteria attached to hyaline or cellular casts are commonly observed (61).

## A Model for Pathogenesis of Infections with *S. saprophyticus*

Infection by microorganisms is often preceded by colonization with the agent. In the case of *S. saprophyticus*, this colonization may require acquisition of the organism via the ingestion of contaminated food. Accidental colonization of the skin may be an alternative. Additional predisposing conditions, such as recent sexual intercourse, may facilitate an ascending infection and may induce microlesions of the mucous membranes. It is not known which surface structures are expressed by *S. saprophyticus* colonizing the skin or the rectum. If one assumes that the conditions are similar to those encountered on dialysis membranes, the cells would express Ssp and the hemagglutinin. It is clear from clinical as well as experimental data that urease, the hemagglutinin, and Ssp are expressed during infection with *S. saprophyticus* (60). Expression of the hemagglutinin might facilitate bacterial attachment to urothelia and to fibronectin in the microlesions. Noteworthy is the observation that intact uroepithelial cells are probably not covered by fibronectin (147). The Ssp might favor intercellular adhesion after initial attachment. This concept would explain the observation that the hemagglutinin is preferentially expressed in liquid media, whereas production of Ssp requires culture on membranes. The finding that surface hydrophobicity is induced by culture in liquid media but is not related to expression of the known appendages also fits this picture. Once a microcolony has been established, hydrolysis of urea yields toxic products that cause further tissue damage and may contribute to the rather severe symptoms commonly seen with *S. saprophyticus* UTI. Expression of the hemagglutinin may promote colonization of the kidneys and cause symptoms of upper urinary tract involvement (30). Urease, extracellular proteins, slime, and adherence to hyaline casts or mucus may give rise to concretions that may cause recurrent or, more rarely, persistent infections.

Although the sequence outlined above is largely hypothetical, evidence for the individual steps is ample. The initial events that turn an asymptomatic colonization into infection are, however, poorly understood. It is my impression that future work should focus on the properties and structures expressed by bacteria in the phase prior to infection.

## STAPHYLOCOCCI OTHER THAN *S. SAPROPHYTICUS*

UTIs caused by staphylococci other than *S. saprophyticus* present with an epidemiology that is clearly distinct from that of *S. saprophyticus* UTI. While *S. saprophyticus* mainly infects young female outpatients with no predisposing underlying conditions, the other staphylococci are usually isolated from hospitalized elderly patients who have undergone manipulations or operations of the urinary tract or who have indwelling catheters (17, 81, 95, 98, 105). In these situations, the relevance of a staphylococcal urinary isolate is often debatable. Some case reports, however, indicate that coagulase-negative staphylococci can cause UTI even in patients who are not severely debilitated. The general paucity of symptoms that is typical of true infections caused by coagulase-negative staphylococci (114) augments the diagnostic problems by making it difficult to differentiate contamination from infection (Table 1).

Even *S. aureus,* which is an accepted pathogen in many clinical situations, only rarely causes UTI in outpatients (17). Methicillin-resistant strains, however, are an established cause of infections or contaminations of the urinary tract in hospitalized patients (21).

The major importance of coagulase-negative staphylococci resides in their ability to colonize indwelling artificial devices such as intravascular catheters or prostheses. Growth of adhering bacteria and detachment of some organisms give rise to systemic and local symptoms, such as fever or loosening of the device, associated with these infections. It is conceivable that the capability of these organisms to colonize artificial surfaces accounts for their frequent isolation from the manipulated or catheterized urinary tract.

### Adhesion

Formation of a bacterial biofilm on an artificial surface requires adhesion to the material, growth, and adhesion between adjacent bacteria to avoid dislodgement of microorganisms. Only recently have tools become available that allow distinguishing between some phases of biofilm formation in staphylococci. In many earlier publications, the ability to produce a biofilm was inadvertently labeled "slime" production.

**TABLE 1** Comparison of UTIs due to *S. saprophyticus* and *S. epidermidis*[a]

| Characteristic | S. saprophyticus | S. epidermidis |
|---|---|---|
| Host | Young, healthy, sexually active female outpatients | Elderly, debilitated, hospitalized |
| Urinary catheter present | No | Yes |
| Urinary instrumentations or manipulations | No | Yes |
| Symptoms | Dysuria, hematuria, upper urinary tract involvement frequent, recurrence common | ± Dysuria, rarely involvement of upper urinary tract |
| Quantitative culture results | Pathogenic organism may be present in low numbers only ($<10^5$/ml) | Organism usually recovered in high numbers ($>10^5$/ml) |
| Adherence to uroepithelial cells | Yes | No |

[a] Data are from reference 114 with modifications.

This approach, measuring only the ultimate outcome, fails to recognize the various influences that alterations of the different phases of biofilm formation may have.

## Initial Attachment

Several studies have shown that bacteria with hydrophobic surfaces adhere better to polymers than do those with hydrophilic surfaces (83). In addition, the composition of the artificial substratum influences the number of adhering bacteria (83). Consequently, chemical modifications of polymer surfaces can be used to decrease bacterial adhesion.

Apart from this nonspecific mechanism, adhesins that mediate the interaction of bacteria with polymers have been described. The best studied is the polysaccharide adhesin (PS/A), which was identified and characterized by Tojo et al. (141). The large (>500,000-Da) molecule consists mainly of galactose and glucosamine. It inhibits binding of PS/A-positive strains to catheters and elicits antibodies that interfere with the attachment of those strains. Later, it was shown that rabbits can be protected against experimental endocarditis caused by a PS/A-positive challenge strain by immunization with purified PS/A or antibody against it (56, 76). Transposon mutagenesis with Tn917 was used to derive PS/A- and slime (i.e., biofilm)-negative mutants from a PS/A-producing wild-type strain. The parent strain caused endocarditis in six of eight rabbits, but no evidence for endocarditis was found in animals who had received the mutant (132). The suggestion that PS/A and the ability to form a biofilm contribute to colonization is corroborated by the finding that, at the end of the experiment, only the parent strain was isolated from the endocardial vegetations and intracardiac catheters, which are an integral part of this animal model.

Although epidemiological data show that most (87%) of the *S. epidermidis* strains capable of biofilm formation are PS/A positive (103), these same data also indicate that PS/A is not the only prerequisite. In addition, many (about 50%) of PS/A-positive strains do not produce biofilms, and strains that attach to silastic catheters but do not express PS/A have been found (141).

A candidate for an additional adhesin implied by these findings is the hemagglutinin described by Rupp and Archer (113). As PS/A, it is more often present in *S. epidermidis* isolated from clinical infections than in control strains. Hemagglutination, a trait whose in vitro detection does not require metabolic activity, correlates with adhesion to polystyrene as measured by biofilm formation. This adhesin is apparently different from PS/A, because PS/A-negative strains may express the hemagglutinin. The nature of this property is not yet clearly established. Hemagglutination is significantly diminished or even abolished by treating the bacteria with periodate, which suggests that carbohydrates are mediating this trait (136). However, treatment with certain proteases also decreases hemagglutination titers, indicating a role for surface proteins. Rupp et al. used phenol extraction to prepare an extract that agglutinated sheep erythrocytes but did not contain detectable protein (115).

While PS/A and the hemagglutinin consist mostly of carbohydrates, another, proteinaceous adhesin has been described by Timmerman et al. (140). Those authors raised monoclonal antibodies against whole cells of S. epidermidis and identified an antibody that specifically inhibits adherence to polystyrene. It reacts with a 220-kDa band on immunoblots that use staphylococcal proteins as antigens. The protein is associated with surface structures identified by electron microscopy.

## Biofilm Formation

After being attached to a surface, bacteria replicate and accumulate into an adherent microcolony. Since staphylococci form multilayered colonies, the process logically requires adherence to the artificial substratum as well as between individual cells. Although surface structures that contribute to initial attachment may form components of the biofilm, this is not necessarily and by no means exclusively so. The slimy substance that embeds staphylococci adhering to catheters appears only after prolonged incubation (108). Current data suggest that distinct structures are responsible for attachment and accumulation (11, 85, 86, 130, 141).

Many publications used formation of a biofilm to measure adherence of S. epidermidis, neglecting the differences between the phases of attachment and accumulation. Consequently, the terms "slime" and "adherence" have meanings that depend on the author using them.

Several attempts have been made to purify and characterize the extracellular material of staphylococci in biofilms. Upon ion-exchange chromatography, the preparation of Ludwicka et al. (84) yielded four major fractions, of which three contained galactose and one contained mannose as the major component. It was later shown that the galactose of slime preparations probably originates from the agar (18, 63, 64). Extracts prepared from media without agar or by degradation of cell walls contain glucose and glucosamine as their major components but do not contain significant galactose (63, 64). Christensen et al. (11) raised an immune serum to whole killed S. epidermidis cells that reacted with crude extracts from strain RP62A but not with extracts prepared from non-biofilm-producing mutants. It was therefore named SAA, for slime-associated antigen. The antigen is heat resistant and protease stable, suggesting carbohydrates as its main components. Chemical analysis revealed glucose to be the most abundant sugar; galactose is present in small amounts only. Comparisons of unrelated strains with known PS/A and SAA status indicate that PS/A mediates initial attachment, whereas the SAA status predicts the ability to produce biofilms (11).

Mack et al. (85) used transposon mutagenesis with Tn917 to generate derivatives that were no longer able to produce biofilms. However, in experiments determining primary attachment, parent and mutant strains adhered to polystyrene spheres in similar numbers. The mutants no longer produced a polysaccharide antigen that the same group had reported to be associated with accumulative growth (86). Antigen extracts from the parent and the isogenic mutant showed striking differences in hexosamine contents, identifying this monosaccharide as the major component of the intercellular adhesin (IA).

Schumacher-Perdreau et al. (130) used chemical mutagenesis with mitomycin to generate a biofilm-negative mutant. Mutant and parent strains showed comparable adherence kinetics in tests for initial adherence; however, only the parent strain was capable of accumulative, surface-associated growth. Crude, extracellular material isolated from both strains grown on dialysis membranes on agar did not differ in their carbohydrate compositions. In contrast, when extracellular protein patterns were compared, the mutant lacked polypeptides of 115 and 18 kDa. Although these findings are suggestive of some contribution to biofilm formation by proteins, they do not provide conclusive evidence, because chemically induced mutants may differ in elusive, yet important properties. In addition, presence of the antigen of Mack et al. (86) or of the SAA has not been checked in this mutant.

## Protective Effects of Slime Production

The extracellular material present in staphylococcal biofilms has been described as decreasing the susceptibility of the bacteria to commonly used antibiotics (42). In addition, the extracellular material inhibits phagocytosis of embedded bacteria (112); i.e., it impairs the defense mechanisms of the host. The decreased phagocytosis rate of slime-producing bacteria probably originates from the lower hydrophobicity slime confers on the bacteria. Hydrophilic particles are less likely to get into close contact with phagocytes, a prerequisite for efficient phagocytosis.

## Secreted Virulence Factors

Although *S. aureus* secretes a plethora of different virulence factors such as toxins and enzymes, these factors appear to be less common in *S. epidermidis* and other coagulase-negative staphylococci. However, these bacteria may produce extracellular enzymes such as nucleases or proteases (34), but the relevance of these enzymes to pathogenesis has not been clearly defined. In 1968, Varadi and Saqueton (144) reported degradation of elastin by *S. epidermidis* isolated from skin lesions. It was later shown that the enzyme is produced by many strains from clinical materials (69). Elastase was found to be inducible by the presence of elastin or some soluble compound present in the elastin preparation. The enzyme was partially characterized and purified in 1990 by Sloot et al. (137), who found that the enzyme is a cysteine protease that has similarities to the elastase from *S. aureus* (109). In addition to cleaving elastase, the enzyme also degrades human immunoglobulins (including immunoglobulin A), fibronectin, albumin, and fibrinogen. Proteases that degrade immunoglobulin A have been described for many bacteria and are thought to play a role in the colonization of mucous membranes (87).

*S. aureus* is known to produce at least four different hemolysins (alpha, beta, gamma, and delta). Alpha-toxin is a well-established virulence factor of this organism (for a review, see reference 5). The pathogenetic relevance of the other toxins is less clear. Hemolytic substances are also produced by coagulase-negative staphylococci, particularly *S. epidermidis*. Hemolytic toxins of these microorganisms usually bear similarities to the delta-toxin of *S. aureus*, a surface-active substance. High-level production of delta-toxin is associated with neonatal necrotizing enterocolitis. Strains that produce enough toxin to cause damage to fibroblasts are more likely to be resistant to multiple antibiotics and are more often isolated from premature infants than from full-term infants (121).

Production of enterotoxins and of the toxic shock toxin by coagulase-negative staphylococci has also been described (6, 16). These strains, however, appear to be very uncommon.

Some strains of S. epidermidis produce and release a neutrophil-inhibitory factor that inhibits the bactericidal activity of human neutrophils (106). Activity is separated into two fractions that differ in molecular mass (>300,000 and 20,000 to 40,000 Da). Since material from inhibitory and noninhibitory strains shows similar carbohydrate and protein concentrations, the chemical nature of this substance remains unknown.

## Pathogenesis of UTIs with Coagulase-Negative Staphylococci

Staphylococci other than S. saprophyticus seem to need indwelling catheters, instrumentation, or other underlying conditions to enable them to persist in this environment. Once a staphylococcal biofilm is established, the protective functions of the biofilm make it difficult, if not impossible, to eradicate the bacteria. Those bacteria that detach from the adherent phase enter the rather static planktonic phase that is typical of urinary tracts with predisposing conditions. This step probably facilitates growth to a dense bacterial suspension.

Coagulase-negative staphylococci (S. epidermidis and S. saprophyticus) have a propensity to preferentially adhere to the intercellular junctions of the uroepithelium (94). It is not clear whether the different adhesins play any role in this attachment. The position at the cellular junctions facilitates access of secreted toxic components to the basolateral pole as well as to the subcellular space. The toxic products generated by the urease of Helicobacter pylori may destroy the tight junctions between epithelial cells (47). This destruction would disrupt the epithelial barrier and give the microorganism access to deeper, nutrient-rich areas. In an animal model of UTI, staphylococci recruited fewer leukocytes than Escherichia coli did, which may reflect the clinical situation in which bacteriuria without pyuria is common with coagulase-negative staphylococci.

The function of the diverse virulence factors of S. epidermidis in UTI, however, remains speculative. Given that clinically relevant UTIs with S. epidermidis are rather uncommon, it will most likely be very difficult and possibly unrewarding to devise clinically relevant animal models to study these infections, although it would be highly desirable to know the conditions that predispose a particular parasite-host combination to clinically overt infection.

## ADHESION AND DESTRUCTION: A UNIFIED VIEW OF GRAM-POSITIVE PATHOGENICITY

The gram-positive urinary pathogens discussed in this chapter share the abilities to adhere to natural or artificial substrata and to secrete compounds that may facilitate their access to nutrients. Enterococci and S. saprophyticus are capable of direct adherence to uroepithelial cells by means of specific surface structures.

Most strains of E. faecalis can produce an aggregation substance that may facilitate attachment to cells that express RGDS-recognizing surface integrins. A subset of E. faecalis strains possess an additional adhesin that is specific for cells from the urinary tract.

S. saprophyticus grown in liquid culture expresses a surface protein that mediates hemagglutination and fibronectin binding. This situation is very likely to occur during UTI. The hemagglutinin may therefore serve as the initial adhesin.

The situation is somewhat different for S. epidermidis. This organism colonizes artificial substrata very efficiently. However, a film of serum proteins deposited on these substrata inhibits adhesion (102). This may explain why S. epidermidis usually adheres poorly to eukaryotic cells. It is therefore unlikely that surface structures known to facilitate attachment to artificial substrata play a role in cellular adherence. Only a few strains that attach more efficiently to covered than to uncoated substrata have been described. It is not known whether these strains are more common colonizers of the urinary tract.

Once an initial colony is established, multiplication ensues, and intercellular adhesion becomes necessary. Factors that may play a role in this phase have been described for staphylococci but are not yet known for enterococci. In enterococci as well as in *S. saprophyticus*, the ability to interact with host proteins may facilitate the formation of a colony.

An adherent microcolony may secrete toxic products that cause damage to the epithelium and facilitate access of the microorganisms to nutrients. The enterococci produce a cytolysin and a protease, *S. saprophyticus* releases toxic products through the action of the urease, and *S. epidermidis* may produce a variety of secreted products, like the delta-lysin or the elastase, that function during this phase. Further events may include modulation of surface factor expression and spread in enterococci or modulation of the host defense mechanisms by all three pathogens discussed here. Systemic infection probably occurs only rarely with UTI caused by *S. epidermidis* and *S. saprophyticus*.

Clearly, more work is needed to elucidate the events that take place during infections with these organisms. Such studies should also address the possible effects of the interplay of the various bacterial and host factors. The tools required for these analyses are gradually becoming available for staphylococci and will likely provide the most rewarding approaches to problems associated with staphylococcal UTIs.

## ACKNOWLEDGMENTS

I thank R. Wirth for critically reading the part of this chapter that deals with enterococci and for his permission to use unpublished data on the relevance of the hemolysin and aggregation substance to endocarditis. I am also greatly indebted to G. Wanner, who prepared and provided the fantastic electron micrographs.

Part of this work was supported by the Deutsche Forschungsgemeinschaft (grant DFG Ga 352/2-1).

## REFERENCES

1. **Almeida, R. J., and J. H. Jorgensen.** 1984. Comparison of adherence and urine growth rate properties of *Staphylococcus saprophyticus* and *Staphylococcus epidermidis*. *Eur. J. Clin. Microbiol.* **3:**542–545.
2. **Arthur, M., and P. Courvalin.** 1993. Genetics and mechanisms of glycopeptide resistance in enterococci *Antimicrob. Agents Chemother.* **37:**1563–1571.
3. **Beachey, E. H., W. A. Simpson, I. Ofek, D. L. Hasty, J. B. Dale, and E. Whitnack.** 1983. Attachment of *Streptococcus pyogenes* to mammalian cells. *Rev. Infect. Dis.* **5**(Suppl. 4)**:**S670–S677.
4. **Beuth, J., L. Ko, F. Schumacher-Perdrau, G. Peters, P. Heczko, and G. Pulverer.** 1988. Hemagglutination by *Staphylococcus saprophyticus* and other coagulase-negative staphylococci. *Microb. Pathog.* **4:**379–383.
5. **Bhakdi, S., and J. Tranum-Jensen.** 1991. Alpha-toxin of *Staphylococcus aureus*. *Microbiol. Rev.* **55:**733–751.
6. **Breckinridge, J. C., and M. S. Bergdoll.** 1971. Outbreak of food-borne gastroenteritis due to a coagulase-negative staphylococcus. *N. Engl. J. Med.* **284:**541–543.
7. **Brunkhorst, B., and R. Niederman.** 1991. Ammonium decreases human polymorphonuclear leukocyte cytoskeletal actin. *Infect. Immun.* **59:**1378–1386.
8. **Carruthers, M. M., and W. J. Kabat.** 1983. Mediation of staphylococcal adherence to mucosal cells by lipoteichoic acid. *Infect. Immun.* **40:**444–446.
9. **Cheung, A. L., and V. A. Fischetti.** 1988. Variation of cell wall proteins of *Staphylococcus aureus* grown on solid and liquid media. *Infect. Immun.* **56:**1061–1065.
10. **Chow, J. W., L. A. Thal, M. B. Perri, J. A. Vazquez, S. M. Donabedian, D. B. Clewell, and M. J. Zervos.** 1993. Plasmid-associated hemolysin and aggregation substance production contribute to virulence in experimental enterococcal endocarditis. *Antimicrob. Agents Chemother.* **37:**2474–2477.
11. **Christensen, G. D., L. P. Barker, T. P. Mawhinney, L. M. Baddour, and W. A. Simpson.** 1990. Identification of an antigenic marker of slime production for *Staphylococcus epidermidis*. *Infect. Immun.* **58:**2906–2911.

12. **Christiansen, G., and P.-A. Mårdh.** 1986. Electron microscopy of negative-stained *Staphylococcus saprophyticus* reveals filamentous surface protrusions, p. 145–147. *In* P.-A. Mårdh and K. H. Schleifer, (ed.), *Coagulase-Negative Staphylococci*. Almqvist & Wicksell, Stockholm.
13. **Clewell, D. B.** 1990. Movable genetic elements and antibiotic resistance in enterococci. *Eur. J. Clin. Microbiol. Infect. Dis.* **9:** 90–102.
14. **Colleen, S., B. Hovelius, A. Wieslander, and P.-A. Mårdh.** 1970. Surface properties of *Staphylococcus saprophyticus* and *Staphylococcus epidermidis* as studied by adherence tests and two-polymer aqueus phase systems. *Acta Pathol. Microbiol. Scand. Sect. B* **87:**321–328.
15. **Colleen, S., and P.-A. Mårdh.** 1981. Bacterial colonization of human urethral mucosa. *Scand. J. Urol. Nephrol.* **15:**181–187.
16. **Crass, B. A., and M. S. Bergdoll.** 1986. Involvement of coagulase-negative staphylococci in toxic shock syndrome. *J. Clin. Microbiol.* **23:**43–45.
17. **Digranes, A., and P. Oeding.** 1975. Characterization of Micrococcaceae from the urinary tract. *Acta Pathol. Microbiol. Scand. Sect. B* **83:**373–381.
18. **Drewry, D. T., L. Galbraith, B. J. Wilkinson, and S. G. Wilkinson.** 1990. Staphylococcal slime: a cautionary tale. *J. Clin. Microbiol.* **28:**1292–1296.
19. **Ember, J. A., and T. E. Hugli.** 1989. Characterization of the human neutrophil response to sex pheromones from *Streptococcus faecalis*. *Am. J. Pathol.* **134:**797–805.
20. **Fischetti, V. A.** 1989. Streptococcal M protein: molecular design and biological behavior. *Clin. Microbiol. Rev.* **2:**285–314.
21. **Flournoy, D. J., and L. J. Davidson.** 1993. Methicillin-resistant *Staphylococcus aureus*—relationship of community-acquired and hospital-acquired infection, colonisation and contamination to body site. *Med. Sci. Res.* **21:**701–702.
22. **Fowler, J. E.** 1985. *Staphylococcus saprophyticus* as the cause of infected urinary calculus. *Ann. Intern. Med.* **102:**342–343.
23. **Fujita, K., T. Yokota, T. Oguri, M. Fujime, and R. Kitagawa.** 1992. In vitro adherence of *Staphylococcus saprophyticus, Staphylococcus epidermidis, Staphylococcus haemolyticus,* and *Staphylococcus aureus* to human ureter. *Urol. Res.* **20:**399–402.
24. **Galli, D., F. Lottspeich, and R. Wirth.** 1990. Sequence analysis of *Enterococcus faecalis* aggregation substance encoded by the sex pheromone plasmid pAD1. *Mol. Microbiol.* **4:**895–904.
25. **Galli, D., R. Wirth, and G. Wanner.** 1989. Identification of aggregation substances of *Enterococcus faecalis* cells after induction by sex pheromones. An immunological and ultrastructural investigation. *Arch. Microbiol.* **151:**486–490.
26. **Gatermann, S., J. John, and R. Marre.** 1989. *Staphylococcus saprophyticus* urease: characterization and contribution to uropathogenicity in unobstructed urinary tract infection of rats. *Infect. Immun.* **57:**110–116.
27. **Gatermann, S., B. Kreft, R. Marre, and G. Wanner.** 1992. Identification and characterization of a surface-associated protein (Ssp) of *Staphylococcus saprophyticus*. *Infect. Immun.* **60:**1055–1060.
28. **Gatermann, S., M. Kretschmar, B. Kreft, E. Straube, H. Schmidt, and R. Marre.** 1991. Adhesion of *Staphylococcus saprophyticus* to renal tubular epithelial cells is mediated by an N-acetyl-galactosamine-specific structure. *Zentralbl. Bakteriol. Int. J. Med. Microbiol.* **275:**358–363.
29. **Gatermann, S., and R. Marre.** 1989. Cloning and expression of *Staphylococcus saprophyticus* urease gene sequences in *Staphylococcus carnosus* and contribution of the enzyme to virulence. *Infect. Immun.* **57:**2998–3002.
30. **Gatermann, S., R. Marre, J. Heesemann, and W. Henkel.** 1988. Hemagglutinating and adherence properties of *Staphylococcus saprophyticus*: epidemiology and virulence in experimental urinary tract infection of rats. *FEMS Microbiol. Immunol.* **47:**179–186.
31. **Gatermann, S., and H.-G. W. Meyer.** 1994. *Staphylococcus saprophyticus* hemagglutinin binds fibronectin. *Infect. Immun.* **62:**4556–4563.
32. **Gatermann, S., H.-G. W. Meyer, R. Marre, and G. Wanner.** 1993. Identification and characterization of surface proteins from *Staphylococcus saprophyticus*. *Zentralb. Bakteriol. Int. J. Med. Microbiol.* **278:**258–274.
33. **Gatermann, S., H.-G. W. Meyer, and G. Wanner.** 1992. *Staphylococcus saprophyticus* hemagglutinin is a 160-kDa surface polypeptide. *Infect. Immun.* **60:**4127–4132.
34. **Gemmell, C. G.** 1983. Extracellular toxins and enzymes of coagulase-negative staphylococci, p. 809–827. *In* C. S. F. Easmon and C. Adlam (ed.), *Staphylococci and Staphylococcal Infections*. Academic Press, London.
35. **Gemmell, C. G., and M. Thelestam.** 1981. Toxinogenicity of clinical isolates of

coagulase-negative staphylococci towards various animal cells. *Acta Pathol. Microbiol. Scand. Sect. B* **89:**417–421.

36. **Gillespie, W. A., M. A. Sellin, P. Gill, M. Stephens, L. A. Tuckwell, and A. L. Hilton.** 1978. Urinary tract infection in young women, with special reference to *Staphylococcus saprophyticus*. *J. Clin. Pathol.* **31:**348–350.

37. **Gilmore, M. S., R. A. Segarra, and M. C. Booth.** 1990. An HlyB-type function is required for expression of the *Enterococcus faecalis* hemolysin/bacteriocin. *Infect. Immun.* **58:**3914–3923.

38. **Golledge, C.** 1988. *Staphylococcus saprophyticus* bacteremia. *J. Infect. Dis.* **157:**215.

39. **Gordon, A. H., P. D'Arcy Hart, and M. R. Young.** 1980. Ammonia inhibits phagosome-lysosome fusion in macrophages. *Nature* (London) **286:**79–80.

40. **Graninger, W., and R. Ragette.** 1992. Nosocomial bacteremia due to *Enterococcus faecalis* without endocarditis. *Clin. Infect. Dis.* **15:**49–57.

41. **Griffith, D. P., D. M. Musher, and C. Itin.** 1976. Urease, the primary cause of infection-induced urinary stones. *Invest. Urol.* **13:**346–350.

42. **Gristina, A. G., R. A. Jennings, P. T. Naylor, Q. N. Myrvik, and L. X. Webb.** 1989. Comparative in vitro antibiotic resistance of surface-colonizing coagulase-negative staphylococci. *Antimicrob. Agents Chemother.* **33:**813–816.

43. **Gross, P. A., L. Messinger Harkavy, G. E. Barden, and M. F. Flower.** 1976. The epidemiology of nosocomial enterococcal urinary tract infection. *Am. J. Med. Sci.* **272:**75–81.

44. **Gunnarsson, A., P.-A. Mårdh, A. Lundblad, and S. Svensson.** 1984. Oligosaccharide structures mediating agglutination of sheep erythrocytes by *Staphylococcus saprophyticus*. *Infect. Immun.* **45:**41–46.

45. **Guzman, C. A., C. Pruzzo, G. LiPira, and L. Calegari.** 1989. Role of adherence in pathogenesis of *Enterococcus faecalis* urinary tract infection and endocarditis. *Infect. Immun.* **57:**1834–1838.

46. **Handley, P. S., P. L. Carter, and J. Fielding.** 1984. *Streptococcus salivarius* strains carry either fibrils or fimbriae on the cell surface. *J. Bacteriol.* **157:**64–72.

47. **Hawtin, P. R., A. R. Stacey, and D. G. Newell.** 1990. Investigation of the structure and localization of the urease of *Helicobacter pylori* using monoclonal antibodies. *J. Gen. Microbiol.* **136:**1995–2000.

48. **Hedman, P., and O. Ringertz.** 1991. Urinary tract infections caused by *Staphylococcus saprophyticus*. A matched case control study. *J. Infect.* **23:**145–153.

49. **Hedman, P., O. Ringertz, M. Lindström, and K. Olsson.** 1991. The origin of *Staphylococcus saprophyticus* from cattle and pigs. *Scand. J. Infect. Dis.* **25:**57–60.

50. **Hedman, P., O. Ringertz, K. Olsson, and R. Wollin.** 1991. Plasmid-identified *Staphylococcus saprophyticus* isolated from the rectum of patients with urinary tract infections. *Scand. J. Infect. Dis.* **23:**569–572.

51. **Hell, W., and S. Gatermann.** Unpublished observations.

52. **Herman, D. J., and D. N. Gerding.** 1991. Antimicrobial resistance among enterococci. *Antimicrob. Agents Chemother.* **35:**1–4.

53. **Hirose, T., Y. Kumamoto, N. Tanaka, M. Yoshioka, and T. Tsukamoto.** 1989. Study on pathogenesis of *Enterococcus faecalis* in urinary tract. *Urol. Res.* **17:**125–129.

54. **Hjelm, E., and I. Lundell-Etherden.** 1989. Effects of extracellular products from *Staphylococcus saprophyticus* on human lymphocytes. *APMIS* **97:**935–940.

55. **Hjelm, E., and I. Lundell-Etherden.** 1991. Slime production by *Staphylococcus saprophyticus*. *Infect. Immun.* **59:**445–448.

56. **Hogt, A., J. Dankert, C. E. Hulstaert, and J. Feijen.** 1986. Cell surface characteristics of coagulase-negative staphylococci and their adherence to fluorinated poly(ethylenepropylene). *Infect. Immun.* **51:**294–301.

57. **Hovelius, B., S. Colleen, and P.-A. Mårdh.** 1984. Urinary tract infections in men caused by *Staphylococcus saprophyticus*. *Scand. J. Infect. Dis.* **16:**37–41.

58. **Hovelius, B., and P.-A. Mårdh.** 1979. Haemagglutination by *Staphylococcus saprophyticus* and other staphylococcal species. *Acta Pathol. Microbiol. Scand. Sect. B* **87:**45–50.

59. **Hovelius, B., and P.-A. Mårdh.** 1984. *Staphylococcus saprophyticus* as a common cause of urinary tract infections. *Rev. Infect. Dis.* **6:**328–337.

60. **Hovelius, B., and P.-A. Mårdh.** 1985. Antibody-coating and haemagglutination by *Staphylococcus saprophyticus*. *Acta Pathol. Microbiol. Immunol. Scand. Sect. B* **93B:**37–40.

61. **Hovelius, B., P.-A. Mårdh, and P. Bygren.** 1979. Urinary tract infections caused by *Staphylococcus saprophyticus*: recurrences and complications. *J. Urol.* **122:**645–647.

62. **Hovelius, B., I. Thelin, and P.-A. Mårdh.** 1979. *Staphylococcus saprophyticus* in

the aetiology of nongonococcal urethritis. *Br. J. Vener. Dis.* **55**:369–374.
63. Hussain, M., J. G. M. Hastings, and P. J. White. 1991. Isolation and composition of the extracellular slime made by coagulase-negative staphylococci in a chemically defined medium. *J. Infect. Dis.* **163**:534–541.
64. Hussain, M., M. H. Wilcox, and P. J. White. 1993. The slime of coagulase-negative staphylococci—biochemistry and relation to adherence. *FEMS Microbiol. Rev.* **104**:191–208.
65. Huycke, M. M., C. A. Spiegel, and M. S. Gilmore. 1991. Bacteremia caused by hemolytic, high-level gentamicin-resistant *Enterococcus faecalis*. *Antimicrob. Agents Chemother.* **35**:1626–1634.
66. Ike, Y., D. B. Clewell, R. A. Segarra, and M. S. Gilmore. 1990. Genetic analysis of the pAD1 hemolysin/bacteriocin determinant in *Enterococcus faecalis*: Tn917 insertional mutagenesis and cloning. *J. Bacteriol.* **172**:155–163.
67. Ike, Y., H. Hashimoto, and D. B. Clewell. 1984. Hemolysin of *Streptococcus faecalis* subspecies *zymogenes* contributes to virulence in mice. *Infect. Immun.* **45**:528–530.
68. Ike, Y., H. Hashimoto, and D. B. Clewell. 1987. High incidence of hemolysin production by *Enterococcus (Streptococcus) faecalis* strains associated with human parenteral infections. *J. Clin. Microbiol.* **25**:1524–1528.
69. Janda, J. M. 1986. Elastolytic activity among staphylococci. *J. Clin. Microbiol.* **24**:945–946.
70. Jansen, B., J. Beuth, and H. L. Ko. 1990. Evidence for lectin-mediated adherence of *S. saprophyticus* and *P. aeruginosa* to polymers. *Zentralbl. Bakteriol.* **272**:437–442.
71. Jett, B. D., H. G. Jensen, R. E. Nordquist, and M. S. Gilmore. 1992. Contribution of the pAD1-encoded cytolysin to the severity of experimental *Enterococcus faecalis* endophthalmitis. *Infect. Immun.* **60**:2445–2452.
72. Jönsson, K., C. Signäs, H.-P. Müller, and M. Lindberg. 1991. Two different genes encode fibronectin binding proteins in *Staphylococcus aureus*. *Eur. J. Biochem.* **202**:1041–1048.
73. Jordan, P. A., A. Irvani, G. A. Richard, and H. Baer. 1980. Urinary tract infections caused by *Staphylococcus saprophyticus*. *J. Infect. Dis.* **142**:510–515.
74. Kasprowicz, A., A. Bialecka, and P. B. Heczko. 1987. Surface properties of *Staphylococcus saprophyticus* strains isolated from various sources. *Zentralbl. Bakteriol. Mikrobiol. Hyg. Suppl.* **16**:77–81.
75. Kerr, H. 1973. Urinary infections caused by Micrococcus subgroup 3. *J. Clin. Pathol.* **26**:918–920.
76. Kojima, Y., M. Tojo, D. A. Goldmann, T. D. Tosteson, and G. B. Pier. 1990. Antibody to the capsular polysaccharide adhesin protects rabbits against catheter-related bacteremia due to coagulase-negative staphylococci. *J. Infect. Dis.* **162**:435–441.
77. Kreft, B., R. Marre, U. Schramm, and R. Wirth. 1992. Aggregation substance of *Enterococcus faecalis* mediates adhesion to cultured renal tubular cells. *Infect. Immun.* **60**:25–30.
78. LeBlanc, D. J., L. N. Lee, D. B. Clewell, and D. Behnke. 1983. Broad geographical distribution of a cytotoxin gene mediating beta-hemolysis and bacteriocin activity among *Streptococcus faecalis* strains. *Infect. Immun.* **40**:1015–1022.
79. Lee, W., R. J. Carpenter, L. E. Phillips, and S. Faro. 1987. Pyelonephritis and sepsis due to *Staphylococcus saprophyticus*. *J. Infect. Dis.* **155**:1079–1080.
80. Lemoine, L., and P. R. Hunter. 1987. Enterococcal urinary tract infections in a teaching hospital. *Eur. J. Clin. Microbiol.* **6**:574–575.
81. Lewis, J. F., S. R. Brake, D. J. Anderson, and G. N. Vredeveld. 1982. Urinary tract infection due to coagulase-negative Staphylococcus. *Am. J. Clin. Pathol.* **77**:736–739.
82. Ljungh, A., S. Hjertén, and T. Wadström. 1985. High surface hydrophobicity of autoaggregating *Staphylococcus aureus* strains isolated from human infections studied with the salt aggregation test. *Infect. Immun.* **47**:522–526.
83. Ludwicka, A., B. Jansen, T. Wadström, and G. Pulverer. 1984. Attachment of staphylococci to various synthetic polymers. *Zentralbl. Bakteriol. Hyg. A* **256**:479–489.
84. Ludwicka, A., G. Uhlenbruck, G. Peters, P. N. Seng, E. D. Gray, J. Jeljaszewicz, and G. Pulverer. 1984. Investigations on extracellular slime substance produced by *Staphylococcus epidermidis*. *Zentralbl. Bakteriol. Hyg. A* **258**:256–267.
85. Mack, D., M. Nedelmann, A. Krokotsch, A. Schwarzkopf, J. Heesemann, and R. Laufs. 1994. Characterization of transposon mutants of biofilm-producing *Staphylococcus epidermidis* impaired in the accumulative phase of biofilm production: genetic identification of a hexosamine-containing polysaccharide intercellular adhesin. *Infect. Immun.* **62**:3244–3253.

86. Mack, D., N. Siemsen, and R. Laufs. 1992. Parallel induction by glucose of adherence and a polysaccharide antigen specific for plastic-adherent *Staphylococcus epidermidis*: evidence for functional relation to intercellular adhesion. *Infect. Immun.* **60:**2048–2057.
87. Maeda, H., and A. Molla. 1989. Pathogenic potentials of bacterial proteases. *Clin. Chim. Acta* **185:**357–368.
88. Maki, D. G., and W. A. Agger. 1988. Enterococcal bacteremia: clinical features, the risk of endocarditis, and management. *Infect. Dis.* **67:**248–269.
89. Mårdh, P.-A., S. Colleen, and B. Hovelius. 1979. Attachment of bacteria to exfoliated cells from the urogenital tract. *Invest. Urol.* **15:**367–371.
90. Mårdh, P.-A., B. Hovelius, K. Hovelius, and P. O. Nilsson. 1978. Coagulase-negative, novobiocin-resistant staphylococci on the skin of animals and man, on meat and in milk. *Acta Vet. Scand.* **19:**243–253.
91. Marrie, T. J., C. Kwan, M. A. Noble, A. West, and L. Duffield. 1982. *Staphylococcus saprophyticus* as a cause of urinary tract infections. *J. Clin. Microbiol.* **16:**427–431.
92. Maskell, R. 1974. Importance of coagulase-negative staphylococci as pathogens in the urinary tract. *Lancet* **i:**1155–1158.
93. McGavin, M. H., D. Krajewska-Pietrasik, C. Ryden, and M. Höök. 1993. Identification of a *Staphylococcus aureus* extracellular matrix-binding protein with broad specificity. *Infect. Immun.* **61:**2479–2485.
94. McTaggert, L. A., R. C. Rigby, and T. S. J. Elliott. 1990. The pathogenesis of urinary tract infections associated with *Escherichia coli*, *Staphylococcus saprophyticus* and *S. epidermidis*. *J. Med. Microbiol.* **32:**135–141.
95. Meers, P. D., W. Whyte, and G. Sandys. 1975. Coagulase-negative staphylococci and micrococci in urinary tract infections. *J. Clin. Pathol.* **28:**270–273.
96. Meyer, H. G. W., and S. Gatermann. 1994. Surface properties of *Staphylococcus saprophyticus*: hydrophobicity, haemagglutination and *Staphylococcus saprophyticus* surface-associated protein (Ssp) represent distinct entities. *APMIS* **102:**538–544.
97. Milagres, L. G., and C. E. A. Melles. 1992. Differencias nas propriedades adesivas de *Staphylococcus saprophyticus* a céllulas HEp-2 e eritrócitos. *Rev. Inst. Med. Trop. Sao Paulo* **34:**315–321.
98. Mitchell, R. G. 1968. Classification of Staphylococcus albus strains isolated from the urinary tract. *J. Clin. Pathol.* **21:**93–96.
99. Mobley, H. L. T., and R. P. Hausinger. 1989. Microbial ureases: significance, regulation, and molecular characterization. *Microbiol. Rev.* **53:**85–108.
100. Montgomerie, J. Z., G. M. Kalmanson, and L. B. Guze. 1977. Virulence of enterococci in experimental pyelonephritis. *Urol. Res.* **5:**99–102.
101. Morrison, A. J., and R. P. Wenzel. 1986. Nosocomial urinary tract infections due to enterococcus. Ten years' experience at a university hospital. *Arch Intern. Med.* **146:**1549–1551.
102. Muller, E., S. Takeda, D. A. Goldman, and G. B. Pier. 1991. Blood proteins do not promote adherence of coagulase-negative staphylococci to biomaterials. *Infect. Immun.* **59:**3323–3326.
103. Muller, E., S. Takeda, H. Shiro, D. Goldmann, and G. B. Pier. 1993. Occurrence of capsular polysaccharide adhesin among clinical isolates of coagulase-negative staphylococci. *J. Infect. Dis.* **168:**1211–1218.
104. Musher, D. M., D. P. Griffith, D. Yawn, and R. D. Rossen. 1975. Role of urease in pyelonephritis resulting from urinary tract infection with Proteus. *J. Infect. Dis.* **131:**177–181.
105. Nicolle, L. E., S. A. Hoban, and G. K. M. Harding. 1983. Characterization of coagulase-negative staphylococci from urinary tract specimens. *J. Clin. Microbiol.* **17:**267–271.
106. Noble, M. A., S. K. Grant, and E. Hajen. 1990. Characterization of a neutrophil-inhibitory factor from clinically significant *Staphylococcus epidermidis*. *J. Infect. Dis.* **162:**909–913.
107. Paulsson, M., A. Ljungh, and T. Wadstrom. 1992. Rapid identification of fibronectin, vitronectin, laminin, and collagen cell surface binding proteins on coagulase-negative staphylococci by particle agglutination assays. *J. Clin. Microbiol.* **30:**2006–2012.
108. Peters, G., R. Locci, and G. Pulverer. 1982. Adherence of coagulase-negative staphylococci on surfaces of intravenous catheters. *J. Infect. Dis.* **156:**479–482.
109. Potempa, J., A. Dubin, G. Korzus, and J. Travis. 1988. Degradation of elastin by a cysteine proteinase from *Staphylococcus aureus*. *J. Biol. Chem.* **263:**2664–2667.
110. Riley, T. V., and P. F. Schneider. 1992. Infrequency of slime production by urinary isolates of *Staphylococcus saprophyticus*. *J. Infect.* **24:**63–66.
111. Ringertz, O., and J. Torssander. 1987. Prevalence of *Staphylococcus saprophyticus* in

patients in a veneral disease clinic. *Eur. J. Clin. Microbiol.* **5**:358–361.
112. **Rodgers, J., F. Phillips, and C. Olliff.** 1994. The effects of extracellular slime from *Staphylococcus epidermidis* on phagocytic ingestion and killing. *FEMS Immunol. Med. Microbiol.* **9**:109–115.
113. **Rupp, M. E., and G. Archer.** 1992. Hemagglutination and adherence to plastic by *Staphylococcus epidermidis*. *Infect. Immun.* **60**:4322–4327.
114. **Rupp, M. E., and G. L. Archer.** 1994. Coagulase-negative staphylococci: pathogens associated with medical progress. *Clin. Infect. Dis.* **19**:231–243.
115. **Rupp, M. E., N. Sloot, H.-G. W. Meyer, and S. G. Gatermann.** Unpublished data.
116. **Rupp, M. E., D. E. Soper, and G. L. Archer.** 1992. Colonization of the female genital tract with *Staphylococcus saprophyticus*. *J. Clin. Microbiol.* **30**:2975–2979.
117. **Sanford, B. A., V. L. Thomas, and M. A. Ramsay.** 1989. Binding of staphylococci to mucus in vivo and in vitro. *Infect. Immun.* **57**:3735–3742.
118. **Sannomiya, P., R. A. Craig, D. B. Clewell, A. Suzuki, M. Fujino, G. O. Till, and W. A. Marasco.** 1990. Characterization of a class of nonformylated *Enterococcus faecalis*-derived neutrophil chemotactic peptides: the sex pheromones. *Proc. Natl. Acad. Sci. USA* **87**:66–70.
119. **Schaeffer, A. J., W. R. Schwan, S. J. Hultgren, and J. L. Duncan.** 1987. Relationship of type 1 pilus expression in *Escherichia coli* to ascending urinary tract infections in mice. *Infect. Immun.* **55**:373–380.
120. **Schafer, U. K., and H. Kaltwasser.** 1994. Urease from *Staphylococcus saprophyticus*: purification, characterization and comparison to *Staphylococcus xylosus* urease. *Arch. Microbiol.* **161**:393–399.
121. **Scheifele, D. W., and G. L. Bjornson.** 1988. Delta toxin activity in coagulase-negative staphylococci from the bowels of neonates. *J. Clin. Microbiol.* **26**:279–282.
122. **Schennings, T., A. Heimdahl, K. Coster, and J. I. Flock.** 1993. Immunization with fibronectin-binding protein from *Staphylococcus aureus* protects against experimental endocarditis in rats. *Microb. Pathog.* **15**:227–236.
123. **Schleifer, K. H., and W. E. Kloos.** 1975. Isolation and characterization of staphylococci from human skin. I. Amended descriptions of *Staphylococcus epidermidis* and *Staphylococcus saprophyticus* and descriptions of three new species: *Staphylococcus cohnii*, *Staphylococcus haemolyticus*, and *Staphylococcus xylosus*. *Int. J. Syst. Bacteriol.* **25**:50–61.
124. **Schmidt, H., G. Bukholm, and M. Holberg-Petersen.** 1989. Adhesiveness and invasiveness of staphylococcal species in a cell culture model. *APMIS* **97**:655–660.
125. **Schmidt, H., G. Naumann, and H.-P. Putzke.** 1988. Detection of different fimbriae-like structures on the surface of *Staphylococcus saprophyticus*. *Zentralbl. Bakteriol. Hyg. A* **268**:228–237.
126. **Schmidt, K. H., K. Mann, J. Cooney, and W. Köhler.** 1993. Multiple binding of type 3 streptococcal M protein to human fibrinogen, albumin, and fibronectin. *FEMS Microbiol. Immunol.* **7**:135–144.
127. **Schneider, P. F., and T. V. Riley.** 1991. Cell-surface hydrophobicity of *Staphylococcus saprophyticus*. *Epidemiol. Infect.* **106**:71–75.
128. **Schulze-Koops, H., H. Burckhardt, J. Heesemann, T. Kirsch, B. Swoboda, C. Bull, S. Goodman, and F. Emmrich.** 1993. Outer membrane protein YadA of enteropathogenic yersiniae mediates specific binding to cellular but not plasma fibronectin. *Infect. Immun.* **61**:2513–2519.
129. **Schulze-Koops, H., H. Burckhardt, J. Heesemann, K. vonderMark, and F. Emmrich.** 1992. Plasmid-encoded outer membrane protein YadA mediates specific binding of enteropathogenic yersiniae to various types of collagen. *Infect. Immun.* **60**:2153–2159.
130. **Schumacher-Perdreau, F., C. Heilmann, G. Peters, F. Gotz, and G. Pulverer.** 1994. Comparative analysis of a biofilm-forming *Staphylococcus epidermidis* strain and its adhesion-positive, accumulation-negative mutant M7. *FEMS Microbiol. Lett.* **117**:71–78.
131. **Segarra, R. A., M. C. Booth, D. A. Morales, M. M. Huycke, and M. S. Gilmore.** 1991. Molecular characterization of the *Enterococcus faecalis* cytolysin activator. *Infect. Immun.* **59**:1239–1246.
132. **Shiro, H., E. Muller, N. Gutierrez, S. Boisot, M. Grout, T. D. Tosteson, D. Goldmann, and G. B. Pier.** 1994. Transposon mutants of *Staphylococcus epidermidis* deficient in elaboration of capsular polysaccharide/adhesin and slime are avirulent in a rabbit model of endocarditis. *J. Infect. Dis.* **169**:1042–1049.
133. **Shlaes, D. M., J. Levy, and E. Wolinsky.** 1981. Enterococcal bacteremia without endocarditis. *Arch. Intern. Med.* **141**:578–581.

134. **Shorrock, P. J., and P. A. Lambert.** 1989. Binding of fibronectin and albumin to *Enterococcus (Streptococcus) faecalis*. *Microb. Pathog.* **6**:61–67.
135. **Singh, V. R., and I. Raad.** 1990. Fatal *Staphylococcus saprophyticus* native valve endocarditis in an intravenous drug addict. *J. Infect. Dis.* **162**:783–784.
136. **Sloot, N., M. E. Rupp, H. G. W. Meyer, and S. G. G. Gatermann.** Unpublished data.
137. **Sloot, N., M. Thomas, R. Marre, and S. Gatermann.** 1992. Purification and characterisation of elastase from *Staphylococcus epidermidis*. *J. Med. Microbiol.* **37**:201–205.
138. **Switalski, L. M., C. Rydén, K. Rubin, A. Ljungh, M. Höök, and T. Wadström.** 1983. Binding of fibronectin to *Staphylococcus* strains. *Infect. Immun.* **42**:628–633.
139. **Teti, G., M. S. Chiofalo, F. Tomasello, C. Fava, and P. Mastroeni.** 1987. Mediation of *Staphylococcus saprophyticus* adherence to uroepithelial cells by lipoteichoic acid. *Infect. Immun.* **55**:839–842.
140. **Timmerman, C. P., A. Fleer, J. M. Besnier, L. Degraaf, F. Cremers, and J. Verhoef.** 1991. Characterization of a proteinaceous adhesin of *Staphylococcus epidermidis* which mediates attachment to polystyrene. *Infect. Immun.* **59**:4187–4192.
141. **Tojo, M., N. Yamashita, D. A. Goldman, and G. B. Pier.** 1988. Isolation and characterization of a capsular polysaccharide adhesin from *Staphylococcus epidermidis*. *J. Infect. Dis.* **157**:713–722.
142. **Torres Pereira, A.** 1962. Coagulase-negative strains of staphylococcus possessing antigen 51 as agents of urinary infection. *J. Clin. Pathol.* **15**:252–253.
143. **Tsuchimori, N., R. Hayashi, A. Shino, T. Yamazaki, and K. Okonogi.** 1994. *Enterococcus faecalis* aggravates pyelonephritis caused by *Pseudomonas aeruginosa* in experimental ascending mixed urinary tract infection in mice. *Infect. Immun.* **62**:4534–4541.
144. **Varadi, D. P., and A. C. Saqueton.** 1968. Elastase from *Staphylococcus epidermidis*. *Nature* (London) **218**:468–470.
145. **Wallmark, G., I. Arremark, and B. Telander.** 1978. *Staphylococcus saprophyticus*: a frequent cause of acute urinary tract infection among female outpatients. *J. Infect. Dis.* **138**:791–797.
146. **Ward, G. K., S. S. Stewart, G. B. Price, and W. J. Mackillop.** 1987. Cellular heterogeneity in normal human urothelium: quantitative studies of lectin binding. *Histochem. J.* **19**:337–344.
147. **Westerlund, B., and T. K. Korhonen.** 1993. Bacterial proteins binding to the mammalian extracellular matrix. *Mol. Microbiol.* **9**:687–694.
148. **Wirth, R.** 1994. The sex pheromone system of *Enterococcus faecalis*—more than just a plasmid-collection mechanism? *Eur. J. Biochem.* **222**:235–246.
149. **Wirth, R.** Personal communication.
150. **Wright, R., and F. N. Judson.** 1978. Relative and seasonal incidences of the sexually transmitted diseases. *Br. J. Vener. Dis.* **54**:433–440.

# IN VITRO MODELS FOR THE STUDY OF UROPATHOGENS

*Bogdan J. Nowicki, M.D., Ph.D.*

# 13

The pathogenesis of ascending urinary tract infection involves endogenous flora spreading from the intestinal tract to the lower urinary tract and then ascending to the upper urinary tract. The search for the mechanisms of ascending urinary tract infection has resulted in the discovery of bacterial and host factors that contribute to the development of the process of ascending. Understanding these mechanisms has been made possible by the establishment of in vivo and in vitro models for the study of the interaction of host and microbial cell. In this chapter, I review the history of and provide new information regarding in vitro systems that allow investigation of fimbrial phase variation, adhesin-ligand-mediated tissue tropism, and invasiveness of uropathogens.

## HISTORY

The discovery of extracellular hairlike appendages on microorganisms (pili, fimbriae, and adhesins) and the hemagglutinating properties of uropathogens that express these extracellular appendages were the first findings related to an in vitro model of bacterial-cell–eukaryotic-cell interaction (11, 12, 20, 21, 34, 46). The contribution of these early findings to our understanding of the pathogenesis of urinary tract infection was, however, not recognized for a long time. Nevertheless, in those studies, *Escherichia coli* induces different hemagglutination patterns of both human and animal erythrocytes, which indicates that microorganisms can detect a variety of cell types and thus a variety of tissue ligands (21). Further studies explored the interaction between bacterial cells and yeast, plant, animal, and human cells (7, 72, 73, 76). For example, *E. coli* carrying type 1 fimbriae attaches to mannans and aggregate yeast cells (72, 73).

The turning point in understanding the uropathogenic properties of urinary pathogens was the use of human uroepithelial cells as targets for the binding of *E. coli*, *Proteus mirabilis,* and other species. *E. coli* isolates from different clinical presentations of urinary tract infection, including asymptomatic bacteriuria, cystitis, and pyelonephritis, display quantitative differences in binding to uroepithelial cells (143, 145–148). The number of bacteria attaching per epithelial cell is lowest for

*Bogdan J. Nowicki,* Department of Obstetrics and Gynecology and Department of Microbiology and Immunology, 301 University Boulevard, University of Texas Medical Branch, Galveston, Texas 77555-1062.

asymptomatic bacteriuria isolates, intermediate for cystitis isolates, and highest for pyelonephritis strains. These studies provided the evidence that in vitro systems using human cells from the urinary tract can serve as a model for testing the potential virulence of urinary isolates and associating these findings with the source of a urinary tract infection isolate. Additionally, the use of human erythrocytes that express various blood group antigens and erythrocytes with the corresponding null phenotypes that do not carry individual blood group antigens (e.g., erythrocytes with P blood group antigen and the corresponding P-negative [p] phenotype) allowed the identification of the binding specificity of the main virulence factor of acute pyelonephritis-associated *E. coli*, the P fimbria; *E. coli* isolated from patients with acute pyelonephritis hemagglutinated erythrocytes of patients in the P blood group but not those from donors that lacked P antigens (55–57, 86, 87). These experiments established the basis for further characterization of the properties of uropathogens and human tissues with respect to their relevance to the pathogenesis of urinary tract infection.

## IN VITRO MODELS FOR STUDYING MULTIFIMBRIAL PHASE VARIATION

In the 1980s, it became evident that individual microorganisms associated with urinary tract infection may express more than one type of colonization factor. A typical uropathogenic *E. coli* strain expresses several fimbrial types (53, 77, 156, 157). Brinton (11, 12) and Duguid et al. (20, 21) showed that *E. coli* expressing type 1 fimbriae may change from a fimbriated to a nonfimbriated phase. The genetic mechanism of the type 1 fimbriae on-off switch was explained by Eisenstein's group, who found evidence for an invertible element in the region upstream of the type 1 fimbrial structural gene (1). Rhen and colleagues, using immunoprecipitation with fimbria-specific immunoglobulin G (IgG), provided the first indirect evidence that P and type 1C fimbriae of uropathogenic *E. coli* do not occur on the same cells and that there is a rapid phase switch between P-fimbriated and type 1C-fimbriated cells (130).

## Direct Immunofluorescence Staining of Fimbriated Cells

To directly study multifimbrial phase variation, a simple immunofluorescence test for assessing the expression of fimbrial antigens on single bacterial cells was developed (104). This method allows us to characterize large populations of *E. coli* cells instead of the small samples that are visualized by electron microscopy. Subpopulations of *E. coli* cells carrying single fimbrial types were detected by using phase-contrast microscopy with double staining with anti-type 1, anti-P, or anti-type 1C IgG labeled with either fluorescein or rhodamine (104). Individual subpopulations were made up of a group of cells (15 to 30%) carrying single fimbrial types, a small fraction of cells (3 to 9%) carrying more than one fimbrial type, and a major group of cells (40 to 50%) that were nonfimbriated (Fig. 1). Therefore, a culture of *E. coli* derived from one progeny cell was composed of several subpopulations. For example, a culture of *E. coli* KS71, which expressed four fimbrial antigens, was composed of at least six cell types: cells with type 1, type 1C, and P (two subtypes) fimbriae; nonfimbriated cells; and several cell types expressing at least two fimbriae. Figure 2 shows *E. coli* cell subpopulations of a hypothetical strain that expresses two fimbrial types.

To investigate whether fimbrial phase variation is a random process, cells were grown at room temperature, a condition under which no fimbriae were expressed. Cells were then transferred to a static broth culture at 37°C, and samples were taken every hour for 26 h. Type 1C-fimbriated cells were first detected at 1 h, and the percentage increased rapidly to 68% in 4 h. P-fimbriated cells were detected at 2 h, and the percentage rose gradually to 21% by 8 h. Type 1-fimbriated cells were not detected until 9 h. The percentage of type 1-fimbria-bearing cells remained low at first but then increased to 21% in 20 h (104). Accordingly, the original percentage of nonfimbriated cells (100%) decreased rapidly to 24% in 4 h. Therefore, fimbrial phase variation was not totally random; a random variation would not explain the rapid increase in the percentage of type 1C-fimbriated cells or the late appearance of type 1-fimbriated cells (Fig. 3).

### In Vitro Model for Fractionation of Fimbriated Cells

A fractionation method for isolation of fimbriated bacterial-cell subpopulations by absorption to erythrocytes and yeast cells was developed to study the kinetics of fimbrial switching (105). This method is useful for obtaining a homogeneous bacterial subpopulation (96 to 98% one cell type) for the study of growth and adherence of cells carrying specific fimbrial antigens. A bacterial culture of *E. coli* 3040, a urinary isolate that expresses type 1 and S fimbriae, was fractionated into subpopulations that either expressed one of the fimbrial types or were nonfimbriated. The isolated subpopulations were inoculated into broth, and the fimbriation of individual cells was assayed by immunofluorescence over time. A reversible shift from a particular fimbrial phase to another fimbrial phase was measured. An intriguing property of multifimbrial phase variation was its extreme rapidity compared to flagellar phase variation in *Salmonella* spp. (140). An overnight culture of fractionated bacteria that expressed only one fimbrial type or that lacked fimbriae produced heterogeneous colonies of all fimbrial types of the strain. The apparent generation time of nonfimbriated cells was 14.6 min, and that of the

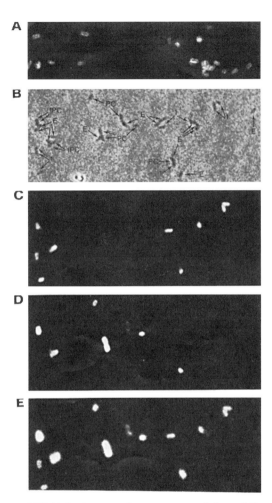

**FIGURE 1** immunoflourescence staining of *E. coli* KS71. (A) Underexposed micrograph of cells stained with anti-type 1 fluorescein isothiocyanate (FITC) conjugate (note the strong staining at cell edges); (B) phase-contrast micrograph of cells; (C) anti-type 1 FITC staining; (D) anti-P- and anti-C TRITC staining; (E) double exposure of FITC and TRITC conjugates. In panel B, nonfimbriated cells are marked E, type 1-fimbriated cells are marked 1, C- and/or P-fimbriated cells are marked PC, and cells stained with both conjugates (FITC and TRITC) are marked 1PC. Magnifications are $\times 2,800$ (A) and $\times 3,400$ (B through E). (From reference 104.)

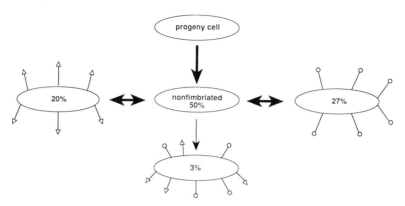

**FIGURE 2** Graphic representation of multifimbrial phase variation for a hypothetical strain that expresses two different fimbrial types. A progeny cell grown at 22°C is nonfimbriated. When transferred to 37°C, this progeny cell expresses two fimbrial types. Thick arrows show directions of preferential switch and cell type frequencies of subpopulations at 37°C.

whole culture was 25.6 min. This difference, which was observed consistently, indicates that a fraction of S-fimbriated cells change into nonfimbriated cells. The rate of phase shift from S-fimbriated to nonfimbriated cells was on the order of $8.2 \times 10^{-3}$ per cell generation. The rate of shift from type 1 fimbriation to nonfimbriation for this period was $1.6 \times 10^{-2}$. This rate was rapid enough to explain the heterogeneity of cells in colonies obtained from overnight growth of fractionated subpopulations. The preferential switch from fimbriated cells to nonfimbriated cells occurred within half an hour, and then cells having the other fimbrial type appeared. However, shifts directly from one fimbrial type to another have also occurred (Fig. 4).

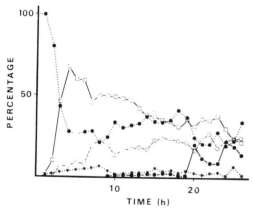

**FIGURE 3** Kinetics of fimbrial phase variation in *E. coli* KS71. Nonfimbriated cells grown on an agar plate at room temperature were transferred to static broth at 37°C and assayed for fimbriation every hour by immunofluorescence. About 2,500 cells were examined each hour. Symbols: ●⋯●, nonfimbriated cells; □, C-fimbriated cells; ○, P-fimbriated cells; ●—●, type 1-fimbriated cells; ★, cells with both P and C fimbriae. (From reference 104.)

The fimbrial phase shift at the level of single cells was visualized by immunofluorescence staining (Fig. 5). Samples taken from an S-fimbriated subpopulation grown for 1.0 to 1.5 h contained dividing cells that showed a special pattern of immunofluorescence staining in which half of the dividing cell was stained with anti-S fimbria IgG and the other portion was not stained. Such cells were probably undergoing a shift change from S fimbriation to nonfimbriation. Cells that were half stained with anti-S and half stained with anti-type 1 conjugates have never been observed. The existence of phase variation in *E. coli* carrying P and other fimbriae was confirmed by other investigators using

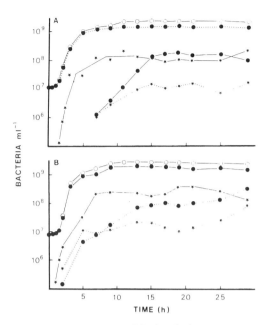

**FIGURE 4** Kinetics of fimbrial phase variation of the S-fimbriated subpopulation (A) and the type 1-fimbriated subpopulation (B). Symbols: ○, total cell number; ●····●, S-fimbriated cells; ●——●, type 1-fimbriated cells; ★——★, nonfimbriated cells; ★····★, cells with both type 1 and S fimbriae. (From reference 106a with permission.)

electron microscopy and molecular genetics (9, 29). Their reported rate of on-off shifting in a strain that expressed only type 1 fimbriae was slower than ours (22). These differences may be explained by the characteristics of individual isolates or by the methods used.

## Model for a Study of Colony Structure and Expression of Fimbriae

An in vitro method for testing the expression of fimbrial types with a colony has been developed (106). A modification of the direct immunofluorescence technique is used to detect the fimbrial subpopulations in bacterial colonies that are grown on nitrocellulose membranes. In general, the use of specific antibodies against several fimbrial types shows that fimbriated cells in the colony are organized into sectors of different shapes and sizes (Fig. 6). Control experiments showed that an overnight culture of a fractionated subpopulation carrying only one fimbrial type produces colonies that are heterogeneous with respect to fimbrial antigens that are detected by agglutination with anti-type 1- and S fimbria-specific IgG.

Colonies of *E. coli* grown on a nitrocellulose membrane were double stained with anti-type 1 fluorescein IgG conjugate and anti-S-fimbria rhodamine IgG conjugate. Colonies that most likely originated from a single cell in a particular fimbrial phase were stained in sectors whose lengths and numbers per colony were dependent on the fimbrial phase of the progeny cells. Short, narrow S-fimbrial sectors represented growth of cells that had switched from a type 1-fimbriated to an S-fimbriated phase. Conversely, colonies originating from the S-fimbriated subpopulation revealed long S-fimbriated sectors and short, narrow type 1 sectors. Nonstained dark sectors probably represented nonfimbriated cells that had switched from fimbrial types to a nonfimbriated phase. Despite various morphologies and numbers of sectors, boundaries of individual sectors were very clear and did not overlap. Similarly, a boundary was observed between two S-type colonies. Sectors of identical fimbrial types in two colonies appeared not to intermingle (Fig. 7). These in vitro studies demonstrated orderly heterogeneity (also called clonal exclusiveness) in colonies of fimbriated *E. coli* (106). Shapiro proposed that clonal exclusiveness depends on surface markers and accounts for the sharp colonial sector and intercolonial boundaries (138). Although the cause of clonal exclusiveness is not clear and clarification of the mechanism of multifimbrial phase variation is in the early stages, this fascinating phenomenon was postulated to contribute to pathogenicity of infection.

## Approaches to the Study of Phase Variation in Vivo

The complexity of phase variation has been further documented by the finding that a single microbial cell isolated directly from a patient or experimental animal usually expresses one fimbrial type but may rapidly switch to another type (50, 108, 125, 136). Patient urine or samples from experimental animals were analyzed directly on glass smears for fimbrial subpopulation types. Fractionated bacterial subpopulations expressing type 1, S, or no fimbriae were inoculated into experimental animals (peritonitis and meningitis models), and the occurrence of multifimbrial phase variation and the kinetics of fimbrial switching were investigated. In this in vivo model of mouse bacteremic peritonitis that was developed with fractionated *E. coli* cells, rapid phase variation occurred (Fig. 8A). The phenomenon observed for the S-fimbrial fraction was much faster than the one observed in vitro. A markedly faster switch occurring in vivo was mimicked in an in vitro system with mouse serum or peritoneal washing (Fig. 8B). An S-fimbrial on-phase inducer was postulated to be a low-molecular-weight dialyzable component of serum or tissue fluid (108). The induction of the S-fimbriated cells was so rapid that practically every new cell had switched to S-fimbria production (90 to 95% of cells independent of fractions). In contrast, the expression of type 1 fimbriae was not influenced by mouse serum or

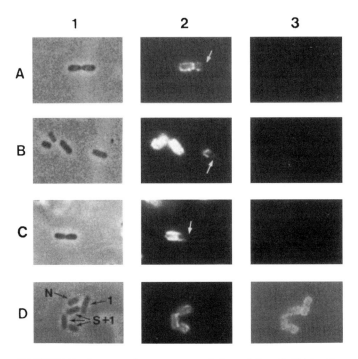

**FIGURE 5** Immunofluorescence staining of *E. coli* 3040 cells. Column 1, phase-contrast micrographs; column 2, anti-S TRITC staining; column 3, anti-type 1 FITC staining. Cells were sampled from the S-fimbriated subpopulation after growth for 1.5 h (A through C) or for 7 h (D). Arrows in A through C indicate non-stained sections of cells. Symbols in panel D: N, nonfimbriated cell; 1, type 1-fimbriated cell; S + 1, cells with both type 1 and S fimbriae. (From reference 106a with permission.)

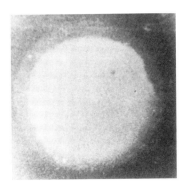
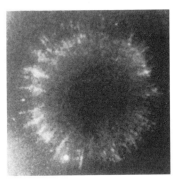
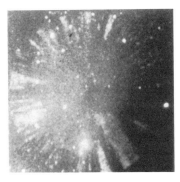

**FIGURE 6** Immunofluorescence staining of colonies of a type 1-fimbriated subpopulation of *E. coli* 3040. The same colony is shown with anti-type-1 FITC staining (a) and anti-S TRITC staining (b). (c) Colony stained with anti-S TRITC conjugate under agitation. (From reference 106 with permission.)

peritoneal washing. Development of the cell fractionation method also allowed investigation of differences in virulence of bacterial cell subpopulations carrying individual fimbrial types. Intraperitoneal infection of selected subpopulations showed that S fimbriae are advantageous to *E. coli* cells in the infectious process. The anti-S fimbria antibodies protect mice from lethal infection due to S-fimbriated *E. coli* subpopulations (108). In contrast, type 1-fimbriated cells are rapidly cleared from the circulation and are less likely to cause lethal infection. This finding is of special importance for dealing with bacteria that are expressing several fimbrial types and undergoing multifimbrial phase variation. The future development of protective measures should therefore accommodate the phenomenon of multiple fimbrial variation and fimbrial types expressed by uropathogenic strains in vivo.

Further modifications of the technique resulted in the development of a highly sensitive indirect immunofluorescence

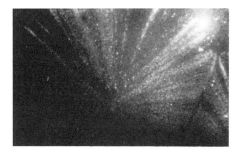

**FIGURE 7** Colonies of an S-fimbriated subpopulation stained with anti-S TRITC conjugate under agitation. (From reference 106 with permission.)

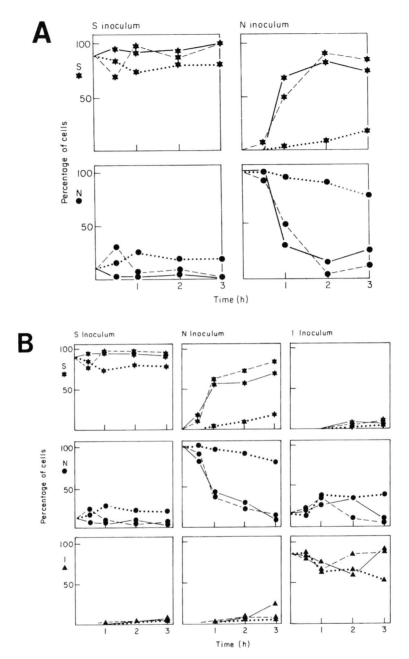

**FIGURE 8** (A) Percentage of bacteria that were S fimbriated (★) or nonfimbriated (●) in the inoculum (time 0), peritoneal cavity (---), or blood (———) at different times after intraperitoneal injection of $10^6$ S-fimbriated or nonfimbriated (N) bacteria (*E. coli* IH3080). Dotted lines indicate fimbriation patterns of the same inocula with continuing growth in Luria broth. (From reference 108 with permission.) (B) Percentage of bacteria (*E. coli* IH3080) that were S fimbriated (★), nonfimbriated (●), or type 1 fimbriated (▲) in the inoculum (time 0) or after different periods of growth in mouse serum (———), peritoneal washing (---), or Luria broth (···). Inocula were the same subpopulations injected in mice for panel A. (From reference 108 with permission.)

assay for the detection and evaluation of expression of P, type 1, and type 1C fimbriae in the urine of patients with acute urinary tract infections (125). Use of indirect immunofluorescence was necessary because of significant variation in expression (41, 109, 150), antigenic epitopes, and limited cross-reactivity between P fimbriae from *E. coli* cells of different O serotypes (125, 126). Using direct smears of urine or urine sediments, we demonstrated heterogeneity of fimbriated bacterial subpopulations in the urine of patients with pyelonephritis or other clinical presentations of urinary tract infection. The presence of cells that express a single fimbrial type is interpreted to be the result of fimbrial phase variation in the urinary tract in vivo. The percentage of P-fimbriated cells in bacterial populations of a given patient varied between 0.1 and 95% in urine and did not correlate with the level of P-fimbria-phase cells the isolates produced on agar plates (Table 1). The expression of type 1 and type 1C fimbriae in vivo is less frequent than the expression of P fimbriae. The association of different subpopulations with uroepithelial cells has been also documented.

Finding this on-off type 1 fimbrial variation and multifimbrial phase variation contributed to our understanding of the properties and tissue tropism of bacteria and the potential mechanisms of ascending urinary tract infection. The presence of multiple *E. coli* populations bearing adhesins of different binding specificities may contribute to preferential colonization and infection of the lower urinary tract, the upper urinary tract (renal tissue), or both (74, 108, 109, 125, 126, 136). The recognition that bacteria can be fimbriated during infection and may differ from bacteria grown on normal laboratory media has many consequences, both for the understanding of pathogenic mechanisms and for the design of preventive measures.

## IN VITRO MODELS OF TISSUE TROPISM OF UROPATHOGENS

The first attempts to investigate interactions between uropathogens and renal tissue were made by Scandinavian and U.S. investigators. Originally, receptors for P-fimbriated *E. coli* were found in the primate kidney (132, 149). Further, Väisänen-Rhen demonstrated an interaction between uropathogenic *E. coli* and human renal tissue: they showed that bacterial cells labeled with fluorochrome attach to cryostat sections of human kidney (158). In those early studies, however, the use of an *E. coli* strain that expressed several fimbrial types resulted in a uniform distribution of the *E. coli* cells binding to the renal tissue and

**TABLE 1** Level of P-fimbria expression by *E. coli* in infected urine and after subculture on agar plates[a]

| Strain | Source | Serogroup | % of P-fimbriated cells in bacterial population | |
|---|---|---|---|---|
| | | | Urine | Subculture |
| AP4 | Pyelonephritis | O2 | 95 | 1 |
| AP5 | Pyelonephritis | O4 | <0.1 | 20 |
| AP7 | Pyelonephritis | O4 | 95 | 50 |
| AP10 | Cystitis | O6 | <0.1 | 10 |
| AP11 | Cystitis | Nontypeable | 95 | 50 |
| AP15 | Cystitis | Nontypeable | <0.1 | 0.5 |
| AP16 | Pyelonephritis | O2 | 20 | 30 |
| AP18 | Pyelonephritis | O6 | 50 | 50 |
| AP19 | Cystitis | Nontypeable | 90 | 0.5 |

[a] Data are from reference 125 with permission.

therefore to a great extent masked the specific differential renal tropism of *E. coli* cell subpopulations bearing distinct fimbriae (53, 77, 156–158).

## Differential Tissue Tropism of Uropathogens

Evidence for differential tissue tropism in various *E. coli* uropathogens expressing different fimbriae was provided by Nowicki et al. (100). The zonal topography of cryostat sections of human kidney was visualized by staining with plant lectins that detect renal substructures (45). Some plant lectins show a very specific pattern of binding to morphologically restricted domains of the kidney and are used as tissue markers (Table 2). Plant lectin-specific binding patterns indicate compartmentalization of glycoconjugates in different parts of the human kidney and therefore suggest the possibility of a related phenomenon for bacterial lectinlike factors. Following lectin staining, tissue sections overlaid with fluorochrome-labeled *E. coli* strains expressing either P fimbriae (type KS71A) or O75X (Dr) fimbriae. These experiments showed that P-fimbriated *E. coli* cells preferentially attach to luminal sites in the renal tubules, while Dr-fimbriated *E. coli* cells attach to the interstitial tissue and Bowman's capsule (Fig. 9 and 10). Extensions of these studies resulted in the use of purified bacterial fimbriae obtained from clinical isolates (71) or recombinant strains (98) in which cloned adhesins were expressed. These observations showed that, depending on fimbrial type, uropathogens interact with different compartments in the kidney. It was concluded that interaction with different tissue compartments is associated with the binding specificity of each fimbrial type. These findings, combined with multifimbrial phase variation, contribute to the general concept that a bacterial culture contains different subsets of cells that can interact with different segments of the urinary tract. The same phenomenon, in combination with tissue enhancers of fimbrial expression, may provide microorganisms with options for displaying differential renal tissue tropism. Escape from the immune attack of a fimbrial subpopulation is also likely, considering the intriguing mechanism of rapid phase switch (104, 130) and the substantial differences in antigenic epitopes of different adhesins (126).

## Binding of P Fimbriae to Human Urinary Tract Tissues

Molecular cloning of different fimbrial types and studies of binding specificities allowed investigators to isolate a family of

**TABLE 2** Lectin markers for nephron domains[a]

| Marker | Abbreviation | Nominal sugar specificity | Nephron site recognized |
|---|---|---|---|
| Lectins | | | |
| *Dolichos biflorus* | DBA | $\alpha$-D-GalNAc | Collecting ducts |
| *Arachis hypogaea* | PNA | $\beta$-D-Gal-D-GalNAc | Distal tubules, Bowman's capsule |
| *Ulex europaeus* | UEAI | $\alpha$-L-Fuc | Vascular endothelium |
| Antibodies to: | | | |
| Proximal tubular brush border | | | Proximal tubules |
| Tamm-Horsfall protein | | | Distal tubules |
| Cytokeratin | | | Collecting ducts |
| Vimentin | | | Peritubular areas |

[a] Data are from reference 100 with permission.

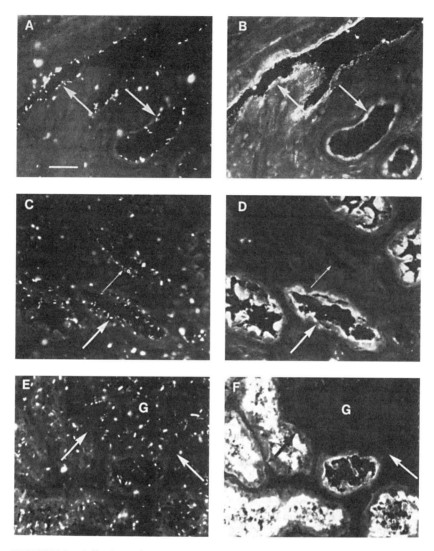

**FIGURE 9** Adhesion of EH824 (A, C, and E) to human kidney. Bacteria adhere specifically to vascular endothelium (thick arrows in panel A), as can be seen from double staining with UEAI, a marker for vascular endothelium (B). The strain also binds to the lumina of proximal tubules (thick arrow in panel C) and to the glomerules (marked by G in panel E), visualized by double staining with anti-brush border antibodies (D and F). The thin arrow in panel C shows bacterial adhesion to the lumen of a distal tubule that is negative for anti-brush border antibodies. Bar, 10 μm. (From reference 100 with permission.)

related P adhesins (49, 60, 61, 65, 66, 88, 160). This in turn allowed the study of tissue tropism and the analysis of subtle differences in binding sites for the several P fimbriae within different segments of the urinary tract.

Differences in adhesion have been analyzed in vitro by using cryostat sections of human kidney, which allows further dissection of receptor specificities and locations of binding sites. The receptor molecules that provide binding sites for P

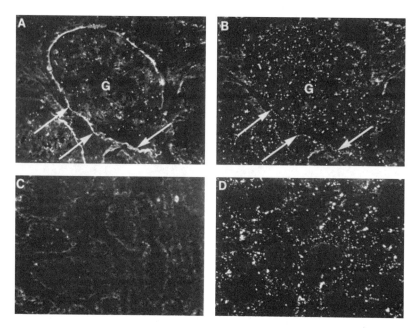

**FIGURE 10** Adhesion of BN53 to the glomerulus (A and B). Marker staining in panel A was with fluorescein isothiocyanate peanut agglutinin. Arrows indicate bacterial adhesion to Bowman's capsule. Effect of anti-O75X (C) and anti-type 1C (D) fimbrial Fab fragments on adhesion by IH11033. Note efficient inhibition by anti-O75X Fab fragments. G, glomerules. Bar, 10 μm. (From reference 100 with permission.)

fimbriae in renal tissue were identified by using specific antibodies and ligand analogs that inhibit adhesin binding. Two genetically related fimbriae, called Pap and Pap-2, or Prs, that were molecularly cloned from *E. coli* J96 detect distinct binding sites within the renal tissue or on erythrocytes of different species (60, 61) (Fig. 11 and 12). Pap fimbriae attach predominantly to luminal sites in collecting ducts, and Pap-2 fimbriae bind to Bowman's capsule. The renal antigen recognized by Pap-2 in this tissue is thought to be the P blood group-related stage-specific embryonic antigen 4 (SSEA-4) (58, 155). The primary structure of SSEA-4 is that of a globoside with terminal NeuAc$\alpha$2 → Gal$\beta$1 → 3GalNAc$\beta$1 → 3Gal$\alpha$1 → 4Gal. Interestingly, GalNAc$\beta$1 → 3Gal inhibits the binding of purified Pap-2 fimbriae to Bowman's capsule (Fig. 13). Studies in which different erythrocyte species were used for characterization of Pap-2 (Prs) adhesin identified Forssman antigen of sheep erythrocytes as the binding molecule for Pap-2 (88). Although Forssman antigen, which contains the terminal structure GalNAc$\beta$1 → 3Gal, seems to be partially related to SSEA-4, only some individuals of blood group A carry this antigen in the kidneys (10, 39). We characterized the binding of monoclonal antibody, anti-SSEA-4, and anti-Forssman antigen with respect to renal binding and attempted to use these reagents to interfere with the attachment of Pap-2 to renal substructures. Anti-SSEA-4, similarly to Pap-2, bound to Bowman's capsule, but in the same individual, anti-Forssman IgG did not. In addition, anti-SSEA-4 blocked binding of Pap-2 fimbriae to Bowman's capsule, while anti-Forssman did not.

13. IN VITRO MODELS OF UROPATHOGENS ■ 353

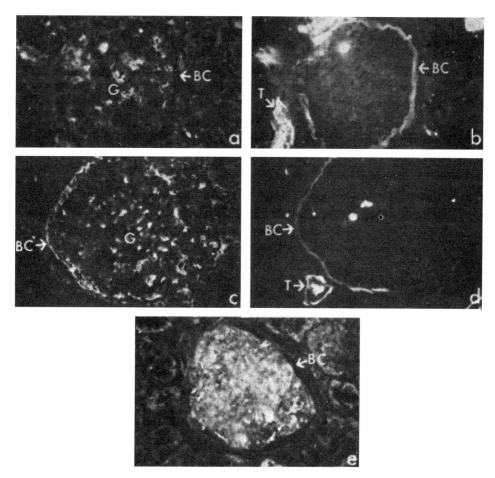

**FIGURE 11** Binding of purified Pap and Pap-2 fimbriae to glomeruli or Bowman's capsule. Pap fimbriae adhered to glomerular elements but not to Bowman's capsule (a), even after overnight incubation (e). Pap-2 fimbriae adhered to Bowman's capsule and some glomerular elements (c). Double staining the sections with peanut agglutinin-fluorescein detected Bowman's capsule and some tubules (b and d). Abbreviations: BC, Bowman's capsule; G, glomerulus; T, tubule. (From reference 60.)

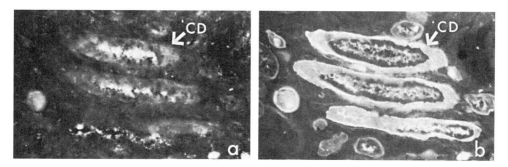

**FIGURE 12** Pap-2 fimbriae bound to the luminal surfaces of collecting ducts (CD) (a) as detected by peanut agglutinin double staining of the same tissue section (b). (From reference 60.)

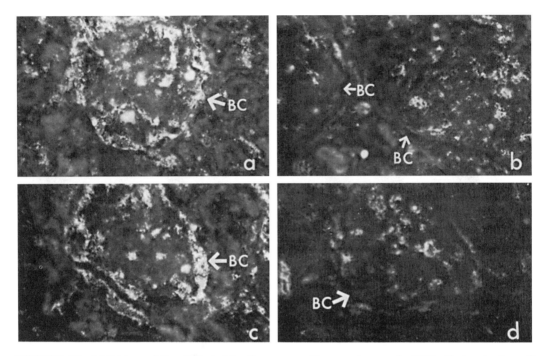

**FIGURE 13** Inhibition of Pap-2 fimbrial adherence to Bowman's capsule (BC). Preincubation of purified fimbriae with 0.75% Gal$\alpha$1 → 4Gal had no inhibitory effect on Pap-2 adherence to Bowman's capsule (a and c), but 0.75% GalNAc$\beta$1 → 3Gal completely blocked this binding (b and d). (From reference 60.)

These observations suggest that the binding epitope recognized by Pap-2-encoded fimbriae is complex, possibly including the long internal structure of SSEA-4. Therefore, on Bowman's capsule of the human kidney, SSEA-4 seems to be a likely receptor for Pap-2 fimbriae.

Finding that *E. coli* pyelonephritis-associated isolates may express two P-related adhesins with different receptor specificities for renal tissue furthered our understanding of the pathogenesis of urogenital infections. It is possible that a specialized subpopulation of cells expressing individual fimbrial types is advantageous for the microorganism, allowing the display of unique tissue tropisms and escape from immune attack.

*E. coli* cells of different serotypes may express antigenically different P fimbriae (123, 126), and one strain may even carry three copies of Pap-related genes (48, 49). Three related P adhesins can hypothetically have different tissue tropisms. An example of such differences between different isolates or P fimbriae displaying diversified renal tropism was investigated. Korhonen and colleagues purified P fimbriae from *E. coli* KS71. P fimbria KS71A is one of the two P-related adhesins expressed by *E. coli* KS71 (79, 129, 131). Interestingly, purified P fimbriae (KS71A) bound to Bowman's capsule and to vascular endothelium in the renal interstitium and the glomeruli. Fimbria KS71A also bound to the luminal aspects of proximal and distal tubules and of collecting ducts. The binding of KS71A-P fimbriae was restricted to epithelial and vascular elements and to the endothelium of the kidney. Apparently, localization of renal binding sites for the Pap and Pap-2 fimbriae was different from that observed for KS71A (Table 3). This P-fimbrial type (KS71A) seemed, to some extent, to display the combined specificities of Pap and Pap-2, binding to both Bowman's capsule and tubular luminal elements. In another study, Hull and colleagues molecularly cloned another copy of the *pap* genes of *E. coli* (66). Although this fimbrial type was not tested with respect to tissue specificity, the hemagglutination patterns represented the combined binding specificities of Pap and Pap-2 fimbriae. In general, these results demonstrate that despite the minimal structure of Galα1 → 4Gal necessary for providing binding sites for P fimbriae, subtle differences between the related adhesins occur. These differences may contribute to the very specific and differential tissue tropisms of individual strains and probably offer the invading microorganism a variety of opportunities for binding to the epithelium in the urinary tract and the kidney. It remains to be seen whether subtle diversity in the receptor specificities of different pyelonephritis-associated *E. coli* strains can determine the development and progress of an individual's urinary tract infection.

## Binding of Dr Fimbriae to Human Urinary Tract Tissues

Studies using cryostat sections of human kidneys and other portions of the urinary tract overlaid with purified fimbrial fibers

**TABLE 3** Tissue-binding specificities of various uropathogenic adhesins[a]

| Tissue substructure | Adhesin binding[b] | | | | | | | | |
|---|---|---|---|---|---|---|---|---|---|
| | P (Pap) | P-2 (Prs) | P (K571A) | Dr | Type 1[c] | Type 1C | S | MR/P | MR/K |
| Kidney | | | | | | | | | |
| Glomerulus | + | + | + | +/− | − | − | + | − | + |
| Bowman's capsule | − | + | + | +++ | − | − | + | − | +++ |
| Basement membrane | − | − | − | +++ | − | − | − | − | +++ |
| Tubule (lumen) | +/− | +/− | ++ | − | +/− | +/− | ++ | ++ | +/− |
| Vescular endothelium | | | +++ | +/− | +++ | − | − | | |
| Urinary bladder | | | | | | | | | |
| Epithelium | +++ | +++ | + | − | +/−★ | − | ++ | | |
| Muscular layer | +++ | +++ | + | + | +++ | + | + | | |
| Connective tissue | +/− | +/− | − | +++ | − | − | ++ | | |
| Urine: sediment cells | | | + | + | − | − | + | +++ | +/− |
| Uterus | | | | | | | | | |
| Endometrial glands | | | | +/− | | | | | |
| Basement membranes | | | | +/− | | | | | |
| Myometrium | | | | − | | | | | |
| Colon: colonic glands (enterocytes) | + | | | +++ | +/− | | | | |

[a] This summary is based on information available in the literature.
[b] +++ to +/−, binding intensity from strong to weak, respectively; −, no binding.
[c] Reports on interaction of type 1-fimbriated *E. coli* with human uroepithelium have not been consistent, showing either strong attachment or complete lack of binding.

resulted in the detection of specific high-density binding sites in different anatomical locations and tissue substructures (Fig. 14).

Comprehensive mapping of the potential binding sites for *E. coli* that carry Dr adhesin types has been achieved with cryostat sections of different organs and tissues, including tissues from the digestive tract, lower and upper urinary tract, anatomically associated genital tract, and respiratory tract (64, 107, 167). For example, ligand binding sites for Dr fimbriae were detected in the luminal portions of the colonic glands, uroepithelium of the bladder, urethras, renal pelvis, kidney, interstitial tissue, and glomerulus (Fig. 14) (107). In the renal tissue, purified Dr adhesin selectively bound to the basement membranes of proximal and distal tubules and with slightly lower efficiency to the basement membranes of collecting ducts (80). In the glomerulus, Dr adhesin bound to Bowman's capsule (80, 107). Binding to exfoliated epithelial cells in human urine was also observed (80). This suggests that Dr adhesin can provide a mechanism for bacterial binding both to epithelial surfaces in the lower urinary tract and to nonepithelial domains of the renal interstitial tissue.

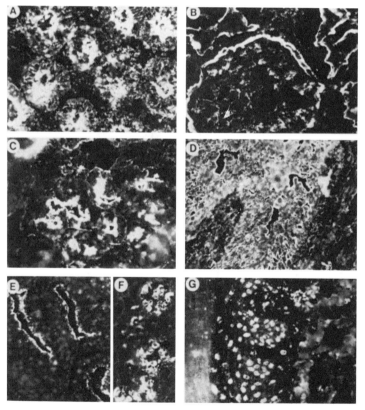

**FIGURE 14** Binding specificity of purified Dr hemagglutinin for human tissues. A, colonic glands; B, renal tubular basement membrane (curved arrows) and Bowman's capsule (straight arrows); C, bronchial glands (arrows indicate basement membrane); D, ureter, transitional epithelial cells (area between arrows); E, endometrial glands; F, fallopian tube; G, skin, nuclei (thin arrows) (asterisk and thick arrows show layers of skin, stratum corneum, and malpighian layer, respectively). (From reference 107 with permission.)

## Binding of Dr Fimbriae to the Genital Tract

Dr binding sites have also been found in other organs and tissues, including endometrial, sweat, and bronchial glands (Fig. 14) (107). Dr binding sites in some structures may not be accessible as potential receptors for colonization; however, expression of these epitopes in the glands, which are directly accessible to bacteria, may be relevant for colonization (64).

Because of the anatomical association of and the functional relationship between the urinary and genital tracts, colonization of the periurethral area and the vaginal introitus is crucial for the development of ascending infection (27, 137). Genitourinary infections are often associated with pregnancy. Pyelonephritis occurring during gestation is recognized as a high-risk infection for preterm labor or intrauterine retardation (96). Unlike the mechanism of ascending infection in the urinary tract, that of ascending infection in the genital tract is not well understood (64). It is very likely that, as in the urinary tract, receptor binding sites for microorganisms colonizing the genital tract are expressed along the epithelial cells of the lower and upper genital tracts and reach the endometrial epithelium. A recent study indicated Dr binding sites in the endometrial glands of several patients (64). Clear variations in the distribution and density of Dr binding sites between individuals were observed. Interestingly, two binding specificities are present in the one structural DraA fimbrial protein (98, 165). A binding site for Dr fimbriae found on Dr blood group antigen (103) was further localized as a portion of decay accelerating factor (DAF) (101, 121, 153), a complement regulatory protein that protects host tissue from the cytotoxic activity of the human complement system (44, 97). Korhonen's group also reported a collagen type IV binding specificity for Dr fimbriae (165).

To resolve the question of whether natural binding sites for Dr fimbriae present in the endometrial glands represent DAF or collagen type IV, we immunohistochemically characterized binding domains in the cryostat section of human endometrium by using purified recombinant fimbriae, DAF-specific monoclonal antibody, and anti-type IV collagen IgG. Inhibition studies indicated blocking of fimbrial binding to endometrial glands by anti-DAF IgG and lack of blocking by anti-type IV collagen IgG. Corresponding experiments on parallel cryostat sections using staining with anti-DAF or anti-type IV collagen indicated positive staining of the same glandular substructures with anti-DAF but negative staining with anti-type IV collagen IgG. This indicates that DAF, not type IV collagen in the endometrial glands, is likely to be the natural receptor for Dr fimbriae (64). In situ hybridization with a DAF cDNA probe in human endometrium demonstrated a strong DAF mRNA signal in the glandular epithelium at the secretory phase and a weak signal at the proliferative phase (62). Interestingly, the availability of Dr ligands for potential colonization also changed. Dr ligands in the secretory phase were present in the apical sites of glandular epithelium, but during the proliferative phase, they were expressed in glandular basement membranes. This study provided evidence that a rapid cyclic change in the Dr ligand density occurs in the female genitourinary tract. (For detailed information, see Methods for Quantitation of Tissue Ligands for Bacterial Colonization below.)

## Binding of Type 1 Fimbriae to Human Urinary Tract Tissues

Type 1 fimbrial genes are present in the majority of E. coli genomes (11–14, 20, 21, 31). The expression of type 1 fimbriae, however, varies depending on the environment (68, 91, 116). The binding specificity of type 1 fimbriae is similar to that of concanavalin A: both recognize $\alpha$-D-mannose, although concanavalin A may also recognize other carbohydrates (25, 26, 33, 40, 47, 82, 112, 115, 127, 139).

Type 1 fimbriae display remarkably different binding patterns within the human kidney and bladder than do P and Dr adhesins (161). In the kidney, weak binding to the luminal and cytoplasmic elements of proximal tubules and to the connective tissue of veins and arteries occurs. Type 1 fimbriae bind to urinary slime or Tamm-Horsfall glycoprotein, a main component of the slime that is available on the surfaces of uroepithelial cells (110, 117, 145). Interestingly, uroepithelial cells of distal tubules may synthesize and secrete Tamm-Horsfall glycoprotein; nevertheless, type 1 fimbriae bind only weakly to the distal part of the nephron (161). In the bladder, muscle layers and vasal walls provide strong binding sites for type 1 fimbriae. Surprisingly, no binding of type 1 fimbriae to uroepithelium in the human bladder has been detected by Korhonen's group (162). Other investigators demonstrated binding of type 1-fimbriated E. coli to the uroepithelium (169).

There are several explanations for the reported discrepancies. In studies by Virkola et al. (162), a lack of type 1 fimbriae binding to the bladder uroepithelium correlated with a lack of antibody staining of Tamm-Horsfall protein. Other investigators who reported type 1 fimbrial binding to the uroepithelium did not always describe similar controls. Differences in the reported studies may have resulted from differences in the sources of tissues, ages and genders of patients, binding assays, and strains used. For example, in one study demonstrating uroepithelial binding of type 1-positive E. coli, uropithelium was obtained from elderly males with prostate cancer (169).

Support for the role of type 1 fimbriae in the infection process has been generated by using animal models. The contribution of type 1 fimbriae to the development of experimental pyelonephritis and the protective effect of mannose compounds strongly support the importance of this adhesin in experimental urinary tract infection (36–38, 52, 89, 111, 144). Bloch et al. (8) used an experimental neonatal mouse model to demonstrate the importance of E. coli type 1 fimbriae in the colonization of the buccal cavity. However, although type 1 fimbriae may be important in human infections, definitive clinical evidence has been limited. Except for a few reports that include studies of the role of type 1 fimbriae in the colonization of catheterized patients and the association of type 1 fimbriae with infection in early pregnancy, extensive data to strongly support this notion are not available (93, 102).

## Binding of S Fimbriae to Human Urinary Tract Tissues

Some uropathogenic E. coli strains, as well as some E. coli strains associated with bacterial meningitis, express S fimbriae (78, 108, 136). Binding of S fimbriae is inhibited by sialolactose, an analog of the receptor necessary for S-fimbrial attachment to epithelial cells (35, 94, 95, 119).

S fimbriae have also been studied: they bind to the epithelial-cell layer in the bladder (162). Weak interaction with interstitial and connective tissue components was observed. S fimbriae also bind to the human kidney, in particular to glomerular structures, including Bowman's capsule (75). Interestingly, S-fimbria-positive E. coli associated with meningitis bind to the endothelium and epithelium of the chorionic plexus of the neonatal rat brain (118). Within the human urinary tract, S fimbriae exhibit binding patterns related to those of P fimbriae. Similarity in the binding patterns of the S and P fimbrial types does not, however, correlate with the virulence of strains expressing these fimbriae (the expression of P fimbriae is most frequently associated with acute renal infections). This discrepancy indicates that the presence of similar binding sites in the urinary tract and the kidney does not alone explain why P fimbriae have a higher pathogenic potential in renal infection than S fimbriae do (120, 135).

## Binding of Type 1C Fimbriae to Human Urinary Tract Tissues

The role of type 1C fimbriae of uropathogenic *E. coli* has only recently been investigated. Interest in this fimbrial type is due to its immunological relatedness to type 1 fimbriae (67, 69, 124, 125). Kohonen's group characterized potential binding sites for type 1C fimbriae in the urinary tract (162). In the kidney, recombinant type 1C fimbriae expressed in a laboratory strain attached to distal tubules and collecting ducts and bound very weakly to glomerular structures. Binding to vascular endothelium of the kidney and bladder was also observed. A type 1C-fimbria-expressing recombinant strain also adhered to cultured renal tubular cells isolated from proximal tubules of a pig (90). Type 1C fimbriae also seemed to bind to interstitial elements, most likely basement membranes (162). The role of type 1C fimbriae in the pathogenesis of pyelonephritis is not clear, especially since type 1C fimbriae do not adhere to epithelial cells from human urine. However, binding to the distal parts of the nephron and to the interstitial space may contribute to the critical steps in renal-tissue invasion. Further studies are necessary for increasing our understanding of the involvement of type 1C fimbriae in the pathogenesis of urinary tract infection.

## Binding of MR/P Fimbria and MR/K Hemagglutin of *P. mirabilis* to Human Urinary Tract Tissues

*P. mirabilis* is a common microorganism found in complicated urinary tract infections in humans. It is associated with urinary tract infections in hospitalized patients and in individuals with anatomic abnormalities and with local damage of the urinary tract, e.g., indwelling catheters (84). Among *P. mirabilis* adhesins, two types have been extensively tested for attachment (2, 92, 113). MR/P fimbriae are associated with the ability to hemagglutinate human erythrocytes in the presence of mannose, and MR/K (also called type 3) hemagglutinin is associated with the ability to agglutinate tannic acid-treated erythrocytes. Similarly to other uropathogens, MR/K hemagglutinin and MR/P fimbriae show different binding patterns in the urinary tract (135). MR/P fimbriae bind poorly to epithelial cells and show no interaction with glomerular elements. MR/P, however, binds sufficiently to tubular epithelial cells of the kidney and to exfoliated epithelial cells from human urine. A limiting factor that potentially restricts the capacity of MR/P fimbriae for bacterial colonization is the fact that normal human urine inhibits the binding of MR/P fimbriae. This inhibition may be a natural protection in the human host against *P. mirabilis* infections (135).

The renal tropism of MR/K hemagglutinin is completely different from that of MR/P. MR/K most likely recognizes areas close to the tubular basement membranes and Bowman's capsules of glomeruli. Poor binding or no attachment to tubular epithelial cells and epithelial cells of the urine sediment was observed. It has been suggested that such tissue tropism is not likely to be useful in the colonization of intact epithelial surfaces. On the other hand, MR/K specificity may help in the colonization of extracellular matrices (ECMs) where these structures are exposed. Binding of the MR/K hemagglutinin is not inhibited by urine and therefore is likely to contribute to *P. mirabilis* tropism toward basement membranes and connective tissue.

## Binding of Uropathogens to ECM Components

Bacterial adhesins may attach to host tissues through complex interactions. Some of the bacterial cell surface adhesins specifically interact with ECM components. These adhesins have generally been designated microbial surface components recognizing adhesive matrix molecules

(MSCRAMM) (122). MSCRAMM recognize fibronectin, fibrinogen, collagen, and heparin-related molecules. The importance of these molecules in host tissue colonization and invasion was reviewed recently (81, 122). Therefore, this chapter introduces these interactions in general and provides a few examples applicable to uropathogens.

The biological significance of bacterial adherence to matrix proteins remains largely speculative. The ECM is a biologically active tissue composed of a complex mixture of molecules that, in addition to serving as structural components, profoundly affects the cellular physiology of these tissues (42). The composition of the ECM affects eukaryotic cell adhesion, migration, proliferation, and differentiation (133). Interactions between eukaryotic cells and ECM components are mediated by specific cellular receptors, among which the integrin-mediated interactions are the best understood (133). The ECM may serve as a target not only for the adhesion of eukaryotic host cells to each other but also for the attachment of colonizing microorganisms, including uropathogens.

The biological importance of microbial interaction with ECMs and the role of this process in pathogenesis are only now beginning to be addressed. Some invasive microorganisms appear to use integrins to invade host cells (51). The ECM may form sheets called basement membranes, which separate different types of cells. Basement membranes, which influence the polarization of the cells and the three-dimensional organization of tissue, may also serve as barriers for eukaryotic cell movement and may participate in the filtration of selected molecules (24, 59, 154, 168). The major components of basement membranes include but are not limited to type IV collagen, laminin, heparin sulfate, and proteoglycans. In 1978, Kuusela was the first to report an interaction between microorganism and matrix protein (85). He found that soluble fibronectin binds to *Staphylococcus aureus*.

Attachment of uropathogens to the individual substructure, e.g., to basement membranes, may be promoted by several different components of the basement membrane. For example, type V collagen binding provides a target for *Klebsiella pneumoniae* (152), whereas Dr fimbriae may mediate *E. coli* binding to type IV collagen (152, 165). It appears that these interactions may be even more complex, because the same *draA*-encoded Dr-fimbrial structural protein seems to display binding to type IV collagen and DAF, both of which are present in selected basement membranes. Subsequent studies showed that Dr fimbriae recognize type IV collagen in a specific manner. The binding site for Dr fimbriae has been localized to the 7S amino-terminal domain of type IV collagen (164, 165).

Type 3 fimbriae are expressed by several uropathogens, including *Klebsiella, Enterobacter, Providencia, Serratia, Morganella, Proteus,* and other species (4, 19, 30, 92, 152). These organelles bind not only to the intracellular matrix but also with increased ability to urinary catheter material (92). It is somewhat surprising that, in a fashion similar to *E. coli* cells that express Dr fimbriae, several other uropathogens, including *Klebsiella* spp., bind to Bowman's capsule. The MrkD minor protein of the type 3 fimbria of *K. pneumoniae* promotes binding to Bowman's capsule, arterial walls, interstitial connective tissue, and, most likely, the tubular basement membranes of the human kidney. The renal binding molecule recognized by type 3 fimbriae of *Klebsiella* spp. was identified as type V collagen (152).

Most uropathogenic species carry genes encoding type 1 fimbriae (13, 14). These fimbriae possess mannose-binding specificities mediated by the *fimH*-encoded adhesin (40, 47, 68, 82, 115, 116). The *fimH* product also exhibits fibronectin binding that is not affected by periodate treatment and therefore may not involve a carbohydrate component (Table 4) (83, 141). This suggests that type 1 fimbriae may have alternative ways of recognizing carbohydrate and protein ligands, as opposed to Dr adhesin, which seems to recognize noncarbohydrate peptide sequences on both type IV collagen and DAF.

P fimbria was initially recognized as the *E. coli* organelle required for binding Galα1 → 4Gal disaccharide. This binding was localized to the PapG tip adhesin protein. Two other minor proteins associated with PapG (PapE and PapF) promote noncarbohydrate-mediated adherence to fibronectin (164, 166). Similarly, *E. coli* curli appendages express fibronectin-binding properties (6). Other ECM components may also be a target for binding by fimbriae. *E. coli* type 1 fimbriae may mediate binding to laminin through the *fimH* gene product (159). Laminin may also be a target for binding by S fimbriae (162) and curli (114).

Research on the biological significance of ECM components and the role of uropathogen attachment to them is in its infancy. Many of the specificities are not yet known, and those already identified need to be further characterized. The limited information gathered to date suggests that there are some interesting structural trends in bacterial binding proteins and that MSCRAMM-ECM ligand interactions may be important steps in the molecular pathogenesis of some infections. It is conceivable that after microbial invasion, ECM components are available for interaction. Similarly, exposure of basement membranes following tissue injury or toxic activity of secreted microbial components may be an additional factor that contributes to infection. Our unpublished experiments on a clinical Dr$^+$ *E. coli* strain and its insertional Dr$^-$ mutant, in which expression of the Dr fimbriae was abolished, suggest an involvement of the Dr-fimbrial coding region in the development of chronic nephritis. Dr fimbriae bind to type IV collagen

**TABLE 4** Fimbrial adherence factors[a]

| Adherence factor | Specific adhesin(s) | Receptor | Carbohydrate or protein | Inhibitor | Organism | Reference(s) |
|---|---|---|---|---|---|---|
| Type 1 | | Fibronectin | Protein | Mannose | *Escherichia coli* | 159 |
| Type 1 | FimH | Laminin | Carbohydrate | Mannose | *Escherichia coli*, *Salmonella enteritidis* | 83, 141 |
| Type 3 | MrkD | Type V collagen | Protein | Spermidine | *Klebsiella pneumoniae* | 152 |
| Dr/O75X | DrA | Type IV collagen, DAF | Protein | Chloramphenicol, N-acetyltyrosine | *Escherichia coli* | 164, 165 |
| S | | Laminin | Carbohydrate | Sialyl (α 2-3) galactose | *Escherichia coli* | 162 |
| Pap | PapE, PapF | Fibronectin | Protein | | *Escherichia coli* | 166 |
| Curli, thin aggregative fimbriae | Crl | Fibronectin, laminin, type I and IV collagen | Protein | | *Escherichia coli* | 6, 114 |

[a] Reproduced with permission from the *Annual Review of Microbiology* (122), © 1994 by Annual Reviews Inc.

and DAF, and therefore, intracellular matrix proteins and other molecules of basement membranes such as DAF could be of crucial importance as targets for adhesion in the selected group of patients in whom a common denominator may be chronic persistent colonization. This hypothesis remains to be investigated.

## METHODS FOR QUANTITATION OF TISSUE LIGANDS FOR BACTERIAL COLONIZATION

Historically, experiments provided evidence that uroepithelial or vaginal cells of patients with chronic infections bind uropathogens more efficiently than do cells from healthy individuals (27). Those early experiments suggested quantitative differences in uroepithelial tissue ligands in infectious processes in tested subjects. Other approaches, e.g., fluorescence-activated cell sorting or enumeration of bacterial cells binding to individual epithelial cells, were also attempted (143, 145–149). However, these studies were at best semiquantitative. Development of purification methods and isolation of recombinant adhesins allowed the use of bacterial adhesins as staining reagents. Consequently, such adhesins, including Dr hemagglutinin (101), were proposed for use in the diagnosis of human diseases and were used as tissue-staining reagents.

Recent progress in microcomputer image analysis offered new options for diagnosis of human diseases (28). An objective measurement of cumulative optical density of estrogen receptors from histological sections of breast cancer was developed and proven to correspond well to receptor density determined by chemical purification (28).

Quantitative methods that measure the number of tissue-binding sites for bacterial adhesins and therefore the potential contribution of these binding sites to colonization and infection were recently explored by Kaul and colleagues (64). Computer image analysis was used for quantitating the densities of tissue-binding sites for bacterial adhesins in the urogenital tract (Fig. 15). An example of such an analysis is the measurement of Dr ligand density in the human uterus (64) and kidney (unpublished data). Interestingly, individual subjects differ dramatically in the receptor density of the Dr ligands. These differences are postulated to contribute to individual sensitivity to colonization. Studies by Rutter et al. showed that lack of binding sites for adhesive *E. coli* correlates with low infection rates in piglets (134). In humans, however, the majority of ligands mediating bacterial colonization are common antigens present in almost all individuals. Consequently, each person should be susceptible to infection at all times. Our group postulated that rapid changes in the density of tissue ligands could occur and could contribute to the development of infection in young noncompromised individuals (62–64).

The rapid cyclic change of Dr ligands in young women occurs in response to hormonal regulation of their menstrual cycles. In the endometrial glands, the expression of Dr ligand increases during the secretory phase of the cycle (days 15 to 28) and decreases during the proliferative phase of the cycle (days 1 to 14). Association with the phases of the menstrual cycle suggests that progesterone may affect the expression of bacterial ligand molecules. The temporal pattern of Dr ligand expression was confirmed by in situ hybridization through the use of DAF cDNA probes (63). The results of these studies, however, need to be correlated with the occurrence of infections, and the potential relevance for pathogenesis of urogenital infections must be determined. In fact, a temporal pattern of genital infection such as that of pelvic inflammatory disease was proposed (54, 70, 151). Pelvic inflammatory disease with gram-negative bacteria develops during the secretory phase. This seems to correlate with cyclic

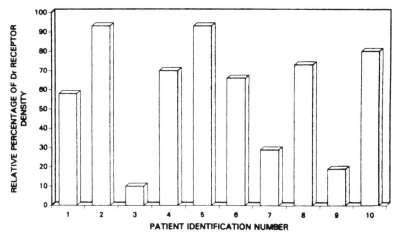

**FIGURE 15** Quantitation of Dr binding site content in endometrial samples by computer image analysis. (From reference 64 with permission.)

changes in Dr ligands. A related phenomenon was recently observed in the kidneys of pregnant mice and rats (61a, 62, 63). Further study should provide evidence as to whether quantitation of tissue ligands for bacterial adhesins is useful in the diagnosis of an individual's susceptibility to infection.

## IN VITRO RECOMBINANT MODELS FOR STUDYING UROPATHOGENS

Studies using cryostat sections of human or animal tissue and purified bacterial adhesins allow detection of organ and tissue substructures that express binding sites for microbial cells and explain the tissue tropisms of different uropathogens. To further develop in vitro systems that would allow us to study uropathogen-host tissue interaction at the molecular level, Nowicki et al. developed a cell-cell interaction system in which both the human ligand molecule and the bacterial adhesin are expressed in laboratory cells and allowed to interact so that the structure-function relationship between the ligand and the bacterial colonization factor can be investigated (99). Chinese hamster ovary (CHO) cells that do not express Dr ligands (DAF) were transformed with human DAF cDNA or DAF recombinant molecules containing deletions of individual short consensus repeat (SCR) domains or anchoring structure (16). E. coli in vitro binding to CHO cells expressing recombinant DAF and DAF deletion mutations allowed identification of the SCR-3 subunit as the possible binding site for Dr fimbriae and the related AFA I, AFA III, and F1845 adhesins (Fig. 16 and 17) (128). A single change, of Ser-165 to Leu-165, in SCR-3 abolished the binding of Dr and related adhesins. CHO-DAF transformants that expressed different quantities (25, 50, 100, and 150%) of DAF were used in vitro to create a model mimicking the variable receptor density of the ligand that may occur in vivo (Fig. 18) (99). Binding of Dr fimbriae and the related adhesins is dose dependent and correlates with increasing concentration of the decay-accelerating molecule expressed. Further studies using this system resulted in identification of a more diversified DAF family in uropathogenic E. coli. Strains positive by *dra*-specific PCR displayed binding to DAF-expressing CHO cells. More important, some isolates showed

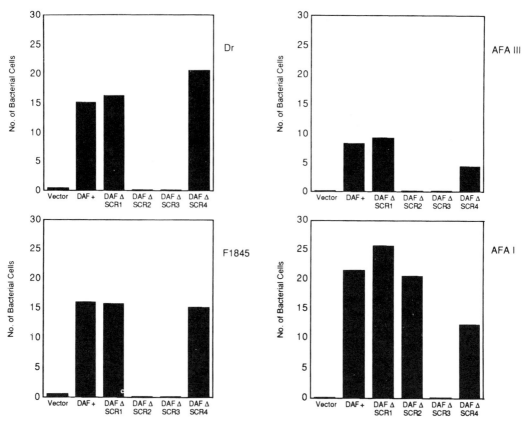

**FIGURE 16** Attachment of *E. coli* strains that express recombinant Dr and related adhesins AFA I, AFA III, and F1845 to CHO transfectants DAFΔ SCR-1, -2, -3, and -4 deletion mutants. (Reproduced from *The Journal of Experimental Medicine* (99) by copyright permission of The Rockefeller University Press.)

lack of binding to an SCR-4 mutant, indicating subtle diversity in binding epitopes on DAF (128). These approaches may facilitate the characterization of the structure-function relationship between bacterial colonization factor and human tissue ligands.

## IN VITRO MODELS FOR STUDYING UROPATHOGEN INVASIVENESS

It has been postulated that, unlike cystitis, infections of the upper urinary tract involve invasion of renal tissue, which results in morbidity and development of pyelonephritis (5, 15, 43). To investigate this aspect of the virulence of uropathogens, an in vitro model of invasiveness using tissue cell lines originating from human kidney was adapted (163). Warren et al. investigated internalization of *E. coli* into human renal tubular epithelial cells (163). These investigators hypothesized that in order to cause pyelonephritis, bacteria must pass either through or between uroepithelial cells to reach interstitial tissue. To investigate these questions, several uropathogenic isolates of *E. coli* were tested. Of the *E. coli* strains characterized, most were internalized into epithelial cells. It was demonstrated that *E. coli* are contained within the membrane-bound vacuoles. However, the invasion mechanism of uropathogens at that stage is not yet clear.

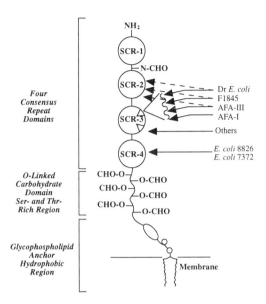

**FIGURE 17** Simplified structure of DAF containing hypothetical ligands for the family of adhesins encoded by *dra* and *dra*-related operons. (Reproduced from reference 128 with permission.)

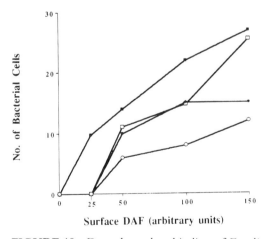

**FIGURE 18** Dose-dependent binding of *E. coli* strains that express recombinant adhesins to CHO transfectants that express increasing amounts of surface DAF. Symbols: ■, AFA I; □, Dr; ●, F1845; ○, AFA III. (Reproduced from *The Journal of Experimental Medicine* (99) by copyright permission of The Rockefeller University Press.)

More recent studies characterized the internalization of *E. coli* strains originating from fecal sources or patients with pyelonephritis (18). This investigation proposed an in vitro model for bacterial internalization that would mimic renal parenchymal invasion in pyelonephritis. A gentamicin survival assay of primary human renal epithelial cells was used. This assay allows bacteria remaining outside the epithelial cells to be killed. The internalized bacteria, however, are not affected by gentamicin (17, 23). Following gentamicin treatment, epithelial cells are lysed, and internalized bacterial cells are released and quantitatively cultured. *E. coli* strains, regardless of their origin, efficiently enter human renal epithelial cells. This process is inhibited by cytochalasin D. Both fecal isolates and pyelonephritis-associated *E. coli* are capable of being internalized by the cell line. Interestingly, nonhemolytic strains are more efficiently internalized than hemolytic strains. This phenomenon is explained by the greater cytotoxicity of hemolytic strains for kidney cells. Interestingly, there is no evidence of intracellular multiplication of *E. coli* (Fig. 19). Overall, these results demonstrate that a primary culture of human renal epithelial cells is capable of efficient uptake of *E. coli*, regardless of the source of the bacteria.

Recently, Straube and colleagues investigated the adhesiveness and internalization of *E. coli* strains that express various pathogenic determinants (142). These investigators used a permanent cell line of porcine tubular epithelial cells, LLC-PK1. Adherence to and invasion of this cell line were tested with *E. coli* O18:K5 and several mutants of this strain that differed in expression of K5 antigen, hemolysin, and fimbriae. A K-negative mutant was more efficiently internalized than the parent K5-antigen-positive strain. Expression of hemolysin by these strains was associated with an increase in adherence and internalization. Straube et al. postulated that internalization of an attached microorganism is

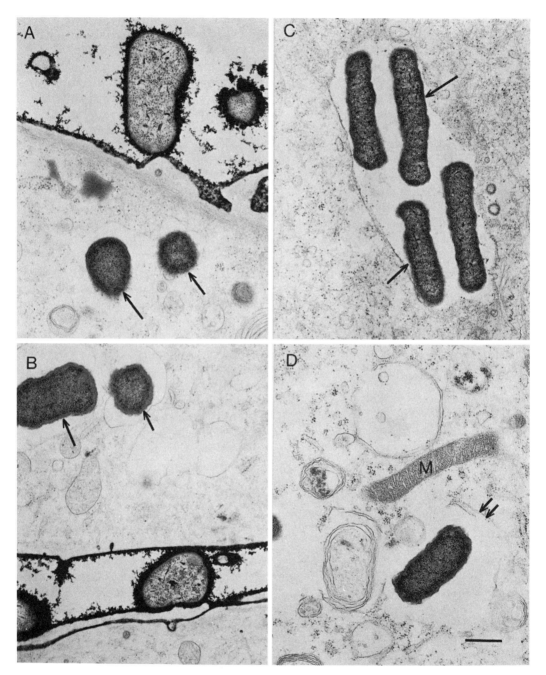

**FIGURE 19** Transmission electron micrographs of cultured human renal tubular epithelial cells after incubation with *E. coli*. (A) *E. coli* CFT204 found extracellularly in close apposition to the epithelial cell surface and stained with ruthenium red and also found intracellularly not stained with ruthenium red; (B) *E. coli* 888 found stained between cells and unstained intracellularly; (C) *E. coli* 884 found intracellularly unstained; (D) *E. coli* 884 found intracellularly unstained. Single arrow, internalized *E. coli*; double arrows, vacuole; m, mitochondrion. Bar = 0.5 μm. (From reference 163 with permission, © The University of Chicago Press.)

endocytosis rather than invasion. This hypothesis was tested by analyzing the influence of cytoskeletal inhibitors (including cytochalasin V, cytochalasin D, colchicine, and chloroquine) on bacterial internalization. The cytoskeletal inhibitors significantly inhibited internalization of the bacteria tested.

Although these experiments seem to be at early stages, the in vitro systems that allow the study of invasiveness have provided some evidence for the internalization of different uropathogens into the types of cells originating from the human or animal urinary tract. The possibility exists that different pathogens preferentially invade or are internalized by different cell types and therefore, in association with fimbria-mediating attachment and the toxic effects of bacteria, contribute to the renal tropism of the pathogen.

## Adhesin-Tissue Ligand-Based Mechanism of Ascending Urinary Tract Infection

Studies of tissue tropism and bacterial pili provided an adhesin-ligand-based explanation for the mechanism of ascending urinary tract infection (107). The presence of receptor binding sites in the colon may be crucial for efficient colonization by endogenous flora (Fig. 20). Specific endogenous microorganisms may use epithelial binding sites to colonize (107, 167) the periurethral area and/or the vaginal introitus and ascend to the lower urinary tract. Following lower genital and urinary tract tract colonization, microorganisms ascend through the ureters to the renal pelvis by using receptor-binding sites expressed in the uroepithelial cells. Anchoring to the epithelial cells could explain persistent colonization and the escape of the uropathogen from flushing by secreted urine and other fluids (27, 111, 137). Further stages of the colonization process may depend on differential tissue tropism. For example, binding sites for P fimbriae are different from those for Dr fimbriae. P-fimbriated *E. coli* strains are associated with acute pyelonephritis and bind to the luminal sites of the tubules. Their interaction is usually associated with a dramatic response in the patient, i.e., inflammatory cytokines and fever reactions (3). Hypothetically, the interstitial location of Dr-fimbrial binding sites (basement membranes and Bowman's capsule) may facilitate interstitial colonization by Dr-fimbria-positive *E. coli* (107). Interstitial localization of Dr binding sites is not directly available; bacteria may require additional factors such as internalization or invasiveness to reach and interact with the Dr-receptor-containing basement membranes. In 1987, Nowicki et al. (98) proposed that the interaction of Dr-bearing *E. coli* with Dr-receptor-containing interstitium may lead to interstitial inflammation and therefore to the development of chronic interstitial nephritis (98, 107). In fact, an experimental model of chronic interstitial nephritis with $Dr^+$ *E. coli* was developed in our laboratory (32, 33a). Together, these studies suggest that differential tissue tropism mediated by an adhesin-tissue ligand interaction may be important in the development of a different clinical form of urinary tract infection.

## SUMMARY

The in vitro models used to study uropathogens, including pathogen-host tissue interactions, have yielded profound insights into the pathogenesis of urinary tract infection. Experimental data have yielded knowledge about the molecular biology of adhesins and the basic adhesin-ligand interaction at the tissue substructural and molecular levels. Specific localization of the ligands serving bacterial attachment in the tissue substructures, temporal changes in ligand density and availability, multifimbrial phase variation, and internalization may contribute to renal tropism and the susceptibility of young noncompromised individuals to bacterial infection.

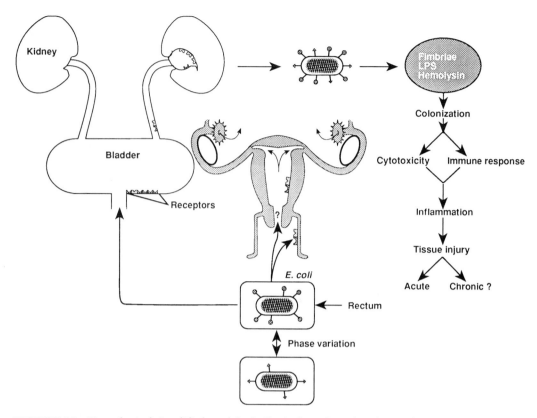

**FIGURE 20** Hypothetical simplified model of adhesin-ligand-mediated ascending genitourinary tract infections. The proposed model includes urinary and genital tract epithelial receptor-binding sites that promote the adherence of fimbriated microorganisms. Arrows indicate directions of bacterial spread and hypothetical outcomes. Different binding specificities are indicated by triangle- or circle-marked adhesins and corresponding tissue-binding sites. LPS, lipopolysaccharide.

Although major progress has been made because of studies performed in recent decades, there is still much to learn about the ways uropathogens cause urogenital diseases. Future investigations may therefore include molecular characterization of adhesive and invasive properties of uropathogens, development of pharmacological means of controlling the expression of bacterial adhesins and tissue ligands, studies of strategies for diagnosing bacterial and host high-risk factors for developing urinary tract infection, and exploration of novel preventive and therapeutic approaches, including vaccines.

### ACKNOWLEDGMENTS

I thank Stella Nowicki, Pawel Goluszko, and Anil Kaul for their helpful comments on the chapter. I acknowledge Linda Morrow Smith, Robert G. McConnell, and his staff in the Department of Obstetrics and Gynecology's Publication, Grant, and Media Support for their assistance in the preparation of this chapter.

The unpublished data and the references from my laboratory between 1991 and 1995 were supported by NIH grant RO1 #DK42029 and the John Sealy Memorial Endowment Fund (to me) and the McLaughlin Fund (to Anil Kaul and Tuan Pham).

### REFERENCES

1. **Abraham, J. M., C. S. Freitag, J. R. Clements, and B. I. Eisenstein.** 1985. An

invertible element of DNA controls phase variation of type 1 fimbriae of *Escherichia coli*. *Proc. Natl. Acad. Sci. USA* **82:**5724–5727.
2. **Adegbola, R. A., D. C. Old, and B. W. Senior.** 1983. The adhesins and fimbriae of *Proteus mirabilis* strains associated with high and low affinity for the urinary tract. *J. Med. Microbiol.* **16:**427–431.
3. **Agace, W. W., S. R. Hedges, M. Ceska, and C. Svanborg.** 1993. Interleukin-8 and the neutrophil response to mucosal gram-negative infection. *J. Clin. Invest.* **92:**780–785.
4. **Allen, B. L., G. F. Gerlach, and S. Clegg.** 1991. Nucleotide sequence and functions of *mrk* determinants necessary for expression of type 3 fimbriae in *Klebsiella pneumoniae*. *J. Bacteriol.* **173:**916–920.
5. **Aoki, S., M. Merkel, M. Aoki, and W. R. McCabe.** 1967. Immunofluorescent localization of bacterial antigen in pyelonephritis. I. The use of antisera against the common enterobacterial antigen in experimental renal lesions. *J. Lab. Clin. Med.* **70:**204–212.
6. **Arnquist, A., A. Olsén, J. Pfeifer, D. Russell, and S. Normark.** 1992. The Crl protein activates cryptic genes for curli formation and fibronectin binding in *Escherichia coli* HB101. *Mol. Microbiol.* **6:**2443–2452.
7. **Beachey, E. H. (ed.).** 1980. *Bacterial Adherence*. Chapman & Hall, Ltd., London.
8. **Bloch, C. B., B. Stocker, and P. Orndorff.** 1992. A key role for type 1 pili in enterobacterial communicability. *Mod. Microbiol.* **6:**697–701.
9. **Braaten, B. A., L. B. Blyn, B. S. Skinner, and D. A. Low.** 1991. Evidence for a methylation-blocking factor (*mbf*) locus involved in *pap* pilus expression and phase variation in *Escherichia coli*. *J. Bacteriol.* **173:**1789–1800.
10. **Breimer, M. E.** 1985. Chemical and immunological identification of the Forssman pentaglycosylceramide in human kidney. *Glycoconjugate J.* **2:**375–385.
11. **Brinton, C. C.** 1959. Non-flagellar appendages of bacteria. *Nature* (London). **183:**782–786.
12. **Brinton, C. C.** 1965. The structure, function, synthesis, and genetic control of bacterial pili and a molecular model for DNA and RNA transport in gram negative bacteria. *Trans. N.Y. Acad. Sci.* **27:**1003–1054.
13. **Buchanan, K., S. Falkow, R. A. Hull, and S. I. Hull.** 1985. Frequency among *Enterobacteriaceae* of the DNA sequences encoding type 1 pili. *J. Bacteriol.* **162:**799–803.

14. **Clegg, S., S. Hull, R. Hull, and J. Pruckler.** 1985. Construction and comparison of recombinant plasmids encoding type 1 fimbriae of members of the family *Enterobacteriaceae*. *Infect. Immun.* **48:**275–279.
15. **Cotran, R. S., L. D. Thrupp, S. N. Hajj, D. P. Sangwill, E. Vivaldi, E. H. Kass.** 1963. Retrograde *E. coli* pyelonephritis in the rat: a bacteriologic, pathologic, and fluorescent antibody study. *J. Lab. Clin. Med.* **61:**987–1004.
16. **Coyne, K. E., S. E. Hall, S. Thompson, M. A. Arce, T. Kinoshita, T. Fujita, D. J. Anstee, W. Rosse, and D. M. Lublin.** 1992. Mapping of epitopes, glycosylation sites, and complement regulatory domains in human decay accelerating factor. *J. Immunol.* **149:**2906–2913.
17. **Donnenberg, M. S., A. Donohun-Rolfe, and G. T. Keusch.** 1989. Epithelial cell invasion: an overlooked property of enteropathogenic *Escherichia coli* (EPEC) associated with the EPEC adherence factor. *J. Infect. Dis.* **160:**452–459.
18. **Donnenberg, M. S., B. Newman, S. J. Utsalo, A. L. Trifillis, J. R. Hebel, and J. W. Warren.** 1994. Internalization of *Escherichia coli* into human kidney epithelial cells: comparison of fecal and pyelonephritis-associated strains. *J. Infect. Dis.* **169:**831–838.
19. **Duguid, J. P.** 1959. Fimbriae and adhesive properties of *Klebsiella* strains. *J. Gen. Microbiol.* **21:**271–286.
20. **Duguid, J. P., and R. R. Gillies.** 1957. Fimbriae and adhesive properties in dysentery bacilli. *J. Pathol. Bacteriol.* **74:**397–341.
21. **Duguid, J. P., L. W. Smith, G. Dempster, and P. N. Edmunds.** 1955. Nonflagellar filamentous appendages ("fimbriae") and haemagglutinating activity in Bacterium coli. *J. Pathol. Bacteriol.* **70:**335–349.
22. **Eisenstein, B. I.** 1981. Phase variation of type 1 fimbriae in *Escherichia coli* is under transcriptional control. *Science* **214:**337–339.
23. **Falkow, S., P. Small, R. Isberg, S. E. Hayes, and D. Corwin.** 1987. A molecular strategy for the study of bacterial invasion. *Rev. Infect. Dis.* **9**(Suppl):S450–S455.
24. **Farquhar, M. G.** 1983. The glomerular basement membrane. A selective macromolecular filter, p. 335–378. *In* E. D. Hay (ed.), *Cell Biology of Extracellular Matrix*. Plenum Press, New York.
25. **Firon, N., S. Ashkenazi, D. Mirelman, I. Ofek, and N. Sharon.** 1987. Aromatic alpha-glycosides of mannose are powerful inhibitors of the adherence of type 1 fimbriated *Escherichia coli* to yeast and intestinal epithelial cells. *Infect. Immun.* **55:**472–476.

26. Firon, N., D. Duksin, and N. Sharon. 1985. Mannose-specific adherence of *Escherichia coli* to BHK cells that differ in their glycosylation patterns. *FEMS Microbiol. Lett.* **27**:161–165.
27. Fowler, J. E., Jr., and T. A. Stamey. 1977. Studies of introital colonization in women with recurrent urinary infections. VII. The role of bacterial adherence. *J. Urol.* **117**:472–476.
28. Franklin, W. A., M. Bibbo, M. I. Doria, H. E. Dytch, J. Toth, E. DeSombre, and G. L. Wied. 1987. Quantitation of estrogen receptor content and Ki67 staining in breast carcinoma by the microTICAS image analysis system. *Anal. Quant. Cytol. Histol.* **9**:279–286.
29. Gander, R. M., and V. L. Thomas. 1987. Distribution of type 1 and P pili on uropathogenic *Escherichia coli* O6. *Infect. Immun.* **55**:293–297.
30. Gerlach, G. F., B. L. Allen, and S. Clegg. 1989. Type 3 fimbriae among enterobacteria and the ability of spermidine to inhibit MR/K hemagglutination. *Infect. Immun.* **57**:219–224.
31. Gerlach, G. F., S. Clegg, and B. L. Allen. 1989. Identification and characterization of the genes encoding the type 3 and type 1 fimbrial adhesins of *Klebsiella pneumoniae*. *J. Bacteriol.* **171**:1262–1270.
32. Girón, J. A., T. Jones, F. Millán-Vellasco, E. Castro-Muñoz, L. Zárate, J. Fry, G. Frankel, S. L. Moseley, B. Baudrey, J. B. Kaper, et al. 1991. Diffuse-adhering *Escherichia coli* (DAEC) as a putative cause of diarrhea in Mayan children in Mexico. *J. Infect. Dis.* **163**:507–513.
33. Goldhar, J., R. Perry, J. R. Golecki, H. Hoschützky, B. Jann, and K. Jann. 1987. Nonfimbrial mannose-resistant adhesins from uropathogenic *Escherichia coli* O83:K1:H4 and O14:K?:H11. *Infect. Immun.* **55**:1837–1842.
33a. Goluszko, P., et al. Unpublished data.
34. Guyot, G. 1908. Uber die bakteriolle Hämagglutination. *Zentralbl. Bakteriol. Abt. 1* **47**:640–653.
35. Hacker, J., H. Hof, L. Emödy, and W. Goebel. 1986. Influence of cloned *Escherichia coli* hemolysin genes, S-fimbriae and serum resistance on pathogenicity in different animal models. *Microb. Pathog.* **1**:533–547.
36. Hagberg, L., I. Enberg, R. Freter, J. Lam, S. Olling, and C. Svanborg Edén. 1983. Ascending, unobstructed urinary tract infection in mice caused by pyelonephritogenic *Escherichia coli* of human origin. *Infect. Immun.* **40**:273–283.
37. Hagberg, L., R. Hull, S. Hull, S. Falkow, R. Freter, and C. Svanborg Edén. 1983. Contribution of adhesion to bacterial persistence in the mouse urinary tract. *Infect. Immun.* **40**:265–272.
38. Hagberg, L., U. Jodal, T. K. Korhonen, G. Lidin-Janson, U. Lindberg, and C. Svanborg Edén. 1981. Adhesion, hemagglutination, and virulence of *Escherichia coli* causing urinary tract infections. *Infect. Immun.* **31**:564–570.
39. Hakomori, S., S. M. Wang, and W. W. Young, Jr. 1977. Isoantigenic expression of Forssman glycolipid in human gastric and colonic mucosa: its possible identity with "A-like antigen" in human cancer. *Proc. Natl. Acad. Sci. USA* **74**:3023–3027.
40. Hanson, M. S., and C. C. Brinton, Jr. 1988. Identification and characterization of *E. coli* type-1 pilus tip adhesion protein. *Nature* (London) **332**:265–268.
41. Harber, M. J., S. Chick, R. Mackenzie, A. W. Asscher. 1982. Lack of adherence to epithelial cells by freshly isolated urinary pathogens. *Lancet* **i**:586–588.
42. Hay, E. D. (ed.). 1991. *Cell Biology of Extracellular Matrix*. Plenum Press, New York.
43. Heptinstall, R. H. 1983. Pyelonephritis: pathologic features, p. 1323–1396. *In* R. Heptinstall (ed.), *Pathology of the Kidney*, 3rd ed. Little, Brown & Co., Boston.
44. Hoffman, E. M. 1969. Inhibition of complement by a substance isolated from human erythrocytes. I. Extraction from human erythrocyte stromata. *Immunochemistry* **6**:391–403.
45. Holthöfer, H., I. Virtanen, E. Pettersson, T. Törnroth, O. Alfthan, E. Linder, and A. Miettinen. 1981. Lectins as fluorescence microscopic markers for saccharides in the human kidney. *Lab. Invest.* **45**:391–399.
46. Houvink, A. L., and W. van Iterson. 1950. Electron microscopical observations on bacterial cytology. II. A study of flagellation. *Biochim. Biophys. Acta* **5**:10–44.
47. Hull, R. A., R. E. Gill, P. Hsu, B. H. Minshew, and S. Falkow. 1981. Construction and expression of recombinant plasmids encoding type 1 or D-mannose-resistant pili from a urinary tract infection *Escherichia coli* isolate. *Infect. Immun.* **33**:933–938.
48. Hull, S., S. Clegg, C. Svanborg Edén, and R. Hull. 1985. Multiple forms of genes

in pyelonephritogenic *Escherichia coli* encoding adhesins binding globoseries glycolipid receptors. *Infect. Immun.* **47**:80–83.
49. Hull, S. I., S. Bieler, and R. A. Hull. 1988. Restriction fragment length polymorphism and multiple copies of DNA sequences homologous with probes for P-fimbriae and hemolysin genes among uropathogenic *Escherichia coli. Can. J. Microbiol.* **34**:307–311.
50. Hultgren, S. J., T. N. Porter, A. J. Schaeffer, and J. L. Duncan. 1985. Role of type1 pili and effects of phase variation on lower urinary tract infections produced by *Escherichia coli. Infect. Immun.* **50**:370–377.
51. Isberg, R. R., and J. M. Leong. 1990. Multiple β1 chain integrins are receptors for invasin, a protein that promotes bacterial penetration into mammalian cells. *Cell* **60**:861–871.
52. Iwahi, T., Y. Abe, M. Nakao, A. Imada, and K. Tsuchiya. 1983. Role of type 1 fimbriae in the pathogenesis of ascending urinary tract infection induced by *Escherichia coli* in mice. *Infect. Immun.* **39**:1307–1315.
53. Jann, K., B. Jann, and G. Schmidt. 1981. SDS polyacrylamide gel electrophoresis and serological analysis of pili from *Escherichia coli* of different pathogenic origin. *FEMS Microbiol. Lett.* **11**:21–25.
54. Johnson, D. W., K. K. Homes, P. A. Kvale, C. W. Haverson, and W. P. Hirsch. 1969. An evaluation of gonorrhea case finding in the chronically infected female. *Am. J. Epidemiol.* **90**:438–448.
55. Kallenius, G., R. Möllby, S. B. Svenson, J. Winberg, and H. Hultberg. 1980. Identification of a carbohydrate receptor recognized by uropathogenic *Escherichia coli. Infection.* **8**(Suppl. 3):288–293.
56. Kallenius, G., R. Mollby, S. B. Svenson, J. Winberg, A. Lundblad, S. Svensson, and B. Cedergren. 1980. The P$^k$ antigen as receptor for the haemagglutinin of pyelonephritic *Escherichia coli. FEMS Microbiol. Lett.* **7**:297–302.
57. Kallenius, G., S. Svenson, R. Möllby, B. Cedergren, H. Hultberg, and J. Winberg. 1981. Structure of carbohydrate part of receptor on human uroepithelial cells for pyelonephritogenic *Escherichia coli. Lancet* **ii**:604–606.
58. Kannagi, R., N. A. Cochran, F. Ishigami, S. Hakomori, P. W. Andrews, B. B. Knowles, and D. Solter. 1983. Stage-specific embryonic antigens (SSEA-3 and -4) are epitopes of a unique globo-series ganglioside isolated from human teratocarcinoma cells. *EMBO J.* **2**:2355–2361.
59. Kanwar, Y. S. 1984. Biophysiology of glomerular filtration and proteinuria. *Lab. Invest.* **51**:7–21.
60. Karr, J. F., B. Nowicki, L. D. Truong, R. A. Hull, and S. I. Hull. 1989. Purified P fimbriae from two cloned gene clusters of a single pyelonephritogenic strain adhere to unique structures in the human kidney. *Infect. Immun.* **57**:3594–3600.
61. Karr, J. F., B. J. Nowicki, L. D. Truong, R. A. Hull, J. J. Moulds, and S. I. Hull. 1990. *pap-2*-encoded fimbriae adhere to the P blood group-related glycosphingolipid stage-specific embryonic antigen 4 in the human kidney. *Infect. Immun.* **58**:4055–4062.
61a. Kaul, A., et al. Unpublished data.
62. Kaul, A., D. Kumar, M. Nagamani, P. Goluszko, S. Nowicki, and B. Nowicki. Cyclic expression of endometrial ligand decay accelerating factor for *Escherichia coli* Dr colonization factor during menstrual phases. Submitted for publication.
63. Kaul, A., D. Kumar, M. Nagamani, P. Goluszko, S. Nowicki, and B. Nowicki. Expression of Dr ligands for Dr fimbriae of *Escherichia coli* in kidneys of pregnant rats. Submitted for publication.
64. Kaul, A., B. Nowicki, M. Martens, P. Goluszko, A. Hart, M. Nagamani, D. Kumar, T. Pham, and S. Nowicki. 1994. Decay-accelerating factor is expressed in the human endometrium and may serve as the attachment ligand for Dr pili of *Escherichia coli. Am. J. Reprod. Immun.* **32**:194–199.
65. Klann, A. G., R. A. Hull, and S. I. Hull. 1992. Sequences of the genes encoding the minor tip components of *pap-3* pili of *Escherichia coli. Gene* **119**:95–100.
66. Klann, A. G., R. A. Hull, T. Palzkill, and S. I. Hull. 1994. Alanine-scanning mutagenesis reveals residues involved in binding of *pap-3*-encoded pili. *J. Bacteriol.* **176**:2312–2317.
67. Klemm, P. 1985. Fimbrial adhesins. *Rev. Infect. Dis.* **7**:321–340.
68. Klemm, P. 1986. Two regulatory fim genes, *fimB* and *fimE*, control the phase variation of type 1 fimbriae in *Escherichia coli*, p. 1389–1393. IRL Press Ltd., Oxford, England.
69. Klemm, P., I. Orskov, and F. Orskov. 1982. F7 and type 1-like fimbriae from three *Escherichia coli* strains isolated from urinary tract infections: protein chemical and immunological aspects. *Infect. Immun.* **36**:462–468.

70. **Kock, M. L.** 1947. A study of cervical cultures taken in cases of acute gonorrhea with special reference to the phases of the menstrual cycle. *Am. J. Obstet. Gynecol.* **54:** 861–866.
71. **Korhonen, T., R. Virkola, V. Väisänen-Rhen, and H. Holthöfer.** 1986. Binding of purified *Escherichia coli* O75X adhesin to frozen sections of human kidney. *FEMS Microbiol. Lett.* **35:**313–318.
72. **Korhonen, T. K.** 1979. Yeast cell agglutination by purified enterobacterial pili. *FEMS Microbiol. Lett.* **6:**421–425.
73. **Korhonen, T. K., H. Leffler, and C. Svanborg Edén.** 1981. Binding specificity of piliated strains of *Escherichia coli* and *Salmonella typhimurium* to epithelial cells, *Saccharomyces cerevisiae* cells, and erythrocytes. *Infect. Immun.* **32:**796–804.
74. **Korhonen, T. K., B. Nowicki, M. Rhen, V. Väisänen-Rhen, A. Pere, R. Virkola, J. Tenhunen, K. Saukkonen, and J. Vuopio-Varkila.** 1986. *Fimbrial Phase Variation in Escherichia coli: a Mechanism of Bacterial Virulence?*, p. 245–251. Academic Press, Inc., London.
75. **Korhonen, T. K., J. Parkkinen, J. Hacker, J. Finne, A. Pere, M. Rhen, and H. Holthöfer.** 1986. Binding of *Escherichia coli* S fimbriae to human kidney epithelium. *Infect. Immun.* **54:**322–327.
76. **Korhonen, T. K., E. Tarkka, H. Ranta, and K. Haahtela.** 1983. Type 3 fimbriae of *Klebsiella* sp.: molecular characterization and role in bacterial adhesion to plant roots. *J. Bacteriol.* **155:**860–865.
77. **Korhonen, T. K., V. Väisänen, H. Saxén, H. Hultberg, and S. B. Svenson.** 1982. P-antigen-recognizing fimbriae from human uropathogenic *Escherichia coli* strains. *Infect. Immun.* **37:**286–291.
78. **Korhonen, T. K., M. V. Valtonen, J. Parkkinen, V. Väisänen-Rhen, J. Finne, F. Orskov, I. Orskov, S. B. Svenson, and P. H. Mäkelä.** 1985. Serotypes, hemolysin production, and receptor recognition of *Escherichia coli* strains associated with neonatal sepsis and meningitis. *Infect. Immun.* **48:**486–491.
79. **Korhonen, T. K., R. Virkola, and H. Holthöfer.** 1986. Localization of binding sites for purified *Escherichia coli* P fimbriae in the human kidney. *Infect. Immun.* **54:**328–332.
80. **Korhonen, T. K., R. Virkola, V. Väisänen-Rhen, and H. Holthöfer.** 1986. Binding of purified *Escherichia coli* O75X adhesin to frozen sections of human kidney. *FEMS Microbiol. Lett.* **35:**313–318.
81. **Korhonen, T. K., B. Westerlund, A.-M. Tarkkanen, T. Sareneva, R. Virkola, P. Kuusela, H. Holthöfer, I. van Die, W. Hoekstra, B. L. Allen, and S. Clegg.** 1991. Binding of enterobacterial fimbriae to proteins of basement membranes and connective tissue: a novel function for fimbriae, p. 11–21. *In* E. Z. Ron and S. Rotten, *Microbial Surface Components and Toxins in Relation to Pathogenesis*. Plenum Press, New York.
82. **Krogfelt, K. A., H. Bergmans, and P. Klemm.** 1990. Direct evidence that the FimH protein is the mannose-specific adhesin of *Escherichia coli* type 1 fimbriae. *Infect. Immun.* **58:**1995–1998.
83. **Kukkonen, M., T. Raunio, R. Virkola, K. Lahteenmaki, P. H. Makela, P. Klemm, S. Clegg, and T. K. Korhonen.** 1993. Basement membrane carbohydrate as a target for bacterial adhesion: binding of type I fimbriae of *Salmonella enterica* and *Escherichia coli* to laminin. *Mol. Microbiol.* **7:** 229–237.
84. **Kunin, C. M.** 1987. *Detection, Prevention and Management of Urinary Tract Infections*. Lea & Febiger, Philadelphia.
85. **Kuusela, P.** 1978. Fibronectin binds to *Staphylococcus aureus*. *Nature* (London) **276:** 718–720.
86. **Leffler, H., H. Lomberg, E. Gotschlich, L. Hagberg, U. Jodal, T. Korhonen, B. E. Samuelsson, G. Schoolnik, and C. Svanborg-Edén.** 1982. Chemical and clinical studies on the interaction of *Escherichia coli* with host glycolipid receptors in urinary tract infection. *Scand. J. Infect. Dis. Suppl.* **33:**46–51.
87. **Leffler, H., and C. Svanborg Edén.** 1980. Chemical identification of a glycosphingolipid receptor for *Escherichia coli* attaching to human urinary tract epithelial cells and agglutinating human erythrocytes. *FEMS Microbiol. Lett.* **8:**127–134.
88. **Lund, B., B. I. Marklund, N. Stromberg, F. Lindberg, K. A. Karlsson, and S. Normark.** 1988. Uropathogenic *Escherichia coli* can express serologically identical pili of different receptor binding specificities. *Mol. Microbiol.* **2:**255–263.
89. **Marre, R., and J. Hacker.** 1987. Role of S- and common-type 1-fimbriae of *Escherichia coli* in experimental upper and lower urinary tract infection. *Microb. Pathog.* **2:** 223–226.
90. **Marre, R., B. Kreft, and J. Hacker.** 1990. Genetically engineered S and F1C fimbriae

differ in their contribution to adherence of *Escherichia coli* to cultured renal tubular cells. *Infect. Immun.* **58:**3434–3437.

91. Mobley, H. L., G. R. Chippendale, J. H. Tenney, R. A. Hull, and J. W. Warren. 1987. Expression of type 1 fimbraie may be required for persistence of *Escherichia coli* in the catheterized urinary tract. *J. Clin. Microbiol.* **25:**2253–2257.

92. Mobley, H. L., G. R. Chippendale, J. H. Tenney, A. R. Mayrer, L. J. Crisp, J. L. Penner, and J. W. Warren. 1988. MR/K hemagglutination of *Providencia stuartii* correlates with adherence to catheters and with persistence in catheter-associated bacteriuria. *J. Infect. Dis.* **157:**264–271.

93. Mobley, H. L. T., G. R. Chippendale, J. H. Tenney, R. A. Hull, and J. W. Warren. Expression of type 1 fimbriae may be required for persistence of *Escherichia coli* in the catheterized urinary tract. *J. Clin. Microbiol.* **25:**2253–2257.

94. Moch, T., H. Hoschützky, J. Hacker, K. D. Kröncke, and K. Jann. 1987. Isolation and characterization of the alpha-sialyl-beta-2,3-galactosyl-specific adhesin from fimbriated *Escherichia coli*. *Proc. Natl. Acad. Sci. USA* **84:**3462–3466.

95. Morschhäuser, J., H. Hoschützky, K. Jann, and J. Hacker. 1990. Functional analysis of the sialic acid-binding adhesin SfaS of pathogenic *Escherichia coli* by site-specific mutagenesis. *Infect. Immun.* **58:**2133–2138.

96. Naeye, R. L. 1979. Causes of excessive rates of perinatal mortality and prematurity in pregnancies complicated by maternal urinary-tract infections. *N. Engl. J. Med.* **300:**819–823.

97. Nicholson-Weller, A., J. Burge, and K. F. Austen. 1981. Purification from guinea pig erythrocyte stroma of a decay-accelerating factor for the classical c3 convertase, C4b,2a. *J. Immunol.* **127:**2035–2039.

98. Nowicki, B., J. P. Barrish, T. Korhonen, R. A. Hull, and S. I. Hull. 1987. Molecular cloning of the *Escherichia coli* O75X adhesin. *Infect. Immun.* **55:**3168–3173.

99. Nowicki, B., A. Hart, K. E. Coyne, D. M. Lublin, and S. Nowicki. 1993. Short consensus repeat-3 domain of recombinant decay-accelerating factor is recognized by *Escherichia coli* recombinant Dr adhesin in a model of a cell-cell interaction. *J. Exp. Med.* **178:**2115–2121.

100. Nowicki, B., H. Holthöfer, T. Saraneva, M. Rhen, V. Väisänen-Rhen, and T. K. Korhonen. 1986. Location of adhesion sites for P-fimbriated and for O75X-positive *Escherichia coli* in the human kidney. *Microb. Pathog.* **1:**169–180.

101. Nowicki, B., R. Hull, and J. Moulds. 1988. Use of the Dr hemagglutinin of uropathogenic *Escherichia coli* to differentiate normal from abnormal red cells in paroxysmal nocturnal hemoglobinuria. *N. Engl. J. Med.* **319:**1289–1290. (Letter.)

102. Nowicki, B., M. Martens, A. Hart, and S. Nowicki. 1994. Gestational age-dependent distribution of *Escherichia coli* fimbriae in pregnant patients with pyelonephritis. *Ann. N.Y. Acad. Sci.* **730:**290–291.

103. Nowicki, B., J. Moulds, R. Hull, and S. Hull. 1988. A hemagglutinin of uropathogenic *Escherichia coli* recognizes the Dr blood group antigen. *Infect. Immun.* **56:**1057–1060.

104. Nowicki, B., M. Rhen, V. Väisänen-Rhen, A. Pere, and T. K. Korhonen. 1984. Immunofluorescence study of fimbrial phase variation in *Escherichia coli* KS71. *J. Bacteriol.* **160:**691–695.

105. Nowicki, B. J., M. Rhen, V. Väisänen-Rhen, A. Pere, and T. K. Korhonen. 1985. Fractionation of a bacterial cell population by adsorption to erythrocytes and yeast cells. *FEMS Microbiol. Lett.* **26:**35–40.

106. Nowicki, B., M. Rhen, V. Väisänen-Rhen, A. Pere, and T. K. Korhonen. 1985. Organization of fimbriate cells in colonies of *Escherichia coli* strain 3040. *J. Gen. Microbiol.* **131:**1263–1266.

106a. Nowicki, B., M. Rhen, V. Väisänen-Rhen, A. Pere, and T. K. Korhonen. 1985. Kinetics of phase variation between S and type 1 fimbriae of *Escherichia coli*. *FEMS Microbiol. Lett.* **28:**237–242.

107. Nowicki, B., L. Truong, J. Moulds, and R. Hull. 1988. Presence of the Dr receptor in normal human tissues and its possible role in the pathogenesis of ascending urinary tract infection. *Am. J. Pathol.* **133:**1–4.

108. Nowicki, B., J. Vuopio-Varkila, P. Viljanen, T. K. Korhonen, and P. H. Mäkelä. 1986. Fimbrial phase variation and systemic *E. coli* infection studied in the mouse peritonitis model. *Microb. Pathog.* **1:**335–347.

109. Ofek, I., A. Mosek, and N. Sharon. 1981. Mannose-specific adherence of *Escherichia coli* freshly excreted in the urine of patients with urinary tract infections, and of isolates subcultured from the infected urine. *Infect. Immun.* **34:**708–711.

110. Ofek, I. L., D. Mirelman, and N. Sharon. 1977. Adherence of *Escherichia*

*coli* to human mucosal cells mediated by mannose receptors. *Nature* (London) **265:** 623–625.
111. **O'Hanley, P., D. Lark, S. Falkow, and G. Schoolnik.** 1985. Molecular basis of *Escherichia coli* colonization of the upper urinary tract in BALB/c mice. *J. Clin. Invest.* **75:**347–360.
112. **Old, D. C.** 1972. Inhibition of the interaction between fimbrial haemagglutinins and erythrocytes by D-mannose and other carbohydrates. *J. Gen. Microbiol.* **71:**149–157.
113. **Old, D. C., and R. A. Adegbola.** 1982. Hemagglutinins and fimbriae of *Morganella, Proteus,* and *Providencia. J. Med. Microbiol.* **15:**551–564.
114. **Olsén, A., A. Jonsson, and S. Normark.** 1989. Fibronectin binding mediated by a novel class of surface organelles on *Escherichia coli. Nature* (London) **338:**652–655.
115. **Orndorff, P. E., and S. Falkow.** 1985. Nucleotide sequence of *pilA*, the gene encoding the structural component of type 1 pili in *Escherichia coli. J. Bacteriol.* **162:** 454–457.
116. **Orndorff, P. E., P. A. Spears, D. Schauer, and S. Falkow.** 1985. Two modes of control of *pilA*, the gene encoding type 1 pilin in *Escherichia coli. J. Bacteriol.* **164:**321–330.
117. **Orskov, I., A. Ferencz, and F. Orskov.** 1980. Tamm-Horsfall protein or uromucoid in the normal urinary slime that traps type 1 fimbriated *Escherichia coli. Lancet* **i:**887. (Letter.)
118. **Parkkinen, J., T. K. Korhonen, A. Pere, J. Hacker, and S. Soinila.** 1988. Binding sites in the rat brain for *Escherichia coli* S fimbriae associated with neonatal meningitis. *J. Clin. Invest.* **81:**860–865.
119. **Parkkinen, J., A. Ristimaki, and B. Westerlund.** 1989. Binding of *Escherichia coli* S fimbriae to cultured human endothelial cells. *Infect. Immun.* **57:**2256–2259.
120. **Parkkinen, J., R. Virkola, and T. K. Korhonen.** 1988. Identification of factors in human urine that inhibit the binding of *Escherichia coli* adhesins. *Infect. Immun.* **56:** 2623–2630.
121. **Parsons, S. F., F. A. Spring, A. H. Merry, M. Uchikawa, G. Mallinson, D. J. Anstee, V. Rawlinson, and M. Daha.** 1988. *Proc. 20th Congr. Int. Soc. Blood Transfusion Br. Blood Transfusion Soc.,* abstr. 116.
122. **Patti, J. M., B. L. Allen, M. J. McGavin, and M. Hook.** 1994. MSCRAMM-mediated adherence of microorganisms to host tissues. *Annu. Rev. Microbiol.* **48:**585–617.

123. **Pere, A.** 1986. P fimbriae on uropathogenic *Escherichia coli* O16:K1 and O18 strains. *FEMS Microbiol. Lett.* **37:**19–26.
124. **Pere, A., M. Leinonen, V. Väisänen-Rhen, M. Rhen, and T. K. Korhonen.** 1985. Occurrence of type-1C fimbriae on *Escherichia coli* strains isolated from human extraintestinal infections. *J. Gen. Microbiol.* **131:**1705–1711.
125. **Pere, A., B. Nowicki, H. Saxen, A. Siitonen, and T. K. Korhonen.** 1987. Expression of P, type-1, and type-1C fimbriae of *Escherichia coli* in the urine of patients with acute urinary tract infection. *J. Infect. Dis.* **156:**567–574.
126. **Pere, A., V. Väisänen-Rhen, M. Rhen, J. Tenhunen, and T. K. Korhonen.** 1986. Analysis of P fimbriae on *Escherichia coli* O2, O4, and O6 strains by immunoprecipitation. *Infect. Immun.* **51:**618–625.
127. **Perry, A., Y. Keisari, and I. Ofek.** 1985. Liver cell and macrophage surface lectins as determinants of recognition in blood clearance and cellular attachment of bacteria. *FEMS Microbiol. Lett.* **27:**345–350.
128. **Pham, T., A. Kaul, A. Hart, P. Goluszko, J. Moulds, S. Nowicki, D. M. Lubin, and B. J. Nowicki.** 1995. *dra*-related X adhesins of gestational pyelonephritis-associated *Escherichia coli* recognize SCR-3 and SCR-4 domains of recombinant decay accelerating factor. *Infect. Immun.* **63:** 1663–1668.
129. **Rhen, M., J. Knowles, M. E. Penttila, M. Sarvas, and T. K. Korhonen.** P fimbriae of *Escherichia coli*: molecular cloning of DNA fragments containing the structural genes. *FEMS Microbiol. Lett.* **19:**119–123.
130. **Rhen, M., P. H. Mäkelä, and T. K. Korhonen.** 1983. P fimbriae of *Escherichia coli* are subject to phase variation. *FEMS Microbiol. Lett.* **19:**267–271.
131. **Rhen, M., E. Wahlström, and T. K. Korhonen.** 1983. P-fimbriae of *Escherichia coli*: fractionation by immune precipitation. *FEMS Microbiol. Lett.* **18:**227–232.
132. **Roberts, J. A., B. Kaack, G. Källenius, R. Möllby, J. Winberg, and S. B. Svenson.** 1984. Receptors for pyelonephritogenic *Escherichia coli* in primates. *J. Urol.* **131:** 163–168.
133. **Ruoslahti, E.** 1991. Integrins as receptors for extracellular matrix, p. 343–363. *In* E. D. Hay (ed.), *Cell Biology of Extracellular Matrix.* Plenum Press, New York.
134. **Rutter, J. M., M. R. Burrows, R. Sellwood, and R. A. Gibbons.** 1975. A genetic

basis for resistance to enteric disease caused by *E. coli. Nature* (London) **257:**135–136.

135. **Sareneva, T., H. Holthöfer, and T. K. Korhonen.** 1990. Tissue-binding affinity of *Proteus mirabilis* fimbriae in the human urinary tract. *Infect. Immun.* **58:**3330–3336.

136. **Saukkonen, K. M., B. Nowicki, M. Leinonen.** 1988. Role of type 1 and S fimbriae in the pathogenesis of *Escherichia coli* O18:K1 bacteremia and meningitis in the infant rat. *Infect. Immun.* **56:**892–897.

137. **Schaeffer, A. J., J. M. Jones, W. S. Falkowski, J. L. Duncan, J. S. Chmiel, and B. J. Plotkin.** 1982. Variable adherence of uropathogenic *Escherichia coli* to epithelial cells from women with recurrent urinary tract infection. *J. Urol.* **128:**1227–1230.

138. **Shapiro, J. A.** 1984. Transposable elements, genome reorganization and cellular differentiation in Gram-negative bacteria, p. 169–193. *In* D. P. Kelly and N. G. Carr (ed.), *The Microbe 1984*, part II. *Prokaryotes and Eukaryotes*. Cambridge University Press, Cambridge.

139. **Sharon, N., and I. Ofek.** 1986. Mannose specific bacterial surface lectins, p. 55–81. *In* D. Mirelman (ed.), *Microbial Lectins and Agglutinins*. John Wiley & Sons, Inc., New York.

140. **Simon, M., J. Zieg, M. Silverman, G. Mandel, and R. Doolittle.** 1980. Phase variation: evolution of a controlling element. *Science* **209:**1370–1374.

141. **Sokurenko, E. V., H. S. Courtney, S. N. Abraham, P. Klemm, and D. L. Hasty.** 1992. Functional heterogeneity of type 1 fimbriae of *Escherichia coli. Infect. Immun.* **60:**4709–4719.

142. **Straube, E., G. Schmidt, R. Marre, and J. Hacker.** 1993. Adhesion and internalization of *E. coli* strains expressing various pathogenicity determinants. *Int. J. Med. Microbiol. Virol. Parasitol. Infect. Dis.* **278:**218–228.

143. **Svanborg-Edén, C., B. Eriksson, and L. A. Hanson.** 1977. Adhesion of *Escherichia coli* to human uroepithelia cells *in vitro*. *Infect. Immun.* **18:**767–774.

144. **Svanborg-Edén, C. R. Freter, L. Hagberg, R. Hull, S. Hull, H. Leffler, and G. Schoolnik.** 1982. Inhibition of experimental ascending urinary tract infection by an epithelial cell-surface receptor analogue. *Nature* (London) **298:**560–562.

145. **Svanborg-Edén, C., and H. A. Hansson.** 1978. *Escherichia coli* pili as possible mediators of attachment to human urinary tract epithelial cells. *Infect. Immun.* **21:**229–237.

146. **Svanborg-Edén, C., and U. Jodal.** 1979. Attachment of *Escherichia coli* to urinary sediment epithelial cells from urinary tract infection-prone and healthy children. *Infect. Immun.* **26:**837–840.

147. **Svanborg-Edén, C., U. Jodal, L. Å. Hanson, V. Lindberg, and A. SohlÅkerlund.** 1976. Variable adhesion to normal human urinary tract epithelial cells of *Escherichia coli* strains associated with various forms of urinary tract infection. *Lancet* **i:**490–492.

148. **Svanborg-Edén, C., P. Larsson, and H. Lomberg.** 1980. Attachment of *Proteus mirabilis* to human urinary sediment epithelial cells in vitro is different from that of *Escherichia coli. Infect. Immun.* **27:**804–807.

149. **Svenson, S. B., and G. Källenius.** 1983. Density and localization of P-fimbriae-specific receptors on mammalian cells: fluorescence-activated cells analysis. *Infection* **11:**6–12.

150. **Svenson, S. B., G. Kallenius, R. Mollby, H. Hultberg, and J. Winberg.** Rapid identification of P-fimbriated *Escherichia coli* by a receptor-specific particle agglutination test. *Infection* **10:**209–214.

151. **Sweet, R. L., M. Blankfort-Doyle, M. O. Robbie, and J. Schacter.** 1986. The occurrence of chlamydial and gonococcal salpingitis during the menstrual cycle. *JAMA* **255:**2062–2064.

152. **Tarkkanen, A. M., B. L. Allen, B. Westerlund, H. Holthöfer, P. Kuusela, L. Risteli, S. Clegg, and T. K. Korhonen.** 1990. Type V collagen as the target for type-3 fimbriae, enterobacterial adherence organelles. *Mol. Microbiol.* **4:**1353–1361.

153. **Telen, M. J., S. E. Hall, A. M. Green, J. J. Moulds, and W. F. Rosse.** 1988. Identification of human erythrocyte blood group antigens on decay-accelerating factor (DAF) and an erythrocyte phenotype negative for DAF. *J. Exp. Med.* **167:**1993–1998.

154. **Timpl, R., H. Wiedemann, V. van Delden, H. Furthmayr, and K. Kühn.** 1981. A network model for the organization of type IV collagen molecules in basement membranes. *Eur. J. Biochem.* **120:**203–211.

155. **Tippett, P., P. W. Andrews, B. B. Knowles, D. Solter, and P. N. Goodfellow.** 1986. Red cell antigens P (globoside) and Luke: identification by monoclonal antibodies defining the murine stage-specific embryonic antigens −3 and −4 (SSEA-3 and SSEA-4). *Vox Sang.* **51:**53–56.

156. **Väisänen, V., J. Elo, L. G. Tallgren, A. Siitonen, P. H. Mäkelä, C. Svanborg-Edén, G. Källenius, S. B. Svenson, H.

Hultberg, and T. K. Korhonen. 1981. Mannose-resistant haemagglutination and P antigen recognition are characteristic of *Escherichia coli* causing primary pyelonephritis. *Lancet* **ii**:1366–1369.
157. Väisänen-Rhen, V., J. Elo, E. Väisänen, A. Siitonen, I. Orskov, F. Orskov, S. B. Svenson, P. H. Mäkelä, and T. K. Korhonen. 1984. P-fimbriated clones among uropathogenic *Escherichia coli* strains. *Infect. Immun.* **43**:149–155.
158. Väisänen-Rhen, V., M. Rhen, E. Linder, and T. K. Korhonen. 1985. Adhesion of *Escherichia coli* to human kidney cryostat sections. *FEMS Microbiol. Lett.* **27**: 179–182.
159. Valkonen, K. H., J. Veijola, B. Dagberg, and B. E. Uhlin. 1991. Binding of basement-membrane laminin by *E. coli*. *Mol. Microbiol.* **5**:2133–2141.
160. Van Die, I., G. Spierings, I. van Megan, E. Zuidweg, W. Hoekstra, and H. Bergmans. 1985. Cloning and genetic organization of the gene cluster encoding $F7_1$ fimbriae of a uropathogenic *Escherichia coli* and comparison with the $F7_2$ gene cluster. *FEMS Microbiol. Lett.* **28**:329–334.
161. Virkola, R. 1987. Binding characteristics of *Escherichia coli* type 1 fimbriae in the human kidney. *FEMS Microbiol. Lett.* **40**:257–262.
162. Virkola, R., B. Westerlund, H. Holthöfer, J. Parkkinen, M. Kelomaki, and T. K. Korhonen. 1988. Binding characteristics of *Escherichia coli* adhesins in human urinary bladder. *Infect. Immun.* **56**:2615–2622.
163. Warren, J. W., H. L. Mobley, and A. L. Trifillis. 1988. Internalization of *Escherichia coli* into human renal tubular epithelial cells. *J. Infect. Dis.* **158**:221–223.
164. Westerlund, B., and T. K. Korhonen. 1993. Bacterial proteins binding to the mammalian extracellular matrix. *Mol. Microbiol.* **9**:687–694.
165. Westerlund, B., P. Kuusela, J. Risteli, L. Risteli, T. Vartio, H. Rauvala, R. Virkola, and T. K. Korhonen. 1989. The O75X adhesin of uropathogenic *Escherichia coli* is a type IV collagen-binding protein. *Mol. Microbiol.* **3**:329–337.
166. Westerlund, B., P. Kuusela, T. Vartio, I. van Die, and T. K. Korhonen. 1989. A novel lectin-independent interaction of P fimbriae of *Escherichia coli* with immobilized fibronectin. *FEBS Lett.* **243**:199–204.
167. Wold, A. E., M. Thorssen, S. Hull, and C. Svanborg Edén. 1988. Attachment of *Escherichia coli* via mannose- or Galα 1 →4Galβ-containing receptors to human colonic epithelial cells. *Infect. Immun.* **56**: 2531–2537.
168. Yamada, K. M., S. K. Akiyama, T. Hasegawa, E. Hasegawa, M. J. Humphries, D. W. Kennedy, K. Nagata, H. Urushihara, K. Olden, and W. T. Chen. 1985. Recent advances in research on fibronectin and other cell attachment proteins. *J. Cell. Biochem.* **28**:79–97.
169. Yamamoto, T., F. Kazuhiko, and T. Yokota. 1990. Adherence characteristics to human small intestinal mucosa of *Escherichia coli* isolated from patients with diarrhea or urinary tract infections. *J. Infect. Dis.* **162**: 896–908.

# ANIMAL MODELS OF URINARY TRACT INFECTION

*David E. Johnson, Ph.D., and Robert G. Russell, D.V.M., Ph.D.*

## 14

Animal models, a critical element in a program assessing mechanisms of pathogenicity, provide vital information not obtainable from in vitro studies. Animal studies provide an opportunity to assess interactions between the pathogen and host, including the critical first step in establishment of infection, attachment of the pathogen to a host surface. The dynamic interplay throughout the infection process that determines the ultimate fate of the pathogen and the host can be studied only in an in vivo system. The opposing elements of the pathogen, including variable expression of attachment organelles and elaboration of toxins and/or other noxious materials, and the host, including nonspecific and pathogen-directed defense mechanisms, can be assessed throughout the dynamic infection process. Use of isogenic mutants of the pathogen and animals genetically deficient in an important defense mechanism are critical to such studies. Additionally, the effects of foreign bodies on enhancement of virulence of the pathogen and modalities of immunization against the pathogen can be assessed only in an in vivo model.

Numerous factors enter into the selection of the appropriate animal for model studies. To successfully conduct any animal experiments, the animal must (i) be healthy and well nourished, (ii) be free of adventitious pathogens, and (iii) be housed in a clean and well-controlled environment. Susceptibility to infection may be dependent on the type, gender, and age of the animal. If a new infection is to be studied, selection of the type of animal may require considerable investigation, since natural resistance to infection is common. Animal size may also be a factor in selection of the proper animal type for the proposed project. For example, although mice are popular because they are inexpensive to purchase and house, some procedures are technically difficult to perform in mice because of their small size and low blood volume. In addition to animal type, animal strain may be an important factor. Use of inbred animals provides the opportunity to study an infection in animals with a homogeneous genetic background, unlike outbred animals, in which the genetic background is variable. If sex hormones affect

---

*David E. Johnson,* Research Service, Veteran's Administration Medical Center, 10 North Green Street, Baltimore, Maryland 21201. *Robert G. Russell,* Department of Comparative Medicine, University of Maryland School of Medicine, Baltimore, Maryland 21201.

establishment of infection, animal gender is an important consideration. Animal gender may also be important because anatomical differences may affect the ability to perform a needed procedure. For example, a catheter can be inserted into the bladder of a female mouse via the urethra, but this procedure cannot be conducted in a male mouse because of the anatomy of its urinary tract. Since animal age affects both animal size and susceptibility to infection, the age of an animal should be carefully considered, and once an age is chosen, care must be taken not to allow age to be a variable. Since age affects animal size, inocula and therapy should be expressed relative to animal weight.

The route of infection must also be carefully considered. Ideally, the route of animal infection should mimic the natural route of the human infection for which the animal studies are modeling. However, this is not always possible because of the natural resistance some animals have to infection. If, because of this natural resistance to infection, a compromising procedure is necessary to render the animal susceptible to infection, then the relationship between the model and the natural infection is jeopardized.

Infection in animals must be dose responsive, and the rate of infection must be high enough to allow statistical assessment of differences while using a small number of animals. The frequency of infection must usually be considerably higher than is seen in the natural human infection. Although this factor is critical to animal studies, it may lead to difficulties in correlation with natural infection. The end point of the infection in animals must also be easily quantifiable and must mimic the end point of the natural human infection.

## CHARACTERISTICS OF ANIMAL MODELS OF UTI

Animals have been used to elucidate many aspects of urinary tract infections (UTIs). The purpose of animal models of UTI, like other animal models, is to closely mimic human infection. In 1982, Kaijser and Larsson (71) reviewed the use of animal models in experimental acute pyelonephritis caused by enterobacteria. Since no animal model perfectly reflects human infection, a number of models have been proposed.

## ANIMAL SPECIES

Dogs, mice, monkeys, pigs (58), rabbits, and rats have been used to study UTI. In the late 1800s and early 1900s, the route of infection of the human urinary tract had not been established but was speculated to be hematogenous, lymphogenous, or ascending. Consequently, many early investigations of experimental UTI involved animals challenged by a variety of routes in the hope that the characteristic of human infection could be duplicated in animals and thus the true route of human infection could be established. Also, in those earlier studies, animal species were selected for susceptibility to the study organism without regard for the mechanism of infection, which generally was not known. In addition, animals were frequently subjected to some kind of manipulation to enhance susceptibility to the study organism. As a consequence, findings from many of those studies are unreliable predictors of events critical to establishment of human infection of the urinary tract by the ascending route. More recently, careful selection of animal species, route of inoculation, and method of challenge has ensured that the models more closely parallel human ascending infection.

## Rabbits
### HEMATOGENOUS PYELONEPHRITIS

Although not specifically documented, early investigators studying UTI probably used rabbits because their size allowed easy challenge and sampling and because rabbits were frequently used to make antiserum.

In 1893, Sherrington (136) conducted a series of studies in which he subcutaneously or intravenously (i.v.) injected a variety of organisms into rabbits and mice and examined secretions from those animals for the challenge organism. The prevailing belief that the body rids itself of infecting microorganisms by releasing them into secretions was not confirmed by Sherrington's experiments. On the contrary, "at a time when every drop of the circulating blood is teeming with micro-organisms there may not be the slightest transit of them into the urinary and biliary fluids then secreted." He concluded from his experiments that only pathogenic organisms have the power to go from the circulation to the urine by damaging the kidney, as evidenced by the appearance in infected urine of blood, hemoglobin, or albumin.

In keeping with the prevailing belief during the early 1900s that UTI resulted from bacteremia, experiments were conducted in an attempt to reproduce the infection in rabbits. Lepper (82), however, observed that rabbits challenged i.v. with *Escherichia coli* did not become bacteriuric but frequently died of bacteremia. She discovered, however, that if urine outflow from the kidney was obstructed by compression of the ureter for as little as 15 min, the kidney became more susceptible to infection with *E. coli* i.v. challenge. She also noted that some *E. coli* strains were more likely to induce renal infection than other strains. Mallory et al. (90) reported that virulence was reduced by repeated passage in vitro but restored by repeated animal passage. Lepper reported that the renal changes described by Sherrington (136) (hematuria, albuminuria, and leukocyturia) were also seen in her animals. Heptinstall and Gorrill (56) created unilateral renal infection by briefly occluding a single ureter. They used this model to study the relationship between pyelonephritis and elevated blood pressure that had been observed in humans. They reported that rabbits became hypertensive if the uninfected kidney was surgically removed but remained normotensive if the uninfected kidney remained intact. This model was somewhat impractical to use, since there was a 40% mortality rate following nephrectomy.

Although renal infections with *E. coli* were difficult to establish in healthy rabbits, infections with *Staphylococcus aureus* were established with little difficulty following i.v. challenge. De Navasquez (27) hypothesized that this ease of infection was due to diffusion of coagulase from plasma into the surrounding renal parenchyma. Surviving animals had renal scars that were similar to those of the underlying chronic pyelonephritis seen in human kidneys surgically removed for intractable and unilateral pyelonephritis. Helmholz and Beeler (52, 53) and Heptinstall and Gorrill (56) reported that *S. aureus* infection enhanced the renal pathogenicity of *E. coli*. Renal infection with *E. coli* was greater when rabbits were challenged with a mixture of *S. aureus* and *E. coli* than when they were challenged with *E. coli* alone (52) or when animals with renal scarring surviving an *S. aureus* infection were subsequently challenged with *E. coli* (27).

## ASCENDING PYELONEPHRITIS

Helmholz and Beeler (53) may have been the first to report establishment of UTI following intravesicular challenge in unmanipulated animals. Prior to challenge, urine was removed from the bladders of their rabbits. Presumably by use of a catheter, the inoculum "was allowed to run into the bladder by gravity." To demonstrate that the inoculum did not reflux into the ureters, they substituted gentian violet for the inoculum and could not find the dye in any ureters. When this technique was used, 10 of 15 rabbits challenged with *E. coli* developed pyelitis. One rabbit developed a renal abscess, and although renal abscesses following i.v. challenge were diffusely scattered, the abscess in the rabbit challenged intravesically was confined to one area of the kidney. More recently, Gnarpe and Olding (41) investigated leukocyturia in rabbits following intravesical challenge with *Proteus vulgaris* and *E. coli*. They found that if urine pH was below 7.75, as in *E. coli* infections, leukocytes were abundant in the urine. In contrast, if urine pH was above 7.75, as was the case with *Proteus* bacteriuria, the number of intact leukocytes in the urine was low despite inflammatory foci, but numerous leukocyte casts confirmed that leukocyte disintegration in vivo occurs in an alkaline environment. These results correlate with the clinical observation that *Proteus* bacteriuria is frequently associated with the absence of leukocytes in the urine (41). Stotter et al. (146) used a catheter inserted in the renal pelvis to induce ascending *E. coli* bacteriuria that resulted in chronic pyelonephritis. In contrast to other models of *E. coli* bacteriuria, in which there is rapid, spontaneous healing of renal damage, their animals exhibited increased renal changes for up to 6 months after challenge.

## ANTIBODIES

Rabbits have been used to study the production of urinary antibodies or protection from infection following i.v. or retrograde challenge. Lehmann et al. (81) and Kaijser and Olling (73) studied antibody production in rabbits in which they induced unilateral pyelonephritis following i.v. challenge with *E. coli* by the procedure described by Lepper (82), in which one ureter was transiently occluded. Lehmann et al. (81), in assessing local antibody production within the urinary tract, observed that the majority of antibody produced by the infected kidney was of the immunoglobulin G (IgG) class; IgA levels in infected kidneys, the contralateral uninfected kidney, and kidneys from uninfected rabbits were similar. Kaijser and Olling (73) and Smith and Kaijser (140) found that antibody to O antigen of *E. coli* was produced in all exposed animals and that it protected against pyelonephritis inducible by hematogenous challenge. Antibody to K antigen was also protective but was only sporadically produced. Antibody to H antigen was not protective. Kunin et al. (78) determined that members of the family *Enterobacteriaceae* share a common cell wall hapten, the enterobacterial common antigen (CA), which may be useful as an immunodiagnostic marker and an immunogen. Aoki et al. injected organisms directly into the kidney and by immunofluorescence studies determined that live organisms that gave positive hemagglutination reactions in vitro stained in vivo with CA but that dead organisms (regardless of whether they contained CA) and organisms not containing CA did not stain (4). Domingue et al. (28) and McLaughlin and Domingue (95) assessed the protective effect of immunization with CA to i.v. or retrograde challenge with *Proteus mirabilis*, *E. coli*, *Klebsiella pneumoniae*, or *Pseudomonas aeruginosa*. The specificity of the immune response was demonstrated by protection against *P. mirabilis* and *E. coli* (expresses CA) challenge but not against *Pseudomonas aeruginosa* (does not express CA) challenge. Antibody also did not protect against challenge with encapsulated *K. pneumoniae*, which was not opsonized by CA antibody in vitro.

## DEVICES

Rabbits have been used to study the effects of indwelling catheters (104) and catheter drainage systems (105) on the development of UTI. Nickel et al. (104) demonstrated that contamination of the catheter drainage system by a nonsterile break in the system at the distal junction of the catheter and proximal drainage system junction results in the rapid (within 32 to 48 h) development of bacteriuria. In this case, bacteria ascend through the catheter lumen from the site of introduction to the bladder. If a sterile closed drainage system is maintained, bacteriuria develops more slowly, taking between 72 and 168 h, and occurs via the extraluminal route. Ascending bacteriuria appears to develop within glycocalyx-enclosed biofilm either within the catheter lumen or on the outside lumen surface. The drainage bag outlet tube is another important source of system contamination. Experimental contamination of the conventional outlet tube with *E. coli* resulted in contamination of the system in 11 of 12 rabbits (mean system contamination rate in days after contamination of outlet tube: drainage bag, 2.5 days; catheter, 4.8 days). Use of a microbicidal outlet tube in a similar experiment prevented system contamination in 12 of 16 animals and delayed system contamination in the other 4 animals. Thus, experiments in rabbits can effectively assess devices used in or proposed for clinical practice.

## Dogs

In the early 1900s, studies in dogs, like other animal studies of the time, were undertaken to duplicate pyelonephritis seen clinically. At the time, it was believed that pyelonephritis in humans resulted from hematogenous infection, ascending infection from the bladder, or spread along periureteral lymphatics from an infected bladder to the subpelvic fat of the kidney with extension into the kidney parenchyma. Since dogs have been used frequently to model human diseases, it is somewhat surprising that the use of dogs as models for UTI has been limited. Dogs have been used to assess the effect of ureteral obstruction on atrophy of the kidney (13) and as models of UTI (16, 25, 37, 126, 143). The difficulty most investigators have had in establishing UTI in dogs by the ascending route most likely explains the limited use of dogs as models of UTI. Brewer (16) and David (25) made numerous, mostly unsuccessful attempts to induce pyelonephritis by the ascending route. When their attempts to induce pyelonephritis in the normal urinary tract failed, attempts were made to establish an upper tract infection by numerous alterations of the urinary tract, including temporary urethral ligation, bruising of the kidney, passing a suture through the renal pelvis several times, using a probe to disrupt the renal parenchyma, and injecting small seeds of blue moss into the renal artery. These alterations also failed to produce pyelonephritis following establishment of cystitis with *E. coli, Streptococcus pyogenes,* or *Neisseria gonorrhoeae.* Pyelonephritis was established only as a result of ligation of the ureter with injection of the challenge organism proximal to the ligation. Since cystitis, which was established in most of those studies, did not progress to pyelonephritis, even with extensive manipulation of the kidney, the ascending route of infection was thought to be less likely to result in pyelonephritis than the hematogenous route.

The fact that Brewer (16) could not establish pyelonephritis by the ascending route in dogs but did establish pyelonephritis by the hematogenous route in rabbits led him to conclude "that during the progress of any acute infectious disease a certain number of microorganisms find their way into the blood-current, and that many of these organisms are excreted through the kidney." In addition, Rocha (126) established *E. coli* pyelonephritis in dogs from hematogenous challenge following cautery injury to the medulla of the kidney. David (25) concluded that in dogs with partially obstructed bladders, in which the infecting organism is frequently recovered from the ureter and renal pelvis, upper urinary tract colonization most likely resulted from travel from the bladder through the ureteral lumen but could have also resulted by way of the periureteral lymphatics. Harrison et al. (51) established a persistent *E. coli* pyelonephritis by creating surgical reflux by ureteral meatotomy.

Ginder (37) proposed that adenovirus infection predisposes the urinary tract to infection with *E. coli*. Sommer and Roberts (143) used a paraffin ball as a foreign body in the bladder to induce chronic *E. coli* cystitis. Using that model, they determined that infection-induced increase in intravesical pressure leads to reflux in 50% of dogs challenged with *E. coli* and 94% of dogs challenged with *P. mirabilis*.

## Rats

By far the majority of animal studies of UTI have been conducted in rats. Studies of UTI in rats started in the mid-1900s and continue today. Rats were chosen because of economic considerations (less costly to purchase and house than rabbits) and because they develop pyelonephritis spontaneously (153). Studies in rats have been used to assess the effect of vaccination, antibiotic therapy, and bacterial factors on the development of UTI. Routes of challenge have included hematogenous, bladder, or directly into the kidney parenchyma.

Although Vivaldi et al. (152) were able to establish ascending *P. vulgaris* infection in normal rats, most investigators have had to use various manipulations to make the rat urinary tract more susceptible to infection, especially with *E. coli*. Various abilities of different bacterial strains and species to establish pyelonephritis have also been observed. Braude et al. (15) reported that *Proteus morganii* (now *Morganella morganii*) produced more severe pyelonephritis than did *Pseudomonas aeruginosa*, *E. coli*, or enterococci, although renal infection with enterococci was the most prolonged. Shapiro et al. (135) noted that the majority of rats sacrificed ≥14 weeks after challenge with *P. morganii* (now *M. morganii*) (23 [88%] of 26) or *Streptococcus zymogenes* (26 [100%] of 26) had kidney cultures positive for the challenge organism, while only 4 (13%) of 31 rats challenged with *E. coli* had positive kidney cultures ≥14 weeks after challenge.

Sommer (142) reported that a higher percentage of rat kidneys were infected with *S. aureus* (19 [79%] of 24) than with *E. coli* (8 [50%] of 16) or *P. mirabilis* (2 [10%] of 21) 1 month after i.v. challenge. Braude et al. (14) observed that the suppuration and pyuria seen in rats after challenge with a highly virulent strain of *E. coli* were severely reduced or absent in rats challenged with an *E. coli* strain in which the virulence had been reduced by repeated in vitro passage.

## HEMATOGENOUS PYELONEPHRITIS

As with other animal models of UTI, it is difficult to establish pyelonephritis in the normal rat, and manipulation of the urinary tract greatly increases the susceptibility of the kidney to infection from a hematogenous focus. Obstruction of urine flow from the kidney by ureteral ligation increases renal infection by allowing multiplication of the organism trapped in the kidney because of the obstruction (44, 145). Since ureteral ligation also results in hydronephrosis (the effects of which are difficult to separate from the effects of infection), other methods for the induction of pyelonephritis in rats were developed. Braude et al. (14, 15) and Shapiro et al. (135) demonstrated that "gentle but firm" massage of the kidneys immediately after intracardiac challenge with *E. coli* results in development of pyelonephritis (20 of 22 kidneys developed microscopic evidence of pyelonephritis) not seen in challenged controls without renal massage (0 of 22 kidneys developed microscopic evidence of pyelonephritis). Multiplication began in the renal interstitium after passage of the infecting organism from the circulation through vessel walls and evoked a leukocyte response (128). Bacteriuria, which occurred late in the infection, represented secondary invasion from outside renal tubules rather than multiplication within tubular cells. Although bacterial growth was not seen in renal tubular cells, ultrastructural studies demonstrate that the initial pathology from E. coli infection occurs in the mitochondria of proximal tubular cells, in which swelling and degeneration occur as early as 3 h after challenge with E. coli or cell-free broth filtrates (34). The rapidity of the ultrastructural change suggests that it is due to a bacterial toxin, most likely endotoxin, since the challenge organism does not express hemolysin. The resulting cellular necrosis and sloughing create focal obstruction of nephrons, which may result in the kidney being more susceptible to infection. Similar focal obstruction is observed in renal collecting ducts of rats fed oxamide (the diamide of oxalic acid) and in kidneys of patients who died of causes other than renal disease (32, 60). When oxamide is fed to rats, it is absorbed from the intestine and excreted unchanged in the urine, but because of limited solubility, it may crystallize in and occlude renal tubules and increase susceptibility to pyelonephritis. In rats challenged with E. coli, pyelonephritis developed in 52 (70%) of 74 rats fed oxamide but in 0 of 31 normal rats (32). Examination of 15 patients who had died of something other than renal disease revealed intraductal crystallization in the kidneys of 10 (67%) of them. Therefore, results from animal studies demonstrate that intraductal obstruction increases susceptibility of the kidney to infection, and clinical studies suggest that transient focal intraductal obstruction does occur (32). This observation may aid in explaining how an otherwise normal human kidney may become susceptible to infection from a hematogenous focus.

## ASCENDING PYELONEPHRITIS

The difficulty that other investigators had with establishing pyelonephritis in other animals was also experienced by investigators who used rats as a model of UTI. Either intentionally or unintentionally, retrograde challenge of rats results in reflux of the inoculum from the bladder into the ureters or the kidneys. Vesicoureteral reflux, which occurs naturally in rats (89, 111), can be increased by numerous manipulations of the rat urinary tract. Cotran et al. (22) reported that reflux routinely occurred with challenge volumes of 0.2 ml and occasionally at lower volumes; Andersen and Jackson (1), using methylene blue as a tracer, reported that "vesicoureteral reflux usually occurred in the range of 0.25 to 0.3 ml and a volume of 0.6 ml or more caused reflux in all of the animals." Retrograde challenge of rats is routinely performed with ≥0.2 ml. Fierer et al. (29) observed that vesicoureteral reflux sufficient to damage the renal fornix produced pyelonephritis that originated at the damage site. Vesicoureteral reflux may also induce bacteremia shortly after challenge. Fierer et al. (29) reported that 55 (81%) of 68 rats were bacteremic 3 min after challenge with 1.0 ml of E. coli suspension. Larsson et al. (79) did not detect bacteremia in 20 rats at 15 to 30 min after intravesical E. coli challenge at volumes of ≤0.5 ml but did detect bacteremia with increased challenge volumes (1 of 6 rats challenged with 0.6 ml, 4 of 9 rats challenged with 0.75 ml, and 15 of 15 rats challenged with ≥1.0 ml). Therefore, pyelonephritis induced by retrograde challenge of rats with concomitant renal damage and bacteremia is mechanistically similar to i.v. challenge.

Cotran et al. (22) and Heptinstall (55) in comparative studies of retrograde and hematogenous challenge techniques did observe differences in the two techniques. At 24 to 48 h after retrograde challenge, organisms appeared first in the renal pelvis, and infection spread to the medulla and cortex through the interstitium and tubules. In contrast, after hematogenous challenge, organisms first appeared in the cortical and medullary blood vessels, from which they spread to the interstitium and produced widespread lesions.

Other techniques have also been used to increase susceptibility of the rat kidney to infection from retrograde challenge. Cotran et al. (21) reported that insertion of a single glass bead in the bladder both enhanced and prolonged renal infection in rats following retrograde challenge with *E. coli*. They theorized that the role of the glass bead was to maintain residual urine in the bladder after micturition. Vivaldi et al. (152) reported that insertion of glass beads in rat bladders enhanced renal infection following both retrograde and hematogenous challenge with *P. mirabilis*. At 4 days after retrograde challenge, pyelonephritis developed in 60% of rats without glass beads and in 95% of rats with glass beads inserted in the bladder. Pyelonephritis was observed in 15% of rats without glass beads and in 40% of rats with glass beads at 4 days after intracardiac challenge.

By ligating one ureter and demonstrating that the corresponding kidney was protected from infection seen in the contralateral kidney, Vivaldi et al. (152) were the first to document that ascending pyelonephritis results from bladder challenge. Arana et al. (5) used multiple urethral challenges to enhance renal infection of *E. coli*. Renal lesions in rats in the "repeated challenge" group (retrograde infusion every other day for three times on alternate weeks throughout the observation period of up to 8 months) lasted longer than those in rats in the "initial challenge only" group (retrograde infusion every other day for three times during the first week of the experiment only). The development of antibodies in the repeated-challenge group appeared to decrease the number of renal lesions and the frequency of positive kidney cultures.

Heptinstall (54) first reported that bladder massage increases vesicoureteral reflux and *E. coli* infection of the rat kidney. After transurethral challenge, the bladder, palpated through the abdominal wall, was gently squeezed between the fingers while the urethral meatus was compressed to prevent escape of the inoculum. Prat et al. (111) confirmed Heptinstall's observation that bladder massage increases kidney infection and further observed that renal damage induced by temporary ureteral ligation for 4 to 6 h prior to retrograde challenge (ligature removed before challenge) both enhances and prolongs *E. coli* renal infection compared to infection in the contralateral, normal kidney. Asscher and Chick (7) undertook experimental studies in rats to determine whether growing kidneys (mimicking those of children) are more susceptible to infection from a retrograde focus in the setting of vesicoureteral reflux than fully grown kidneys. Using the bladder massage technique after retrograde challenge, they reported that unilateral nephrectomy enhances *E. coli* infection in the remaining kidney compared to renal infection in sham nephrectomized rats and that the enhanced renal infection corresponds to compensatory renal hypertrophy.

Brooks et al. (17) described a method of retrograde challenge in which vesicoureteral reflux was induced but bacteremia and hematogenous pyelonephritis were avoided. Immediately after a refluxing inoculum of 0.4 ml was introduced into the bladder, the left ureter, previously exposed through a midline abdominal incision, was partially occluded for approximately 20 h. This technique induced in the left, partially occluded kidney a higher incidence and a more prolonged *E. coli* infection than in the right, normal kidney.

To increase retention of bacteria in the urinary tract after challenge, Balish et al. (9) and Davis et al. (26) obstructed the urethra after challenge, and Reid et al. (113) challenged rats with organisms incorporated within agar beads. Urethral obstruction was accomplished by application of a wax seal to the urethral meatus (9) or by clamping the meatus with a hemostat (26). Bacteria were incorporated into agar beads (20 to 150 $\mu$m in diameter) when a combination of bacterial suspension, molten 2% agar, and peanut oil was vortexed, and the agar was solidified into beads by placing the mixture in an ice bath.

**Direct Kidney Inoculation.** Several investigators used direct inoculation of the kidney to establish a more persistent *E. coli* pyelonephritis (98, 110, 132). However, even with this method of challenge, not all kidneys become infected. Schmidt et al. (132), who occluded the ureter for 15 min after direct renal injection, reported that histologic evidence of infection was present in only 31 (67%) of 46 kidneys 6 to 8 weeks after challenge. Prat et al. (110), who infected rats by delivering 0.02 ml to three sites within the kidney, obtained a consistent and reproducible pyelonephritis for up to 7 weeks after challenge without abscess formation. Miller and Robinson (98), using the challenge method of Prat et al. (110), obtained a consistent and reproducible *E. coli* pyelonephritis for up to 100 days after challenge with as few as $3 \times 10^2$ bacteria.

**Water Diuresis.** Since increased consumption of liquids has been used clinically to treat bacteriuric patients, the effect of water diuresis on UTI has been investigated experimentally in animals. If rats are given water containing 5% glucose or sucrose, water consumption is greatly increased compared to that of rats given tap water. After i.v. challenge of rats, renal infection begins in the medulla (45, 126). However, Andriole and Epstein (3) reported that water diuresis prevented pyelonephritis from i.v. challenge with *S. aureus* and *Candida albicans,* possibly by reducing medullary osmolality and/or by reducing the sodium and urea concentrations in the medulla. Andriole (2) also reported that water restriction increased the incidence of *E. coli* pyelonephritis following i.v. challenge. Levison and Kaye (83) noted that the combination of ampicillin and water diuresis prevented enterococcal pyelonephritis following i.v. challenge better than either alone. Mahoney and Persky (89) demonstrated that after injection of *P. vulgaris* into the bladder lumen, water diuresis reduced pyelonephritis by 48%.

However, Freedman (31) reported that following bladder challenge, water diuresis increased susceptibility to *E. coli* bacteriuria 1 million-fold. Danzig and Freedman (24) further reported that diuresis increased susceptibility of the kidney to *E. coli* pyelonephritis following direct inoculation into the kidney. Kaye (75) demonstrated that after direct left-kidney challenge, diuresis protected against enterococcal and *S. aureus* pyelonephritis but enhanced susceptibility to *E. coli* pyelonephritis in the contralateral (right) kidney induced by the ascending route from the infectious focus in the left kidney. A possible explanation of those results could be that concentrated urine is more inhibitory for *E. coli* than for enterococci or *S. aureus*. The discrepancy between studies may be the result of differences in the route of bacterial challenge and the resultant pyelonephritis, differences in the susceptibility of organisms to the inhibitory effects of solutes in the urinary tract, or differences in the abilities of organisms to resist phagocytosis or antibody-induced killing. Increased susceptibility to experimental pyelonephritis may be a unique feature of the rat, in which naturally occurring vesicoureteral reflux may be intensified by diuresis through increased bladder volume. The resulting increased intravesical pressure could induce renal damage and increased susceptibility to infection.

## INTERACTIONS BETWEEN BACTERIA AND HOST

Rat studies have been used extensively to elucidate the interaction between bacteria and the host during infection of the urinary tract. The inability to concentrate urine appears to be an early functional abnormality in the development of pyelonephritis (84). Spitznagel and Schroeder (145) demonstrated that arterial hypertension develops in rats with chronic pyelonephritis.

Fried and Wong (33) observed that while hemolytic *E. coli* strains produce pyelonephritis in up to 54% of rats challenged, pyelonephritis was not induced by nonhemolytic strains. They speculated that hemolysin may rupture the lysosomal membranes of renal parenchymal cells, leading to renal-cell death. In assessing the role of fimbriae in *P. mirabilis* UTI, Silverblatt (137) reported that fimbrial type change during the course of ascending pyelonephritis. While bacterial cells in the inoculum expressed fimbriae 40 Å (4.0 nm) in diameter (Brinton's type III), those adhering to renal pelvic epithelium 24 h after challenge expressed fimbriae 70 Å (7.0 nm) in diameter (Brinton's type IV). Results from subsequent experiments demonstrated that bacteria expressing type IV fimbriae were significantly more uropathogenic than bacteria expressing type III fimbriae. However, *P. mirabilis* heavily fimbriated with type IV fimbriae was less uropathogenic than lightly fimbriated organisms after i.v. challenge. Cortical abscesses were seen in 13 of 24 rats challenged with the lightly fimbriated strain but in none of 24 rats challenged with the heavily fimbriated strain (139). Hughes et al. (60) observed that cell wall-deficient variants of *P. mirabilis* are as uropathogenic as the parent strain if the variant easily reverts to the parental form; stable variants have limited uropathogenicity.

Fukushi et al. (35), using electron microscopy to study the interaction between bacteria and host urinary bladder, noted that the initial attachment of *E. coli* to the luminal membrane is followed by infolding of the membrane to envelope the organism, destruction of the membrane, apparent killing of the bacteria, desquamation of infected epithelial cells, and prompt regeneration of the desquamated epithelial layers. Bladder mucin appears to play a protective role against bacterial infection by enmeshing and subsequently removing the infecting organisms from the urinary tract (9). Establishment of cystitis is associated with disruption of the mucin layer, bacterial adherence to the uroepithelium, and swelling of the epithelial folds. Host response to infection appears to be exfoliation of damaged epithelial cells and subsequent regeneration of the epithelial layers (26). Nonfimbriated *Pseudomonas aeruginosa* was shown by scanning electron microscopy to adhere to rat bladders pretreated with a weak acid solution that removes surface mucin but not to untreated bladders (141, 149). The results underscore the importance of bladder mucin in protection against bacterial colonization and suggest that fibrinlike strands or other mechanisms aid in bacterial adherence to bladder epithelial cells.

Michaels et al. (97) observed that *E. coli* bacteriuria is reduced when the challenge dose is suspended in D-mannose, possibly because of inhibition of *E. coli* adherence to bladder epithelium, and to a lesser degree when the dose is suspended in D-glucose, possibly because of repression of the fimbrial operon. Keith et al. (77), using isogenic mutants of a clinical *E. coli* isolate that expressed type I fimbriae, reported that a similar inhibition of bacteriuria was obtained when organisms lacking the receptor-binding function or organisms that did not express type I fimbriae were used to challenge rats. Marre et al. (91), using mutants of a clinical isolate into which cloned virulence factor genes were reintroduced, demonstrated that S fimbriae, hemolysin, and serum resistance all individually contributed to *E. coli* pyelonephritis in rats. Parenteral administration of low-molecular-weight iron complexes (which pass the glomerulus) but not high-molecular-weight iron complexes promoted renal growth and subsequent development of renal abscess in rats and mice challenged with *E. coli, Staphylococcus albus,* and *Mycobacterium fortuitum* (30).

Raffel et al. (112) reported that renal colonization and renal inflammation were greater in diabetic rats than in normal rats after challenge with *C. albicans* and *S. aureus* but not with enterococci. Results could be partially explained by the fact that the inhibitory effect for those organisms in the urine of nondiuresing, normal rats could be overcome by adding glucose or water to the urine.

Animal studies have demonstrated that acute renal infection may lead to chronic pyelonephritis in which the kidneys are scarred, shrunken, and frequently sterile. Studies were initiated to investigate whether products of bacterial growth or host response to that growth is responsible for the development of chronic pyelonephritis. Glauser et al. (38) and Meylan et al. (96), using different antibiotic regimens at different stages of acute renal infection with *E. coli,* demonstrated that antibiotic sterilization of the kidneys early in acute infection prevented the development of chronic pyelonephritis. They further demonstrated that partial antibiotic therapy that suppressed acute suppuration but allowed persistent bacterial growth in the kidney also prevented chronic pyelonephritis, which suggests that renal damage was due to suppuration rather than to products of bacterial growth. Bille and Glauser (11), using either colchicine therapy prior to bacterial challenge to depress leukocyte mobility or cyclophosphamide to induce neutropenia, confirmed that chronic pyelonephritis resulted from infiltration of polymorphonuclear leukocytes into the site of acute infection, even though bacterial counts in kidneys from treated rats were higher than those in untreated controls.

## UREA, UROLITHIASIS, AND UREASE INHIBITORS

While urease is most frequently associated with apatite and struvite stone formation, urease alone also promotes renal invasion of *P. mirabilis*. Musher et al. (102) used acetohydroxamic acid, a potent urease inhibitor, to demonstrate that urease-induced alkalinization of urine damaged rat renal epithelium and promoted tissue damage by *P. mirabilis*.

Without using bacterial challenge, Vermeulen and Goetz (150) reported that the presence of a zinc disk as a foreign body in the rat urinary tract promoted the development of urinary stones: calcium phosphate stones in Holtzman rats (stones in female rats had a higher calcium content than those in male rats) and magnesium ammonium phosphate (struvite) stones in Harlan Sprague-Dawley rats. Struvite stones also develop in the urinary tracts of rats as the result of urease elaboration from *Corynebacterium* group D2 (144) or *P. mirabilis* (106) infection, possibly following disruption of the bladder mucous coat (43). The *P. mirabilis*-infected rat model has been used to assess the in vivo efficacy of urease inhibitors such as *N*-(pivaloyl)glycinohydroxamic acid (130) and *N*-(diaminophosphinyl)isopentenoylamide (129) and of antibiotic therapy (151) in preventing urolithiasis.

Although numerous animal studies have been conducted to assess the in vivo efficacy of antibiotic therapy for UTI, a few examples will suffice to demonstrate the utility of these models. Despite the absence of detectable levels in urine, the accumulation and storage of aminoglycosides in kidneys, characteristics of those compounds that may lead to nephrotoxicity, were effective in preventing acute *E. coli* ascending pyelonephritis and the resulting chronic pyelonephritis (10, 39). An antibiotic combination that is synergistic in vitro was significantly more effective in vivo in treating obstructive pyelonephritis than was either drug alone (40). The combination was the only regimen that sterilized the infected kidneys.

The immune response to UTI has been considered not only to protect against subsequent bacterial challenge but also to contribute to the development of chronic pyelonephritis. Cotran et al. (22) speculated that bacterial antigen, which persisted in the kidney for 20 weeks after the kidney became sterile, contributed to continued chronic renal inflammation by the persistent local appearance of antibody-producing cells. Uehling and Wolf (148) demonstrated that the protective effect of parenteral immunization against *E. coli* cystitis did not correlate with levels of circulating antibody. Vesical immunization was not protective and did not induce circulating antibody. Pazin and Braude (108), using an intrarenal infection model to study ascending infection of the contralateral kidney, reported that antibody induced by formalin-killed *E. coli* cells (containing both O and H antigens) protected against ascending infection, but immunization with boiled cells containing only O antigen did not protect. They further demonstrated that the protective antibody immobilized the infecting organism, suggesting motility as a bacterial virulence factor. Brooks et al. (18) demonstrated that immunization with formalin-killed and boiled cells protected against *E. coli* pyelonephritis with all but the most virulent (Riffle) strain. Protection correlated with the development of high serum titers to lipopolysaccharide; no antibody was found in the urine. They noted that infection caused an acute drop in antibody titer and speculated that lack of protection against challenge with the Riffle strain was due to inadequate antibody titer. Immunization also resulted in less parenchymal destruction and renal shrinkage (19). Kaijser et al. (72) observed that although serum and urinary antibodies were produced against O and K antigens following acute pyelonephritis, intravesical immunization with formalin-killed *E. coli* cells resulted mostly in the production of urine antibodies.

Intravesical immunization resulted in protection from pyelonephritis by homologous but not heterologous challenge. Passive intravesical immunization with sterile urine from infected rats protected against pyelonephritis, and antibody to K antigen appeared to be particularly important in that protection. Antibody response in both bladder and kidney appears to be biphasic, i.e., IgM followed by a stronger IgG response (57). Silverblatt and Cohen (138) reported that antifimbrial antibodies from both active and passive immunization protected against homologous but not heterologous ascending *E. coli* pyelonephritis.

Peroral (p.o.) immunization with live *E. coli* produced IgG anti-O and IgM anti-K serum antibodies; IgG anti-O urine antibody; and IgG, IgM, and IgA anti-O bronchopulmonary antibodies, and it protected against pyelonephritis from homologous challenge. Since p.o. immunization produces urinary antibody, results suggest that the urinary tract forms part of the common mucosal immune system. Peroral immunization did not produce antibody to lipid A, and passive immunization with anti-lipid A did not protect against pyelonephritis (94). In long-term studies lasting up to 1 year after challenge, even though urinary and high serum anti-O titers persisted, kidneys remained culture positive (93).

## Mice

i.v. CHALLENGE
As was observed in experiments with rats, investigators had difficulty establishing infection in the urinary tracts of normal mice challenged with gram-negative bacilli. Following i.v. challenge of mice with *Pseudomonas aeruginosa, E. coli,* or *P. mirabilis,* Gorrill and De Navasquez (42) had difficulty producing UTI in mice because the kidney-infecting dose was very close to the lethal dose. They obtained a descending infection that was first detected by lesions in

the glomeruli and progressed to papillary necrosis with subsequent infection of ureters and bladder and no evidence of ascending infection. Lesions produced by the three organisms were morphologically similar, but there was no discussion of urolithiasis following challenge with *P. mirabilis*. MacLaren (88) reported that treatment of mice with acetohydroxamic acid, a potent inhibitor of bacterial urease, prior to and after i.v. challenge with *P. mirabilis* reduced the severity of renal infection, as demonstrated by smaller abscesses, lower serum lactic dehydrogenase levels (suggesting less tissue damage), and longer survival times than those of untreated mice. He states that "renal infection with *Proteus* is not associated in mice with the development of renal calculi." Legnani-Fajardo et al. (80a) reported that immunization of mice with *P. mirabilis* fimbrial preparations but not flagellar preparations conferred homologous and heterologous protection from pyelonephritis after subsequent i.v. challenge as judged by significantly fewer immunized mice with renal abscesses (9 of 48 immunized, 38 of 40 control). Again, there was no mention of urolithiasis.

## WATER DIURESIS

Mouse studies were initiated by Keane and Freedman (76) in an attempt to reproduce results in rats which suggested that water diuresis impaired bacterial clearance from the urinary tract following bladder challenge. They found that *E. coli* clearance from the urinary tracts of mice undergoing diuresis was also impaired. In addition, severe pyelonephritis and papillary necrosis, which are not seen in diuresing rats, were seen 3 weeks after bladder challenge in 9 of 19 diuresing mice and 0 of 16 mice drinking tap water. Furtado and Freedman (36), noting that the effect of diuresis on establishment of UTI may depend on the organism, inoculation route, and animal species, investigated the effect of diuresis on development of UTI in mice following hematogenous and retrograde challenge with *Pseudomonas aeruginosa* and *S. aureus* and retrograde challenge with *E. coli*. Since bacterial challenge resulted in an interruption of drinking, the effect of diuresis on UTI could not be tested. Pyelonephritis seen after i.v. challenge (in 34% challenged with *Pseudomonas aeruginosa* and $\geq$80% challenged with *S. aureus*) also occurred in 17% of normal mice challenged by the retrograde route with *Pseudomonas aeruginosa* but was not seen after retrograde challenge with *S. aureus*. Kalmanson et al. (74), extending the observations of Keane and Freedman (76), observed that *E. coli* persisted in the urine and kidneys for up to 32 weeks after retrograde challenge in diuresing mice. Necrotizing abscesses, mononuclear infiltration, tubular atrophy, and interstitial scarring seen at 32 weeks after challenge are extensions of the pyelitis first seen 1 week after challenge. Guze et al. (46) used the retrograde challenged, diuresis mouse model to correlate uropathogenicity of 22 *E. coli* strains with possible virulence factors. Nephropathogenicity, the ability to produce renal lesions, correlated with the presence of K antigen, resistance to phagocytosis and serum bactericidal activity, ability to ferment dulcitol, and ability to multiply in urine and minimal medium but not with the ability to adhere to mouse bladder epithelial cells or with the presence of fimbriae (101).

The effect of urease inhibitors on the uropathogenicity of *P. mirabilis* was also studied in retrograde challenged diuresing mice. Aronson et al. (6), using mice challenged with a mixture of *P. mirabilis* and *E. coli,* found that hydroxyurea treatment led to a reduction in *P. mirabilis* renal and urine colonization and a reduction in renal pathology score but had no effect on *E. coli* colonization of urine. Thiourea, a less potent urease inhibitor than hydroxyurea, also had less of an effect on *P. mirabilis* uropathogenicity as demonstrated by reduced renal colonization, less effect on renal pathology score, and no effect on urine colonization. The urease inhibitors were effective prophylactically but ineffective therapeutically.

Antibody titers to the challenge *E. coli* strain were significantly higher in infected mice than in uninfected controls, but emergence of antibody did not arrest the progressive chronic infection or prevent apparent reinfection, as evidenced by acute inflammation 32 weeks after challenge (74). At 4 weeks after bladder challenge of diuresing mice with *E. coli*, Bluestone et al. (12) detected increases in serum IgG and IgM, including IgG-specific antibody to the infecting organism, but did not detect increases in urinary immunoglobulins over levels in uninfected controls. Serum antibodies did not appear to protect against renal infection. In contrast, Layton and Smithyman (80) demonstrated an approximately 5-log reduction in *E. coli* bladder colonization in mice immunized with an outer membrane protein (intramuscularly [i.m.] with Freund's complete adjuvant followed by a p.o. boost) compared to that in unimmunized mice. Histologically, bladders from vaccinated mice appeared normal, while inflammation, mucosal hypertrophy, edema, and thickening of blood vessel walls were seen in bladders from unimmunized mice. High levels of immunoglobulins in serum and low levels in urine resulted from i.m.-p.o. immunization. A p.o.-p.o. immunization resulted in significant increases in serum and urine immunoglobulins, but protection from infection was less effective than with i.m.-p.o. immunization resulting in a 2-log reduction in bladder colonization compared to that in unimmunized controls. Results suggest that outer membrane protein of *E. coli* is an effective immunogen and that the urinary tract is part of the common mucosal immune system.

The diuresis mouse model has also been used to evaluate the importance of fimbrial phase variation during *K. pneumoniae* infection, to study the effect of moderate stress on susceptibility to *E. coli* UTI, and to assess the efficacy of antimicrobial therapy. Maayan et al. (86) reported that the rate of UTI in mice infected with *K. pneumoniae* expressing type 1 (mannose-sensitive [$MS^+$]) fimbriae was 85% and that all isolates recovered during the infection were $MS^+$. However, when mice were challenged with an $MS^-$ phenotype of the same strain, heterogeneous results were obtained. One group, in which shedding of $MS^+$ organisms was ≥70%, had an infection rate of 68%; a second group, in which shedding of $MS^+$ organisms was ≤30%, had a significantly lower infection rate of 28%. Challenge of mice with an $MS^-$ variant that had lost its ability to undergo the phase variation shift to $MS^+$ in vitro resulted in an infection rate of 14% and recovery of only $MS^-$ isolates. In urine, the $MS^+$ phenotype organisms outgrew the $MS^-$ phenotype organisms, but the $MS^-$ phenotype cells predominated in the kidneys. Results suggest that expression of type 1 fimbriae provides a selective advantage for *K. pneumoniae* colonization of the bladder but that phase variation to $MS^-$ confers a selective advantage for renal colonization. Dalal et al. (23) observed that female but not male mice subjected to moderate stress by exposure to constant illumination for 96 h or to 37°C heat for 24 h displayed increased uroepithelial cell shedding, increased migration of polymorphonuclear cells into the bladder following chemotactic stimuli, and reduced susceptibility to *E. coli* UTI as judged by bacteriuria. Stress-induced uroepithelial shedding continued at a constant rate for at least 2 weeks after the stimulus. Hubert et al. (59) noted that therapy for 3 weeks with ampicillin or penicillin cured established *E. coli* UTI, but 6 weeks of therapy was required with cephalothin and kanamycin. Delay in initiation of therapy reduced therapeutic efficacy.

## ASCENDING PYELONEPHRITIS

In studies designed to mimic the ascending route of infection, thought to be the most important mode of human UTI, mice have been challenged intravesically either with other manipulations of the urinary tract or without additional manipulations. Hagberg et al. (48) carefully described ascending *E. coli* UTI in mice challenged transurethrally without additional manipulation of the urinary tract. Renal infection was dependent on the mouse strain used and the expression of P fimbriae (*pap*) but not type 1 fimbriae (*pil*) by the challenge organism. When mice were challenged with a mixture of $pap^+$ $pil^-$ and $pap^-$ $pil^+$ organisms (mutants derived from N-methyl-N-nitro-N-nitrosoguanidine treatment of *E. coli* HU734, which is a *lac* mutant nitrous acid-treated derivative of strain GR12, which was isolated from a patient with acute pyelonephritis), $pap^+$ $pil^-$ dominated over $pap^-$ $pil^+$ more in CBA mouse kidneys than in BALB/c mice, possibly because of a higher glycolipid composition of the CBA mouse kidney (47). Bladder colonization by the two mutants was similar in the two mouse strains. Pyelitis was present in one-third of mice sacrificed 3 weeks after challenge with $pap^+$, but pyelonephritis was seen in only 2 (5%) of 42 of mice studied. Culture of urine, a potentially simple and convenient method for monitoring animals for UTI, was unreliable. Animals frequently had sterile urine while bladder and kidney cultures were positive (48), or urine contained nonfimbriated organisms when the bladder was colonized with fimbriated organisms (61). *E. coli* FN414, a fecal isolate from a healthy child that expresses neither P fimbriae nor type 1 fimbriae, was cleared from the urinary tract by 7 days after challenge, a time when 20 of 20 bladders and 6 of 20 kidneys from mice challenged with *E. coli* HU734 ($pap^+$ $pil^+$) were positive for the challenge organism. Thus, the model distinguishes between pyelonephritogenic and nonuropathogenic fecal *E. coli* strains on the basis of renal colonization and pathology mediated by P fimbria, which has been determined epidemiologically to be an important *E. coli* virulence factor in strains isolated from patients with pyelonephritis. The model provides the opportunity of conducting a detailed histopathological analysis that can greatly enhance the assessment of uropathogenicity (67, 68), of screening *E. coli* strains isolated from patients with acute pyelonephritis for the ability to cause pyelonephritis (99), and of studying the expression of virulence factors.

The model has also been useful in defining the role of *E. coli* fimbriation in the establishment of UTI. Receptors for *E. coli* type 1 and Gal-Gal-binding P fimbriae were found throughout the urogenital system of BALB/c mice, including the squamous epithelium of the vagina; the transitional epithelium of the bladder, ureter, and renal pelvis; and epithelial cells of the proximal tubules, loop of Henle, and collecting ducts but not the glomeruli (107). Some *E. coli* strains undergo phase variation in their expression of fimbriae. When the cells were grown in broth, expression of type 1 fimbriae was enhanced and expression of P fimbriae was suppressed; growth on agar has the opposite effect. When mice were challenged with phase-variant *E. coli* strains, significantly better bladder colonization was obtained with broth-grown (type 1-enhanced) cultures than with agar-grown (type 1-suppressed) cultures (61). Examination by immunocytochemistry demonstrated large numbers of type 1-fimbriated organisms adhering to bladder transitional epithelial cells. Antibody to type 1 fimbriae blocked adherence of broth-grown cultures to mouse bladder epithelial cells. However, organisms colonizing the kidney lost their abilities to express type 1 fimbriae (131). Results suggest that expression of type 1 fimbriae promotes *E. coli* bladder colonization, that nonfimbriated strains are significantly less able to establish cystitis, that *E. coli* fimbrial phase variation occurs in vivo, and that expression of P fimbriae may be important in *E. coli* renal colonization. Since antibody to P fimbriae protects mice from renal colonization and invasion following both homologous and heterologous challenge with pyelonephritogenic *E. coli* strains that express P fimbriae, results provide additional in vivo evidence that P fimbriae are important in *E. coli* renal colonization and suggest that a P-fimbria vaccine may be effective clinically in preventing *E. coli* pyelonephritis (109, 133). However, when both distinct copies of the *pap* operon were deleted by molecular genetic techniques from a highly virulent *E. coli* strain that also expresses *pil*, *foc* (F1C fimbriae), and *hly* (hemolysin), pyelonephritogenicity was retained (100). Results suggest that this *E. coli* strain, in addition to expressing P fimbriae, may possess other virulence factors sufficient to cause acute pyelonephritis in the absence of binding to the P blood group antigen.

The model has also been used to demonstrate that lipopolysaccharide-induced phagocyte activation is a major defense mechanism against *E. coli* (147) but not against gram-positive organisms (49). Results from a later study indicated that inhibition of inflammation not dependent on inhibition of interleukin-6 or phagocyte recruitment impaired bacterial renal clearance (85). Studies using scanning electron microscopy documented that pyelonephritogenic *E. coli* adheres to both bladder and renal mucosal surfaces and within 24 h after challenge, forms on those surfaces microcolonies that are associated with large amounts of amorphous extracellular material (50).

Hagberg et al. (48) demonstrated the utility of the intravesically challenged mouse model for studying *E. coli* UTI in an unobstructed, nonmanipulated urinary tract, but the model has also been useful in studying the uropathogenicity of other microorganisms and the effect of clinically relevant manipulations of the urinary tract on bacterial uropathogenicity. The mouse model has been used to document the uropathogenicity of *Providencia stuartii*, a species found commonly in long-term catheterized patients, and to distinguish between uropathogenic and nonuropathogenic strains (63). Results from previous studies suggest that elaboration of urease is a *P. mirabilis* virulence factor. The importance of urease as a *P. mirabilis* urovirulence factor was confirmed by a comparison in the mouse model of the uropathogenicity of the parent strain (urease positive) with that of its isogenic mutant (urease negative) containing an insertion mutation within *ureC*, the gene that encodes the large subunit of the enzyme (66).

*P. mirabilis* produces at least four types of fimbriae. Molecular genetic techniques were used to prepare isogenic mutants so that the contributions of two of those fimbriae, PMF (*P. mirabilis* fimbriae) and MR/P (mannose-resistant *Proteus*-like), to *P. mirabilis* uropathogenicity could be determined in the mouse model. The *pmfA* mutant colonized the bladders of transurethrally challenged CBA mice in numbers 83-fold lower than those of the parent strain (92). However, the mutant colonized the kidneys in numbers similar to those of the parent strain. Therefore, these data suggest a role for PMF in colonization of the bladder but not of kidney tissue. On the other hand, MR/P significantly contributed to both bladder and renal colonization in CBA mice.

An advantage of the mouse model described by Hagberg et al. (48) is that since uropathogenicity is achieved in an unobstructed, nonmanipulated urinary tract, the mouse urinary tract can be intentionally altered to study conditions that appear to be important clinically in the development of UTI. Catheter-associated bacteriuria is the most common infection occurring in hospitals, where urethral catheters are generally in place for a few days, and in nursing homes, where catheters may be in place for months and years. *P. mirabilis*, frequently isolated from the urinary tracts of patients with urethral catheters, is an infrequent isolate from patients without urethral catheters. Placement of catheters in the bladders of mice, simulating the bladder segments of human urinary catheters, resulted in the spontaneous development of *P. mirabilis* bacteriuria, acute pyelonephritis, chronic renal inflammation, and struvite stone formation (64). Since those complications are similar to the complications common in patients with long-term catheters, results suggest that the mouse model may be useful in investigating the mechanism(s) by which catheterization causes enhanced susceptibility of the urinary tract to *P. mirabilis* infection.

Obstruction of urine outflow may be caused by prostatic hypertrophy, urethral stricture, or encrustation of a urethral-catheter lumen. The sequelae include fever, acute pyelonephritis, chronic renal inflammation, and death. Studies were initiated to determine whether even brief obstruction of the urinary tract containing a nonvirulent bacterium would result in these complications. Mice were challenged transurethrally with *E. coli* FN414, which in normal mice is rapidly eliminated from the urinary tract and is nonuropathogenic (48), and urine outflow was temporarily obstructed for 1, 3, or 6 h by application of collodion to the urethral meatus. The collodion was removed with acetone at the appropriate time (65). The majority of mice obstructed for 1 h demonstrated parenchymal renal inflammation 48 h later. After a 3-h obstruction, 9 of 10 mice were bacteremic; some bacteremias were present at 48 h after removal of the obstruction. As little as 6 h of obstruction resulted not only in acute renal changes but also in chronic renal inflammation and fibrosis in the majority of animals sacrificed 3 and 6 weeks later. Obstruction enhanced the renal lesions produced by *E. coli* CFT073, a uropathogen in normal mice that was originally isolated from a patient with symptoms of pyelonephritis. Results demonstrate that brief urethral obstruction may (i) induce organisms that are cleared rapidly from the normal urinary tract to cause bacteriuria, bacteremia, and pyelonephritis, and (ii) intensify the renal lesions caused by a uropathogen.

A number of investigations have been conducted to determine whether the inoculation procedure used to challenge mice induces vesicoureteral reflux. Hagberg et al. (48) monitored deposition of the inoculum in the mouse urinary tract with India ink and [$^{14}$C]mannose and found that vesicoureteral reflux was minimized by use of a challenge volume of 50 $\mu$l delivered over 20 s. Larger volumes or more rapid delivery of the inoculum result in an increase in vesicoureteral reflux. O'Hanley et al. (107), using methylene blue as a tracer, reported that an inoculum volume of 100 $\mu$l did not cause ureteric reflux, but a 250-$\mu$l inoculum did cause reflux. Schaeffer et al. (131), using an intraurethral inoculation technique to minimize artifactual retrograde intraureteral inoculation, obtained positive kidney cultures in 5% of mice 1 h after a 50-$\mu$l challenge. Pecha et al. (109) reported that a 100-$\mu$l inoculum did not cause acute ureteric reflux. Johnson and Manivel (69), using an unusually high rate of delivery of 10 $\mu$l/s, conducted a detailed study of the effect of varying the inoculum volumes on vesicoureteral reflux and found that reflux increased with increasing volumes. Mobley et al. (100), using an infusion pump set to deliver an inoculum of 50 $\mu$l over a period of 30 s, traced the disposition of the inoculum with India ink and culture of kidney homogenates. Of 10 mice sacrificed immediately after challenge, 10 had bladders filled with India ink, but the India ink was not visualized in ureters or the renal pelvis. The challenge organism was not cultured from homogenates of the 20 kidneys, and renal lesions were not seen by light microscopy (62). Results from these studies indicate that mice could be unnaturally compromised by vesicoureteral reflux if inoculum volumes exceeded 100 $\mu$l and/or the rate of delivery was faster than 20 s/50 $\mu$l of inoculum. However, careful control of the challenge procedure minimizes or eliminates the complication of vesicoureteral reflux and results in clinically relevant findings in which uropathogenicity is dependent only on the interplay between bacterial virulence factors and host defense mechanisms.

## Nonhuman Primates

Studies in nonhuman primates, although limited by high cost and the small number of animals, have confirmed many important aspects of UTI. UTI in nonhuman primates has been studied as a model of human infection because of the similarities between monkeys and humans: renal and ureteral physiology, natural occurrence of pyelonephritis, and vesicoureteral reflux that is common in infants but uncommon in adults (114–116). In the monkey, *E. coli* strains expressing type 1 fimbriae colonize the vagina but do not cause ascending UTI (120); in the absence of vesicoureteral reflux, pyelonephritis is caused by organisms expressing P fimbriae (125). The ascent of organisms may be aided by a decrease in ureteral peristalsis (115). Results from those studies suggest that the monkey urinary tract, similar to that of humans, contains digalactoside receptors to which the P fimbriae expressed by pyelonephritogenic *E. coli* strains bind (122). The presence of digalactoside receptors in the monkey urinary tract is further suggested by results of experiments that document that immunization with purified P fimbriae protects against pyelonephritis (118). In addition, infection with *E. coli* expressing P fimbriae prompts development of antibodies that are protective against rechallenge; antibiotic therapy begun 72 h after initiation of the primary challenge prevents development of protective antibody (103). This immune response also does not lead to renal damage (117).

Results from monkey studies indicate that pyelonephritis is caused by complement-activated granulocytic aggregation (70), the inflammatory response from bacterial infection, and the release of superoxide during phagocytosis (123), since renal damage is prevented by complement depletion, which decreases the number of inflammatory cells and the number of phagocytic events (124), and pretreatment with allopurinol, which prevents toxicity from superoxide (121). Vaccination with O8 oligosaccharide-protein conjugate does not alter bacteriuria but does protect against renal scarring during *E. coli* infection (119). However, immunization with enterobacterial CA does not protect monkeys infected with *E. coli* from developing pyelonephritis (134).

## HISTOPATHOLOGIC EVALUATION OF UTI IN RATS AND MICE

Evaluation of histopathologic changes in the urinary tract have provided valuable insights into the virulence of uropathogenic bacteria. Histologic changes in the kidneys of rats with acute or chronic pyelonephritis after retrograde UTI with *Klebsiella* spp., *E. coli,* and other gram-negative bacteria include cortical abscesses and wedges of inflammation radiating from the medulla or fibrosis, depending on the severity and duration of damage. Acute lesions are usually healed in 2 weeks, with scarring and destruction of renal parenchyma (1, 22, 54, 55). Pyelitis is the primary lesion in acute infections. In animals with pyelitis, the pelvic epithelium is thickened and infiltrated with inflammatory cells. In the early stages of acute infection, neutrophils are the predominant inflammatory cell. Subsequently, in subacute and chronic lesions, mononuclear cells infiltrate the epithelium and subepithelium. Extension of infection into the parenchyma begins in the fornices, which are fingerlike extensions of the pelvic lumen to the cortex. As infection spreads out toward the perihilar cortex, inflammatory cell infiltration occurs predominantly adjacent to the fornix. Neutrophils accumulate in the tubules. Abscesses develop within 2 to 4 days. Wedge-shaped areas extend into the central part of the papilla. The cortex over the greater curvature of the cortex may be involved. The renal lesions in animals challenged by the intravenous route are basically abscesses or microabscesses caused by bacteremia.

The sequence of histologic changes following ascending infection in mice is similar to that in rats. The severity of pyelonephritis is determined by the virulence of the organism, dose, duration postinfection, and strain of mouse (47, 65–68, 100). The mouse infection model of ascending infection discriminates between uropathogenic isolates cultured from human UTIs and human fecal strains in the severity of renal and urinary bladder pathology (47, 68). Different clinical isolates from human UTIs also vary in virulence in the mouse model (68, 99). The correlation between quantitative renal culture results and severity of renal histopathology is highly significant. Nevertheless, histopathologic evaluation adds to the culture results in determining UTI in experimentally infected mice and in understanding the virulence of uropathogenic bacteria. Histopathology demonstrates inflammation in animals that are culture negative and shows significant between-strain differences in virulence that are not apparent from culture results alone (68).

Johnson et al. (67, 68) used detailed descriptions of histopathologic abnormalities to evaluate renal and urinary bladder damage in mice challenged with different isolates of uropathogenic *E. coli*. The criteria used could also be categorized to indicate either pyelitis (inflammation and epithelial damage restricted to the pelvic cavity, the uroepithelium lining the pelvic cavity, and the immediate subepithelium) or pyelonephritis (inflammation and damage involving the medulla and cortex in addition to pyelitis in ascending infections). A semiquantitative score of severity of renal damage gave findings consistent with the detailed histopathologic criteria (67). The kidneys with higher scores exhibited pyelonephritis. When renal lesions were classified as either pyelonephritis, pyelitis, or no lesions and compared to culture results, the categories could not be distinguished strictly on the basis of renal bacterial concentration (67). Based on the correlation between a detailed histopathologic description and semiquantitative scores, a semiquantitative severity score in which specific histopathologic criteria are used is practical for the evaluation of histologic damage in the kidney and urinary bladder (8, 9, 65, 92). The time of sacrifice of animals for histopathologic evaluation may be selected depending on the objective of the study. However, evaluation at 24 to 48 h in particular indicates acute infection, which in part is associated with large numbers of neutrophils in the pelvic cavity associated with clearance of bacteria in the urine. The renal cultures at this time also probably reflect clearance as well as colonization. Bacterial cultures and histologic examination at later times, such as 1 week postchallenge, indicate effective colonization and significant host inflammatory response. At those times, the mean bacterial titer per group of infected mice is indicative of the percentage of animals with positive titers ($>10^3$ CFU of bacteria per g of tissue or per ml of urine).

The severity of renal damage is markedly lower in mice infected with a urease-negative mutant of *P. mirabilis* than in those infected with the parent strain (66). Similarly, mice challenged with an MR/P isogenic fimbrial mutant of *P. mirabilis* show reduced renal pathology, indicating that the MR/P fimbrial mutant is important in the pathogenesis of pyelonephritis caused by *P. mirabilis*.

The morphologic features of renal pathology in experimental *P. mirabilis* infection are somewhat different from those of *E. coli* kidney infection. This indicates that *P. mirabilis* has virulence mechanisms different from those of *E. coli*. An *E. coli* infection in the mouse or rat model is characterized by inflammatory cell infiltration in the medulla and cortex, with abscesses or pronounced inflammation in the cortex of some animals and low to high numbers of neutrophils in the pelvic cavity. Infection with *P. mirabilis* can cause extensive papillary necrosis in the kidney. The area of acute necrosis is delineated by an intense leukocyte infiltration. *P. mirabilis* causes erosion and ulceration of the uroepithelium lining the pelvic cavity. Struvite crystals are present in the lumen of the pelvic cavity and in areas of uroepithelial damage where there is ulceration and locally intense neutrophil infiltration (66, 68). Papillary necrosis is not seen in mice inoculated with urease-negative mutants via either the i.v. route or the ascending route of infection (66, 87).

In the mouse model, cystitis following *E. coli* infection is characterized by various numbers (low to high) of neutrophils in the lamina propria and necrosis of superficial transitional epithelial cells, sometimes resulting in erosion or ulceration of the epithelium. Bacteria may be adherent to the uroepithelium (67). As with the kidney, a semiquantitative severity score using defined criteria of severity of inflammation and epithelial damage can be used for practical evaluation of cystitis.

## RECOMMENDATIONS FOR THE STUDY OF ASCENDING UTI

Although a wide variety of animals have been used to study UTI, only mice and nonhuman primates appear to model human infection. The urinary tracts of both mice and nonhuman primates contain digalactoside receptors similar to those in the human urinary tract (47, 107, 122). These receptors are the binding sites for the P fimbriae expressed by pyelonephritogenic *E. coli* strains. *E. coli* strains that do not express P fimbriae or similar attachment organelles are not uropathogenic in humans, mice, or nonhuman primates.

Ascending infection is thought to be the most frequent route of human UTI. Unlike other animal species, mice and nonhuman primates may be successfully infected with virulent bacterial strains by ascending routes without further manipulation of the urinary tract. In mice, ascending infection may be induced by either intravesicular or intraurethral challenge. In nonhuman primates, ascending infection follows intraureteral challenge.

The mouse model of ascending infection has been used to assess the uropathogenicity of *E. coli*, *Providencia stuartii*, and *P. mirabilis* strains. The mouse model has also been used successfully to identify the urovirulence factors expressed by those bacterial species. Since UTIs in mice model those infections in humans, and since mice are relatively inexpensive to purchase and house and are available from numerous commercial breeders, the mouse model should be used as the primary model for ascending-UTI studies. Nonhuman primates, which are relatively expensive to purchase and house and are in limited supply from only a few sources, should be used in confirmatory studies of ascending UTIs.

## CONCLUSIONS

The study of UTIs in animal models has confirmed clinical observations, provided insight into the mechanisms of bacterial uropathogenicity, and provided a mechanism for understanding host response to infection, including inflammation and the resulting tissue destruction and antibody response. Mouse models also provided a mechanism by which molecular genetic alterations of uropathogens conducted in vitro may be evaluated in vivo, and they have been useful in assessing antimicrobial efficacy.

Unfortunately, results from a large portion of the studies conducted in animals are not reliable predictors of clinical infection, since unnatural routes of challenge and extensive urinary tract manipulation were used to establish infection. However, experience gained in the use of those models has resulted in the development of models that more closely reflect clinical infection.

Some areas of disagreement remain. The effect of vesicoureteral reflux remains the subject of controversy. While reflux occurs naturally in rats and may be important in establishing ascending infection in those animals, it appears to affect susceptibility to ascending infection in mice and nonhuman primates only if it is severe enough to inflict renal damage. Also unresolved is whether antibody, resulting from either infection or immunization, protects from infection and/or renal tissue damage.

Interestingly, very few studies of the development and prevention of cystitis, the important first step in the development of renal infection, have been conducted. Although type 1 fimbria, which is expressed by most strains of *E. coli,* has been identified by numerous investigators as important in bladder colonization, the mechanisms by which cystitis develops have not been studied extensively and are poorly understood. Animal studies will most likely be important in elucidating the complex interactions between pathogen and host during the development of cystitis.

## REFERENCES

1. **Andersen, B. R., and G. G. Jackson.** 1961. Pyelitis, an important factor in the pathogenesis of retrograde pyelonephritis. *J. Exp. Med.* **114:**375–384.
2. **Andriole, V. T.** 1970. Water, acidosis, and experimental pyelonephritis. *J. Clin. Invest.* **49:**21–30.
3. **Andriole, V. T., and F. H. Epstein.** 1965. Prevention of pyelonephritis by water diuresis: evidence for the role of medullary hypertonicity in promoting renal infection. *J. Clin. Invest.* **44:**73–79.
4. **Aoki, S., M. Merkel, M. Akoi, and W. R. McCabe.** 1967. Immunofluorescent localization of bacterial antigen in pyelonephritis. I. The use of antisera against the common enterobacterial antigen in experimental lesions. *J. Lab. Clin. Med.* **70:**204–212.
5. **Arana, J. A., V. M. Kozij, and G. G. Jackson.** 1964. Retrograde *E. coli* urinary tract infection in rats. *Arch. Pathol.* **78:**558–567.
6. **Aronson, M., O. Medalia, and B. Griffel.** 1974. Prevention of ascending pyelonephritis in mice by urease inhibitors. *Nephron* **12:**94–104.
7. **Asscher, A. W., and S. Chick.** 1972. Increased susceptibility of the kidney to ascending *Escherichia coli* infection following unilateral nephrectomy. *Br. J. Urol.* **44:**202–206.
8. **Bahrani, F. K., G. Massad, C. V. Lockatell, D. E. Johnson, R. G. Russell, J. W. Warren, and H. L. T. Mobley.** 1994. Construction of an MR/P fimbrial mutant of *Proteus mirabilis:* role of virulence in a mouse model of ascending urinary tract infection. *Infect. Immun.* **62:**3363–3371.
9. **Balish, M. J., J. Jensen, and D. T. Uehling.** 1982. Bladder mucin: a scanning electron microscopy study in experimental cystitis. *J. Urol.* **128:**1060–1063.
10. **Bille, J., and M. P. Glauser.** 1981. Prevention of acute and chronic ascending pyelonephritis in rats by amimoglycoside antibiotics accmulated and persistent in kidneys. *Antimicrob. Agents Chemother.* **19:**381–385.
11. **Bille, J., and M. P. Glauser.** 1982. Protection against chronic pyelonephritis in rats by

suppression of acute suppuration: effect of colchicine and neutropenia. *J. Infect. Dis.* **146:**220–226.
12. **Bluestone, R., L. S. Goldberg, G. M. Kalmanson, and L. B. Guze.** 1973. Systemic and urinary immune response in experimental *E. coli* pyelonephritis in mice. *Int. Arch. Allergy* **45:**571–581.
13. **Bradford, R.** 1987. Observations made upon dogs to determine whether obstruction of the ureter would cause atrophy of the kidney. *Br. Med. J.* **2:**1720.
14. **Braude, A. I., A. P. Shapiro, and J. Siemienski.** 1955. Hematogenous pyelonephritis in rats. I. Its pathogenesis when produced by a simple new method. *J. Clin. Invest.* **34:**1489–1497.
15. **Braude, A. I., A. P. Shapiro, and J. Siemienski.** 1959. Hematogenous pyelonephritis in rats. *J. Bacteriol.* **77:**270–280.
16. **Brewer, G. E.** 1911. The present state of our knowledge of acute renal infections: with a report of some animal experiments. *JAMA* **57:**179–187.
17. **Brooks, S. J. D., J. M. Lyons, and A. I. Braude.** 1974. Immunization against retrograde pyelonephritis. *Am. J. Pathol.* **74:**345–358.
18. **Brooks, S. J. D., J. M. Lyons, and A. I. Braude.** 1974. Immunization against retrograde pyelonephritis. II. Prevention of retrograde *Escherichia coli* pyelonephritis with vaccines. *Am. J. Pathol.* **74:**359–364.
19. **Brooks, S. J. D., J. M. Lyons, and A. I. Braude.** 1977. Immunization against retrograde pyelonepheitis. III. Vaccination against chronic pyelonephritis due to *E. coli*. *J. Infect. Dis.* **136:**633–639.
20. **Cotran, R. S.** 1963. Retrograde Proteus pyelonephritis in rats. *J. Exp. Med.* **117:**813–822.
21. **Cotran, R. S., L. D. Thrupp, S. N. Hajj, D. P. Zangwill, E. Vivaldi, and E. H. Kass.** 1963. Retrograde *E. coli* pyelonephritis in the rat: a bacteriologic, pathological, and fluorescent antibody study. *J. Lab. Clin. Med.* **61:**987–1004.
22. **Cotran, R. S., E. Vivaldi, D. P. Zangwill, and E. H. Kass.** 1963. Retrograde Proteus pyelonephritis in rats. *Am. J. Pathol.* **43:**1–31.
23. **Dalal, E., O. Medalia, O. Harari, and M. Aronson.** 1994. Moderate stress protects female mice against bacterial infection of the bladder by eliciting uroepithelial sheeding. *Infect. Immun.* **62:**5505–5510.
24. **Danzig, M. D., and L. R. Freedman.** 1972. Experimental pyelonephritis. XVII. Enhancement of pyelonephritis by water diuresis following direct inoculation of E. coli in the renal medulla of the rat. *Yale J. Biol. Med.* **45:**1–11.
25. **David, V. C.** 1918. Ascending urinary infections. *Surg. Gynecol. Obstet.* **26:**159–170.
26. **Davis, C. P., E. Balish, K. Mizutani, and D. T. Uehling.** 1977. Bladder response to Klebsiella infection. *Invest. Urol.* **15:**227–231.
27. **De Navasquez, S.** 1956. Further studies in experimental pyelonephtitis produced by various bacteria, with special reference to renal scarring as a factor in pathogenesis. *J. Pathol. Bacteriol.* **71:**27–32.
28. **Domingue, G., A. Salhi, C. Rountree, and W. Little.** 1970. Prevention of experimental hematogenous and retrograde pyelonephritis by antibodies against enterobacterial common antigen. *Infect. Immun.* **2:**175–182.
29. **Fierer, J., L. Talner, and A. I. Braude.** 1971. Bacteremia in the pathogenesis of retrograde *E. coli* pyelonephritis in the rat. *Am. J. Pathol.* **64:**443–454.
30. **Fletcher J., and E. Goldstein.** 1970. The effect of parenteral iron preparations on experimental pyelonephritis. *Br. J. Exp. Pathol.* **51:**280–285.
31. **Freedman, L. R.** 1967. Experimental pyelonephritis. XIII. On the ability of water diuresis to induce susceptibility to *E. coli* bacteriuria in the normal rat. *Yale J. Biol. Med.* **39:**255–266.
32. **Fried, F. A., and R. J. Wong.** 1969. Etiology of pyelonephritis: intraductal crystallization as a co-factor. *J. Urol.* **101:**786–790.
33. **Fried, F. A., and R. J. Wong.** 1970. Etiology of pyelonephritis: significance of hemolytic *Escherichia coli*. *J. Urol.* **103:**718–721.
34. **Fry, T. L., F. A. Fried, and B. A. Goven.** 1975. Evidence of obstructive etiology in intravenous bacterial pyelonephritis. *J. Surg. Res.* **18:**277–284.
35. **Fukushi, Y., S. Orikasa, and M. Kagaylama.** 1979. An electron microscopic study of the interaction between visceral epithelium and *E. coli*. *J. Urol.* **17:**61–68.
36. **Furtado, D., and L. R. Freedman.** 1970. Experimental pyelonephritis. XVI. *Pseudomonas aeruginosa, Escherichia coli,* and *Staphylococcus aureus* infections in mice and the effect of "water diuresis." *Yale J. Biol. Med.* **43:**177–193.
37. **Ginder, D. R.** 1974. Urinary tract infection and pyelonephritis due to *Escherichia coli* in dogs infected with canine adenovirus. *J. Infect. Dis.* **129:**715–719.

38. **Glauser, M. P., J. M. Lyons, and A. I. Braude.** 1978. Prevention of chronic experimental pyelonephritis by supression of acute suppuration. *J. Clin. Invest.* **61**:403–407.
39. **Glauser, M. P., J. M. Lyons, and A. I. Braude.** 1979. Synergism of ampicillin and gentamicin against obstructive pyelonephritis due to *E. coli* in rats. *J. Infect. Dis.* **139**:133–140.
40. **Glauser, M. P., J. M. Lyons, and A. I. Braude.** 1979. Prevention of pyelonephritis due to *Escherichia coli* in rats with gentamicin stored in kidney tissue. *J. Infect. Dis.* **139**:172–177.
41. **Gnarpe, H., and L. Olding.** 1970. The inflammatory reaction and urinary leucocytes in ascending urinary-tract infections. *Acta Pathol. Microbiol. Scand. Sect. B* **78**:208–214.
42. **Gorrill, R. H., and S. J. De Navasquez.** 1964. Experimental pyelonephritis in the mouse produced by *Escherichia coli*, *Pseudomonas aeruginosa* and *Proteus mirabilis*. *J. Pathol. Bacteriol.* **87**:79–87.
43. **Grenabo, L., H. Hedelin, J. Hugosson, and S. Pettersson.** 1988. Adherence of urease-induced crystals to rat bladder epithelium following acute infection with different uropathogenic organisms. *J. Urol.* **140**:428–430.
44. **Guze, L. B., and P. B. Beeson.** 1956. Experimental pyelonephritis. I. Effect of ureteral ligation on the course of bacterial infection in the kidney of the rat. *J. Exp. Med.* **104**:803–815.
45. **Guze, L. B., B. H. Goldner, and G. M. Kalmanson.** 1961. Pyelonephritis. I. Observations on the course of chronic non-obstructed enterococcal infection in the kidney of the rat. *Yale J. Biol. Med.* **33**:372–385.
46. **Guze, L. B., J. Z. Montgomerie, C. S. Potter, and G. M. Kalmanson.** 1973. Pyelonephritis XVI. Correlates of parasite virulence in acute ascending *Escherichia coli* pyelonephritis in mice undergoing diuresis. *Yale J. Biol. Med.* **46**:203–211.
47. **Hagberg, L., I. Engberg, R. Freter, J. Lam, S. Olling, and C. Svanborg-Eden.** 1983. Ascending unobstructed urinary tract infection in mice caused by pyelonephritogenic *Escherichia coli* of human origin. *Infect. Immun.* **40**:273–283.
48. **Hagberg, L., R. Hull, S. Hull, S. Falkow, R. Freter, and C. Svanborg-Eden.** 1983. Contribution of adhesion to bacterial persistence in the mouse urinary tract. *Infect. Immun.* **40**:265–272.
49. **Hagberg, L., R. Hull, S. Hull, J. R. McGhee, S. M. Michaelek, and C. Svanborg-Eden.** 1984. Differences in susceptibility to gram-negative urinary tract infection between C3H/HeJ and C3H/HeN mice. *Infect. Immun.* **46**:839–844.
50. **Hagberg, L., J. Lam, C. Svanborg-Eden, and J. W. Costerton.** 1986. Interaction of a pyenlonephritogenic *Escherichia coli* strain with the tissue components of the mouse urinary tract. *J. Urol.* **136**:165–172.
51. **Harrison, L. H., A. S. Cass, B. C. Bullock, and C. E. Clark.** 1973. Experimental pyelonephritis in dogs. I. Confirmation by antibody response. *J. Urol.* **109**:163–166.
52. **Helmholz, H. F., and C. Beeler.** 1917. Focal lesions produced in the rabbit by colon bacilli isolated from pyelocystitis cases. *Am. J. Dis. Child.* **14**:5–24.
53. **Helmholz, H. F., and C. Beeler.** 1918. Experimental pyelitis in the rabbit. *J. Urol.* **2**:395–418.
54. **Heptinstall, R. H.** 1964. Experimental pyelonephritis. *Nephron* **1**:73–92.
55. **Heptinstall, R. H.** 1965. Experimental pyelonephritis: a comparison of blood-borne and ascending patterns of infection. *J. Pathol. Bacteriol.* **89**:71–80.
56. **Heptinstall, R. H., and R. H. Gorrill.** 1955. Experimental pyelonephritis and its effect on the blood pressure. *J. Pathol. Bacteriol.* **69**:191–198.
57. **Hilz, M. E., M. S. Cohen, C. P. Davis, and M. M. Warren.** 1988. Acute and chronic bacterial infection in the rat urinary tract: immunofluorescent localization of immunoglobulins. *J. Urol.* **139**:840–843.
58. **Hodson, J., T. M. J. Maling, P. J. McManamon, and M. G. Lewis.** 1975. Reflux nephropathy. *Kidney Int.* **8**:S50.
59. **Hubert, E. G., G. M. Kalmanson, and L. B. Guze.** 1969. Antibiotic therapy of *Escherichia coli* pyelonephritis produced in mice undergoing chronic diuresis. *Antimicrob. Agents Chemother.* **8**:507–510.
60. **Hughes, B. F., H. Schwarz, and D. Gomolka.** 1972. Evaluation of a rat model for induction of pyelonephritis with cell wall deficient variants of *Proteus mirabilis*. *Invest. Urol.* **10**:10–13.
61. **Hultgren, S. J., T. N. Portner, A. J. Schaeffer, and J. L. Duncan.** 1985. Role of type 1 pili and effects of phase variation on lower urinary tract infections produced by *Escherichia coli*. *Infect. Immun.* **50**:370–377.
62. **Johnson, D. E.** Unpublished results.
63. **Johnson, D. E., C. V. Lockatell, M. Hall-Craggs, H. L. T. Mobley, and J. W.**

Warren. 1987. Uropathogenicity in rats and mice of *Providencia stuartii* from long-term catheterized patients. *J. Urol.* **138**:632–635.

64. Johnson, D. E., C. V. Lockatell, M. Hall-Craggs, and J. W. Warren. 1991. Mouse model of short- and long-term foreign body in the urinary bladder: analogies to the bladder segment of urinary catheters. *Lab. Anim. Sci.* **41**:451–455.

65. Johnson, D. E., R. G. Russell, C. V. Lockatell, J. C. Zulty, and J. W. Warren. 1993. Urethral obstruction of 6 hours or less causes bacteriuria, bacteremia, and pyelonephritis in mice challenged with "nonuropathogenic" *Escherichia coli*. *Infect. Immun.* **61**:3422–3428.

66. Johnson, D. E., R. G. Russell, C. V. Lockatell, J. C. Zulty, J. W. Warren, and H. L. T. Mobley. 1993. Contribution of *Proteus mirabilis* urease to persistence, urolithiasis, and acute pyelonephritis in a mouse model of ascending urinary tract infection. *Infect. Immun.* **61**:2748–2754.

67. Johnson, J. R., T. Berggren, and J. C. Manivel. 1992. Histopathologic-microbiologic correlates of invasiveness in a mouse model of ascending unobstructed urinary tract infection. *J. Infect. Dis.* **165**:299–305.

68. Johnson, J. R., T. Berggren, D. S. Newburg, R. H. McCluer, and J. C. Manivel. 1992. Detailed histopathological examination contributes to the assessment of *Escherichia coli* urovirulence. *J. Urol.* **147**:1160–1166.

69. Johnson, J. R., and J. C. Manivel. 1991. Vesicoureteral reflux induces renal trauma in a mouse model of ascending, unobstructed pyelonephritis. *J. Urol.* **145**:1306–1311.

70. Kaack, M. B., K. J. Dowling, G. M. Patterson, and J. A. Roberts. 1986. Immunology of pyelonephritis. VIII. *E. coli* causes granulocytic aggregation and renal ischemia. *J. Urol.* **136**:1117–1122.

71. Kaijser, B., and P. Larsson. 1982. Experimental acute pyelonephritis caused by enterobacteria in animals. A review. *J. Urol.* **127**:786–790.

72. Kaijser, B., P. Larsson, and S. Olling. 1978. Protection against ascending *Escherichia coli* pyelonephritis in rats and significance of local immunity. *Infect. Immun.* **20**:78–81.

73. Kaijser, B., and S. Olling. 1973. Experimental hematogenous pyelonephritis due to *Escherichia coli* in rabbits: the antibody response and its protective capacity. *J. Infect. Dis.* **128**:41–49.

74. Kalmanson, G. M., J. Z. Montgomerie, E. G. Hubert, L. Barajas, and L. B. Guze. 1973. Pyelonephritis. XV. Long-term study of ascending *Escherichia coli* pyelonephritis in mice. *Yale J. Biol. Med.* **46**:196–202.

75. Kaye, D. 1971. The effect of water diuresis on spread of bacteria through the urinary tract. *J. Infect. Dis.* **124**:297–305.

76. Keane, W. F., and L. R. Freedman. 1967. Experimental pyelonephritis. XIV. Pyelonephritis in normal mice produced by inoculation of *E. coli* into the bladder lumen during water diuresis. *Yale J. Biol. Med.* **40**:231–237.

77. Keith, B. R., L. Maurer, P. A. Spears, and P. A. Orndorff. 1986. Receptor-binding function of type 1 pili effects bladder colonization by a clinical isolate of *Escherichia coli*. *Infect. Immun.* **53**:693–696.

78. Kunin, C. M., M. V. Beard, and N. E. Halmagyi. 1962. Evidence for a common hapten associated with endotoxin fractions of *E. coli* and other Enterobacteriaceae. *Proc. Soc. Exp. Biol. Med.* **111**:160–166.

79. Larsson, P., B. Kaijser, I. Mattsby Baltzer, and S. Olling. 1980. An experimental model for ascending acute pyelonephritis caused by *Escherichia coli* or *Proteus* in rats. *J. Clin. Pathol.* **33**:408–412.

80a. Legnani-Fajardo, C., P. Zunino, G. Algorta, and H. F. Laborde. 1991. Antigenic and immunogenic activity of flagella and fimbriae preparations from uropathogenic *Proteus mirabilis*. *Can. J. Microbiol.* **37**:325–328.

80. Layton, G. T., and A. M. Smithyman. 1983. The effects of oral and combined parenteral/oral immunization against experimental *Escherichia coli* urinary tract infection in mice. *Clin. Exp. Immunol.* **54**:305–312.

81. Lehmann, J. D., J. W. Smith, T. E. Miller, J. A. Barnett, and J. P. Sanford. 1968. Local immune response in experimental pyelonephritis. *J. Clin. Invest.* **47**:2541–2550.

82. Lepper, E. H. 1921. The production of coliform infection in the urinary tract of rabbits. *J. Pathol. Bacteriol.* **24**:192–204.

83. Levinson, S. P., and D. Kaye. 1972. Influence of water diuresis on antimicrobial treatment of enterococcal pyelonephritis. *J. Clin. Invest.* **51**:2408–2413.

84. Levinson, S. P., P. G. Pitsakis, and M. E. Levison. 1982. Free water reabsorption during diuresis in experimental enterococcal pyelonephritis in rats. *J. Lab. Clin. Med.* **99**:474–480.

85. Linder, H., I. Engberg, C. vanKooten, P. deMan, and C. Svanborg-Eden. 1990. Effects of anti-inflammatory agents on mucosal inflammation induced by infection with gram-negative bacteria. *Infect. Immun.* **58:**2056–2060.

86. Maayan, M. C., I. Ofek, O. Medalia, and M. Aronson. 1985. Population shift in mannose-specific fimbriated phase of *Klebsiella pneumoniae* during experimental urinary tract infection in mice. *Infect. Immun.* **49:**785–789.

87. MacLaren, D. M. 1969. The significance of urease in *Proteus* pyelonephritis: a histological and biochemical study. *J. Pathol.* **97:**43–49.

88. MacLaren, D. M. 1974. The influence of acetohydroxamic acid on experimental Proteus pyelonephritis. *Invest. Urol.* **12:**146–149.

89. Mahoney, S. A., and L. Persky. 1963. Observations on experimental ascending pyelonephritis in the rat. *J. Urol.* **89:**779–783.

90. Mallory, G. K., A. R. Crane, and J. E. Edwards. 1940. Pathology of acute and of healed experimental pyelonephritis. *Arch. Pathol.* **30:**330–347.

91. Marre, R., J. Hacker, W. Henkel, and W. Goebel. 1986. Contribution of cloned virulence factors from uropathogenic *Escherichia coli* strains to nephropathogenicity in an experimental rat pyelonephritis model. *Infect. Immun.* **54:**761–767.

92. Massad, G., C. V. Lockatell, D. E. Johnson, and H. L. T. Mobley. 1994. *Proteus mirabilis* fimbriae: construction of an isogenic *pmfA* mutant and analysis of virulence in a CBA mouse model of ascending urinary tract infection. *Infect. Immun.* **62:**536–542.

93. Mattsby-Baltzer I., L. A. Hanson, B. Kaijser, P. Larsson, S. Olling, and C. Svanborg-Eden. 1982. Experimental *Escherichia coli* ascending pyelonephritis in rats: changes in bacterial properties and the immune response of surface antigens. *Infect. Immun.* **35:**639–646.

94. Mattsby-Baltzer, I., L. A. Hanson, S. Olling, and B. Kaijser. 1982. Experimental *Escherichia coli* ascending pyelonephritis in rats: active peroral immunization with live *Escherichia coli*. *Infect. Immun.* **35:**647–653.

95. McLaughlin, J. C., and G. L. Domingue. 1974. The immunologic role of the ethanol-soluble enterobacterial common antigen versus experimental renal infection. *Immunol. Commun.* **3:**51–75.

96. Meylan, P. R., G. Braoudakis, and M. P. Glauser. 1986. Influence of inflammation on the efficacy of antibiotic treatment of experimental pyelonephritis. *Antimicrob. Agents Chemother.* **29:**760–764.

97. Michaels, E. K., J. S. Chimel, B. J. Plotkin, and A. J. Schaffer. 1983. Effect of D-mannose and D-glucose on *Escherichia coli* bacteriuria in rats. *Urol. Res.* **11:**97–102.

98. Miller, T. E., and K. B. Robinson. 1973. Experimental pyelonephritis: a new method for inducing pyelonephritis in the rat. *J. Infect. Dis.* **127:**307–310.

99. Mobley, H. L. T., D. M. Green, A. L. Trifillis, D. E. Johnson, G. R. Chippendale, C. V. Lockatell, B. D. Jones, and J. W. Warren. 1990. Pyelonephritogenic *Escherichia coli* and killing of cultured human renal proximal tubular epithelial cells: role of hemolysin in some strains. *Infect. Immun.* **58:**1281–1289.

100. Mobley, H. L. T., K. G. Jarvis, J. P. Elwood, D. I. Whittle, C. V. Lockatell, R. G. Russell, D. E. Johnson, M. S. Donnenberg, and J. W. Warren. 1993. Isogenic P-fimbrial deletion mutants of pyelonephritogenic *Escherichia coli:* the role of $\alpha$Gal (1-4) $\beta$Gal binding in virulence of a wild-type strain. *Mol. Microbiol.* **10:**143–155.

101. Montgomerie, J. Z., S. Turkel, G. M. Kalmanson, and L. B. Guze. 1980. *E. coli* adherence to bladder epithelial cells of mice. *Urol. Res.* **8:**163–165.

102. Musher, D. M., D. P. Griffith, D. Yawn, and R. D. Rossen. 1975. Role of urease in pyelonephritis resulting from urinary tract infection with Proteus. *J. Infect. Dis.* **131:**177–181.

103. Neal, D. E., M. B. Kaack, G. Baskin, and J. A. Robert. 1991. Attenuation of antibody response to acute pyelonephritis by treatment with antibiotics. *Antimicrob. Agents Chemother.* **35:**2340–2344.

104. Nickel, J. C., S. K. Grant, and J. W. Costerton. 1985. Catheter-associated bacteriuria. *Urology* **26:**369–375.

105. Nickel, J. C., S. K. Grant, K. Lam, M. E. Olson, and J. W. Costerton. 1991. Bacteriologically stressed animal model of new closed catheter drainage system with microbicidal outlet tube. *Urology* **38:**280–289.

106. Nickel, J. C., M. Olson, R. J. C. McLean, S. K. Grant, and J. W. Costerton. 1987. An ecological study of infected urinary stone genesis in an animal model. *Br. J. Urol.* **59:**21–30.

107. O'Hanley, P., D. Lark, S. Falkow, and G. Schoolnik. 1985. Molecular basis of *Escherichia coli* colonization of the upper urinary tract in Balb/c mice. *J. Clin. Invest.* **75:**347–360.

108. Pazin, G. J., and A. I. Braude. 1974. Immobilizing antibodies in urine. II. Prevention of ascending spread of *Proteus mirabilis*. *Invest. Urol.* **12**:129–133.
109. Pecha, B., D. Low, and P. O'Hanley. 1989. Gal-Gal vaccines prevent pyelonephritis by piliated *Escherichia coli* in a murine model. *J. Clin. Invest.* **83**:2102–2108.
110. Prat, V., M. Hatala, and H.-J. Mohr. 1975. Bacterial renal infection in rats produced by direct injection of bacteria into renal tissue—an experimental model. *Acta Biol. Med. Ger. Band* **34**:1499–1508.
111. Prat, V., H. Losse, L. Konickoca, and W. Ritzerfeldd. 1970. Experimental ascending *Escherichia coli* pyelonephritis in the rat. *Invest. Urol.* **8**:311–317.
112. Raffel, L., P. Pitsakis, S. P. Levinson, and M. E. Levinson. 1981. Experimental *Candida albicans*, *Staphylococcus aureus*, and *Streptococcus faecalis* pyelonephritis in diabetic rats. *Infect. Immun.* **34**:773–779.
113. Reid, G., R. C. Y. Chan, A. W. Bruce, and J. W. Costerton. 1985. Prevention of urinary tract infection in rats with an indigenous *Lactobacillus casei* strain. *Infect. Immun.* **49**:320–324.
114. Roberts, J. A. 1978. Studies of vesicoureteral reflux: a review of work in a primate model. *South. Med. J.* **71**:28–30.
115. Roberts, J. A. 1992. Vesicoureteral reflux and pyelonephritis in the monkey: a review. *J. Urol.* **148**:1721–1725.
116. Roberts, J. A., J. D. Clayton, and H. R. Seibold. 1972. The natural incidence of pyelonephritis in the nonhuman primate. *Invest. Urol.* **9**:276–281.
117. Roberts, J. A., G. J. Domingue, L. N. Martin, and C. S. Kim. 1981. Immunology of pyelonephritis in the primate model: live versus heat-killed bacteria. *Kidney Int.* **19**:297–305.
118. Roberts, J. A., K. Hardaway, B. Kaack, E. N. Fussell, and G. Baskin. 1984. Prevention of pyelonephritis by immunization with P-fimbriae. *J. Urol.* **131**:602–607.
119. Roberts, J. A., M. B. Kaack, G. Baskin, and S. B. Svenson. 1993. Prevention of renal scarring from pyelonephritis in nonhuman primates by vaccination with a synthetic *Escherichia coli* serotype O8 oligosaccharide-protein conjugate. *Infect. Immun.* **61**:5214–5218.
120. Roberts, J. A., M. B. Kaack, and E. N. Fussell. 1989. Bacterial adherence in urinary tract infections: preliminary studies in a primate model. *Infection* **17**:401–404.
121. Roberts, J. A., M. B. Kaack, E. N. Fussell, and G. Baskin. 1986. Immunology of pyelonephritis. VII. Effect of allopurinol. *J. Urol.* **136**:960–963.
122. Roberts, J. A., B. Kaack, G. Kallenius, R. Mollby, J. Winberg, and S. B. Svenson. 1984. Receptors for pyelonephritogenic *Escherichia coli* in primates. *J. Urol.* **131**:163–168.
123. Roberts, J. A., J. E. Roth, G. Domingue, R. W. Lewis, B. Kaack, and G. Baskin. 1982. Immunology of pyelonephritis in the primate model. V. Effect of superoxide dismutase. *J. Urol.* **128**:1394–1400.
124. Roberts, J. A., J. K. Roth, G. Domingue, R. W. Lewis, B. Kaack, and G. Baskin. 1983. Immunology of pyelonephritis in the primate model. VI. Effect of complement depletion. *J. Urol.* **129**:193–196.
125. Roberts, J. A., G. M. Suarez, B. Kaack, G. Kallenius, and S. B. Svenson. 1985. Experimental pyelonephritis in the monkey. VII. Ascending pyelonephritis in the absence of vesicoureteral reflux. *J. Urol.* **133**:1068–1075.
126. Rocha, H. 1963. Experimental pyelonephritis. Characteristic of the infection in dogs. *Yale J. Biol. Med.* **36**:183–190.
127. Rocha, H., L. B. Guze, L. R. Freeman, and P. B. Beeson. 1958. Experimental pyelonephritis. III. The influence of localized injury in different parts of the kidney on susceptibility to bacillary infection. *Yale J. Biol. Med.* **30**:341–354.
128. Sanford, J. P., B. W. Hunter, and P. Donaldson. 1963. Localization and fate of *Escherichia coli* in hematogenous pyelonephritis. *J. Exp. Med.* **116**:285–294.
129. Satoh, M., K. Munakata, H. Takeuchi, O. Yoshida, S. Takebe, and K. Kobashi. 1991. Evaluation of effects of novel urease inhibitor, N-(pivaloyl)glycinohydroxamic acid on the formation of an infection bladder stone using a newly designed urolithiasis model in rats. *Chem. Pharm. Bull.* **39**:894–896.
130. Satoh, M., K. Munakata, H. Takeuchi, O. Yoshida, S. Takebe, and K. Kobashi. 1991. Effects of a novel urease inhibitor, N-(diaminophosphinyl)isopentinoylamide on the infection stone in rats. *Chem. Pharm. Bull.* **39**:897–899.
131. Schaeffer, A. J., W. R. Schwan, S. J. Hultgren, and J. L. Duncan. 1987. Relationship of type 1 pilus expression in *Escherichia coli* to ascending urinary tract infection in mice. *Infect. Immun.* **55**:373–380.
132. Schmidt, B. J., A. O. Ramos, D. Monteiro, and L. R. Trabulsi. 1967. Experimental pyelonephritis and bacteriuria,

pyuria and renal injury. *J. Pediatr.* **70:** 281–284.

133. **Schmidt, M. A., P. O'Hanley, D. Lark, and G. K. Schoolnik.** 1988. Synthetic peptides corresponding to protective epitopes of *Escherichia coli* digalactoside-binding pilin prevent infection in a murine pyelonephritis model. *Proc. Natl. Acad. Sci. USA* **85:** 1247–1251.

134. **Schoonees, R., E. Neter, and G. P. Murphy.** 1972. Experimental pyelonephritis in primates. *J. Med.* **3:**363–372.

135. **Shapiro, A. P., A. I. Braude, and J. Siemienski.** 1959. Hematogenous pyelonephritis in rats. IV. Relationship of bacterial species to the pathogenesis and sequelae of chronic pyelonephritis. *J. Clin. Invest.* **38:** 1228–1240.

136. **Sherrington, C. S.** 1893. Experiments on the escape of bacteria with the secretions. *J. Pathol. Bacteriol.* **1:**258–278.

137. **Silverblatt, F. J.** 1974. Host-parasite interaction in the rat renal pelvis. A possible role for pili in the pathogenesis of pyelonephritis. *J. Exp. Med.* **140:**1696–1711.

138. **Silverblatt, F. J., and L. S. Cohen.** 1979. Anti-pili antibody affords protection against experimental ascending pyelonephritis. *J. Clin. Invest.* **64:**333–336.

139. **Silverblatt, F. J., and I. Ofek.** 1978. Influence of pili on the virulence of *Proteus mirabilis* in experimental hematogenous pyelonephritis. *J. Infect. Dis.* **138:**664–667.

140. **Smith, J. W., and B. Kaijser.** 1976. The local immune response to *Escherichia coli* O and K antigen in experimental pyelonephritis. *J. Clin. Invest.* **58:**276–281.

141. **Sobel, J. D., and Y. Vardi.** 1982. Scanning electron microscopy study of *P. aeruginosa in vivo* adherence to rat bladder epithelium. *J. Urol.* **128:**414–417.

142. **Sommer, J. L.** 1961. Experimental pyelonephritis in the rat with observations on ureteral reflux. *J. Urol.* **86:**375–381.

143. **Sommer, J. L., and J. A. Roberts.** 1966. Ureteral reflux resulting from chronic urinary infection in dogs: long-term studies. *J. Urol.* **95:**502–510.

144. **Soriano, F., C. Ponte, M. Santamaria, C. Castilla, and R. F. Robelas.** 1986. In vitro and in vivo study of stone formation by *Corynebacterium* group D2 (*Corynebacterium urealyticum*). *J. Clin. Microbiol.* **23:**691–694.

145. **Spitznagel, J. K., and H. A. Schroeder.** 1951. Experimental pyelonephritis and hypertension in rats. *Proc. Soc. Exp. Biol. Med.* **77:**762–764.

146. **Stotter, L., L. S. Fischer, M. Stock, I. Braveny, U. Hagele, G. Grunberg, and H. P. Schulze.** 1975. A new method for producing a chronic *E. coli* pyelonephritis in rabbits. *Nephron* **15:**444–455.

147. **Svanborg-Eden C., L. Hagberg, R. Hull, S. Hull, K. E. Magnusson, and L. Ohman.** 1987. Bacterial virulence versus host resistance in the urinary tracts of mice. *Infect. Immun.* **55:**1224–1232.

148. **Uehling, D. T., and L. Wolf.** 1969. Enhancement of the bladder defense mechanism by immunization. *Invest. Urol.* **6:** 520–526.

149. **Vardi, Y., T. Meshulam, N. Obedeanu, D. Marzbach, and J. D. Sobel.** 1983. In vivo adherence of *P. aeruginosa* to rat bladder epithelium. *Proc. Soc. Exp. Biol. Med.* **172:** 449–456.

150. **Vermeulen, C. W., and R. Goetz.** 1954. Experimental urolithiasis. VII. Role of sex and genetic strain in determining chemical composition of stones in rats. *J. Urol.* **72:** 93–98.

151. **Vermeulen, C. W., and R. Goetz.** 1954. Experimental urolithiasis. VIII. Furadantin in treatment of experimental *Proteus* infection with stone formation. *J. Urol.* **72:** 99–104.

152. **Vivaldi, E., R. Cotran, D. P. Zangwill, and E. H. Kass.** 1959. Ascending infection as a mechanism in pathogenesis of experimental non-obstructive pyelonephritis. *Proc. Soc. Exp. Biol. Med.* **102:**242–244.

153. **Wilens, S. L., and E. E. Sproul.** 1938. Spontaneous cardiovascular disease in the rat. II. Lesions of the vascular system. *Am. J. Pathol.* **14:**201.

# PROSPECTS FOR URINARY TRACT INFECTION VACCINES

*Peter O'Hanley, M.D., Ph.D.*

# 15

From a scientific perspective, the prospects are excellent that a number of promising defined vaccines for the prevention of ascending bacterial urinary tract infections could now be assessed in human clinical trials. There are convincing data to justify testing of P pili and/or their PapA serotypes plus denatured alpha-hemolysin for the prevention of pyelonephritis caused by *Escherichia coli* strains in children and women with normal urinary tract anatomy. This enthusiastic assessment is based on a number of factors that are relevant for testing any worthwhile vaccine strategy in humans. These are (i) knowledge of the epidemiology, of pathogenesis at a molecular level, of distribution and diversity of microbial virulence factors, and of host immune responses in the natural course of disease, (ii) demonstration of the safety and immunogenicity of the prototype vaccinal reagents in laboratory animals, (iii) confirmation of the efficacy of the vaccinal reagents in preventing disease in relevant animal models, and (iv) existence of practical means to produce prototype vaccines. It is remarkable that these conditions have been fulfilled only within the last decade. A primary reason for this accomplishment could be attributed to the approach of characterizing the pathogenesis of bacterial infections at the molecular level. This provided for the identification of a number of microbial virulence factors, which provide bacteria the ability to cause disease. The practical benefit of these investigations is that they have provided the opportunity to develop specific anti-virulence factor vaccines to prevent infection. Although complex vaccines (e.g., heat-killed or chemically treated, killed bacteria) might eventually prove to be efficacious, the prevailing opinion in vaccinology is that these vaccines elicit unacceptable adverse reactions and many untoward or nonprotective immune responses. Table 1 provides a summary of potential anti-urovirulence factor interventions based on our current understanding of the pathogenesis of ascending bacterial urinary tract infections.

It remains uncertain whether this basic knowledge and technology will ever be used for any practical clinical interven-

*Peter O'Hanley,* Homeless Veterans Rehabilitation Program, Medicine Service, Palo Alto Veterans Affairs Medical Center, Palo Alto, California 94306, and Department of Medicine, Division of Infectious Diseases and Geographic Medicine, and Department of Microbiology and Immunology, Stanford University School of Medicine, Stanford, California 94305.

**TABLE 1** Proposed anti-urovirulence factors vaccines for the prevention of bacterial urinary tract infections: anticipated interference with uropathogenic steps

| Pathogenic step | Urovirulence factor | Comments |
| --- | --- | --- |
| Adherence | Pili<br>Afimbrial adhesins | P pili vaccines are efficacious against *E. coli* renal infections by preventing bacteria-to-host epithelial attachment. |
| Colonization/ proliferation | Aerobactin<br>Outer membrane proteins | Outer membrane protein vaccine is efficacious against *P. mirabilis* infection; these vaccines should interfere with microbial iron acquisition for most gram-negative uropathogens. |
| Cellular injury | Alpha-hemolysin<br>Lipopolysaccharide | Anti-hemolysin vaccines diminish tissue injury and decrease mortality but not infection; anti-LPS vaccines do not prevent infection but might decrease renal inflammation. |
| Cellular invasion | Cytotoxic necrotizing factors | No experimental vaccines have been developed. |
| Dissemination | Serum resistance<br>IgA protease<br>Capsular polysaccharide | Anti-K vaccines prevent both infection and tissue injury; no IgA protease or serum-resistant specific vaccines have been developed. |

tions. There are currently no licensed vaccines in the United States marketplace for any type of urinary tract infection, although there are two complex urinary tract vaccines available in Europe (SolcoUrovac and Uro-Vaxom). There are justifiable reasons why these vaccines have not been approved by the U.S. Food and Drug Administration: there have been no rigorous clinical trials to assess their efficacy and preliminary clinical data suggest that they are not sufficiently efficacious to justify their usage. There is currently only one ongoing phase I/II clinical trial in the United States that is evaluating P pili vaccines for the prevention of pyelonephritis in young women (i.e., at Stanford University under my direction and supported by North American Vaccine, Inc., Beltsville, Md.). There are no imminent plans by investigators in academia or industry in the United States or elsewhere to test any other potentially efficacious vaccines (either complex or comprised of a defined urovirulence factor[s]) in the prevention of urinary tract infections. The reality is that potentially worthwhile immunoprophylactic vaccines for urinary tract infections, as well as other non-life-threatening infectious diseases, will probably not even be tested in humans after appropriate basic science knowledge has been acquired. This situation will not change until the pharmaceutical industry, physicians, and the general public recognize that, from both health and cost-effectiveness standpoints, it is better to prevent infections than to treat them.

There is a sense of complacency with regard to the current management of urinary tract infections. It is assumed that the present paradigm of management strategies, which are designed for specific groups of patients (e.g., those with uncomplicated cystitis, uncomplicated acute pyelonephritis, and recurrent cystitis and pyelonephritis), provides maximal therapeutic benefits in a cost-effective and safe fashion (71). The most common therapeutic intervention for urinary tract infections is currently the use of antibiotics. It provides pharmaceutical companies with significant fiscal benefits, accounting for more than two billion dollars in drug purchases annually. Pharmaceutical companies thus have no obvious incentive to develop prophylactic vaccines for urinary tract infections. In addition, the cost and liability of conducting vaccine trials are not trivial for the pharmaceutical industry to absorb, especially if the vaccine under development or testing proves to have no therapeutic value. It is not unusual for vaccine efficacy trials in the United States to cost two million dollars or more. This amount of money usually represents less than 5% of all costs associated with pre-licensure expenses for a subsequently approved vaccine. Unfortunately, these fiscal realities establish barriers to the development of a more-comprehensive strategy to manage urinary tract infections. However, the use of antibiotics in the treatment of bacterial urinary tract infections and for chemoprophylactic purposes is not without untoward consequences. It allows for extensive antibiotic usage, which selects for more-resistant microorganisms which will eventually cause even more serious health care consequences. In addition, antibiotic usage is not without adverse effects for the individual patient and can be associated with secondary infections, toxicity, and symptomatic complaints. The failure of physicians and the public to encourage development of preventive medical measures contributes to the lack of progress in developing a comprehensive plan to manage a number of common illnesses, including the majority of ascending bacterial urinary tract infections.

The purpose of this chapter is to provide a review of attempts to develop vaccines for the prevention of ascending bacterial urinary tract infections. The previous chapters, concerning the epidemiology of urinary tract infections and the genetics, structure, and function of urovirulence factors, provide the scientific foundation for development of vaccines for bacterial ascending urinary tract infections. It will not be necessary, therefore, to repeat this information in detail, but merely to highlight certain aspects of this information in order to identify the logic of vaccine strategies. The major focuses of the chapter are to provide insights regarding the need for vaccines against ascending urinary tract infections for specific patient populations, to review the data of potentially efficacious experimental vaccines, and to suggest future directions for vaccine research for the prevention of bacterial ascending urinary tract infections.

## SHOULD BACTERIAL URINARY TRACT INFECTION VACCINES BE DEVELOPED?

Decreased morbidity, prevention of renal scarring, and cost-effective interventions are compelling reasons to develop bacterial urinary tract vaccines to prevent ascending tract infections. It is well recognized that individuals at high risk for symptomatic urinary tract infection include neonates, preschool girls, sexually active women of childbearing age, and elderly women and men. It is, however, important to mention the expected major limitations to developing certain urinary tract vaccines. On the basis of our current understanding of the epidemiology of urinary tract infections and the distribution of urovirulence factors in specific syndromes, it is currently not feasible to develop broadly cross-reactive urovirulence factor vaccines to prevent all types of infections for every patient population. For example, acknowledged urovirulence factors (e.g., P pili, alpha-hemolysin, aerobactin, and $K_1$) are of less importance in *E. coli* urinary tract infections in compromised hosts (see review in reference 24). Table 2 further illustrates this issue by summarizing the distribution of urovirulence factors from specific patient populations. It can be readily appreciated that certain urinary tract syndromes are more likely to be caused by similar or homologous strains, whereas the strains differ in other syndromes (24). It is also not anticipated that vaccines will be developed

**TABLE 2** Accumulative relative frequency of urovirulence factor expression in a variety of *E. coli* urinary tract infections in adult populations and normal feces based on published literature

| Patient group | % of strains with the following attribute: | | | | |
| --- | --- | --- | --- | --- | --- |
| | P pili | Hemolysin | Aerobactin | $K_1$ | Common O serogroup[a] |
| Females, uncomplicated pyelonephritis | 82 | 70 | 73 | 32 | >70 |
| Females, complicated pyelonephritis | 45 | 40 | ND[b] | ND | <30 |
| Males, uncomplicated pyelonephritis | 50 | 70 | 50 | 14 | >80 |
| Females, uncomplicated cystitis | 35 | 40 | 50 | 24 | 60 |
| Normal stool | 20 | 12 | 40 | 23 | <35 |

[a] Common O serogroups: O2, O4, O6, O7, O15, O18, O23, O25, O50, and O75.
[b] ND, not determined.

against every possible bacterial uropathogen, since essentially any strain could cause disease under appropriate compromised conditions. However, the remarkably narrow spectrum of etiologic agents responsible for bacterial urinary tract infections in otherwise healthy, noncompromised hosts facilitates the development of a feasible number of vaccines. *E. coli* strains are responsible for 80% of urinary tract infections in otherwise healthy individuals with normal urinary tract anatomy, *Staphylococcus saprophyticus* is responsible for 5 to 15 percent, and other gram-negative enteric bacteria, like *Proteus* and *Klebsiella* species, comprise the balance (27). With the exception of rare cases of *E. coli* pyelonephritis in young children, only the renal infections due to *Proteus* species, *Klebsiella* species, and other rare gram-negative enteric strains are associated with serious sequelae. In contrast, compromised hosts, including those who are catheterized or recently instrumented, are infected by a greater variety of bacterial pathogens and usually suffer more serious sequelae (71, 83). Therefore, the development of efficacious vaccines for urinary tract infections in individuals who have a functionally, metabolically, or anatomically abnormal urinary tract, including patients who are catheterized or instrumented, does not appear to be readily feasible. It seems most prudent to first develop *E. coli* urinary tract infection vaccines for otherwise healthy individuals, since they could effect the greater public health benefit.

The morbidity of lower or upper urinary tract infections is not trivial in otherwise healthy individuals. Patients with cystitis complain of symptoms for an average of 6.2 days which regularly confines them to bed for an average of 0.4 days and restricts activity for 1.2 days, irrespective of medicine usage (11). In addition to the pain associated with infection, compromises in work productivity, possible loss of salary or reliance on sick leave, and hassles associated with seeking medical care and following therapeutic regimens constitute significant injury and pain to the afflicted individual. In general, urinary tract infections are not life-threatening and do not lead to sequelae except under certain conditions. The major exception is bacterial pyelonephritis. It is the most common cause of bacteremia and sepsis (15 to 30% of all episodes) (53). It is also an important cause of death in high-risk groups (e.g., noncompromised elderly individuals [i.e., greater than 60 years of age]) (60). It should also be noted that certain bacterial species (*Proteus* species, *Klebsiella pneumoniae,* and *Pseudomonas* species) that cause pyelonephritis portend a greater risk for death than most *E. coli* strains (12).

Another major cause of morbidity associated with urinary tract infection involves a subset of women who have recurrent *E. coli* infections. Although the majority of otherwise healthy women experience only one symptomatic episode of urinary tract infection in their life span, 20% of such women suffer three or more reoccurrences of bladder and/or kidney infections per annum. The repetitive nature of these infections causes significant hardship on the afflicted women. The increased susceptibility among these urinary tract infection-prone women cannot be explained by underlying immunological defects. It may be due to fewer soluble receptor compounds, a factor which is associated with bacterial adherence, in their secretions. These individuals are identified as nonsecretors (4). The risk for recurrent *E. coli* urinary tract infection is higher in these women because they have increased susceptibility to vaginal colonization with uropathogenic strains. This risk is linked to a nonsecretor status (Lewis blood group [Le $(a^+b^-)$] and recessive [Le $(a^-b^-)$] phenotypes) (69). At a molecular level, the presence of sialosyl gal-globoside (SGG) and disialosyl gal-globoside (DSGG) on urogenital epithelial cells provides exposed binding sites for P-piliated uropathogenic *E. coli* strains (72). This may account for the increased susceptibility of nonsecretors to recurrent urinary tract infections. In contrast, these globo-series glycosphingolipids are fucosylated and processed to ABH antigens in secretors. These substances are rich in secretions and bathe epithelial surfaces of secretors, thereby diminishing binding sites for uropathogenic P-piliated *E. coli* strains. Also, if transmission of nonsecretor status were understood at a genetic level, this would facilitate screening for this risk factor for recurrent *E. coli* urinary tract infections.

The majority of symptomatic bacterial urinary tract infections are associated with uncomplicated bladder infections and are without any sequelae; however, approximately 10% of these infections clearly involve the kidney. It should also be noted that a high proportion of symptomatic patients with apparent localized acute cystitis have subclinical pyelonephritis (71). The frequency of this phenomenon varies from 8 to 80% (average 30%), depending upon the population studied and the localization technique employed to diagnose renal infection (27). The major therapeutic goal in all patients with urinary tract infections is to prevent renal damage, since renal scarring as a consequence of the bacterial infection may lead to progressive chronic renal failure similar to glomerulonephritis. The urovirulence factors of bacteria that are responsible for renal damage have yet to be identified, although strains that produce urease (e.g., a small percentage of uropathogenic *E. coli* strains, all *Proteus* species and *Pseudomonas* species, and a majority of *Klebsiella* species) are most likely to cause renal scarring even after a single episode of infection. There are individual host parameters which have been identified as being associated with the development of renal scarring: very young and old age, female gender, the presence of gross anomalies of the urinary tract (e.g., vesicoureteral reflux), previous kidney infections, an extended period of time elapsing until diagnosis and subsequent treatment, and unsuccessful antimicrobial therapy (36). Among these risk factors, it has been clearly demonstrated that renal infection in young children constitutes a high risk for renal sequelae. This is because the kidney appears to be more vulnerable to the damaging effects of bacterial infection during the first 3 years of life (2). In a study of 30 adults who had their first infection during infancy, hypertension was documented in one-third and end-stage renal disease was seen in 10%. Of the 27 without end-stage renal disease, renal function, measured in several ways, was on average significantly less than the control (21). Chronic pyelonephritis has been reported as the cause in 15 to 25% of children coming to end-stage renal disease, irrespective of the presence or grade of vesicoureteral reflux (29). It is presumed that renal failure occurs in this patient group if there is sufficient injury to one kidney in childhood that the remnant kidney cannot maintain the increased need for renal function occurring during adolescence. This results in glomerular hyperinfiltration and hypertension of the remaining nephrons (5), which in turn leads to progressive destruction of the remaining nephrons, with focal glomerulosclerosis and further tubulointerstitial disease (55).

The sheer number of urinary tract infections justifies attempts to develop efficacious vaccines, from a cost-effectiveness perspective alone. Bacterial urinary tract infections are one of the most common infections affecting humans, especially among otherwise healthy young women of childbearing age. The incidence of bacterial urinary tract infection correlates directly with age: 1% in neonates and 30% for those over 60 years of age. It is estimated that 12% of men and up to 40% of women experience a symptomatic urinary tract infection during their life span (10, 39). Each year, 5% of visits for primary care in the United States are prompted by symptoms suggestive of bacteriuria (80). It is also estimated that there are more than 8 million episodes of urinary tract infection annually in the United States, with the majority involving the bladder. Furthermore, there are more than 1.5 million hospital discharges that record urinary tract infection as the reason for admission. Among these infections, pyelonephritis accounts for more than 125,000 cases per annum. In addition, urinary tract infections are the most common cause of bacterial nosocomial infections. They account for significant morbidity and mortality and account for considerable financial outlays because of the need for extended hospital stays and additional diagnostic studies and more expensive therapy. There have been no definitive studies to estimate the direct costs for management of urinary tract infections in the United States. It is, however, reasonable to presume that the overall cost for the physician visit, diagnostic tests, and antimicrobial treatment associated with management of urinary tract infections exceeds 8 billion dollars annually in the United States. The costs associated with management of patients who have renal insufficiency or failure as a consequence of previous bacterial infections have also not been systematically determined. However, the costs of physician visits, diagnostic studies, and dialysis are exorbitant. If safe and inexpensive efficacious vaccines could be developed for the prevention of renal infections in particular, this would be a worthwhile preventive modality in the management of urinary tract infections and one that would provide considerable cost-effectiveness.

## RECOMMENDATIONS FOR URINARY TRACT INFECTION VACCINE STRATEGIES

Rational guidelines for the development of efficacious bacterial urinary tract infection vaccines should consider the following factors. (i) Vaccines against uropathogenic *E. coli* strains are considered to be most in need of development, since these bacteria are the etiologic agents in 80% of urinary tract infections in otherwise healthy individuals. (ii) Vaccines for *E. coli* urinary tract infections would be desirable for the following syndromes or patient groups: pyelonephritis in children less than 3 years of age (to decrease the risk of associated renal failure after infection), cystitis and pyelonephritis in young, otherwise healthy women (to reduce the burden on the health care budget), recurrent urinary tract infection among women of a nonsecretor status (to decrease their morbidity and the high costs for care), and pyelonephritis in adults greater than 60 years of age (to decrease their risks of bacteremia and sepsis). (iii) Although *Proteus, Klebsiella,* and *Pseudomonas* species are not a predominant cause of urinary tract infections, vaccines against these species are justified because these uropathogens can cause significant renal damage after a single episode of infection and are associated with greater mortality than *E. coli* strains that cause pyelonephritis.

## IMMUNOLOGICAL ASPECTS RELEVANT TO URINARY TRACT INFECTION VACCINE DEVELOPMENT

Although there are many reports characterizing immune responses after bacterial urinary tract infections, our knowledge remains limited. Immune responses which occur during and after a urinary tract infection are important because they may contribute to resolution of the infection and because naturally occurring protective immune responses are potentially amenable to boosting by immunization. There have been no systematic efforts to evaluate the role of T-cell immunity in bacterial ascending urinary tract infections. It is not anticipated that they would provide significant protection against the invading bacterial uropathogen, although sensitized T cells are critical for the host to elaborate specific antibody responses to microbial determinants of a protein nature. Systemic and local antibody responses to uropathogenic *E. coli* strains have been fairly well characterized in humans (17, 74); however, the antibody responses to other uropathogenic bacteria have not been characterized to any extensive degree. The protective value of these antibody responses remains to be established, although they are considered to be pivotal for protection of the urinary tract against infection (19). Conversely, patients with recurrent urinary tract infections have low levels of urinary and cervicovaginal antibodies (9, 70).

Evaluating antibody responses after infection by uropathogenic bacteria has a number of useful purposes. The production of antibody to specific antigens suggests that they might have a role in uropathogenesis. The presence of circulating or local specific antibody could conceivably prevent clinically apparent urinary tract infection, whereas the presence of specific antibody at the time of infection suggests a lack of relevance of a particular antigen in protection. It is apparent then that analysis of antibody responses can be useful in designing rational vaccines against bacterial ascending urinary tract infection. It would be worthwhile if such studies were prospectively performed so that a protective immunological phenotype could be characterized. It would be best to screen local urinary antibodies, since it is well recognized that circulating antibodies do not correlate with protection (79). To date, no such studies have been conducted.

In general, serum and local antibody titers against the infecting organism are higher after upper urinary tract infection than when the infection is limited to the bladder (82). For example, 90% of the patients with upper urinary tract infection develop a diagnostic change in titer, whereas this occurs only 5% of the time after cystitis (51). Under normal conditions, the kidney is not a significant site of immunoglobulin synthesis. In contrast, a significant immune response is engendered in the pyelonephritic kidney. The predominant specific immunoglobulin is the immunoglobulin G (IgG) class, although specific IgA synthesis also occurs to a minor extent in the pyelonephritic kidney (38). After *E. coli* pyelonephritis, antibody is formed to the O antigen of the infecting strain (62). Antibodies to K antigens, outer membrane proteins, flagella, alpha-hemolysin, and pili are also detectable in the serum. Because of the apparent critical importance of P pili in the pathogenesis of *E. coli* urinary tract infections, the serological responses to this determinant have been more extensively studied than others. In a number of studies, specific antibodies to P pili have been detected in the serum following pyelonephritis (8, 64, 75). There are no published reports indicating that specific antibodies to P pili have been detected in serum following acute cystitis; however, we have found serum antibodies of the IgG class specific against P pili serotypes that are expressed by the causative strain in 4 of 10 female patients with acute cystitis (44). It is interesting that there are no published reports in which specific antibodies to P pili have been detected in the urine following either pyelonephritis or cystitis due to uropathogenic *E. coli* strains. This finding should be further explored. The possibility remains that individuals might not be protected against uropathogenic *E. coli* strains because antibody to the major microbial determinant responsible for uroepithelial adherence is not present in the urine. Vaccine strategies might therefore be efficacious if they elicited sufficient immunity that anti-P antibodies are translocated into the urine and vaginal secretions.

## STATUS OF COMPLEX URINARY TRACT INFECTION VACCINES

There are two complex vaccines available in Europe which are used primarily for the prevention of recurrent urinary tract infections: SolcoUrovac and Uro-Vaxom. These vaccines have not been rigorously assessed in clinical trials for safety, immunogenicity, or efficacy. The U.S. Food and Drug Administration has not licensed these vaccines because of these obvious deficiencies. It is prudent that these vaccines should not be used indiscriminately by the public until they are more carefully scrutinized. Specific information about each of these preparations is provided below for the sake of providing complete details about recent attempts to prevent bacterial urinary tract infections by immunization of humans. Unfortunately, there is limited evidence to suggest that these vaccines are efficacious.

### SolcoUrovac

SolcoUrovac (Solco Basle, Ltd., Basel, Switzerland) is a whole-cell urinary tract vaccine containing heat-killed bacteria from 10 different human uropathogenic isolates: *Proteus mirabilis*, *Morganella morganii*, *Streptococcus faecalis*, *K. pneumoniae*, and 6 different *E. coli* strains (61). Unfortunately, there has been no systematic assessment of the presence of antigens remaining after heat treatment nor has there been characterization of elicited specific antibody responses after immunization. It is anticipated that the major antigens present in sufficient amounts to elicit an immune response after heat treatment would be lipopolysaccharide moieties. If this is the case, this vaccine preparation may not elicit protective immunity, as the data that anti-O antibodies are protective in animal models of UTI is conflicting (31, 33, 46, 56).

SolcoUrovac usage has been generally confined to Europe, where it is administered intramuscularly and orally in attempts to decrease recurrent urinary tract infections. Preliminary studies indicated that after intramuscular injection with SolcoUrovac, there was a decrease in the relapse rate among women with a history of symptomatic recurrent urinary tract infections: 28 infections occurred in 23 vaccinated women, whereas 84 infections occurred in 47 nonimmunized women (13). This apparent protection was short lived (<6 months after immunization). It was, however, impossible to appreciate whether the vaccine stimulated any specific immunological responses, since only total immunoglobulin levels in clinical specimens were measured. The detectable increases in total IgG and secretory IgA levels in urine and serum (61) could be explained by the nonspecific immunostimulatory effects of interleukin-6, which was provoked by administering the lipopolysaccharide-rich mixture contained in the vaccine. In the absence of any detectable specific antibody to the vaccinal strains, it seems improbable that this vaccine would have any efficacy in the prevention of ascending urinary tract infections.

A phase I trial that evaluated the safety and immunogenicity of SolcoUrovac instilled into the vagina has recently been completed in the United States by Uehling and colleagues (77). The rationale for vaginal instillation is that this mode of administration has been associated with increasing antibodies in vaginal secretions. Theoretically, increased antibodies in vaginal secretions might interfere with the colonization of potential uropathogenic bacteria at this site and their effective translocation to periurethral tissues or the urethra. In addition, vaginal instillation of this vaccine does elicit systemic immune effects. Confirmation of an elicited systemic immune effect has been established by identifying splenic antibody-forming cells against the vaccinal strains in laboratory animals administered this vaccine via a vaginal route. However, this systemic antibody response is approximately one-half that produced by parenteral immunization in experimental animals (78). In the recent phase I trial, 25 women who were 45 to 71 years of age and had recurrent urinary tract infections (two or more symptomatic urinary tract infections in the previous year) were enrolled. Five women were administered via vaginal instillation one dose of $2 \times 10^9$ bacteria in a 1-ml stock solution, with individual strains having a concentration of approximately $2 \times 10^8$ each. None of these women had evidence of local irritation or systemic complaints after vaccine instillation. Therefore, 20 women received a total of three weekly doses of the stock vaccine, and total IgG and secretory IgA antibody levels were measured in the vaginal secretions, urine, and sera of these women. Data indicate that only total vaginal and urinary IgG and IgA levels increased significantly by day 80 after the first immunization; they then returned to pretreatment levels. There were no attempts to detect specific IgG or IgA to any of the *E. coli* strains or 2 of the 4 non-*E. coli* strains in the clinical specimens. Subjective reports of 9 of the 20 women who received three doses of the vaccine suggested that the vaccine decreased bladder irritative symptoms. Further study is required to assess whether this complex vaccine has immunoprophylactic benefit.

**Uro-Vaxom**

Uro-Vaxom (OM Laboratories, Meyrin, Geneva, Switzerland) is comprised of a lyophilized proteinaceous mixture obtained by fractionating the alkaline hydrolysate of selected *E. coli* strains. These fractions consist essentially of membrane proteins (glycolipoproteins). Electrophoretic analysis shows a mixture of polypeptides of medium to high molecular mass (approximately 10 to 700 kDa) and an acidic nature (isoelectric point of 4). The concentration in endotoxin is less than 0.1 $\mu$g/mg. Quality controls include biochemical standardization of the glycolipoprotein content and immunobiological efficacy (i.e., standardization of metabolic activation of macrophages and plaque-forming cells). The extract is administered orally in a 6-mg capsule on a daily basis.

A limited number of clinical trials have been conducted in Europe to evaluate the safety and efficacy of Uro-Vaxom in preventing recurrent urinary tract infections (14, 68, 76). Each of these trials involved a double-blind, placebo-controlled, crossover design, although there were other important methodological problems with these studies. In general, despite daily administration of the "immunotherapeutic agent" for 3 months, side effects were few (<5%) among the 356 recipients. These complaints were of a minor nature: pruritus, diarrhea, nausea, vertigo, headache with flushing, and a bad taste in the mouth. In each of the three trials, involving 70 paraplegics and 286 patients from two different groups of males and females with recurrent urinary tract infections, there was a reported significant decrease in the degree of bacteriuria, decreased incidence of symptomatic recurrent infection, and a lesser requirement for antibiotics after 3 months of continuous Uro-Vaxom administration. These studies were flawed by the lack of uniform concomitant antibiotic usage among study subjects, making it difficult to interpret results. In addition, the immunotherapeutic effects were short lived among all recipients (e.g., <5 months after taking daily doses of the *E. coli* lysate for 3 months). The characteristics of the study participants, microbiological data of the urinary tract infections encountered by the study subjects, and immunological characterizations were not provided by these studies. Overall, the methodological design and absence of clinically relevant data in these studies make it difficult to assess this product.

## DEVELOPMENT OF EXPERIMENTAL ANTI-UROVIRULENCE FACTOR URINARY TRACT INFECTION VACCINES

The ability of bacterial strains to cause urinary tract infections requires an array of virulence factors to mediate specific pathogenic steps. It is certain that the presence of a specific urovirulence factor does not absolutely correlate with virulence, irrespective of the bacterial species. Evaluation of urovirulence factors in model systems and assessment of their potential immunoprophylactic efficacy in relevant experimental animal models of human infection provide a rational basis to develop urinary tract vaccines. There have been necessarily different strategies employed to identify urovirulence factors among uropathogenic bacteria because of the nature of microbial uropathogenicity.

Uropathogenic *E. coli* strains constitute a limited number of genetically related groups or clones within the total *E. coli* population. This relationship has given rise to the "clone concept," since certain strains possess properties that uniquely enable them to colonize and invade or injure the urinary tract. Such groups can be identified by their expression of specific surface antigens (26); it is therefore not surprising that uropathogenic *E. coli* strains belong to a restricted number of O, K, and H serogroups and have a conserved carboxylesterase B pattern, unlike other *E. coli* strains. Uropathogenic *E. coli* strains express well-established urovirulence factors which include P pili, alpha-hemolysin, cytotoxic necrotizing factor, $K_1$, aerobactin, and resistance to the bactericidal action of normal human serum. This conclusion is based on the epidemiological observation that these properties are overrepresented among isolates from patients with *E. coli* urinary tract infection compared with other extraintestinal isolates and nonpathogenic fecal isolates, confirmation in animal models that these determinants directly contribute to virulence, and demonstration by assays that these determinants are responsible per se for injury or evasion of host defenses (24).

In contrast, most other uropathogenic bacterial species have not been systematically evaluated for urovirulence factors like uropathogenic *E. coli* strains. An exception is *P. mirabilis*. It appears that most *P. mirabilis* strains, whether isolated from patients with pyelonephritis or catheter-associated bacteriuria or isolated from the feces of healthy individuals, express the factors associated with virulence. These virulence factors include pili, flagella, hemolysin,

IgA protease, iron acquisition via outer membranes, ability to invade uroepithelial cells, and urease (42). Of these factors that have been evaluated in an animal model, urease is the most potent (23, 28). Studies are in progress that are evaluating the prophylactic potential of a number of *Proteus* virulence factors in the prevention of urinary tract infections (41).

There remains a need for further discovery and characterization of other as-yet-unidentified virulence properties among uropathogenic *E. coli* strains and other uropathogenic bacterial species. This will provide the basis for identifying additional potentially worthwhile vaccine candidates. To date, the following virulence factors have been screened as potentially efficacious immunoprophylactic reagents in relevant animal models of urinary tract infection: P pili, alpha-hemolysin, $K_1$ antigen for uropathogenic *E. coli,* and outer membrane proteins for *P. mirabilis*. The results and implications of these studies will be discussed after describing the importance of the most frequently utilized experimental animal models of urinary tract infection.

## Animal Models

A variety of animal models have played an important role in defining virulence factors of uropathogenic *E. coli* strains and mechanisms of host resistance and in assessing the efficacy of potential vaccine candidates. The three most commonly used include the BALB/c mouse model of unobstructive experimental pyelonephritis after bladder challenge (15) and monkey models of unobstructive bladder challenge and unobstructive ureteral challenge (54, 58). It is relevant in this discussion to mention the experimental criteria that establish these animal models as relevant to human disease, as well as the advantages and disadvantages for each model, since the challenge results in these models have been the basis for determining whether a particular vaccine or urovirulence factor vaccine is efficacious and appropriate for further testing in humans.

Characteristics of a valid animal model of human ascending urinary tract infection should include the following: (i) uroepithelial surfaces which qualitatively and quantitatively exhibit the same adhesin receptors for the invading organism as humans, (ii) natural host factors in the animal's urine equivalent to those in humans, (iii) no obstruction to urine flow or traumatic manipulation of tissue, and (iv) simulation of an ascending infection mode.

BALB/c mice and monkeys each possess and exhibit mannose and Gal-Gal pilus receptor compounds similar to those in humans on their genitourinary epithelial cells and associated stromal constituents (46, 56, 57). These receptors are crucial for genitourinary epithelial attachment and subsequent colonization by type 1 and P-piliated uropathogenic *E. coli* strains. With the exception of pigs, none of the other conventional laboratory animals express both of these pili receptor compounds within genitourinary tissues (e.g., rats, guinea pigs, cats, dogs, and rabbits do not express Gal-Gal pili receptor compounds on any of their cellular surfaces within the genitourinary tract, whereas mannose pilus receptor compounds in these animals are homologous to that observed in humans) (37). If an investigator wants to study the pathogenic role of other bacterial adhesins (e.g., Dr or S binding pili) in an animal model, it is obviously critical to demonstrate that the receptor compounds are present on relevant genitourinary cells. It would therefore be imperative to confirm the similarities in receptor compounds between the designated animal species and humans prior to initiating challenge studies.

Like all placental vertebrate animals, mice and monkeys secrete the Tamm-Horsfall protein into the urine. This highly mannosylated uroprotein does have the ability to block colonization of mannose-binding bacteria and is considered a natural human host factor for modulating bacterial colonization of the urinary tract by these microorganisms (48). The major difference between these two animal species is that the mouse secretes 5- to 20-fold-higher amounts of Tamm-Horsfall protein per milliliter of urine than monkeys. It is conceivable, therefore, that the higher urinary concentration of this substance in mice might have greater effects on subsequent colonization of the urinary tract by mannose-binding *E. coli* strains than that seen in monkeys.

Neither of these models entails obstruction to urine flow or traumatic manipulation of tissue, and each simulates an ascending mode of urinary tract infection. The subsequent histological abnormalities and experimental course of infection mimic those observed in human disease (46, 56).

From the outset, there is no question that the use of nonhuman primates as experimental models of any human infection more closely mimics the human condition than use of any other animal species. This is because of their similarity to humans in anatomy, urodynamics, pathophysiology, and immunology. However, there are also fiscal and practical problems in dealing with these animals under laboratory conditions. Costs of the purchase, quarantine requirements, special shipping needs, and boarding are high. The majority of investigators can simply not afford to pursue research involving monkeys. In addition, it is crucial that there is constant veterinary supervision and monitoring during the quarantine period to safeguard personnel from contracting serious unexpected infectious diseases from these animals. Presence of experienced veterinarians is also crucial to maintain humane standards for these animals once the quarantine period terminates and experimental procedures are undertaken with the monkeys. More sophisticated animal husbandry is required for their boarding and care, which entails considerable costs and specially trained personnel. Another issue of considerable importance involves ethical concerns about using a primate when other animals can be used.

The BALB/c mouse appears to be a reasonable substitute for the monkey in experimental urinary tract infections. The major drawback to using mice instead of monkeys is their high incidence of spontaneous reflux of urine. In the monkey, reflux is believed to be abnormal, as it is in humans (54). Although monkeys commonly have reflux in the first months of life, it gradually decreases in frequency until it resolves by 3 years of life. In mice, however, the incidence of reflux is almost universal throughout their lifespan. The consequence of reflux is a greater risk for renal infections. This risk is increased if there is high-grade reflux (i.e., reflux to the kidney with ureteral dilation). It should therefore be taken into consideration that mice are at greater risk for renal infection after bacteria are inoculated into the lower urinary tract than humans or monkeys. This concern does not represent a serious problem, especially if bladder inoculation of mice with uropathogenic bacteria does not produce acute high-grade reflux and/or renal trauma. Recent reports by Johnson and colleagues (25) and Hopkins and colleagues (20) have stressed the importance that intrabladder inoculation volumes can produce investigator-induced reflux to the kidney and occasionally renal trauma in well-hydrated mice if the inoculation volume is too large. These concerns can be minimized by utilizing dehydrated mice (e.g., mice that weigh ~10% less than their recent body weight) and inoculating the bladder after gentle pressure on the abdomen (46). Documented experimental renal infections varied between 59 and 83% among well-hydrated mice (20, 25) versus >95% among dehydrated mice (45, 46) that were challenged by equivalent doses of bacteria in intrabladder inoculations of 100 µl. The experimental renal infection rate was decreased to 20% in well-hydrated mice if the intrabladder inoculation volumes are less than 100 µl (i.e., the upper volume limit that does not produce acute reflux in 16- to 24-week-old BALB/c mice). Because of the greater variability in the rate of experimental renal infections among well-hydrated mice, especially if the bacterial inoculum is <100 µl, it is preferable to employ dehydrated mice in vaccine trials and to use challenge volumes slightly less than the upper volume limit that does not cause acute reflux for the sake of reliability. These experimental concerns about the BALB/c mouse model of unobstructive pyelonephritis do not diminish the importance of utilizing this animal species for evaluating uropathogenicity or for assessing the efficacy of prototype vaccines.

## Anti-P Pili Parenteral Vaccines

Bacterial adherence to uroepithelial cells is a prerequisite for ascending urinary tract infections. P pili are important in the pathogenesis of urinary tract infections because they mediate Gal-Gal-specific bacterial adherence to epithelial cells within the human urinary tract (56). They permit bacterial colonization of the urinary tract and allow other microbial determinants to produce injury or allow invasion of the uroepithelium and deeper tissues, thereby causing inflammation and symptoms of disease. Recent data by Roberts and colleagues suggest that the PapG tip adhesin of P pili is essential in the pathogenesis of human kidney infection, on the basis of the use of genetically well-defined strains in the experimental monkey model (58). Most investigators would agree that vaccines comprised exclusively of PapG peptides should be effective in the immunoprophylaxis against P-piliated urinary tract infections;

however, there is no proof that they work. In addition, practical issues of poor immunogenicity of the PapG moiety and the lack of PapG purification protocols have not been addressed. In contrast, there are convincing data that whole P pili are highly immunogenic and protective in both the BALB/c mouse model of unobstructive experimental pyelonephritis and the monkey model of experimental pyelonephritis after intrabladder or intraureteral administration challenge (45, 46, 49, 56).

Parenteral immunization with both homologous and heterologous purified P pili protected against experimental pyelonephritis after either bladder (mouse) (45, 46, 49) or intraureteral (monkey) (56) inoculation. Among murine parenteral P pili vaccine recipients, protection against subsequent bacterial urinary tract colonization and renal infection by the challenge strains correlated with a primary PapA urine IgG titer of ≥20 (49) and/or a PapA serum IgG titer of ≥100 (46, 49). It is interesting to note that protection correlated with the presence of specific IgG antibodies in the urine and serum that bind to the major pilin structural polypeptide (PapA) and not to the Gal-Gal tip adhesin (PapG) per se. This result is compatible with the finding that the specific antibody in these clinical specimens does not prevent Gal-Gal agglutination of the challenge strains to their receptor moiety under in vitro conditions. The basis of immunological protection among pili recipients has not been addressed in this model. We speculate that the benefit of specific pili antibodies is antibody selection for nonpiliated variants that are unable to adhere to uromucosal cells, thereby facilitating rapid clearance of uropathogenic *E. coli* strains from the urinary tract. Protection against experimental pyelonephritis in monkeys immunized with enriched P pili endotoxin-contaminated preparations correlated with anti-P pili titers of >20,000 and did not correlate with anti-O titers to the homologous and heterologous challenge strains (56). These results support the concept that immunization with a bacterial surface coat constituent can prevent mucosal infection by interfering with colonization.

Synthetic PapA pilin vaccines have further established the protective capacity of anti-PapA serum IgG antibodies (66). This strategy is particularly worthwhile on theoretical grounds since nonimmunogenic epitopes within the native molecule can be selected. This will avoid antibody pressure that might eventually select for antigenic variants. On the basis of the immunochemistry of a prototype PapA F13 serotype (67) (Fig. 1), peptides were synthesized that corresponded to highly conserved and variable linear regions and linear immunogenic and antigenic epitopes. Parenteral immunization of mice with these synthetic peptides elicited specific antibodies that were detectable in the serum. Thereafter, mice were challenged with a wild-type pyelonephritic strain that expressed P pili that corresponded to the primary structure of synthetic PapA peptides. Results indicate that the immunogenic dominant region of the PapA pilin (i.e., residues 65 to 75) and the antigenic region corresponding to residues 5 to 12 elicited protective IgG antibodies that prevented subsequent bacterial colonization of the urinary tract and renal infection. Vaccine failures with the other synthetic peptides were not due to lack of immunogenicity among these analogs; however, these elicited antibodies do not bind to intact pili. Therefore, protective epitopes reside in two separate regions of the PapA pili that elicit antibodies that bind intact pili (66). The basis of efficacy of synthetic peptide residues 5 through 12 and 65 through 75 has not been addressed. Explanations for protection include the ability of specific antibody to select for nonpiliated mutants or

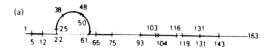
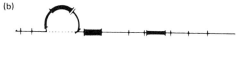
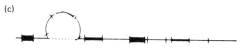
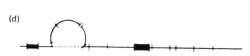

**FIGURE 1** Mapping of linear immunogenic and antigenic epitopes for a prototype PapA pilin (66). The linear depiction shows the location of synthesized peptides (a), location of immunogenic epitopes (b), location of antigenic epitopes (c), and the recognition of denatured PapA by antisera elicited by synthetic peptides, detected by Western immunoblotting (d). The thickness of the bar represents the relative amount of binding.

the loss of pilus function in situ by antibody binding as a result of steric hindrance, allosteric effects, or agglutination of filaments. In additional studies (44), immunization with the synthetic peptide corresponding to the linear immunogenic dominant region of any of the established F serotypes afforded protection against experimental pyelonephritis in the BALB/c mouse model when challenged by piliated wild-type strains expressing homologous F serotypes. Furthermore, cross-reacting protection against heterologous serotypes in this model is uniformly afforded by immunizing mice with combinations of synthetic peptides that correspond to the primary structure of F71, F72, and F8 through F13, residues 5 through 12 or 4 through

13. These data support the previous observation (66) that this region of the PapA pilin specifies a cross-reacting protective epitope.

P pili immunization, as well as immunization with the 7 to 10 amino acids corresponding to the antigenic linear epitope at the amino-terminal end of PapA pilins (66), elicits cross-protection against heterologous piliated strains (49, 56) in relevant models of human urinary tract infection. These results are compatible with in vitro studies that confirm that elicited specific IgG antibody to one P pilus serotype is cross-reactive to heterologous P pili under many circumstances (1, 8, 16, 24, 36, 52, 62–65). This is undoubtedly due to a high degree of conservation among PapA pilins at both genetic and protein levels (6, 7, 24). However, there are numerous reports that indicate that anti-P antibody preparations do not uniformly cross-react with P pili preparations or P piliated strains (8, 24, 63), and no antibody preparation has been identified that will cross-react with all F serotypes associated with Gal-Gal binding. These data are interpreted by some to suggest that it will be difficult to design clinically effective P pili vaccines. This conclusion might be unnecessarily pessimistic. In one report, more than 85% of *E. coli* renal infections in otherwise healthy women are the consequence of uropathogenic *E. coli* strains expressing P pili of the F13 serotype (6). It is anticipated that further characterization of the F serotypes among uropathogenic *E. coli* strains that cause specific syndromes will provide a rational basis for determining which P pili types should be incorporated into a vaccine for a particular patient population in geographically diverse locales. Additionally, this vaccine formulation could readily be improved by supplementing it with synthetic peptides that elicit cross-reacting protective antibodies.

## Anti-Alpha-Hemolysin Parenteral Vaccines

The role of alpha-hemolysin in the pathogenesis of *E. coli* urinary tract infection and its contribution to virulence remain controversial. There are experimental data in relevant animal models that suggest that alpha-hemolysin contributes to the severity of urinary tract infections (45, 81, 84). It is presumed that alpha-hemolysin causes cellular injury by disruption of cell membranes by pore formation; cell death follows if sufficient damage occurs (3). Strains that express a combination of P pili and alpha-hemolysin cause greater mortality and renal parenchymal injury in mice than strains that express none or only one of these determinants (45, 85). In fact, recombinant strains that express P pili and alpha-hemolysin are sufficient to produce disease in the BALB/c mouse model of unobstructive experimental pyelonephritis (45). Their efficacy as vaccines for the prevention of experimental pyelonephritis was also assessed (45). As expected, parenteral P pili immunization prevented subsequent colonization by a challenge wild-type strain that exhibited homologous pili. The purified, denatured alpha-hemolysin parenteral vaccine did not abrogate bacterial renal colonization on challenge, but it did protect mice from subsequent renal injury compared with mice immunized with lipopolysaccharide or saline. Protection was correlated with a specific anti-alpha hemolysin serum IgG titer of ≥1,000. This is a novel result. On the basis of the antigenic topology of alpha-hemolysin (22, 50), it is presumed that specific IgG antibodies that bind to the amino-terminal 2 to 160 residues, residues 626 to 726, and residues within the $Ca^{2+}$-binding domain (i.e., residues 425 to 892) account for in vivo neutralization of hemolytic injury. The vaccine combination of P pili and alpha-hemolysin was also protective. In fact, this combination in a urinary tract vaccine might represent a potentially worthwhile strategy for human immunoprophylaxis against pyelonephritis by interdicting several steps in the pathogenesis of a bacterial mucosal infection (Table 1).

It is anticipated that it would be extremely easy to produce alpha-hemolysin vaccines, although they will be combined with anti-colonization vaccines since they alone will not afford protection against infection. Alpha-hemolysin can be readily produced by use of recombinant DNA technology. Incorporation of the *hly* gene into a nonpathogenic *E. coli* K-12 strain allowed for milligram amounts of alpha-hemolysin to be produced and purified from culture supernatants from a 5-liter fermentor (22). Alpha-hemolysin denaturation with detergent completely destroys its cytotoxic potential without diminishing its immunoprotective capacity. In view of the highly conserved nature of hemolysin at both the genetic and serological levels (47, 86, 87), it is expected that a broadly cross-reactive alpha-hemolysin vaccine can be developed from only one prototype strain.

### Anti-K Parenteral Vaccines

Acidic capsular polysaccharides, of which *E. coli* has >80 types, and the $K_1$ capsule, in particular, are considered to afford bacterial antiphagocytic and anticomplementary activities (24). The protocol for the isolation and purification of acidic capsular polysaccharides is straightforward, and it is feasible to produce large quantities. A limited number of capsular types account for most cases of human pyelonephritis: $K_1$ and $K_5$ types account for 60% of the isolates from women with pyelonephritis and $K_1$, $K_2$, $K_3$, $K_{12}$, and $K_{13}$ types account for 70% of the isolates from young girls with pyelonephritis (24, 30). It is therefore considered feasible that a vaccine comprised of these antigens could be formulated. It will probably be necessary to conjugate this antigen to a peptide carrier since these antigens are per se poor immunogens in humans (17). For example, there were no detectable serum or urine titers of antibody found in 15 of 17 patients with acute pyelonephritis due to $K_1$ strains when screened during the periods of symptomatic infection or convalescence.

The presence and the amount of capsular polysaccharide and of $K_1$ in particular correlate with lethality, bladder and kidney colonization, and renal pathology in experimental animal models of infection (34) and in humans (30). Considerable literature has been generated by Kaijser and colleagues that has demonstrated that actively or passively acquired anticapsular immunity to $K_1$, $K_2$, $K_6$, and $K_{13}$ polysaccharides protects animals from experimental ascending and hematogenous pyelonephritis when challenged by bacteria expressing a homologous K serotype (32, 33, 35). It is presumed that the basis of protection relates to the binding of specific IgG antibody to the capsule, thereby nullifying its antiphagocytic and anticomplementary activities. K vaccines comprised of the predominate types associated with pyelonephritis would seem to have considerable therapeutic advantage. There are no obvious reasons why these vaccinal reagents are not incorporated into a multivalent vaccine formulation which contains a number of other promising urovirulence factors (e.g., P pili and alpha-hemolysin) and tested in clinical trials for safety and efficacy.

### Anti-Outer Membrane Protein Parenteral Vaccines

The role of outer membrane proteins (OMPs) in the pathogenesis of ascending *P. mirabilis* pyelonephritis has not been rigorously studied. They are, however, thought to mediate a number of important pathogenic steps: attachment to cells, invasion, and iron sequestration for optimal bacterial growth (59). They are also responsible for escaping host immunity by reducing the bactericidal activity of normal serum. There are two major protein moieties (39 and 36 kDa) and a minor constituent (33 kDa) within the envelope. These proteins comprise the major OMP complex for this genus (43). The 39- and 36-kDa OMPs exhibit porin properties, thereby providing channels through which aqueous solutes can penetrate the envelope and structures for bacterium-to-host cell attachment. The function of the 33-kDa OMP is completely unknown. In view of the pathogenic potential of OMPs and the feasibility of purifying them under denaturing conditions, the possibility that a vaccine comprised of OMPs might have immunoprophylactic benefits was considered.

Moayeri and colleagues demonstrated in a BALB/c mouse model of unobstructive *P. mirabilis* pyelonephritis that parenteral immunization with OMPs prevents experimental renal infection by a homologous challenge strain (40). Furthermore, OMP vaccination enhanced bacterial renal clearance of three of four heterologous challenge strains in this model. Despite the fact that three of these heterologous challenge strains could be cultured in high numbers from the kidney in a cohort of mice at 3 days after intravesicular inoculation, there was no histological evidence of renal injury at this time. There was also no evidence of any histological damage among cohorts at 7 days after intravesicular inoculation, when these bacteria had been cleared from the urinary tract. These results are novel and establish the importance of OMP in *Proteus* uropathogenesis. These results also support the concept that immunization with selected bacterial protein surface coat constituents can prevent uromucosal infection by interfering with colonization, thereby preventing renal infection.

The finding that OMPs of *P. mirabilis* exhibit some serological cross-reactivity is consistent with the many observations demonstrating immunogenic conservation of major OMPs among members of the family *Enterobacteriaceae* (18). This would suggest that the protection afforded by *P. mirabilis* OMP immunization in this model might be cross-reactive against many other uropathogenic enteric gram-negative bacteria (e.g., *E. coli* and *K. pneumoniae*). If additional OMP antigens could be identified to encompass the majority of all OMPs associated with uropathogens among this family of bacteria, it might be possible to immunize patient populations at risk for bacterial urinary tract infections with a limited number of antigens. Further research in this pursuit is justified and potentially of great immunoprophylactic value.

## SUMMARY OF UROVIRULENCE FACTOR PARENTERAL VACCINES

Collectively, anti-P pili, alpha-hemolysin, and K parenteral vaccines should afford significant immunoprophylactic benefits against a number of urinary tract infections in otherwise healthy children, young women, and elderly persons. This opinion is based on epidemiological criteria and the fact that considerable experimental data exist that confirm their efficacy in relevant animal models of human urinary tract infection. P pili and K vaccines might be sufficient alone to afford protection in a sizable proportion of otherwise healthy individuals at risk for specific urinary tract infections. However, alpha-hemolysin vaccines are not expected to prevent urinary tract infections per se, but to modulate the severity of urinary tract infections caused by any alpha-hemolytic *E. coli* strain. Therefore, alpha-hemolysin vaccines are not intended be administered as a single vaccinal reagent. On the basis of animal studies, it would be prudent to formulate alpha-hemolysin vaccines with P pili parenteral vaccines. In addition, specific antibodies to each of these three microbial determinants elicited after parenteral immunization have broadly cross-reactive potential against wild-type uropathogenic strains. Each of these determinants can readily be produced and in sufficient quantity to begin early phase clinical trials; none are considered particularly toxic.

The OMP parenteral vaccine that was derived from a *P. mirabilis* strain should be further studied prior to initiating human trials. It would be ideal first to identify additional other prototype OMPs from uropathogenic gram-negative enteric species in order to increase the vaccine's spectrum of protection. Thereafter, it would be necessary to conduct a series of bacterial challenge studies in a relevant animal model of human urinary tract infection to assess whether parenteral immunization with a limited number of antigens might protect recipients against a wide range of uropathogenic species and strains (e.g., *E. coli, Proteus* species, *K. pneumoniae,* and *Pseudomonas* species).

## REFERENCES

1. **Abe, C., S. Schmit, I. Moser, G. Boulnois, H. High, I. Orskov, F. Orskov, B. Jann, and K. Jann.** 1987. Monoclonal antibodies with fimbrial F1C, F12, F13, and F14 specificities obtained with fimbriae from E. coli O4:K12:H$^-$. *Microb. Pathog.* **2:**71–77.
2. **Berg, U., and S. Johasson.** 1982. Age as a main determinant of renal functional damage in urinary tract infection. *Arch. Dis. Child.* **55:**963–969.
3. **Bhakdi, S., and J. Tranum-Jensen.** 1988. Damage to cell membranes by pore-forming bacterial cytolysins. *Prog. Allergy* **40:**1–43.
4. **Blackwell, C., S. May, and R. Brettle.** 1986. Host-parasite interactions underlying non-secretion of blood group antigens and susceptibility to recurrent urinary tract infections, p. 229–230. *In* D. Lark (ed.), *Protein Carbohydrate in Interactions in Biological Systems.* Academic Press, London.
5. **Brenner, B.** 1983. Hemodynamically mediated glomerular injury and the progressive nature of kidney disease. *Kidney Int.* **23:**647–655.
6. **Denich, K., L. B. Blyn, A. Craiu, B. A. Braaten, J. Hardy, D. A. Low, and P. D. O'Hanley.** 1991. DNA sequences of three *papA* genes from uropathogenic *Escherichia coli* strains: evidence of structural and serological conservation. *Infect. Immun.* **59:**3849–3858.
7. **Denich, K., A. Craiu, H. Rugo, G. Muralidhar, and P. O'Hanley.** 1991. Frequency and organization of *papA* homologous DNA sequences among uropathogenic digalactoside-binding *Escherichia coli* strains. *Infect. Immun.* **59:**2089–2096.
8. **DeRee, J. M., and J. F. van den Bosch.** 1987. Serological response to the P fimbriae of uropathogenic *Escherichia coli* in pyelonephritis. *Infect. Immun.* **55:**2204–2207.
9. **Fliedner, M., O. Mehis, E. Rautrerberg, and E. Ritz.** 1986. Urinary sIgA in children with urinary tract infection. *J. Pediatr.* **109:**416–421.
10. **Fowler, J.** 1986. Urinary tract infections in women. *Urol. Clin. North Am.* **13:**673–683.
11. **Foxman, B., and S. Frerichs.** 1985. Epidemiology of urinary tract infection. I. Diaphragm use and sexual intercourse. *Am. J. Public Health* **75:**1308–1313.
12. **Gleckman, R., N. Blagg, D. Hilbert, A. Hall, M. Crowley, A. Pritchard, and J. Warren.** 1982. Symptomatic pyelonephritis in elderly men. *J. Am. Geriatr. Soc.* **30:**690–693.
13. **Grischke, E., and H. Ruttgers.** 1987. Treatment of bacterial infections of the female urinary tract by immunization of the patients. *Urol. Int.* **42:**338–342.
14. **Hachen, H.** 1990. Oral immunotherapy in paraplegic patients with chronic urinary tract infections: a double-blind, placebo-controlled trial. *J. Urol.* **143:**760–763.
15. **Hagberg, I., I. Engberg, R. Freter, J. Lam, S. Olling, and C. Svanborg-Eden.** 1983. Ascending, unobstructive urinary tract infection in mice caused by pyelonephritogenic *Escherichia coli* of human origin. *Infect. Immun.* **40:**273–283.
16. **Hanley, J., I. Salit, and T. Hoffman.** 1985. Immunochemical characterization of pili from invasive *Escherichia coli*. *Infect. Immun.* **49:**581–586.
17. **Hanson, L., A. Fasth, U. Jodal, B. Kaijser, P. Larson, U. Lindberg, S. Olling, A. Sohl-Akerlund, and C. Svanborg-Eden.**

1977. Antigens of *Escherichia coli*, human immune response, and the pathogenesis of urinary tract infections. *J. Infect. Dis.* **136:** 144–149.
18. Hofstra, H., and T. Dankert. 1980. Major outer membrane proteins: common antigens in Enterobacteriaceae species. *J. Gen. Microbiol.* **119:**123–131.
19. Hopkins, W., D. Uehling, and E. Balish. 1987. Local and systemic antibody responses accompany spontaneous resolution of experimental cystitis in cynomologus monkeys. *Infect. Immun.* **55:**1951–1956.
20. Hopkins, W., H. Hall, B. Conway, and D. Uehling. 1995. Induction of urinary tract infection by intraurethral inoculation with *Escherichia coli*: refining the murine model. *J. Infect. Dis.* **171:**462–465.
21. Jacobson, S., O. Eklof, and C. Eriksson. 1989. Development of hypertension and uremia after pyelonephritis in childhood: 27 year follow up. *Br. Med. J.* **299:**703–706.
22. Ji, G., and P. O'Hanley. 1990. Epitopes of *Escherichia coli* alpha hemolysin: identification of monoclonal antibodies that prevent hemolysis. *Infect. Immun.* **58:**3029–3035.
23. Johnson, D., R. Russell, C. Lockatell, J. Zulty, J. Warren, and H. Mobley. 1993. Contribution of *Proteus mirabilis* urease to persistence, urolithiasis, and acute pyelonephritis in a mouse model of ascending urinary tract infection. *Infect. Immun.* **61:** 2748–2754.
24. Johnson, J. 1991. Virulence factors in *Escherichia coli* urinary tract infection. *Clin. Microbiol. Rev.* **4:**80–128.
25. Johnson, J., T. Berggren, and J. Manivel. 1992. Histologic-microbiologic correlates of invasiveness in a mouse model of ascending unobstructed urinary tract infection. *J. Infect. Dis.* **165:**299–305.
26. Johnson, J., I. Orskov, F. Orskov, P. Goullet, B. Picard, S. Moseley, P. Roberts, and W. Stamm. 1994. O, K, and H antigens predict virulence factors, carboxylesterase B pattern, antimicrobial resistance, and host compromise among *Escherichia coli* strains causing urosepsis. *J. Infect. Dis.* **169:** 119–126.
27. Johnson, J., and W. Stamm. 1987. Diagnosis and treatment of acute urinary tract infections. *Infect. Dis. Clin. North Am.* **1:**773–791.
28. Jones, B., C. Lockatell, D. Johnson, J. Warren, and H. Mobley. 1990. Construction of a urease-negative mutant of *Proteus mirabilis*: analysis of virulence in a mouse model of ascending urinary tract infection. *Infect. Immun.* **58:**1120–1123.
29. **Journal of the American Medical Associaton.** 1985. Twelfth report of the Human Renal Transplant Registry. *JAMA* **233:** 787–796.
30. Kaijser, B. 1973. Immunology of *Escherichia coli*: K antigen and its relation to urinary tract infection. *J. Infect. Dis.* **127:**670–677.
31. Kaijser, B., and S. Ahlstedt. 1977. Protective capacity of antibodies against *Escherichia coli* O and K antigens. *Infect. Immun.* **17:** 286–289.
32. Kaijser, B., P. Larsson, W. Nimmich, and T. Soderstrom. 1983. Antibodies of *Escherichia coli* K and O antigens in protection against acute pyelonephritis. *Prog. Allergy* **33:** 275–288.
33. Kaijser, B., P. Larsson, and S. Olling. 1978. Protection against ascending *Escherichia coli* pyelonephritis in rats and significance of local immunity. *Infect. Immun.* **20:**78–81.
34. Kaijser, B., P. Larsson, S. Olling, and R. Schneerson. 1983. Protection against acute, ascending pyelonephritis caused by *Escherichia coli* in rats, using isolated capsular antigen conjugated to bovine serum albumin. *Infect. Immun.* **39:**142–146.
35. Kaijser, B., and S. Olling. 1973. Experimental hematogenous pyelonephritis due to *Escherichia coli* in rabbits: the antibody response and its protective capacity. *J. Infect. Dis.* **128:**41–49.
36. Kallenius, G., S. Jacobson, K. Tullus, and S. Svenson. 1985. P fimbriae studies on the diagnosis and prevention of acute pyelonephritis. *Infection* **13:**159–162.
37. Lark, D. Unpublished data.
38. Lehman, J., J. Smith, T. Miller, J. Barnett, and J. Sanford. 1968. Local immune response in experimental pyelonephritis. *J. Clin. Invest.* **47:**2541–2550.
39. Lipsky, B. 1968. Urinary tract infections in men: epidemiology, pathophysiology, diagnosis, and treatment. *Ann. Intern. Med.* **110:** 138–150.
40. Moayeri, N., C. M. Collins, and P. O'Hanley. 1991. Efficacy of a *Proteus mirabilis* outer membrane protein vaccine in preventing experimental *Proteus* pyelonephritis in a BALB/c mouse model. *Infect. Immun.* **59:** 3778–3786.
41. Mobley, H. Personal communication.
42. Mobley, H., M. Island, and G. Massad. 1994. Virulence determinants of uropathogenic *Escherichia coli* and *Proteus mirabilis*. *Kidney Int.* **46:**129–136.
43. Nixdorff, K., H. Fitzer, J. Gmeiner, and H. Martin. 1977. Reconstitution of model

membranes from phospholipid and outer membrane proteins of *Proteus mirabiliis:* role of proteins in the formation of hydrophilic pores and protection of membranes against detergents. *Eur. J. Biochem.* **81**:63–69.
44. O'Hanley, P. Unpublished data.
45. O'Hanley, P., G. Lalonde, and G. Ji. 1991. Alpha-hemolysin contributes to the pathogenicity of piliated digalactoside-binding *Escherichia coli* in the kidney: efficacy of an alpha-hemolysin vaccine in preventing renal injury in the BALB/c mouse model of pyelonephritis. *Infect. Immun.* **59**:1153–1161.
46. O'Hanley, P., D Lark, S. Falkow, and G. Schoolnik. 1985. Molecular basis of *Escherichia coli* colonization of the upper urinary tract in BALB/c mice. *J. Clin. Invest.* **75**:347–360.
47. O'Hanley, P., R. Marcus, K. H. Baek, K. Denich, and G. E. Ji. 1993. Genetic conservaton of *hlyA* determinants and serological conservation of HlyA: basis for developing a broadly cross-reactive subunit *Escherichia coli* alpha-hemolysin vaccine. *Infect. Immun.* **61**:1091–1097.
48. Orskov, I., A. Frenencz, and F. Orskov. 1980. Tamm-Horsfall protein or uromucoid in the normal urinary slime that traps type 1-fimbriated *Escherichia coli. Lancet* **i**:887.
49. Pecha, B., D. Low, and P. O'Hanley. 1989. Gal-Gal pili vaccines prevent pyelonephritis by piliated *Escherichia coli* in a murine model: single-component Gal-Gal pili vaccines prevent pyelonephritis by homologous and heterologous piliated *Escherichia coli* strains. *J. Clin. Invest.* **83**:2102–2108.
50. Pellet, S., D. Boehm, I. Synder, G. Rowe, and R. Welch. 1990. Characterization of monoclonal antibodies against the *Escherichia coli* hemolysin. *Infect. Immun.* **58**:822–827.
51. Percival, A., W. Brumfitt, and J. DeLouvois. 1964. Serum antibody levels as an indication of clinically inapparent pyelonephritis. *Lancet* **ii**:1027–1033.
52. Pere, A., V. Vaisanen-Rhen, M. Rhen, J. Tenhunen, and T. Korhonon. 1986. Analysis of P fimbriae on *Escherichia coli* O2, O4, and O6 strains by immunoprecipitation. *Infect Immun.* **51**:618–625.
53. Roberts, F., Geere, I., and A. Coldman. 1991. A three-year study of positive blood cultures, with emphasis on prognosis. *J. Infect. Dis.* **13**:34–46.
54. Roberts J. 1992. Vesicoureteral reflux and pyelonephritis in the monkey: a review. *J. Urol.* **148**:1721–1725.
55. Roberts, J. 1991. Etiology and pathophysiology of pyelonephritis. *Am. J. Kidney Dis.* **17**:1–9.
56. Roberts, J., K. Hardaway, B. Kaack, E. Fussell, and G. Baskin. 1984. Prevention of pyelonephritis by immunization with P-fimbriae. *J. Urol.* **131**:602–607.
57. Roberts, J., B. Kaack, G. Kallenius, R. Mollby, J. Winberg, and S. Svenson. 1984. Receptors for pyelonephritogenic *Escherichia coli* in primates. *J. Urol.* **131**:163–168.
58. Roberts, J., B. Marklund, D. Ilver, D. Haslam, M. Kaack, G. Baskin, M. Louis, R. Mollby, J. Winberg, and S. Normark. 1994. The Gal(alpha1–4) Gal-specific tip adhesin of *Escherichia coli* P-fimbriae is needed for pyelonephritis to occur in the normal urinary tract. *Proc. Natl. Acad. Sci. USA* **91**:11889–11893.
59. Robledo, J., A. Serrano, and G. Domingue. 1990. Outer membrane proteins of *E. coli* in the host-pathogen interaction in urinary tract infection. *J. Urol.* **143**:386–396.
60. Rubin, R., N. Tolkoff-Rubin, and R. Cotran. 1986. Urinary tract infection, pyelonephritis, and reflux nephropathy, p. 1085–1411. *In* B. Brenner and F. Rector (ed.), *The Kidney.* W.B. Saunders Co., Philadelphia.
61. Ruttgers, H., and E. Grischke. 1987. Elevation of secretory IgA antibodies in the urinary tract by immunostimulation for the preoperative treatment and post-operative prevention of urinary tract infections. *Urol. Int.* **42**:424–426.
62. Salit, I. E., J. Hanley, L. Clubb, and S. Fanning. 1988. Detection of pilus subunits (pilins) and filaments by using anti-P pilin antisera. *Infect. Immun.* **56**:2330–2335.
63. Salit, I., J. Hanley, L. Clubb, and S. Fanning. 1988. The human antibody response to uropathogenic *Escherichia coli:* a review. *Can. J. Microbiol.* **34**:312–318.
64. Salit, I., J. Hanley, C. Superina, L. Nicolle, and M. Gribble. 1988. The human serum antibody response to infections with uropathogenic *Escherichia coli,* p. 231–241. *In Host-Parasite Interaction in Urinary Tract Infections.* University of Chicago Press, Chicago.
65. Salit, I., J. Vavougios, and T. Hoffman. 1983. Isolation and characterization of *Escherichia coli* pili from diverse clinical sources. *Infect. Immun.* **42**:755–762.
66. Schmidt, M., P. O'Hanley, D. Lark, and G. K. Schoolnik. 1988. Synthetic peptides corresponding to protective epitopes of *Escherichia coli* digalactoside-binding pilin prevent infection in a murine pyelonephritis model. *Proc. Natl. Acad. Sci. USA* **85**:1247–1251.
67. Schmidt, M., P. O'Hanley, and G. Schoolnik. 1985. Gal-Gal pyelonephritis

*Escherichia coli* pili linear immunogenic and antigenic epitopes. *J. Exp. Med.* **161**:705–717.
68. **Schulman, S., A. Corbusier, M. Michiels, and H. Taenzer.** 1993. Oral immunotherapy of recurrent urinary tract infections: a double-blind placebo-controlled multicenter study. *J. Urol.* **150**:917–921.
69. **Sheinfeld, J., A. Schaeffer, C. Cordon-Cardo, A. Rogatko, and W. Fair.** 1989. Association of the Lewis blood-group phenotype with recurrent urinary tract infections in women. *N. Engl. J. Med.* **320**:773–777.
70. **Stamey, T., N. Wehner, G. Mihata, and M. Condy.** 1978. The immunological basis for recurrent bacteriuria: cervicovaginal antibody in enterobacterial colonization of the introital mucosa. *Medicine* **57**:47–57.
71. **Stamm, W., and T. Hooton.** 1993. Management of urinary tract infection in adults. *N. Engl. J. Med.* **329**:1328–1334.
72. **Stapleton, A., E. Nudelman, H. Clausen, S.-I. Hakomori, and W. Stamm.** 1992. Binding of uropathogenic *Escherichia coli* R45 to glycolipids extracted from vaginal epithelial cells is dependent on histo-blood group secretor status. *J. Clin. Invest.* **90**:965–972.
73. **Svanborg-Eden, C., and P. DeMan.** 1987. Bacterial virulence in urinary tract infection. *Infect. Dis. Clin. North Am.* **1**:713–750.
74. **Svanborg-Eden, C., R. Kulhavy, S. Marild, S. Prince, and J. Mestechy.** 1985. Urinary immunoglobulins in healthy individuals and children with acute pyelonephritis. *Scand. J. Immunol.* **28**:305–313.
75. **Svanborg-Edén, C., and A.-M. Svennerholm.** 1978. Secretory immunoglobulin A and G antibodies prevent adhesion of *Escherichia coli* to human urinary tract epitheial cells. *Infect. Immun.* **22**:790–797.
76. **Tammen, H., and The German Urinary Tract Infection Study Group.** 1990. Immunobiotherapy with Uro-Vaxom in recurrent urinary tract infection. *Br. J. Urol.* **65**:6–9.
77. **Uehling, D., W. Hopkins, L. Dahmer, and E. Balish.** 1994. Phase I clinical trial of vaginal mucosal immunization for recurrent urinary tract infections. *J. Urol.* **152**:2308–2311.
78. **Uehling, D., I. James, W. Hopkins, and E. Balish.** 1991. Immunization against urinary tract infection with a multi-valent vaginal vaccine. *J. Urol.* **146**:223–226.
79. **Uehling, D., and E. Steihm.** 1971. Elevated urinary secretory IgA in children with urinary tract infection. *Pediatrics* **47**:40–46.
80. **United States Department of Health and Human Services National Kidney and Urologic Diseases Advisory Board.** 1990. *Long-Range Plan: Window of the 21st Century.* NIH Publication number 90-583. U.S. Department of Health and Human Services, Washington, D.C.
81. **Van den Bosch, J., L. Emody, and I. Ketyi.** 1982. I. Virulence factors. Virulence of hemolytic strains of *Escherichia coli* in various animal models. *FEMS Microbiol. Lett.* **13**:427–430.
82. **Vosti, K., A. Monto, and L. Rantz.** 1965. Host-parasite interaction in patients with infections due to *Escherichia coli*. II. Serologic response of the host. *J. Lab. Clin. Med.* **666**:613–626.
83. **Warren, J.** 1987. Catheter-associated urinary tract infections. *Infect. Dis. Clin. North Am.* **1**:823–854.
84. **Welch, R., E. Dellinger, B. Minshew, and S. Falkow.** 1981. Hemolysin contributes to virulence of extra-intestinal *E. coli* infections. *Nature* (London) **294**:664–667.
85. **Welch, R., and S. Falkow.** 1984. Characterization of *Escherichia coli* hemolysins conferring quantitative differences in virulence. *Infect. Immun.* **43**:153–160.
86. **Welch, R., R. Hull, and S. Falkow.** 1983. The molecular cloning and physical characterization of a chromosomal hemolysin from *Escherichia coli*. *Infect. Immun.* **42**:178–186.
87. **Welch, R., and S. Pellet.** 1988. The transcriptional organization of the *Escherichia coli* hemolysin. *J. Bacteriol.* **170**:1622–1630.

# INDEX

*aad* genes, 250, 261
AAF/1, 177
Abacterial cystitis, 30
ABO blood group, 13, 74–75, 224–225
Abscess
    intrarenal, 39
    perinephric, 39
Accretion process, 136
Acetohydroxamic acid, 387, 389
N-Acetylgalactosamine, 320–321
N-Acetylglucosamine, 321
N-Acetyllactosamine, 321
N-Acetylneuraminic acid, 321
Acridine orange stain, 44
Activated segmented neutrophils, 42
Acute dysuria syndrome, 31
Acute urethral syndrome, 30, 38
Adherence, 68–71, 138–139, 222–225
    competitive inhibitors, 84–85
    enterococci, 315–316
    *K. pneumoniae*, 300
    *P. mirabilis*, 253–254
    *S. epidermidis*, 329–331
    *S. saprophyticus*, 319–321
    secreted inhibitors, 227–228
Adhesin, 136, 148, *see also specific fimbriae*
    *E. coli*, 138–150
    enterococci, 313–318
    interaction with tissue ligand, 367
    *K. pneumoniae*, 300–301
    *P. mirabilis*, 253–258
    *S. epidermidis*, 330–331
ADP-L-glycero-D-mannoheptose-6-epimerase, 285
Adult men, *see also* Elderly
    asymptomatic bacteriuria, 16, 31–32
    normal urinary tract, 15–16
    prostate conditions, 16
    urinary tract infection, 15–16
Adult women, *see also* Elderly; Postmenopausal women; Pregnancy
    asymptomatic bacteriuria, 13–15
    cystitis, 10–12
    sexual activity, 11–12
    urinary tract infection, 10–15
    vaginal flora, 67–68
Aerobactin, 136, 154–156, 221, 304–305
Afa proteins, 177
AFA-I fimbriae, 147–148
AFA-III fimbriae, 147–148
Agg proteins, 177
Aggregation substance, enterococci, 313–315, 317–318
AIDS, 20
Amikacin, 307
Amino acid deaminase, *P. mirabilis*, 260–261, 263
Aminoglycosides, 98–101
Amoxicillin, 80, 98–99, 307
Amoxicillin-clavulanate, 98–99
Amphotericin B, 108, 125–129
Ampicillin, 80, 97–99, 103–105, 307
Ampicillin-sulbactam, 98–99
Animal models, 377–403
    animal species, 378
    characteristics, 378
    dog, 381–382
    mouse, 388–389
    nonhuman primate, 394, 415–417
    rabbit, 378–381
    rat, 382–388
    route of infection, 378

Animal models (*continued*)
  selection of animal type, 377–378
  type 1 fimbriae in urinary tract infection, 150–151
  vaccine development, 415–417
Antibody(ies), urinary, 232–233, 380, 388, 390, 412
Antibody response
  in pregnancy, 235
  protection against infection, 233–234
  serum, 233
  to urinary tract infection, 411–412
Antibody-coated bacteria, urinary, 54–55
Antifimbrial antibody, 233
Antiflagellar antibody, 280
Antigenic variation, flagella of *P. mirabilis*, 260
Antimicrobial agents
  effect on vaginal flora, 79–81
  prophylactic, 79–81
  resistance in *K. pneumoniae*, 307–308
  treatment of urinary tract infections, 97–103
Antimicrobial susceptibility testing, 50–58
  dilution methods, 57–58
  disk diffusion method, 56–58
  principles, 56
Antimycotic agents, 126–128
*asa1* gene, 314
Ascending urinary tract infection, 3–4, 341
  adhesin-tissue ligand-based mechanism, 367
  dog model, 381–382
  mouse model, 391–394
  rabbit model, 379–380
  rat model, 383–385
Asymptomatic bacteriuria, 5, 31, 96, 222–223
  adherence of bacteria and, 69
  adult men, 16, 31–32
  adult women, 13–15
  child, 10, 31, 107
  elderly, 14–15, 106
  pregnant women, 14, 31, 106–107
  treatment, 102, 105–107
Asymptomatic candiduria, 123, 128
ATF fimbriae, *P. mirabilis*, 254–255, 257–258, 262
*atf* genes, 250, 258
Autotrak, 44
Aztreonam, 98–101

BAC-T Screen, 46
BACTEC culture, 50
Bacteremia, 33
  catheter-associated, 33
Bacteria
  antibody-coated, urinary, 54–55
  culture methods
    dipslide, 49
    filter paper method, 49
    pour plate, 48
    quantitative, 48
    roll tube method, 49
    semiquantitative, 48–49
    surface streak procedure, 48–49
  diagnostic microbiology, 29–66
  growth in urine, 156, 160–161
  isolation and identification, 50–55
Bacterial adherence, *see* Adherence
Bacterial urinary tract infection, 38–40
Bactericidal factors, urinary tract mucosa, 226–227
Bacteriuria, 3
  asymptomatic, *see* Asymptomatic bacteriuria
  low-count, 30–31
  microscopic detection, 43–44
  quantitative, 4
  significant, 29–32
Basement membrane, 360–361
B-D Urine Collection Kit, 37
β barrel, 196–197
Beta-lactams, 103
Biofilm, *S. epidermidis*, 330–332
Bioluminescence screening method, 46–47
BiP chaperone, 201
BiP-like motif, 198
Blood culture, 33
Blood group antigens, 13, 74–75
Bma proteins, 177
Bone marrow transplant, 19
Boric acid transport media, 37

Caf1 proteins, 177
Calibrated loop, 48
*Candida*, 40, 77–78
  culture methods, 49–50
*Candida* infection, 119–131
  catheter-associated, 120
  clinical manifestations, 123–124
  cystitis, 122–125, 128
  diagnosis, 124–126
  epidemiology, 119–121
  localization of site of, 125–126
  lower urinary tract, 120–123
  microbiology, 119
  pathogenesis, 121–123
  pyelonephritis, 120, 124
  renal, 120, 128–129
    clinical manifestations, 124
    diagnosis, 125
    epidemiology, 120–121
    pathogenesis, 121–122
  risk factors, 120
  treatment, 107–108, 126–129
  urethritis, 123, 128
Candiduria
  asymptomatic, 123, 128
  significant, 124–125

Capsular polysaccharide, 221
  cell-free, 303
  *K. pneumoniae*, 301–304
  *P. mirabilis*, 284–285, 289–291
Capsule
  *E. coli*, 159–160
  *S. saprophyticus*, 328
Catabolite activator protein, 186–187
Catalase test, 45–46
Catheter, urethral, *see* Urethral catheter
Catheter-associated bacteremia, 33
Catheter-associated funguria, 107–108
Catheter-associated infection
  *Candida*, 120
  *P. mirabilis*, 246, 252, 271, 393
  prevention, 111
  rabbit model, 380–381
  *Staphylococcus*, 329
  treatment, 107–108
Catheterization, intermittent, 19, 32, 246
Catheterized urine specimen, significant bacteriuria, 32
Cell adhesion molecules, 230
Cell division genes, *P. mirabilis*, 285–286
Cell membrane, swimmer and swarmer cells, 275–277
Cell wall, swimmer and swarmer cells, 275–277
Cell-mediated immunity, 232
Cephadroxil, 80
Cephalosporin, 98–101, 104, 109
Cervicovaginal antibody, local, 76
Chaperone, periplasmic, 175–176, 194–196
  carboxyl-terminal assembly domain, 198–199
  function, 200–204
    capping of associative surfaces, 203
    complex formation, 201–202
    periplasmic import, 201
    protein folding, 202–203
  recognition paradigm, 199–200
  second-site interactions, 200
  structure, 196–198
Chemstrip 9 dipstick, 46
Chemstrip LN, 45–46
Child
  asymptomatic bacteriuria, 10, 31, 107
  significant bacteriuria, 32
  urinary tract infection, 5–10
    boys, 6–9
    girls, 6–7
    microbiology, 39
    prevention, 111
    recurrent, 111
    renal scarring, 7–10
    symptomatic infection, 6–10
    treatment, 107
Chloramphenicol, 80
Chronic granulomatous disease, 20
Ciprofloxacin, 110

Circumcision, 6, 15
*cld* locus, 284
Clinical presentation, 3–27
Clinical studies
  P fimbriae, 144
  vaginal flora, 71–73
Clinical syndromes, 4–5
Clonal exclusiveness, 345
"Clone concept," 414
ClpE protein, 176
CNF, *see* Cytotoxic necrotizing factor
Colistimethate, 307
Collagen
  type IV, 148, 357, 360–362
  type V, 301, 360
Colonization
  *K. pneumoniae*, 299
  *P. mirabilis*, 262–263
  tissue ligands, 362–363, 367
Colony formation, *P. mirabilis*, 272
Colony structure, expression of fimbriae and, 345, 347
Competitive exclusion
  with lactobacilli, 83–84
  with nonpathogenic *E. coli*, 84
Complicated urinary tract, 17–19
Complicated urinary tract infection, 4, 16–20, 38, 96
  *P. mirabilis*, 245–269, 271
  prevention, 109–110
  treatment, 100, 105–108
Computer image analysis, tissue ligands for adhesins, 362–363
Condom, 76–77
Contraceptive, 76–77, 108
Cost, management of urinary tract infections, 410
Counting chamber, detection of pyuria, 43
*cpsF* gene, 284–285, 290
Cranberry juice, 110
CS3, 177
Cs3–1 protein, 177
CS31A fimbriae, 176
CS6 fimbriae, 177
Css proteins, 177
Curli appendages, 361
Cystine lactose electrolyte-deficient agar, 49
Cystitis, 4, 38–39, 47, 95–96
  adult men, 15
  adult women, 10–12
  *Candida*, 122–125, 128
  elderly, 106
  *K. pneumoniae*, 299
  pathogenesis, 222
  pregnancy, 107
  prevention of recurrent disease, 108–109
  treatment, 100, 105–107
    single-dose therapy, 102–103
    three-day therapy, 103

Cytokine
  functions in urinary tract infection, 229–230
  modifying epithelial-cell response to bacteria, 230–231
  response to urinary tract infection, 228–229
  urinary, 228–229
Cytolysin, enterococci, 316–317
Cytoscopy, with ureteral sampling, 37
Cytospin preparation, 44
Cytotoxic necrotizing factor 1 (CNF1), 136, 156–157

DAF, see Decay-accelerating factor
*dapE* gene, 284–285
Decay-accelerating factor (DAF), 147–148, 177, 357, 360–365
DegP protease, 201, 203
Diabetes mellitus, 14, 19, 299
Diagnostic microbiology, 29–66
*N*-(Diaminophosphinyl)isopentenoylamide, 387
Diaphragm (birth control), 11–12, 76–78, 108
Digalactoside moiety, see Gal-Gal glycolipids
Dilution method, antimicrobial susceptibility testing, 57–58
Dipstick tests, 44–46, 96
Direct tandem repeat sequence, 286–287
Disk diffusion method, antimicrobial susceptibility testing, 56–58
Disulfide isomerase, 203–204
Dog model, 381–382
Dr adhesins, 147–148, 177, 362
Dr blood group antigen, 147, 357
Dr fimbriae, 221
  binding to extracellular matrix, 360–362
  binding to genital tract tissues, 357
  binding to urinary tract tissues, 355–356
  in vitro models, 350
  recombinant models for studying, 363–364
Dra proteins, 177
Drug resistance, 97, 101–102, 313
Dsb proteins, 203–204, 206

EcpD protein, 177, 195–196
Elastase, 332
Elderly
  asymptomatic bacteriuria, 14–15, 106
  cranberry juice cocktail, 110
  cystitis, 106
  prevention of urinary tract infections, 109–110
  pyelonephritis, 106
  susceptibility to urinary tract infection, 235–236
  treatment of urinary tract infection, 105–106
  women, estrogen replacement therapy, 110
Electrical conductance screening method, 47
Electrochemical detection screening method, 47
Enterobacterial common antigen, 380

Enterochelin, 304–305
Enterococci
  adhesins, 313–318
  pathogenesis of infections, 317–318
  surface factors, 313–316
  toxins, 316–317
  virulence determinants, 313–318
*Enterococcus faecalis*, 313–318
*Enterococcus faecium*, 313–318
Envelope antigen F1, 177
Enzymatic screening methods, 44–46
Epidemiology, 3–27
  *Candida* infection, 119–121
  extraintestinal *E. coli* disease, 136–137
  hemolysin of *E. coli*, 152–153
  infections with *S. saprophyticus*, 319
  lower urinary tract infection, *Candida*, 121
  P fimbria in pyelonephritis, 139–141
  renal candidiasis, 120–121
  type 1 fimbriae in urinary tract infection, 149
Epithelial cells, 223–224, 320
  adherence of uropathogens, 68–71
  cytokine modification, 230–231
  cytokine production, 229
*Escherichia coli*
  adherence, 68–69
  adhesins, 138–150
  capsule, 159–160
  compatible solutes, 161
  competitive exclusion of other vaginal flora, 84
  cytotoxic necrotizing factor, 156–157
  Dr family of adhesins, 147–148
  extraintestinal disease
    epidemiology, 136–137
    significance, 135–136
  fimbriae, 138–150, 342–349
  growth in urine, 160–161
  hemolysin, 151–154, 157
  identification of virulence genes, 161
  invasiveness, 364–367
  iron siderophores, 154–156
  mannose-resistant hemagglutination, 148–149
  mannose-sensitive hemagglutination, 149–151
  P fimbriae, 139–144
  recurrent urinary tract infections, 12
  S family of fimbriae, 145–147
  serogroups and serotypes, 157–159
  serum resistance, 159–160
  tissue tropisms, 349–362
  type 1 fimbriae, 149–151
  vaccine against, 405–425
  virulence determinants, 135–174
  virulence gene blocks, 136–138
Esterase test, white blood cell, 44–45
Estrogen
  effect on vaginal flora, 13, 81–82
  vaginal, 67

Estrogen replacement therapy, 110, 235–236
External urine collection device, 19, 36
Extracellular matrix
    binding of S fimbriae, 186
    binding of *S. saprophyticus*, 321–322
    binding of uropathogens, 359–362

F adhesin, 70
F fimbriae, 74
F17 fimbriae, 176
F17D protein, 176
F17papC protein, 176
F1845 fimbriae, 147–148
F1C fimbriae, 145–147, 176
Fae proteins, 176, 202
Fairley washout technique, 51–54
Family history, 12
Fan proteins, 176, 200
Fat bodies, urine, 42
Fecal flora, 67, 72, 223
Fibrinogen, 360
Fibronectin, 186, 316, 321–323, 329, 360–361
Fibronectin-binding protein, *S. saprophyticus*, 323
Filter paper method, bacterial culture, 49
Filtracheck-UTI, 46
Filtration-based rapid screening method, 46
*fim* genes, 187, 197–198
    *fimH* gene, 185, 360–361
Fim proteins, 176, 182, 188–192, 194, 197–198
    FimH protein, 176, 182–183, 185–186, 189–192, 198, 202
Fimbriae, 69, *see also specific fimbriae*
    assembly, 186–195
    *E. coli*, 138–150
    fractionation of fimbriated cells, 343–345
    immunofluorescence staining, 342–343
    impact on colony structure, 345, 357
    *K. pneumoniae*, 300–301
    multifimbrial phase variation, 342–349
    *P. mirabilis*, 253–258
    subunit-subunit interactions, 194–195
Fimbriosome, 190
*fla* genes, 250, 259–260, 263, 280–287, 292
Flagella
    *P. mirabilis*, 258–260
        antigenic variation, 260
        role in virulence, 259–260
        rotational tethering, 280
        swarmer cells, 273–274
Flagellin, 259, 273, 281–283, 292
*flgH* gene, 259, 284
*flhA* gene, 284, 286
*fli* genes, 259, 281–284
FLORA-STAT Urine Transport System, 37
Fluconazole, 108, 127–129
Flucytosine, 127
Fluoroquinolone, 79–81, 97–101, 103, 105

*foc* operon, 145–147
Foc proteins, 176
Forssman antigen, 181, 224, 352
Frequency/dysuric syndrome, 30
Fungal urinary tract infection, 40, 56, *see also Candida* infection
    treatment, 107–108
Fungi, culture methods, 49–50
Fungus ball, 124–125

G adhesin, 224
G fimbriae, 149
Gal-Gal glycolipids, 69–71, 84–85, 141, 176–183, 223–224, 352, 415
*galU* gene, 284–285
Genital tract tissue, binding of Dr fimbriae, 357
Gentamicin, 104–105
*gidA* gene, 284, 286
Glitter cells, *see* Activated segmented neutrophils
Globo-A glycolipid, 224
Globoseries glycolipids, 69–70, 74–75, 84–85, 141, 178–183, 186, 223–224
Globoside, 352
Globotetraose, 234
Glucose-1-phosphate uridyltransferase, 285
Glutamine, surface signal in *P. mirabilis*, 280–281, 290–291
Glycine betaine, 161
Glycolipids, globoseries, *see* Globoseries glycolipids
Glycophorin A, 146
Glycosyltransferase, 74, 225
Gram stain, 43–44
Gram-positive pathogenicity, 333–334
Granulocytopenia, 19–20
Griess test, *see* Nitrite test
Gross examination, urine, 40

H antigen, 13, 157–159, 380, 388
Hemagglutination, *P. mirabilis*, 253–254
Hemagglutinin
    *S. epidermidis*, 330–331
    *S. saprophyticus*, 320–323, 328–329
Hematogenous urinary tract infection, 3–4, 119
    rabbit model, 378–379
    rat model, 382–383
Hematuria, 41–42
Hemocytometer, detection of pyuria, 43
Hemolysin, 136, 221
    *E. coli*, 151–154, 157
    enterococci, 317
    *S. epidermidis*, 332
    *S. saprophyticus*, 323–324
α-Hemolysin, 151
    anti-hemolysin parenteral vaccine, 406, 419–420
β-Hemolysin, 151

Heparin sulfate, 360
Heparin-related molecules, 360
Heptosyltransferase I, 285
*hha* gene, 152
Hif fimbriae, 176
Histopathologic evaluation, animal models, 394–396
*hlyCABD* genes, 151–152
H-NS protein, 187–188
Hospital admissions, 3
Host factors
   adapting treatment to match, 96
   influencing colonization, 222–228
Host resistance, 221–243
*hpm* genes, 250, 252–253
HpmA hemolysin, *P. mirabilis*
   clinical strains, 252
   cytotoxicity, 252–253
   genetics, 253
   role in virulence, 253, 263, 291–292
HSP70 protein, 201
*htrE* gene, 195–196
HtrE protein, 177
Human leukocyte antigen, 75
Hyperammonemia with encephalopathy, 246

ICAM-1, 230
IEL, *see* Intraepithelial lymphocytes
Ig, *see* Immunoglobulin
IL, *see* Interleukin
Ileal conduit-urostomy urine specimen, 36
Imipenem-cilastatin, 98–101, 105
Immunity, 232–234
   antibody response to urinary tract infection, 232–233
   cell-mediated, 232
Immunobiotherapy, 112
Immunocompromised patient, 120
Immunofluorescence test, fimbriated cells, 342–343
Immunoglobulin (Ig) fold, 196
Immunoglobulin A (IgA), 232–233
   secretory, 228, 232
Immunoglobulin A (IgA) protease, 261, 263, 290, 332
Immunoglobulin G (IgG), 76, 232–233, 380
Immunoglobulin M (IgM), 232–233
Immunoglobulin-like periplasmic chaperones, 195–204
Immunological aspects, vaccine development, 411–412
Immunosuppression, 19, 110, 235
"In-and-out" catheterization, urine specimen, 35
In vitro models, 341–376
   history, 341–342
   invasiveness, 364–367
   multifimbrial phase variation, 342–349
   recombinant models, 363–364
   tissue tropism of uropathogens, 349–362

Incidence of urinary tract infection, 29, 410
Indolylpyruvic acid, 261
Inflammatory mediators, interaction with FimH, 185–186
Inflammatory response, to urinary tract infection, 228–231
Inoculating loop, 48
Integrative host factor protein, 188
Interferon gamma, 231
Interleukin 1 (IL-1), 229
Interleukin 4 (IL-4), 231
Interleukin 5 (IL-5), 231
Interleukin 6 (IL-6), 228–229, 231, 235
Interleukin 8 (IL-8), 229–231
Interleukin 10 (IL-10), 231
Interleukin 12 (IL-12), 231
Interleukin 13 (IL-13), 231
Intermittent catheterization, 19, 32, 246
Intraepithelial lymphocytes (IEL), 230–232
Intrarenal abscess, 39
Invasive (febrile) urinary tract infection, 95
Invasiveness
   in vitro models, 364–367
   *P. mirabilis*, 262, 291
Iron
   availability in urinary tract, 260
   acquisition
      *E. coli*, 154–156
      *K. pneumoniae*, 304–305
      *P. mirabilis*, 260–261, 263
Itraconazole, 127

K antigen, 157–159, 234, 302–303, 380
   anti-K parenteral vaccine, 406, 420
K1 capsule, 159
K88 fimbriae, 176, 202
K99 fimbriae, 176
α-Keto acids, as siderophores, 260–261, 263
Ketoconazole, 127
Kidney
   renal candidiasis, 120
      clinical manifestations, 124
      diagnosis, 125
      epidemiology, 120–121
      pathogenesis, 121–122
      treatment, 128–129
   renal scarring, 7–10, 222, 409
   renal tissue tropism, 349–350
   transplant, 110
*Klebsiella pneumoniae*
   adhesins, 300–301
   antibiotic resistance, 307–308
   binding to extracellular matrix, 360
   capsular polysaccharide, 301–304
   fimbriae, 300–301
   iron acquisition, 304–305
   lipopolysaccharide, 304
   urease, 305–307

vaccine against, 411
virulence determinants, 299–312
KOVA slide, 43

Labeling, urine specimen, 33
Laboratory evaluation, 96–97
β-Lactamase, 104, 307
Lactobacillus
  competitive exclusion of other vaginal flora, 83–84
  therapy, prevention of urinary tract infections, 111–112
Laminin, 146, 186, 321, 360–361
Lectinophagocytosis, 303
LEE, see Locus of enterocyte effacement
Leucine response protein, 186–187
Leukocyte adhesin molecule, 184
Lewis antigens, 13, 74–75
Lipopolysaccharide, 151–152, 221, 392
  K. pneumoniae, 304
  P. mirabilis, 275–277, 284–285
Lipoteichoic acids, 320–321
Localization of urinary tract infection, 51–56
Locus of enterocyte effacement (LEE), 136–137
Lower urinary tract infection, 29, 51–56
  Candida, 120–123

M adhesin, 177
M blood group, 149, 177
Malthus system, 47
α-D-Mannose, 357
Mannose-resistant hemagglutination (MRHA), 139, 148–149, 178, 300
Mannose-sensitive hemagglutination, 70, 149–151, 178, 300
Mannoside-binding lectin, 185
Meat handlers, 319
Medical illness, predisposing to urinary tract infections, 19–20
Menstrual cycle, 68, 81–82, 319, 362
Metabolism, swimmer and swarmer cells, 277
Metalloprotease, P. mirabilis, 261, 263, 290–292
Methyl-α-D-mannopyranoside, 84
Methylene blue stain, 44
Miconazole, 128
Microbiology, urinary tract infections, 38–40
Microscopic screening methods, 41–42, 96
  detection of bacteriuria, 43–44
  detection of pyuria, 42
Midstream clean-voided urine specimen, 34
Monkey model, vaccine development, 415–417
Morbidity, urinary tract infections, 408–410
Mouse model
  ascending pyelonephritis, 391–394
  histopathologic evaluation, 394–396
  i.v. challenge, 388–389
  vaccine development, 415–417
  water diuresis, 389–391

MRHA, see Mannose-resistant hemagglutination
MR/K fimbriae, 176, 300–301, 355, 359
mrk genes, 300–301
Mrk proteins, 176, 360
MR/P fimbriae, 176
  binding to urinary tract tissues, 359
  mouse model, 392
  P. mirabilis, 254–256, 262, 359, 392
    genetic organization, 254–256
    properties, 254
    role in virulence, 256
  tissue-binding specificity, 355
mrp genes, 250, 254–256
Mrp proteins, 176
MS-2 system, 37
MSCRAMM, 359–362
M-specific hemagglutinin, 149
Mucosal cytokine network, 229–230
Multicellular migration, P. mirabilis, 287–291
Mycobacteria
  culture methods, 50
  urinary tract infection, 40
Myf proteins, 177

nac gene, 306
NAF fimbriae, P. mirabilis, 254–255, 258, 262
Nephropathy, reflux, 10
Neurogenic bladder, 17
Neutrophil(s)
  chemoattractants, 230
  cytokine production, 229
  influx in urinary tract infection, 230
  interaction with type 1 fimbriae, 185
  oxidative burst, 185–186
  transepithelial migration, 230
Neutrophil-inhibitory factor, 333
Nfa proteins, 177
NFA1–6 adhesin, 177
Nitrite test, 45
  with white blood cell esterase test, 45
Nitrofurantoin, 79–80, 98–102
  prophylactic, 109
Nitrogen regulation system, global, 306
Nonhuman primate models, 394
  vaccine development, 415–417
Nonoxynol-9, 11–12, 78–79
Nonsecretor, see Secretor status
Norfloxacin, 109
Nosocomial infection, 29, 38, 120, 135, 410
  enterococci, 313
  K. pneumoniae, 299, 307
  P. mirabilis, 246
ntr system, 306

O antigen, 136, 157–159, 234, 284–285, 304, 380, 388
Oligosaccharides, inhibitors of bacterial adherence, 228

Oral contraceptive, 76–77, 81
Organ transplant recipient, 19, 110
Osmolarity, urine, 226
Osmoprotective substances, 161, 226
Outer membrane assembly protein, 175–176, 204–205
  anti-outer membrane protein vaccine, 406, 420–421
  family and structure, 204
  function, 204–205
Oxalate crystals, urine, 41
Oxidative burst, 185–186

P blood group, 74–75, 148–149, 224, 342, 352
$P_1$ blood group, 224
P fimbriae, 70–71, 74–75, 80, 136, 139–144, 175–219, 221–224, *see also* PapG protein
  adherence, 178–179
  antibodies against, 411–412
  anti-P pili vaccine, 406, 417–419
  binding to extracellular matrix, 361
  binding to urinary tract tissues, 350–355
  biogenesis, 206–207
  effect of cloned P-fimbrial determinants, 142
  epidemiology in pyelonephritis, 139–141
  historical aspects, 177–178
  in vitro models, 342, 344, 349–350
  isogenic mutants, 142–143
  mouse model, 391–392
  nonhuman primate models, 394
  in pathogenesis of urinary tract infection, 141–144
  pilus rod, 192–194
  receptor, 141–142, 224
  receptor analogs, 234
  serum antibodies, 233
  vaccine, 144, 234
  volunteer studies, 144
PAI, *see* Pathogenicity-associated island
Pap fimbriae, 352–353, 355
*pap* genes, 143, 186–187, 223
PapA protein, 187, 189, 192–195, 201–203, 207
  vaccine against, 417–419
*papB* gene, 186
PapC protein, 176, 187, 204, 206–207
PapD protein, 176, 181, 187, 194–204, 206–207
PapE protein, 186–189, 192, 195, 199, 201–203, 207, 361
PapF protein, 182, 186–190, 192, 199, 206, 361
PapG protein, 141–142, 176, 179, 187–189, 192, 195–206, 361
  adhesin-binding paradigm, 182–183
  binding specificity, 179–181
  class I, 180–181, 183
  class II, 180–181, 183
  class III, 180–181
  domain structure, 181–182
  vaccine against, 417
  as virulence determinant, 183–184

PapH protein, 187, 207
PapJ protein, 187
PapK protein, 187–189, 192, 195, 199, 201–202, 207
Pathogenesis of urinary tract infection
  *Candida*, 122–123
  coagulase-negative staphylococci, 333
  enterococci, 317–318
  P fimbriae in, 141–144
  *P. mirabilis*, 245–248
  S fimbriae in, 186
  *S. saprophyticus*, 328–329
  steps in, 221–222
  type 1 fimbriae in, 150–151, 184–185
Pathogenicity-associated island (PAI), 136–137, 141, 146–147, 161
Pef fimbriae, 176
*pepQ* gene, 284, 290–291
Peptidoglycan, *P. mirabilis*, 285–286
Perinephric abscess, 39
Periplasmic import, 201
Periurethral washing, 34
pH
  urine, 226
  vaginal, 67–68, 75–76, 235–236
PH6 antigen, 177
Phase variation, 139, 149, 188, 263, 300, 390
  multifimbrial, in vitro models, 342–349
Phenylalanine deaminase, *P. mirabilis*, 277
Phenylpyruvic acid, 261
Pili, *see specific fimbriae*
Pilus rod, 187, 192–194, 203, 207
Piperacillin-tazobactam, 98–99
*N*-(Pivaloyl)glycinohydroxamic acid, 387
Plasmid-mediated drug resistance, 56
PMF fimbriae, 176
  mouse model, 392
  *P. mirabilis*, 254–258, 262, 392
    genetic organization, 257
    properties, 256–257
    role in virulence, 257
*pmf* genes, 250, 257
Pmf proteins, 176
Polyamines, urine, 227
Polymicrobial urinary tract infection, 38
Polysaccharide adhesin, *S. epidermidis*, 330–331
Postcoital prophylaxis, 109
Postmenopausal women
  estrogen status, 82
  susceptibility to urinary tract infection, 235–236
  urinary tract infection, 13
  vaginal flora, 68, 82
Pour plate method, bacterial culture, 48
Pregnancy
  asymptomatic bacteriuria, 14, 31, 106–107
  cystitis, 107
  prevention of urinary tract infection, 110–111

pyelonephritis, 107, 235
  susceptibility to urinary tract infection, 235
  treatment of urinary tract infection, 106–107
P-related fimbriae, 141
Preservative-containing transport device, 37
Preterm delivery, 14, 235
Prevention of urinary tract infection, 108–112
  alternative approaches, 234–235
  catheter-associated, 111
  children, 111
  competitive exclusion
    with lactobacilli, 83–84, 111–112
    with nonpathogenic *E. coli*, 84
  competitive inhibitors of bacterial attachment, 84–85
  complicated infections, 109–110
  cranberry juice, 110
  elderly, 109–110
  estrogen replacement therapy, 110
  immunobiotherapy, 112
  modification of vaginal flora, 82–85
  pregnancy, 110–111
  receptor analog treatment, 234
  recurrent cystitis, 108–109
  renal transplant recipient, 110
  spinal cord injury, 109–110
  vaccine, *see* Vaccine
*pro* genes, 161
Proline betaine, 161
Proline peptidase, *P. mirabilis*, 290–291
Prophylaxis of urinary tract infection, 109–111
Prostatic hypertrophy, 16–17
Prostatitis, 16, 39, 42, 55–56, 106
Proteoglycan, 360
*Proteus mirabilis*
  adherence, 253–254
  adhesins, 253–258
  amino acid deaminase, 260–261, 263
  ATF, 254–255, 257–258, 262
  capsular polysaccharide, 284–285, 289–291
  cell division genes, 285–286
  colonization, 262–263
  damage to host tissue, 263
  deaminase activity, 260–261
  determinants of swarming, 279–291
    flagellar genes, 281–284
    flagellar rotational tethering, 280
    genes and proteins, 281–287
    glutamine, 280–281, 290–291
    surface signal, 280
  evasion of host defense, 263
  fimbriae, 253–258
  flagella, 258–260
  hemagglutination, 253–254
  HpmA hemolysin, 252–253, 263, 291–292
  invasiveness, 262, 291
  iron acquisition, 260–261, 263
  lipopolysaccharide, 284–285
  metalloprotease, 261, 263, 290–292
  model for pathogenesis, 262–264
  MR/K hemagglutinin, 359
  MR/P fimbriae, 254–256, 262, 359, 392
  multicellular migration, 287–291
  NAF, 254–255, 258, 262
  pathology of infection, 245–248
  peptidoglycan, 285–286
  phenylalanine deaminase, 277
  PMF, 254–258, 262, 392
  proline peptidase, 290–291
  sigma factors, 286–287
  swarmer cell differentiation, 259, 262–263
    description, 271–275
    genetics, 259
    spatial cycling, 274–275
    temporal cycling, 274, 276
    uropathogenicity and, 291–293
  swarmer vs. swimmer cells, 275–278
  swarming crippled mutants, 287–291
  swarming motility, 247, 258–259, 278–279
  tryptophanase, 277
  upstream regulatory sequences, 286–287
  urease, 248–252, 277, 291–292, 392
  vaccine against, 264, 411, 414
  virulence determinants, 245–269
Prs fimbriae, 176, 178, 180, 352–355
Prs proteins, 176, 181
*prs*G$_{J96}$-positive strains, 224
PsaB protein, 177
*putP* gene, 161
Pyelitis, 394–395
Pyelonephritis, 95–96
  acute, 3–5, 29, 39, 72
    adult men, 15
    pregnant woman, 14
    renal scarring, 7–10
  ascending
    dog model, 381–382
    mouse model, 391–394
    rabbit model, 379–380
    rat model, 383–385
  *Candida*, 120, 124
  chronic, 410
  elderly, 106
  hematogenous
    rabbit model, 378–379
    rat model, 382–383
  incidence, 410
  P$_1$ blood group and, 224
  P fimbriae in, 139–141
  pathogenesis, 221–222
  in pregnancy, 107, 235
  recurrent, 10
  subclinical, 409
  treatment, 100, 103–107
Pyuria, 29, 42, 230, 380

QUALTURE, 38
Quantitative bacteriuria, 4
Quantitative culture, of urine, 29–32, 48

Rabbit model
  antibodies, 380
  ascending pyelonephritis, 379–380
  catheter-associated infections, 380–381
  hematogenous pyelonephritis, 378–379
Rapid detection, urinary tract infection, 40–46
Rapid urinary screening, see Screening methods
Rat model
  ascending pyelonephritis, 383–385
  direct kidney inoculation, 385
  hematogenous pyelonephritis, 382–383
  histopathologic evaluation, 394–396
  interactions between bacteria and host, 385–387
  urea, urolithiasis, and urease inhibitors, 387–388
  water diuresis, 385
Receptor
  P fimbriae, 70, 141–142, 224
  type 1 fimbriae, 149–150
  variation in expression, 223–225
Receptor analogs, 84–85, 234
Recurrent urinary tract infection, 12–13, 38, 71–73, 77–78, 221
  child, 111
  morbidity, 409
  *P. mirabilis*, 246
  prevention, 108–109
Red blood cells, urinary, 41–42
Reflux nephropathy, 10
Renal culture, 51
Resistance to urinary tract infection
  immunity and, 232–234
  inflammation and, 231
*rfaCD* gene, 284–285
RfaH protein, 152
*rfb* gene, 285
Rho protein, 156
Risk factors, urinary tract infection, 54, 120
  adult men, 15–16
  nonsexual factors, 12
  sexual activity, see Sexual activity
*rmp* genes, 303–304
Roll tube method, bacterial culture, 49

S fimbriae, 145–147, 175–176, 178, 221
  binding to extracellular matrix, 186, 361
  binding to urinary tract tissues, 358
  in vitro models, 342–349
  minor pilins, 191
  in pathogenesis, 186
  phase variation, 342–349
  tissue-binding specificity, 355
S/F1C-related fimbriae, 145–147

Sage Products Urine Culture Tube, 37
Screening methods
  bioluminescence, 46–47
  electrical conductance, 47
  electrochemical detection, 47
  enzymatic, 44–46
  filtration-based, 46
  impact on treatment decisions, 96
  microscopic, see Microscopic screening method
SecD protein, 201
Secretor status, 13, 74–75, 224–225, 409
Secretory IgA, 228, 232
Sef proteins, 177
Segmental urine collection, 55–56
Self-initiated treatment, 109
Serogroups, *E. coli*, 157–158
Serotypes, *E. coli*, 157–158
Serum antibody response, 233
Serum resistance, *E. coli*, 159–160
Sex pheromone, enterococci, 313–314, 317
Sexual activity, 76–79, 108, 319
  adult men, 15–16
  adult women, 11–12
Sexually transmitted disease, urinary tract infections as, 12
*sfa* genes, 145–147, 187
Sfa proteins, 176, 184, 191–192
*sfr* operon, 145–147
Sialolactose, 358
Siderophore, see Iron, acquisition
Sigma factor, 286–287, 306
Significant bacteriuria, 29–32
Significant candiduria, 124–125
Slime
  *P. mirabilis*, 279, 285
  *S. epidermidis*, 332
  *S. saprophyticus*, 328–329
  urinary, 358
*smfA* gene, 257
Sodium chloride-polyvinylpyrrolidone preservative, 37
Solco-Urovac, 406, 412–413
Specific gravity, urine, 44
Specimen, see Urine specimen
Spermicide, 76–79, 108
Spinal cord injury, 109–110
Squamous epithelial cells, 74, 138, 225
SSEA, see Stage-specific embryonic antigen
Ssp protein, 323–324, 328
Stage-specific embryonic antigen 4 (SSEA-4), 352–354
Stamey test, 51
*Staphylococcus aureus*, 329–333
*Staphylococcus epidermidis*
  adhesion, 329–331
  biofilm, 330–332
  hemagglutinin, 330–331

hemolysin, 332
neutrophil-inhibitory factor, 333
pathogenesis of infection, 333
polysaccharide adhesin, 330–331
slime, 332
virulence determinants, 329–333
*Staphylococcus saprophyticus*
  adherence, 319–321
  binding to extracellular matrix, 321–322
  capsule, 328
  epidemiology of infections, 319
  fibronectin-binding protein, 323
  hemagglutinin, 320–323, 328–329
  hemolysin, 323–324
  pathogenesis of infections, 328–329
  secreted factors and toxic products, 323–328
  slime, 328–329
  surface factors, 319–323
  surface hydrophobicity, 321, 329
  surface-associated protein, 322–324, 328
  urease, 319, 324–329
  virulence determinants, 318–329
Stone formation, 17, 246–248, 305–307, 325–326
  rat model, 387–388
Stress fiber, 156
Struvite stones, 305–307, 387
N-Succinyl-L-diaminopimelic acid desuccinylase, 285
Suprapubic aspiration, 33–34
Surface factors
  enterococci, 313–316
  *S. saprophyticus*, 319–323
Surface streak procedure, bacterial culture, 48–49
Surface-associated protein, *S. saprophyticus*, 322–324, 328
Susceptibility testing, *see* Antimicrobial susceptibility testing
Susceptibility to urinary tract infections, 221–243
Swarmer cell differentiation, *see Proteus mirabilis*, swarmer cell differentiation
Swarmer cells, 247, 259, 273
  morphology, 272
  slime, 279
  swimmer cells vs., 275–278
Swarming crippled mutants, 287–291
Swarming motility, *P. mirabilis*, 247, 258–259, 271–274, 278–279
Swimmer cells, 247, 259, 273
  swarmer cells vs., 275–278

T cells, 230–232
Tamm-Horsfall glycoprotein, 184–186, 227–228, 358, 415–416
Ticarcillin-clavulanate, 98–99
Tip fibrillum, 141, 175, 182, 187–192, 195, 203, 207

Tissue ligands, for bacterial colonization, 362–363, 367
Tissue tropism of uropathogens, 349–362
TMP-SMX, *see* Trimethoprim-sulfamethoxazole
TNF, *see* Tumor necrosis factor
Toxin, enterococci, 316–317
*tra* genes, 152
Transforming growth factor β, 231
Transitional cells, 74, 138
Transport culture system, 37–38
Transport system, urine specimen, 37–38
Treatment of urinary tract infection, 95–108
  antimicrobial agents, 97–102
  asymptomatic bacteriuria, 102, 105–107
  asymptomatic candiduria, 128
  *Candida*, 126–129
  catheter-associated infection, 107–108
  child, 107
  by clinical syndrome, 95–96
  complicated infections, 100, 105–108
  cystitis, 100, 102–103, 105–107, 128
  defining the problem, 95
  duration of therapy, 102
  elderly, 105–106
  fungal, 107–108
  host status and, 96
  laboratory evaluation and, 96–97
  pregnancy, 106–107
  pyelonephritis, 100, 103–107
  renal candidiasis, 128–129
  self-initiated, 109
  urethritis, 128
Trimethoprim, 80, 98–101, 103
  prophylactic, 109
Trimethoprim-sulfamethoxazole (TMP-SMX), 79–81, 97–101, 103–104, 307
  prophylactic, 109–110
Tryptophanase, *P. mirabilis*, 277
Tumor necrosis factor (TNF), 229
Type 1 fimbriae, 70–71, 175–179, 188, 221, 300–301, *see also* Fim proteins
  binding to extracellular matrix, 360–361
  binding to urinary tract tissues, 357–358
  epidemiology in urinary tract infection, 149
  in vitro models, 342–349
  minor pilins, 189–191
  mouse model, 390–392
  nonhuman primate models, 394
  in pathogenesis, 150–151, 184–185
  phase variation, 342–349
  rat model, 386
  receptors, 149–150
  structure, 194
  tissue-binding specificity, 355
Type 1C fimbriae
  binding to urinary tract tissues, 359
  in vitro models, 342–343
  tissue-binding specificity, 355

Type 2 fimbriae, 176
Type 3 fimbriae, 176, 300–301
  binding to extracellular matrix, 360
  rat model, 386
Type 4 fimbriae, 386

UDP-glucose dehydrogenase, 284–285
Uncleaned initial-voided urine specimen, 34–35
Uncomplicated urinary tract infection, 4
Upper urinary tract infection, 30, 51–56
  P. mirabilis, 246
  risk factors, 54
Upstream regulatory sequences, P. mirabilis, 286–287
ure genes, 250–251, 306
Urease
  enzymatic reaction, 248–249
  K. pneumoniae, 305–307
  P. mirabilis, 248–249, 263, 277, 291–292, 392
    genetic organization, 249–251
    induction, 250–251
    properties, 249
    role in virulence, 251–252, 263
  S. saprophyticus, 319, 324–329
Urease inhibitors, rat model, 387–388
Ureteral catheter, indwelling, 38
Ureteral sampling, 37
Urethral catheter, 17–19
  intermittent catheterization, 19
  specimen collection, 35
Urethral stricture, 17
Urethritis, 4, 15, 31, 38, 55
  Candida, 123, 128
Urinary antibodies, 232–233, 380, 388, 390, 412
Urinary incontinence, 19
Urinary slime, 185, 358
Urinary tract tissue
  bactericidal factors, 226–227
  binding of Dr fimbriae, 355–356
  binding of MR/K hemagglutinin, 359
  binding of MR/P fimbriae, 359
  binding of P fimbriae, 350–355
  binding of S fimbriae, 358
  binding of type 1 fimbriae, 357–358
  binding of type 1C fimbriae, 359
Urine
  bacterial growth in, 156, 160–161
  gross examination, 40
  osmolarity, 226
  pH, 226
Urine culture, 47–50
  bacterial culture
    dipslide, 49
    filter paper method, 49
    pour plate method, 48
    quantitative, 48
    roll tube method, 49
    semiquantitative, 48–49
    surface streak procedure, 48–49
  fungal culture, 49–50
  mycobacterial culture, 50
  quantitative, 29–32
  transport culture system, 37–38
  treatment decisions and, 96
Urine outflow, obstructed, 225–226, 393
Urine specimen
  catheterized, significant bacteriuria, 32
  collection, 32–37
    segmental, 55–56
  contamination, 33
  external collection device, 19, 36
  ileal conduit-urostomy specimen, 36
  "in-and-out" catheterization, 35
  indwelling urethral catheterization, 35
  labeling, 33
  midstream clean-voided, 34
  suprapubic aspiration, 33–34
  transport, 37–38
  uncleaned initial-voided, 34–35
  unusable, 41, 44
  volume, 32–33
URISCREEN catalase detection system, 46
Uroepithelial cells, see Epithelial cells
Urologic malignancy, 17
Uromodulin, see Tamm-Horsfall glycoprotein
Uro-Vaxom, 406, 412–414
Usher, see Outer membrane assembly protein
UTIScreen, 46–47

Vaccine, 85, 112, 205, 233–234, 405–425
  animal models, 415–417
  anti-alpha-hemolysin, 406, 419–420
  anti-K, 406, 420
  anti-outer membrane protein, 406, 420–421
  anti-P pili, 144, 406, 417–419
  anti-virulence factor, 414–421
  cost-effectiveness, 407
  current status, 412–414
  efficacy trials, 406–407
  immunological aspects, 411–412
  P. mirabilis, 264
  reasons to develop, 407–410
  recommendations for vaccine strategies, 410–411
Vagina, pH, 67–68, 75–76, 235–236
Vaginal cells, adherence of uropathogens, 68–71
Vaginal flora, 67–94
  background, 67
  clinical studies, 71–73
  colonization with and without recurrent urinary tract infection, 72–73
  factors influencing colonization
    antimicrobial agents, 79–81
    blood group antigens, 74–75
    estrogen, 81–82
    exogenous agents, 76–82

host factors, 74–76
human leukocyte antigens, 75
local cervicovaginal antibody, 76
secretor status, 74–75
sexual activity, 76–79
type of cell, 74
vaginal pH, 75–76
healthy women, 67–68
modification to prevent urinary tract infection, 82–85
temporal association of colonization and urinary tract infections, 71–72
Vaginitis, 38
Vascular catheter, *Candida* infection, 120
Vesicoureteral reflux, 7–10, 111, 222, 225–226, 383–384, 393–394, 409
Virulence determinants
anti-virulence factor vaccine, 405–425
*E. coli*, 135–174
enterococci, 313–318
*K. pneumoniae*, 299–312
*P. mirabilis*, 245–269
PapG, 183–184
*S. epidermidis*, 329–333
*S. saprophyticus*, 318–329
Virulence gene(s), *E. coli*, 161
Virulence gene block (linkage), 136–138
Virulence gene clusters, 250

Water diuresis
mouse model, 389–391
rat model, 385
Wet mount, 42
White blood cell esterase test, 44–45
with nitrite test, 45
White blood cells, urine, *see* Pyuria

X adhesins, 148

Yeast, 40, *see also Candida*
culture methods, 49–50
diagnostic microbiology, 29–66